MEDICAL RECORDS DEPT.
COMMUNITY MEDICAL CENTER
99 HWY. 37 W.
TOMS RIVER, NJ 08755

Coding

INCLUDES 12 MONTHS WORTH OF CODE UPDATES

Download a free trial of Encoder Pro 2001 at www.medicode.com/encoderpro or call the toll-free number above.

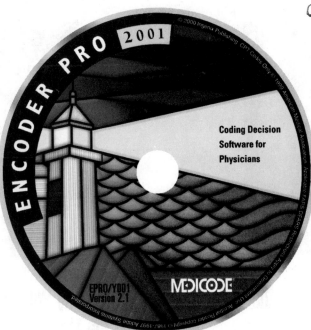

W9-DDH-027

No More Paper Cuts

Encoder Pro

(Item #2717)

$499⁹⁵

No more flipping through code book indexes trying to find the correct code. With Encoder Pro 2001, all the coding and reference books you need are on your PC's desktop – not your desk. This software not only helps you get rid of the stack of code books on your desk, it helps you save time, increase productivity, and improve overall coding accuracy.

This powerful, one-of-a-kind software enables you to search all 3 coding systems simultaneously with just a click of your mouse. Simply type in a key word—it can be an acronym or lay term(and your tabular results are displayed instantaneously, on one screen, with the most likely codes appearing at the top. Each search integrates all outpatient codes so you save time by only entering your search criteria once.

And Encoder Pro 2001 doesn't stop there, for each keyword search you get:

1. **NEW! CCI Unbundle Edits, Plus the Reason Behind the Edit.** Stop billing errors by seeing which CPT codes should not be billed together—both Medicare CCI edits and commercial payer unbundling edits.

2. **NEW! Additional Color Code Symbols for ICD-9 Codes.** Ensure coding accuracy by identifying codes with age and sex edits, and comorbidity/complication flags.

3. **NEW! View Codes According to Status.** Quickly reference new, revised, and deleted codes.

4. **NEW! Primary Procedure Codes.** Improve coding accuracy by knowing the primary procedure codes that are appropriate for CPT add-on codes.

5. **Surgical Cross Coding Information.** Justify code selection and verify a match between code sets.

6. **Medicare Payment Rules, RVUs, Conversion Factors, and Global Surgery Information.** Increase rate of compliance and reduce audit liability.

7. **Lay Descriptions(from our popular CDR and I-9 and HCPCS Annotations.** Improve code selection.

8. **CPT and HCPCS Modifiers.** Ensure coding accuracy by seeing what modifiers are appropriate for a certain code.

Put our complete reference library on your PC desktop — right at your fingertips!

Pricing for single user license only. Call for multi-user and developer pricing. Windows 95 B, Windows 98 and Windows NT 4.x, with service pack 3; 8 MB RAM; 32 MB available hard disk space required. Pentium recommended. 1 MB printer memory required to print HCFA-1500 form. Includes software and data updates for 1 year.

8 CEUs from AAPC

MAKE LIFE A LITTLE EASIER WITH THESE EASY TO USE FEATURES:
- Sticky Notes. No more transferring of notes from year to year.
- Bookmarks. Create your own "cheat-sheet" of frequently referenced codes
- Global Notes. Communicate coding policy to all network users.

MEDICODE®

Medicode, 5225 Wiley Post Way, Suite 500, Salt Lake City, UT 84116 • 801.536.1000 • FAX 801.536.1011

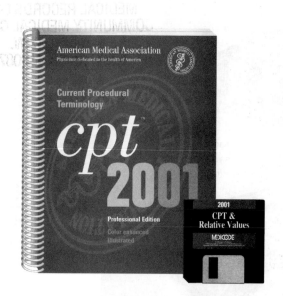
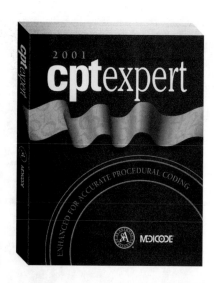
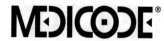

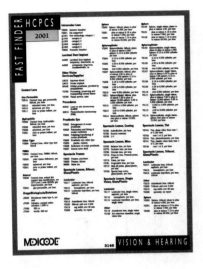
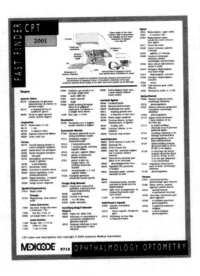
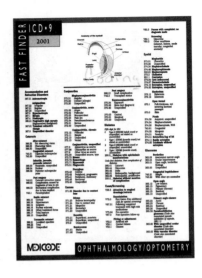
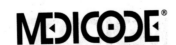

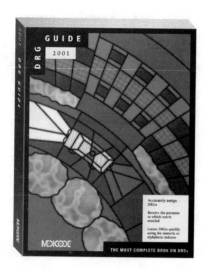
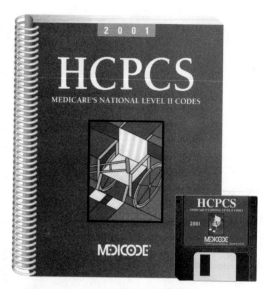
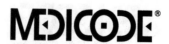

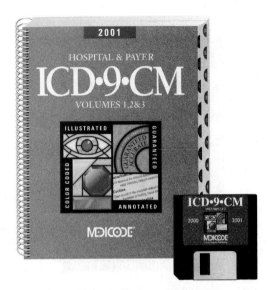
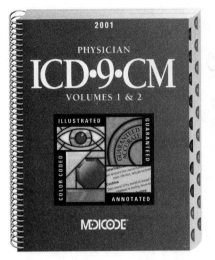
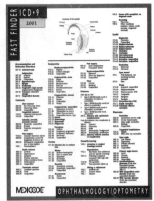
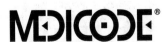

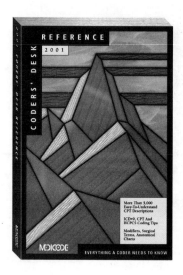

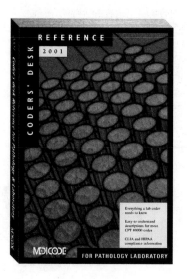

Get Instant Answers to Your Tough Coding Questions

2001 Coders' Desk Reference

ISBN 1-56337-315-7

(Item #5760)   **$99⁹⁵**

Available December 2000

Get instant answers to your tough coding questions. This essential desk reference answers all you toughest coding questions and provides critical, expertly written information on CPT, ICD-9-CM and HCPCS coding.

↪ **EXCLUSIVE Easy-to-Understand, Lay Descriptions for Over 5000 Surgical Procedures.** Helps you more accurately understand and determine the appropriate 2001 CPT code for claim submission.

↪ **NEW CPT 5, ICD-10-CM, and ICD-10-PCS Preparation.** Learn how each coding system will affect you and discover ways to make the transition as smooth as possible.

↪ **NEW Official CPT Headings and Subheadings.** Indicates anatomical and procedural sections so you can determine which CPT codes are associated with what description.

↪ **NEW Updated Glossary of Syndromes with Cross-References to the Applicable CPT Code.** Understand and identify more than 1000 medical and emotional syndromes found in ICD-9-CM.

↪ **Eponyms Defined and Cross-Referenced to Applicable CPT codes.** Understand commonly used eponyms and find out what CPT code uses them.

Have the Definitive Resource Dedicated to Path/Lab Coding at your Fingertips

2001 Coders' Desk Reference for Pathology and Laboratory Services

ISBN 1-56337-317-3

(Item #5856)   **$99⁹⁵**

Available February 2001

The *2001 Coder's Desk Reference for Path/Lab Services* helps you find the code you need with cross-referenced lay descriptions and their associated CPT codes, fully-informed CLIA and HIPAA compliance resources, and an extensive glossary for abbreviations, acronyms, and synonyms to help you fine the path/lab code you need — fast!

↪ **NEW CPT-5, PCS, and ICD-10 Preparation.** Learn how each coding system will affect you and discover ways to make a smooth transition.

↪ **NEW CLIA Preparation and Auditing Information.** Develop a compliance program for a lab of any size.

↪ **FREE *CPT Fast Finder* for Path/Lab.** Easily find the appropriate path/lab code with this popular laminated, quick reference sheet.

↪ **Updated with 2001 CPT Codes.** Easy-to-Understand Explanations of Path/Lab Procedures. Helps you quickly determine the appropriate CPT code.

↪ **Coding Comments for Hundreds of Procedures.** Points you to more specific codes or other procedures that could apply, enabling you to code more accurately.

↪ **HIPPA Compliance Information Including Detailed Information on What Constitutes Fraud & Abuse.** You can be confident that you are coding by the rules.

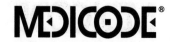

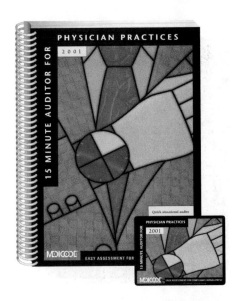

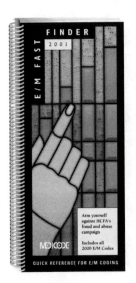

Quick and Easy Billing Audit Templates and Tips

2001 15-Minute Auditor for Physician Practices

ISBN 1-56337-356-4

(Item #3108)

$89⁹⁵

This portable, easy-to-use workbook provides templates and tips for front line health care professionals who want to make quick, random audits of coding and documentation operations to ensure their practice stays in compliance. You'll be able to spot activities that may result in fines or delayed reimbursement and initiate corrective action.

�! **NEW** **Forms and Templates on Diskette.** Now you can organize your auditing data via preformatted electronic templates.

➡ **EXCLUSIVE** **Updated With Case Studies for 2001.** Real-life situations illustrate common and unusual circumstances to help you perform effective audits quickly.

➡ **NEW** **Expanded Key Issues Section.** Prompts you with questions to ask yourself during a self-audit.

➡ **Chart Auditing Instructions.** Cuts training time and provides your employees with a resource to reference other then you.

➡ **EXCLUSIVE** **Your Written Audit History.** Located conveniently within the Table of Contents, your personal audit history will serve as proof of your ongoing efforts to stay compliant.

➡ **Sample Worksheets.** Within each chapter are audit and post audit worksheets to guide you through each element of an audit and track trends.

Ensure the E/M Codes You are Reporting are Correct

2001 E/M Fast Finder

ISBN 1-56337-357-2

(Item #2852)

$29⁹⁵

Available December 2000

With this portable, easy-to-use, reference you can be assured E/M codes are correct before reporting patient encounters. Quick reference graphs make selecting the correct level of service easy. And the convenient size means you can take it wherever you go to make compliance a part of your daily activity.

➡ **Fully Updated.** Make sure you are using the most current E/Mcodes.

➡ **Organized by Site of Service (Office, Hospital, Emergency).** Quickly find the exact range of E/M codes you need.

➡ **Quick Reference Graphs.** Easily check the level of history, exam, and medical decision-making to find the right E/M code.

➡ **Convenient.** Pocket size and durable pages make it ideal for the examination room.

➡ **Step-By-Step Instructions.** Easy to follow instructions and a sample worksheet walk you through the steps needed to properly use the fast finder.

➡ **Abbreviation Key.** A listing of commonly used and accepted medical abbreviations make this a perfect tool for a beginner or an experienced physician.

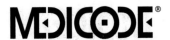

Medicode, 5225 Wiley Post Way, Suite 500, Salt Lake City, UT 84116 • 801.536.1000 • FAX 801.536.1011

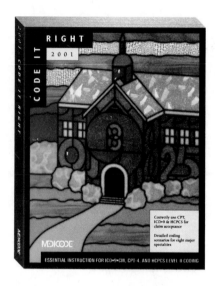
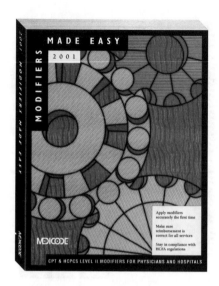
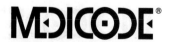

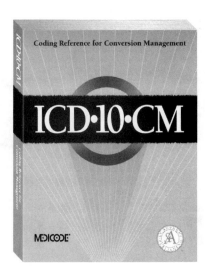
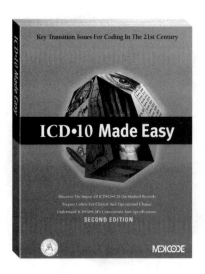
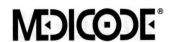

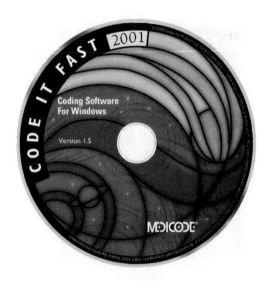
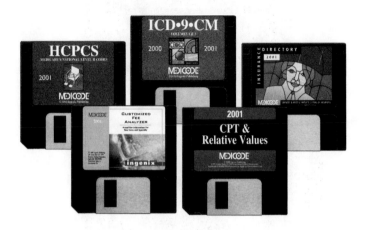
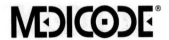

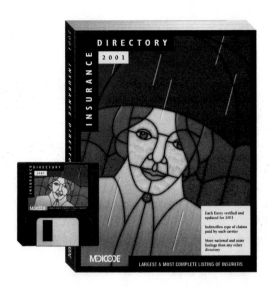
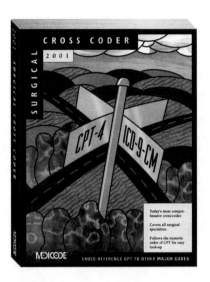
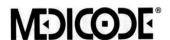

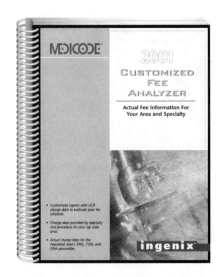
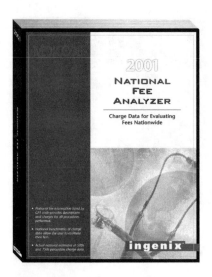
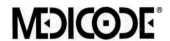

Diagnostic Coding Essentials

MEDICODE®

Notice

Diagnostic Coding Essentials is designed to be an accurate and authoritative source regarding coding and every reasonable effort has been made to ensure accuracy and completeness of the content. However, Medicode makes no guarantee, warranty, or representation that this publication is accurate, complete, or without errors. It is understood that Medicode is not rendering any legal or other professional services or advice in this publication and that Medicode bears no liability for any results or consequences which may arise from the use of this book. Please address all correspondence to:

Ingenix Publishing Group
5225 Wiley Post Way, Suite 500
Salt Lake City, UT 84116-2889

Acknowledgements

Elizabeth Boudrie, *Publisher*
Lynn Speirs, *Senior Director of Publishing*
Sheri Poe Bernard, CPC, *Director Essential Regulatory Products*
Christine B. Fraizer, MA, CPC, *Project Editor*
Charlene Neeshan, *Clinical Editor*
Kerrie Hornsby, *Desktop Publishing Manager*
Kathy Goebel, *Desktop Publishing Specialist*

Copyright

Contents

Introduction

Diagnostic Coding Essentials is a comprehensive ICD-9-CM coding reference designed for the medical office, hospital, or health insurance company, educator, or student who seeks to expand his or her understanding of diagnostic coding. Its goal is to enrich the reader's clinical understanding of ICD-9-CM, so code selection becomes more accurate.

Unlike other ICD-9-CM references, *Diagnostic Coding Essentials* includes all numeric codes in ICD-9-CM, from 001 to 999. In some cases, its narrative discusses clinical issues affecting code selection for comprehensive categories (diabetes, fractures) and in other cases provides code-specific information (sudden infant death syndrome, hydatidiform mole). Because the book does not include the comprehensive index found in the official ICD-9-CM, it does not replace use of an official code book. However, used in conjunction with your code book, *Diagnostic Coding Essentials* will provide you an unparalleled clinical roadmap to code selection.

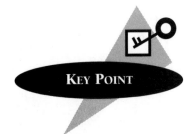

KEY POINT

V codes and E codes are excluded from the first edition of *Diagnostic Coding Essentials*, but are sometimes included as adjunct information with codes with which they would be reported.

Format

Diagnostic Coding Essentials begins with a section on the history and conventions of ICD-9-CM coding. It then follows the organization of ICD-9, looking at diseases and their codes beginning with Infectious and Parasitic Diseases (chapter 1) through Injury and Poisoning (chapter 17), in numeric order. The basic format of the book is to provide clinical coding support, with illustrations, narrative, definitions, and other resources that will help the coder working from the medical record. For quick identification, the name of each chapter appears at the top of each page spread, along with codes found within that chapter. Tabs at the side of the page further simplify your code search.

ICD-9-CM CODES AND DESCRIPTIONS

The codes in *Diagnostic Coding Essentials* are organized in their hierarchical context, appearing within their appropriate three-digit rubric. All three-digit rubrics appear in a capitalized format. If the three-digit code is valid, an icon (**OK**) appears next to the code so that you know it is a valid code for use on a claim form.

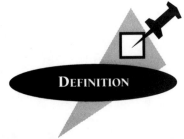

DEFINITION

Rubric: a grouping of similar conditions. In ICD-9-CM, "rubric" denotes a three-digit category, and all codes that begin with that three-digit number are part of a common disease grouping. There are nearly 100 rubrics that represent valid codes because there are no subclassifications within those rubrics. Those rubrics can be used as valid codes in diagnostic reporting.

129 INTESTINAL PARASITISM, UNSPECIFIED **OK**

Use this code only if the disease is known to be parasitic and the parasite is unknown. If the parasite is known, use the appropriate "not elsewhere classified" code from other rubrics in this section.

Note that (**OK**) next to the description with 129 indicates that code 129 represents a valid ICD-9 code. There are less than 100 valid three-digit codes in ICD-9.

Though all three-digit categories appear in *Diagnostic Coding Essentials*, invalid four-digit categories have been eliminated to reduce confusion regarding valid code choices. With the exception of valid three-digit codes, which are displayed above, all other valid codes in *Diagnostic Coding Essentials* appear at the same indent, unlike the presentation in ICD-9 itself. For example, all valid codes that occur in rubric 088 *Other Arthropod-borne diseases*, appear as follows:

088.0	Bartonellosis — *Bartonella bacilliformis; sandflies; Andes*
088.81	Lyme disease — *Borrelia burgdorferi; ticks, United States*
088.82	Babesiosis — *Babesia; ticks*
088.89	Other specified arthropod-borne diseases — *not elsewhere classified*
088.9	Unspecified arthropod-borne disease — *unknown*

Note that some valid codes in rubric 088 are four-digit codes, and some valid codes in this rubric are five-digit codes. Only valid codes are included.

Should there be information within a four-digit subclassification that applies to all five-digit codes within that subclassification, the invalid four-digit code will appear in a different format, to distinguish it from the valid five-digit codes that follow. For example:

722.8 Postlaminectomy syndrome
Postlaminectomy syndrome is a complex of symptoms following laminectomy surgery. It includes conditions and syndromes described as postfusion, postmicrosurgery, and postchemonucleolysis.

722.80	Postlaminectomy syndrome, unspecified region — *unknown site on spine*
722.81	Postlaminectomy syndrome, cervical region — *neck, C1-C7*
722.82	Postlaminectomy syndrome, thoracic region — *upper back, T1-T12*
722.83	Postlaminectomy syndrome, lumbar region — *lower back, L1-L5*

Because the elimination of invalid four-digit codes could compromise the completeness of the code descriptions as they appear in ICD-9, complete descriptions are used with each code in *Diagnostic Coding Essentials*. Therefore, while a code would read in your ICD-9 book like this:

239	Neoplasms of unspecified nature
239.0	Digestive system

In *Diagnostic Coding Essentials*, the codes would read like this:

239	Neoplasms of unspecified nature
239.0	Neoplasms of unspecified nature of digestive system

Note that the information from ICD-9's description for 239 has been combined with the information from ICD-9's description for 239.0 to create the description for *Diagnostic Coding Essentials'* 239.0.

ITALICIZED DESCRIPTORS

Following most codes in *Diagnostic Coding Essentials* are brief descriptors that will help you differentiate the codes and determine which code is best suited for your clinical situation. For example:

701.9	Unspecified hypertrophic and atrophic condition of skin — *including skin tag, atrophoderma, pendulous abdomen, redundant skin, or unknown*

In this example, the term "atrophoderma" appears as a descriptive term under 701.9 in ICD-9; and the other terms are indexed to 701.9 in the official ICD-9 index. In other cases, clinical research provided the synonyms or support information that appears as an italicized descriptor after a code, as in the case of:

001.0	Cholera due to Vibrio cholerae — *Inaba, Ogawa, Hikojima serotypes; classical*
001.1	Cholera due to Vibrio cholerae el tor — *commonly less severe or asymptomatic*
001.9	Unspecified cholera — *unknown whether Vibrio cholerae or Vibrio cholerae el tor*

None of the italicized information above appears in the official ICD-9-CM text.

NARRATIVE

Diagnostic Coding Essentials provides valuable background information on thousands of medical conditions. Information that appears directly after a three-digit category applies to all codes within that rubric. Information that appears following a four-digit subclassification applies to all codes in that subclassification, and information following a fifth-digit code applies only to that code.

MARGINS

Diagnostic Coding Essentials is presented in an educational format that provides additional information in the margins, as well as leaves room in the margins for reader notes. Information in the margins is not a repeat of information in the text. Instead, it augments the text, providing abbreviations commonly seen in the medical record, defintions of medical terms, and other data points that will help the reader to make accurate code selections based on the medical record. See the example in the margin on the previous page.

Also provided in the book'smargins is fifth-digit information for some codes. Codes that require a fifth digit appear with a 5th icon, and the fifth digit information can be found in the margins within the same page spread:

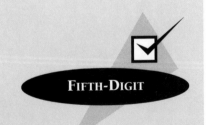

FIFTH-DIGIT

346 MIGRAINE

346.0 5th Classical migraine — *migraine preceded or accompanied by transient focal neurological symptoms; migraine with aura*
346.1 5th Common migraine — *including atypical migraine; sick headache*
346.2 5th Variants of migraine — *including cluster headache; histamine cephalgia; abdominal migraine; migrainous or ciliary neuralgia*
346.8 5th Other forms of migraine — *including hemiplegic or ophthalmoplegic migraine*
346.9 5th Unspecified migraine — *unspecified*

The following fifth-digit subclassification is for use with category 346:

0 without mention of intractable migraine

1 with intractable migraine, so stated

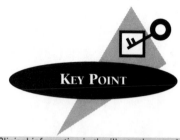

KEY POINT

Clinical information in the illustrations and narrations of *Diagnostic Coding Essentials* is drafted by consultants and technical editors at Ingenix, and draws from a broad spectrum of surgical, clinical and anatomic publications.

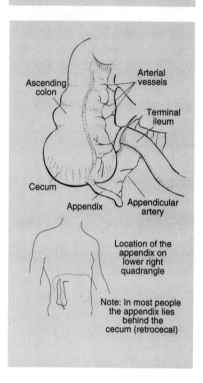

Ascending colon

Arterial vessels

Terminal ileum

Cecum

Appendix

Appendicular artery

Location of the appendix on lower right quadrangle

Note: In most people the appendix lies behind the cecum (retrocecal)

Illustrations

Illustrations in the margins should provide readers a better understanding of the anatomical nuances associated with specific codes. The illustrations usually include a labeled anatomical view, and may include narrative that discusses specific conditions or anatomic sites. The illustrations are almost always simplified schematic representations. In many instances, some detail is eliminated in order to make a clear point about the anatomic site that is the focus of the depiction.

Also, in Chapter 2 of *Diagnostic Coding Essentials*, ICD-O, Morphology of Neoplasms, is printed on alternating pages to provide an additional coding resource to cancer registries and others using ICD-O codes to classify neoplasms.

History of Diagnostic Coding

International Standards of Classification

GATHERING STATISTICS

As commonplace as diagnostic coding appears today, such was not the case 50 years ago when public health professionals were debating the merits of standardized reporting. Wilson G. Smillie, MD and former professor of public health and preventive medicine at Cornell University in New York, advocated giving all physicians a copy of the *International List of Causes of Death* (circa 1891) for guidance in reporting vital statistics. But as far as reporting every disease and where it is occurring? "Why require that?" Dr. Smillie asks in the 1943 publication of his book *Public Health Administration in the United States*. "It's interesting from a statistical point of view," he admits, though unnecessary for diseases that do not present as public health problems. Such a task accomplishes nothing but more work for medical team, he concludes.

Statistics, however, were and remain paramount to the World Health Organization's (WHO) point of view. The (WHO) Charter of 1948 places the overriding objective on attaining among all people the "highest possible level of health." So why require data collection? Because morbidity (illness) and mortality (death) statistics tell how nations live and die and, when tracked, show the diseases causing the highest rates of death, according to the provisions of the WHO Constitution. The information derived from statistics indicates the types of programs and services essential to maintaining and improving the public health.

REPORTING STATISTICS

The *International List of Causes of Death* was revised five times over nearly 60 years (1900, 1910, 1920, 1929, and 1938). The sixth revision, in 1948, resulted in the *International Statistical Classification of Diseases, Injuries and Causes of Death*, which was formally adopted the same year by the First World Health Assembly, together with WHO regulations for compiling mortality and morbidity statistics by cause, age, and sex. The sixth edition was based on anatomical sites, similar to its predecessors. But unlike earlier editions, the sixth revision broke ground with an appendix listing groups of causes:

- Cause groups (001 Tuberculosis of respiratory system through 780-793 and 795 Ill-defined and unknown causes of morbidity and mortality)

- E codes classifying the external cause of accidents, poisonings, and violence (E810-E835 Motor Vehicle Accidents through E990-E999 Injury resulting from operation of war)

OBJECTIVES

Vital and health statistics serve three primary purposes:

1. **Diagnostic Research** - statistical inquiry establishes relationships such as research linking solar radiation to cancers of the skin

2. **Organization** - statistical organization provides clues as to what causes a disease and what preventive measures work best to maintain public health

3. **Planning** - statistical research and organization go into developing the programs and services most suited to the health needs of a specific population

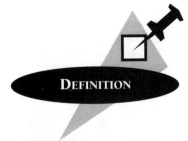

DEFINITION

Nomenclature - A system of standardized names. Nomenclature in ICD-9 refers to the classification system used to track the causes of illness and death.

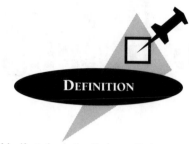

DEFINITION

Manifestation is the display or disclosure of characteristic signs or symptoms of an illness.

Morbidity describes the disease rate or number of cases of a particular disease - in a given age range, gender, occupation, or other relevant population based grouping.

Mortality describes the death rate reflected by the population in a given region, age range, or other relevant statistical grouping.

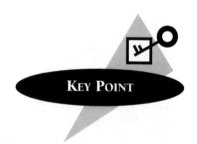

KEY POINT

The reported conditions on the death certificate are translated into medical codes through use of the classification structure and the selection and modification rules contained in the applicable revision of the ICD. These coding rules improve the usefulness of mortality statistics by giving preference to certain categories, by consolidating conditions, and by systematically selecting a single cause of death from a reported sequence of conditions. The single selected cause for tabulation is called the underlying cause of death, and the other reported causes are the nonunderlying causes of death. The combination of underlying and nonunderlying causes is the multiple causes of death.

- N codes classifying the nature of injury resulting from accidents, poisonings and violence (N800-N804 Fracture of skull through N950-N959 and N980-N999 All other and unspecified effects of external causes)

WHO published the Manual of the *International Statistical Classification of Diseases, Injuries, and Causes of Death,* including its appendices, in three languages (English, French, and Spanish). The following year, WHO established the Centre for Classification of Diseases in the General Register Office in London to help in the interpretation and application of the international classification system in coordination with separate national committees on vital and health statistics.

WHO "Regulations No. 1" emphasized the reporting of vital statistics and placed the greatest emphasis on the underlying cause of death as the most useful single element in the analysis of mortality, according to the report *The Second Ten Years of the World Health Organization* (1958-1967). The international law required all countries to adopt a form of medical death certificate that clearly stated the underlying cause of death, as verified by the attending physician. The provision not only validated death certificates, but also made it possible to compare mortality data among nations.

Regulations No. 1 also contained a number of articles governing groupings by age, cause, and area of residence and charged the Expert Committee on Health Statistics with the "study of problems concerning the registration of cases of cancer as well as their statistical presentation." Regulations No. 1 was modified over the next several years to draw attention to the registration, compilation, and transmission of statistics. Subsequent amendments adopted definitions of "live birth" and "foetal (British variance of fetal) death" for purposes of determining rates of infant mortality. No member of the World Health Assembly could vary the groupings without going through a formal process to revise the information.

Financial reports from the same period underline the significance WHO placed on the "development and strengthening of systematic procedures for the securing of adequate vital and health statistics" for the good of public health. In 1957, the WHO Publications Revolving Fund showed an increase in revenue from the sale of the manual and, in a report to the WHO Executive Board, requested funding above the present balance of $35,680 to print additional copies.

In 1958, the World Health Assembly adopted the *Seventh Revision of the Manual of the International Statistical Classification of Diseases, Injuries and Causes of Death.* The seventh revision (in use from 1958 to 1967) introduced improved methods for compiling morbidity data, which had lagged behind mortality data collection partly due to the lack of international definitions of terms used to describe and measure morbidity. The eighth revision adopted by the Nineteenth World Health Assembly in 1966 incorporated definitions for measuring morbidity as well as the type of information necessary for compiling morbidity statistics (i.e., clearly stating either the people affected or the relevant diagnosis and occurrence of illness). The official name was abbreviated to the *International Classification of Diseases* (ICD). Data reservoirs considered for future statistical collection included the possibility of analyzing the medical records of general practitioners, as recommended by WHO Expert Committee on Health Statistics.

The World Health Assembly adopted the familiar International Classification of Diseases, Ninth Revision (ICD-9) in 1976 for projected international application by January 1979. The ninth revision was intended to be much more useful to the clinician than previous

� 5th   Needs fifth-digit   **OK**   Valid three-digit code

revisions, which were oriented more towards the medical statistician. It included new definitions and recommendations concerning material and perinatal morbidity and mortality, and a proposed form of certificate of cause of perinatal death By the end of 1977, ICD-9 had been published in English, French, and Spanish and the Russian edition was in preparation.

In early 1980 work commenced on the tenth revision of ICD. A decision at that time to base the tenth revision on a thorough evaluation of the ninth revision delayed the anticipated 1985 deadline to 1990 for submitting to the World Health Assembly. The proposed revision was called a "radically new coding system" as presented in 1989 at the *International Conference for the Tenth Revision of the International Classification of Diseases.* The tenth revision would allow for the coding of almost twice as many conditions as the basic three-character level to accommodate "the degree of specificity now required for the application of the classification to hospital inpatient morbidity and general medical practice," according to a 1980-1981 report on WHO accomplishments. The official name was changed to the *International Statistical Classification of Diseases and Related Health Problems* to indicate the added scope of the tenth revision. Plans were to submit the revised edition at the 43rd World Health Assembly in 1990 and, if approved, for international application in 1993.

Actual publication of ICD-10 began in 1992 for the English version and in 1993 for the French. Volume 2 (instruction manual) was published in English in 1993, while volume 3 (alphabetical index) was still on the presses. In addition, a three-character version of ICD-10 containing the rules, definitions, standards, and its own index was published in English and French to meet the needs of developing countries. Concurrently with publication, WHO developed a new timetable for updating ICD-10. Changes in the tabular list are made with intervals of between two to three years rather than yearly as has been the practice with ICD-9 and earlier versions. However, the alphabetic index of ICD-10 continues on a yearly schedule with revisions available on the WHO ICD-10 web site.

TABULATING STATISTICS

The advances in collecting and recording data created the need to train people in tabulating statistics. These early "coders," predominantly employed as record officers in hospitals or statisticians in public health departments, were advised to participate in one-week seminars, sponsored by the WHO Centre for Classification of Diseases, focusing on the following subjects:

- Beginnings and endings of medical terms
- Names of the principle bones
- Layout of classification
- Descriptive arrangement of the notes of exceptions and conventions for colons and brackets
- Undesirable terms
- Use of code numbers that vary according to circumstance (the appendix of causes)

Each new revision required additional courses to familiarize coders with the provisions of the latest version. In 1977, for example, courses in ICD-9 were organized by the WHO regional offices for Africa (Accra), Europe (London, Moscow, and Paris) and the Western Pacific (Kuala Lumpur, Singapore, and Sydney). Trained coders attending the first

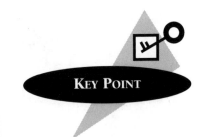

KEY POINT

ICD-10, *International Statistical Classification of Diseases and Related Health Problems, Tenth Revision,* is a list of diagnostic codes, published by WHO, that doubles the number of three-character categories found in ICD-9. ICD-10 is a 3-volume set that contains:

- Tabular lists containing cause-of-death titles and codes (Volume 1)
- Inclusion and exclusion terms for cause-of-death titles (Volume 1)
- Alphabetical index to diseases and nature of injury, external causes of injury, table of drugs and chemicals (Volume 3)
- Description, guidelines, and coding rules (Volume 2)

The ICD-10 system has replaced ICD-9 in most parts of the world and will be the diagnostic coding system in place in the United States once clinically modified and tested.

The Need for Trained Coders
"To lay people unacquainted with medical terminology, ignorant of the structure and physiology of the body, and prejudiced by private theories and popular superstitions, the study of the international classification can be an exacting task, but one which leads to satisfaction in work and a surprising accuracy of application."

Fraser Brockington from his book *World Health,* published in 1958

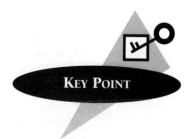

international computer-based course for an orientation to ICD-10, held in 1982, also received instructions on providing similar training to other national coders. Regional training courses were in the making.

National Standards of Classification

CLINICAL MODIFICATION

The *International Classification of Diseases, Ninth Revision, Clinical Modification, Fifth Edition*, commonly referred to ICD-9-CM, is the classification system used by physician offices as well as inpatient and outpatient facilities for the purpose of coding and indexing disease data. The modified version of ICD-9 presents a more precise clinical picture of the patient than was needed for statistical groupings and trend analysis. The United States National Center for Health Statistics (NCHS) added clinical information that allows a more thorough indexing of medical records, medical case reviews, and ambulatory and other medical care groups. In the United States, ICD-9-CM codes are updated every year (with the exception in the year 2000 due to electronic data concerns related to the millennium). Volumes 1 and 2 are used in coding diagnosis information. Volume 3 is used in coding inpatient and outpatient facility procedures.

The medical coder's role in the process is to translate written diagnoses into numeric and alphanumeric (E codes and V codes) codes, similar to the task of the coder working with the international ICD-9. The coded information is used by the physician's office primarily as a means of communicating the reason for the medical services to the commercial and government payers (i.e., Medicare, Medicaid, State Children's Health Insurance Program). As a communication tool, ICD-9-CM diagnosis codes relate the disease, condition, complaint, sign, symptom, or other reason for the medical services provided. In addition to being a means of communication between provider and payer, ICD-9-CM codes are used similarly to the international ICD-9 classification system for purposes such as research and financial analysis. In the United States, the National Committee on Quality Assurance (NCQA) and the Healthplan Employer Data and Information Set (HEDIS) require diagnostic coding to meet compliance standards.

As in the past for earlier editions of ICD, the United States planned a clinical modification of ICD-10 prior to implementation. As agreed upon by the NCHS, all modifications must conform to WHO conventions. The Center for Health Policy Studies (CHIPS) was contracted by NCHS to analyze ICD-10 and to develop the appropriate clinical modifications. Except in rare instances, no modifications have been made to existing codes three-digit categories and four-digit codes, with the exception of title changes in ICD-10-CM that do not change the meaning of the category or code.

The current draft of ICD-10-CM contains a significantly increased number of codes compared to either ICD-10 or ICD-9-CM. Notable revisions in ICD-10-CM, including features not found in ICD-9-CM, include the following:

- Adding information relevant to ambulatory and managed care encounters
- Expanding injury codes
- Creating combination diagnosis/symptom codes to reduce the number of the codes needed to fully describe a condition
- Adding a sixth character (ICD-9-CM goes up to five-character codes)

✔5th   Needs fifth-digit   **OK**   Valid three-digit code

- Incorporating common 4th and 5th digit classifications
- Laterality (i.e., right, left, or bilateral) ICD-10-CM does not add laterality in all cases, though the modification enhances particularly the Neoplasm and Injury chapters. For example, with the reporting of laterality, providers will need to document where the injury occurred.
- Granularity (greater specificity in code assignment)

There is not yet an anticipated implementation date for the ICD-10-CM. There will be a two-year implementation window once the final notice to implement has been published in the Federal Register.

ICD-9 Conventions

The following section summarizes the coding conventions found in ICD-9-CM and the coding conventions that will be found in ICD-10-CM. We start with ICD-9-CM. The overview compares the following features:

1. Format

2. Typeface

3. Punctuation

4. Notes

5. Instructional Notes

6. Modifiers

7. Abbreviations

8. Cross References

THREE VOLUME SET

1. Volume 1 of ICD-9 is a tabular listing of disease and injury divided into 17 sections, generally along anatomic sites. Two supplementary classifications contain alphanumeric codes to report factors influencing health status and other contact with health services (V codes) and causes of injury and poisoning (E codes). Appendixes to Volume 1 provide additional information and references.

2. Volume 2 is an alphabetic index of codes contained in Volume 1 and is important in locating proper diagnoses. An index to external causes of injury (E codes) is included. Three tables are included to assist in the selection of proper codes for hypertension, neoplasms, and drugs and chemicals.

3. A third volume of ICD-9 contains codes developed for coding inpatient facility procedures and is not ordinarily consulted for physician or outpatient services. Volume 3 contains both a tabular listing, arranged along anatomic lines, and an alphabetic index. Volume 3 coding issues are outside the framework of this reference manual.

SUPPLEMENTAL CLASSIFICATIONS

Volume 1 contains two supplemental code classifications: V codes and E codes. V codes can be used as primary diagnoses when reporting services not related to current medical problems or conditions such as periodic or routine medical exams. Whereas, E codes are never used as primary diagnoses, providing supplemental information only on the causes of injury and poisoning. See the individual listings for more information.

V codes (V01-V82), describe circumstances that influence a patient's health status and identify reasons for medical encounters resulting from circumstances other than a disease or injury classified in the main part of ICD-9.

V codes are generally used in three instances:

- When a physician identifies a circumstance or problem in a person who is not currently sick but has nonetheless come in contact with health services (to act as an organ donor or to receive a prophylactic vaccination, for example)
- When an ill or injured patient requires specific treatment (such as chemotherapy for malignancy or removal of pins or rods in postoperative orthopedic care)
- When a problem or circumstance that influences the patient's health is not itself a current illness but may affect future medical treatment

The second set of supplemental codes in Volume 1 is the *Supplementary Classification of External Causes of Injury and Poisoning* (E800-E999), also known as E codes. The E codes are never listed as the primary diagnosis; they are adjunctive. You may need to use more than one E code to describe fully the circumstances of an accident. Use them to establish medical necessity to indicate a secondary payer responsible for payment of the service, identify causes of injury and poisoning, and to identify drugs. The index for the E codes is found in Volume 2, following the Table of Drugs and Chemicals.

APPROACHES TO ICD-9-CM CODING

Determining a diagnostic code begins with analysis of the encounter form, operative report, or diagnostic statement for those words or main terms that best identify the patient's current condition or symptoms. Once the current condition or symptom is identified, consult Volume 2, the alphabetic index, to identify the main term associated with the condition or symptom. Next, identify any modifying terms listed below the main term to more specifically describe the condition or symptom. After the most specific main term and modifiers have been identified, look up the corresponding code in Volume 1, the tabular list. Follow any instructions or notes in both the alphabetic index and the tabular list.

RULES OF ICD-9-CM REFERENCE

An ironclad rule in diagnostic coding is to never derive a code by consulting only the Volume 2 alphabetic index. It is a reference index to the full tabular listing of Volume 1, which often yields a different code, additional codes, or a more specific code.

The six-step process for assigning diagnostic codes can be summarized as follows:

1. Determine the main terms that describe the patient's condition or symptoms.

2. Look up the main term in Volume 2 where the condition is alphabetized as a noun or adjective.

✓5th Needs fifth-digit   **OK** Valid three-digit code

3. If indicated, follow cross-references such as see, see also, and see category to find the correct code.

4. Review subterms and modifying words. Refer to any indented terms under the main term to further clarify the code selection.

5. Verify the code as listed in Volume 2, the alphabetic index, by checking it against Volume 1, the tabular listing.

6. Review all instructions and notes in Volume 1 such as includes, excludes, code first underlying disease or use additional code to assure that the correct code has been selected.

In outpatient coding, do not attempt to code "rule out," "probable," "suspect," or "questionable" descriptions in the documentation. While acceptable in a patient's medical record and for inpatient coding, coding rules do not allow their use in outpatient coding. Rather, code the condition, symptoms, signs, test results, or other reasons that can be documented for the medical encounter. (Consult American Hospital Association [AHA] guidelines for specifics on inpatient hospital coding.)

FORMAT
ICD-9 has an indented format. Subterms are indented two spaces to the right of the term to which they are linked. Continuations of lines too long for columns are indented four spaces.

251.2	Hypoglycemia, unspecified
	Hypoglycemia: Hypoglycemia:
	NOS spontaneous
	reactive

TYPEFACE
Bold type identifies all codes and main terms in the Tabular List (Volume 1), separating it from subordinate information or notes.

Italicized type identifies those categories that cannot be reported as primary diagnosis and also for all exclusion notes.

PUNCTUATION
- Braces (}) enclose a series of terms modified by the statement or terms appearing to the right of the brace.
- Brackets ([ ]) enclose synonyms, alternative wordings, or explanatory phrases. The brackets may be square [ ] or italicized [ ].
- Colon (:) is used in Volume 1 of ICD-9 to identify a term that is incomplete without one or more of the descriptors following it. Do not assign the code unless one or more of the descriptors is present in the physician's diagnostic statement.
- Parentheses ( ) enclose supplementary (nonessential) modifiers and do not generally affect code assignment. However, they do serve to confirm for the coder that the correct code was selected when the nonessential modifier is present in both ICD-9 and

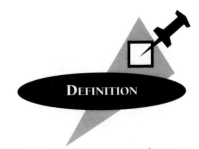

DEFINITION

Category: In ICD-9, a category refers to the three-digit form of each code, such as 384 other disorders of tympanic membrane. Category codes can be further broken down into subcategories (fourth digits) 384.2 Perforation of tympanic membrane, and subcategories can be broken down into subclassifications (fifth digits) 384.21 Central perforation of tympanic membrane. There are approximately 100 valid 3-digit categories listed in ICD-9.

Rubric: In ICD-10-CM rubric (a grouping of similar conditions) denotes either a three-character category or a four-character subcategory.

the physician's documented diagnosis. Parentheses also enclose many see also references.

NOTES

Notes are found in Volumes 1 and 2 and have no fixed length. They give general coding instructions. Notes in Volume 1 are indented and printed in plain type, while those in Volume 2 are boxed and italicized. The placement of these notes is as important as their content. Notes at the beginning of a section apply to all categories within the section. Those at the beginning of a subsection apply to all categories within the subsection. Likewise, notes preceding three-digit categories apply to all fourth-digit and fifth-digit codes within that category.

- *Code Also* dictates the use of two diagnostic codes. List the etiology (cause) first, followed by the manifestation. The two codes combined represent the primary diagnosis.

- *Code First Underlying Disease* identifies diagnoses that are not primary and are incomplete when used alone. In such cases the code, its title, and instructions are italicized. This type of instructional note appears only in Volume 1. A code with this instructional note should be recorded second, with the underlying cause recorded first. Italicized brackets identify this situation in Volume 2.

INSTRUCTIONAL NOTES

To assign diagnostic codes at the highest level of specificity, there are additional notes to follow.

- *Excludes* indicates terms that are not ordinarily coded under the referenced term. The word "Excludes" is surrounded by a box for easy identification and the corresponding note is italicized. This note does not prevent you from using the excluded code in addition to the code from which it was excluded when both conditions are present.

- *Includes* appear immediately under a three-digit code title to provide further definition or to give an example of the category contents.

- *Use Additional Code* in Volume 1 indicates those categories where an additional code is available to provide further information and to give a more complete picture of the diagnosis. The additional code should identify other aspects of the disease, including manifestation, cause, associated condition, and nature of the condition itself.

MODIFIERS

- Essential modifiers are indented two spaces just below the main terms. They are generally presented in alphabetical order, with the exceptions of with and without, which appear before the alphabetized modifiers. Each additional essential modifier clarifies the previous one and is indented two additional spaces to the right. These descriptive terms affect code selection since they describe essential differences in site, etiology, and symptoms. When a main term in the tabular Volume 1 has only one essential modifier, it appears on the same line as the main term, separated by a comma.

- Nonessential modifiers are listed immediately to the right of the main term and are enclosed in parentheses. They serve as examples to help you translate written terminology into numeric codes and may be present or absent in the diagnostic without affecting code assignment.

✓5th Needs fifth-digit   **OK** Valid three-digit code

ABBREVIATIONS

- NEC (not elsewhere classifiable) indicates the main term is broad or not well defined. Use an NEC code only when more information is unavailable. This term is used only in Volume 2.

- NOS (not otherwise specified) is the equivalent of NEC and is used only in Volume 1.

CROSS-REFERENCES

In Volume 2, several types of cross-references are encountered:

- See indicates that you should see the condition listed instead of the term you've found in order to assign the correct diagnostic code.

- See also indicates that additional information is available. This cross-reference may provide a more specific code or an additional code.

- See category directs you to an additional three-digit category, not just a single code. Again, you cannot assign an appropriate code unless you follow this instruction.

I-10 Conventions

THREE VOLUME SET

Similar to ICD-9-CM, the tenth revision is divided into three volumes:

1. Volume 1 (Tabular List) is comprised of 21 chapters that contain the listing of alphanumeric codes. The same hierarchical organization of ICD-9 applies to ICD-10: All codes with the same first three digits have common traits. Each digit beyond three adds more specificity. In ICD-10, valid codes can contain anywhere from three to five digits. In ICD-10-CM, valid codes may contain a sixth digit.

2. If Volume 2 remains the title of the instructional manual after clinical modification in the United States, coders will need to remember that Volume 2 in ICD-10-CM refers to instructions, and not the index, which is what Volume 2 provides in ICD-9-CM.

3. Volume 3 provides the index to the codes in the Tabular List. As in the ICD-9-CM index, terms in the ICD-10 index are found alphabetically, by diagnosis.

All codes in ICD-10 are alphanumeric (i.e., one letter followed by two numbers at the three-character level) as opposed to three numeric characters in the main classification of ICD-9-CM. Of the 26 available letters, all but the letter U is used. Some three-character categories have been left vacant for future expansion and revision.

AXIS OF CLASSIFICATION

ICD-10-CM is an arrangement of similar entities, diseases, and other conventions on the basis of specific criteria. Diseases can be arranged in a variety of ways: according to etiology, anatomy, or severity. The particular criteria chosen is called the axis of classification. Anatomy is the primary axis of classification of ICD-10-CM.

Different axes, such as etiology, site, type or morphology, are used in classifying different diseases within the same chapters. The choice is based upon the most important aspects of the disease from both a statistical and clinical point of view. For example:

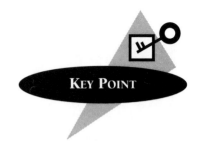

KEY POINT

Contrasts between ICD-9-CM and ICD-10-CM will become more obvious as the United States switches to the tenth revision of the diagnostic classification system. Among the basic differences:

- All codes in ICD-10 are alphanumeric as opposed to three numeric characters in the main classification of ICD-9-CM.

- The Tabular List for ICD-10-CM is comprised of 21 chapters vs. the 17 main chapters and two supplemental classifications (V and E codes) for ICD-9-CM. As in ICD-9-CM, many of the chapters classify diseases of an organ system. Others are devoted to specific types of conditions grouped according to etiology or nature, e.g., neoplasms, referred to in ICD-10 as "special group" chapters.

- ICD-9-CM has a fifth digit for coding to the highest level of specificity, whereas ICD-10-CM has both fifth and sixth digit categories for coding to the highest level of specificity.

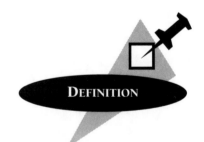

DEFINITION

Deactivated codes: To meet data-gathering goals desired by the federal government for coding in the United States, some codes that are valid in ICD-9 have been deactivated for ICD-10-CM. These codes fall into several categories: procedure codes, death codes, and codes considered to be highly unspecific.

- Pneumonia: etiology or of the pneumonia
- Malignant neoplasm: site
- Cardiac arrhythmia: type
- Leukemia: morphology

SUPPLEMENTAL CLASSIFICATIONS

Many of the chapters in ICD-10-CM classify diseases of an organ system. Others are devoted to specific types of conditions grouped according to etiology or nature, e.g., neoplasms, referred to in ICD-10 as "special group" chapters. Three chapters do not fall into either of these categories: Symptoms, Signs and Abnormal Clinical and Laboratory Findings, Not Elsewhere Classified; External Causes of Morbidity and Mortality; and Factors Influencing Health Status and Contact with Health Services.

A residual category is a place for classifying a specified form of a condition that does not have its own specific subdivision.

FORMAT

Similar to ICD-9-CM, the format in ICD-10-CM depends on indentation. For example, individual five-character subdivisions of four-character subcategories represent the etiology of the disease and, as such, appear like the following:

A02.2	Localized salmonella infections	
	A02.20	Localized salmonella infection, unspecified
	A02.21	Salmonella meningitis
	A02.22	Salmonella pneumonia
	A02.23	Salmonella arthritis
	A02.24	Salmonella osteomyelitis
	A02.25	Salmonella pyelonephritis

ICD-10-CM also includes a sixth character for classification for the most precise subdivision, which appears like the following:

S61.4	Open wound of hand		
	S61.40	Unspecifed open wound of hand	
		S61.401	Unspecified open wound, right hand
		S61.402	Unspecified open wound, left hand
		S61.403	Unspecified open wound, unspecified hand

TYPEFACE

Codes and titles in the Tabular List and main terms in the Alphabetic Index are in bold typeface. Exclusion notes and rubrics not used for primary tabulations of disease are in an italicized typeface.

PUNCTUATION

The ICD-10-CM Tabular list employs certain punctuation that must be clearly understood to use the classification correctly. These include:

- Braces ({ }) enclose a series of terms, each of which is modified by the word(s) following the brace.

✔5th Needs fifth-digit   **OK** Valid three-digit code

- Brackets ([ ]) enclose synonyms, alternative wordings or explanatory phrases.
- Colon (:) is applied rather than a comma for a term that has more than one essential modifier.
- Comma (,) distinguishes modifiers. Words following a comma are essential modifiers.
- Parentheses (( ))enclose supplementary words that are present or absent in the statement of a disease or procedure, but do not affect the code.
- Point Dash (.-) instructs you to turn to the category or subcategory referenced to review the subdivisions available for coding.

NOTES

The tenth revision contains notes that describe the general content of the succeeding categories and provide instructions for using the codes. These include:

- A "code first" note tells you that two codes are necessary to describe the condition. Code first notes may identify the added code - or examples of the added code - required, a range of codes, or instructions to code the underlying disease.
- A "use" note gives specific instructions for using an additional code to completely describe a condition. Depending on the additional information to be encoded, a use note may give a specific code or range of codes or examples of the codes applies. No codes may be specified though the notes describe the information to be encoded.

INSTRUCTIONAL NOTES

Throughout the Tabular List in ICD-9-CM, notes describe the general content of the succeeding categories and provide instructions for using codes. The same holds true for ICD-10-CM.

- Inclusion terms carry the same meaning in ICD-10-CM as they do in ICD-9-CM. The Tabular List contains inclusion notes to clarify the content of the chapter, subchapter, three-character, four-character, or five-character category to which the note applies. The inclusion terms describe other conditions classified to that code, such as synonyms of the condition listed in the code title or for an entirely different condition.
- Exclusion notes always appear with the word "excludes" and, similar to ICD-9-CM, the instructional exclusion note prevents a code from being applied incorrectly. ICD-10-CM expands the usage of exclusion notes, which are found at the beginning of a chapter, block, or category title. For example, exclusion notes are found in certain categories that represent diseases in combination and instruct the coder not to use the code if the condition mentioned in the exclusion note is also present.

After the appropriate instructional notes, each chapter ICD-10-CM starts with a list of subchapters or "blocks" of three-character categories. These blocks provide an overview of the structure of the chapter.

MODIFIERS

Two types of descriptors, called modifiers, are found in the Alphabetic Index:

- Essential modifiers affect code selection for a given diagnosis, due to the axis of classification.

- Non-essential modifiers may be present or absent for the diagnosis to be codes. Either way, the code stays the same.

ABBREVIATIONS

Two abbreviations are found in the tabular list:

NEC means "not elsewhere classified" and tells the coder than certain specified forms are classified elsewhere.

NOS means "not otherwise specified" and applies to residual categories that do not appear in sequence with (i.e., immediately following) the pertinent specific categories. These residual categories are entitled "Other specified." The abbreviation is equivalent to "unspecified." The term is assigned when documentation does not provide the detail for a specific code.

CROSS REFERENCES

In the Alphabetic Index, cross references point to all the possible information for a term or its synonyms.

✔5th   Needs fifth-digit   **OK**   Valid three-digit code

001-139
Infectious and Parasitic Diseases

This section of ICD-9 includes communicable diseases as well as disease of unknown origin but possibly due to infectious organisms. Infective organisms classified to this chapter include bacteria, chlamydia, fungi, helminths, mycoplasmas, protozoans, rickettsias, and viruses. The diseases may be further divided in the ICD-9 classification by anatomic site.

Infectious and parasitic agents live in soil, water, and in the air — virtually everywhere. When these agents infect a host, there are three possible outcomes. The host's immune system can successfully defeat the infective agent. In this outcome, the host may test positive for exposure to the infective agent, but show no symptoms of active disease. In the second outcome, the host can lose ground against the agent, and an equalized state in which the host cannot eradicate the low-grade infection stabilizes. This is generally considered a chronic condition. In its acute form of infection, the infective agent can prevail, causing a multiplication of organisms and an overwhelming infection in the patient. Care must be taken to determine the status of the host before assigning codes. A patient testing positive for tuberculosis, for instance, but exhibiting no symptoms of active disease, would be classified to 795.5 *Nonspecific reaction to tuberculin skin test without active tuberculosis*, rather than to an active TB infection in the 010-018 (active tuberculosis) codes.

In some cases, infectious and parasitic diseases are classified by anatomical site rather than source of infection and found in other chapters of ICD-9. Examples of this include pneumonia and other respiratory infections (460-466), influenza (487), and certain other localized infections. Also, codes reporting contact with infectious diseases, suspected carriers of infectious diseases, and prophylactic vaccination against infectious disease can be found in the supplementary classification of factors influencing health status (V01-V06).

To look up an infectious or parasitic disease in the ICD-9-CM Index To Diseases, don't just look under the main term (e.g., typhoid, shigellosis). A more comprehensive index listing is often found under the heading "Infection" or "Infestation", and then the main term.

001-009 Intestinal Infectious Diseases

001 CHOLERA

Cholera is an infection of the entire bowel due to *V. cholerae* and presents with profuse diarrhea, cramps, and vomiting. It is spread through the ingestion of food or water contaminated with feces of an infected person. Cholera is endemic to parts of Asia, Africa, the Middle East, and also portions of the Gulf Coast of the United States. In endemic areas, outbreaks are usually limited to warm seasons. If the infection is imported to other locales, an outbreak can occur in any season.

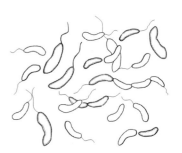

Vibrio cholerae bacteria is a highly motile organism that causes cholera when sufficient numbers reach the small intestine where they multiply and colonize. A biotype known as "eltor" or V. eltor has been identified in the U.S.

Symptoms of cholera can be mild or life threatening. Hypovolemia poses the greatest risk, as it can lead to severe metabolic acidosis and even renal tubular necrosis. Cholera responds to antibiotics, and with treatment, the mortality rate from cholera is less than 1 percent.

A toxic effect of antimony is called "antimonial cholera," but has no relation to a *Vibrio cholerae* infection. Antimonial cholera is reported with 985.4. Report suspected carrier of cholera with V02.0, and exposure to cholera with V01.0. Vaccination against cholera is reported with 003.0.

001.0	Cholera due to Vibrio cholerae — *Inaba, Ogawa, Hikojima serotypes; classical*
001.1	Cholera due to Vibrio cholerae el tor — *commonly less severe or asymptomatic*
001.9	Unspecified cholera — *unknown whether Vibrio cholerae or Vibrio cholerae el tor*

002 TYPHOID AND PARATYPHOID FEVERS

Typhoid fever is a systemic bacterial disease caused by the unique human strain of salmonella, *Salmonella typhi*. Outbreaks of typhoid are rare, because most of the cases are acquired during foreign travel to underdeveloped countries. Paratyphoid is similar in presentation to typhoid, though usually milder, caused by any of several organisms: *Salmonella paratyphi* (paratyphoid A), *S. schottmulleri* (paratyphoid B), or *S. hirschfeldii* (paratyphoid C). The means of infection, clinical course, pathology, and treatment are similar to those for typhoid.

Typhoid and paratyphoid cause high fever, abdominal pain, and rash. Intestinal hemorrhage may occur in severe cases of typhoid. The bacilli are generally transmitted by the ingestion of food or water that is contaminated with feces from an infected person. While typhoid and paratyphoid A are strictly human diseases, paratyphoid B and C have been found in other animals and fowl. Contamination of food and water by infected animals or fowl can spread paratyphoid B and C. In either case, the organism moves through the gastrointestinal tract and enters the bloodstream through the lymphatic system.

Report a suspected carrier of typhoid with V02.1 and vaccination against typhoid with V03.1. When typhoid presents with specific manifestations, report those manifestations secondary to the typhoid infection (endocarditis, 421.1; pneumonia, 484.8; perichondritis, 478.71; osteomyelitis, 730.8 category; spine, 720.81).

002.0	Typhoid fever — *Widal negative*
002.1	Paratyphoid fever A — *serotype paratyphi A*
002.2	Paratyphoid fever B — *serotype schottmulleri*
002.3	Paratyphoid fever C — *serotype hirschfeldii*
002.9	Unspecified paratyphoid fever — *unknown paratyphoid serotype*

003 OTHER SALMONELLA INFECTIONS

This classification is called "other" salmonella infections because typhoid and paratyphoid infections are caused by strains of salmonella. This classification includes all other salmonellas — more than 2000 serotypes — except congenital salmonella, which is reported with 771.8. Salmonella remains a significant health problem in the United States. About 85 percent of salmonella infections present as gastroenteritis. The other 15 percent present as septicemia or as focal disease.

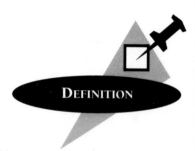

DEFINITION

Metabolic acidosis: a condition that may accompany severe dehydration, in which the chemistry of the blood is skewed, causing dangerous imbalances that can lead to cardiac, kidney, and other complications.

Tenesmus: painful straining, often considered ineffectual, during a bowel movement.

⤶5th   Needs fifth-digit   **OK**   Valid three-digit code

Salmonella gastroenteritis, also known as enteritis, is caused by the ingestion of contaminated foods. Meat, poultry, and raw milk and eggs are the most common sources. Other reported sources include infected pet turtles or lizards, infected dyes, or contaminated marijuana. Immunosuppressed patients are most susceptible to localized salmonella infection.

Suspected carrier of salmonella is reported with V02.3.

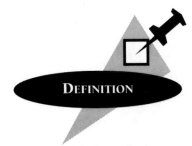

DEFINITION

Focal disease: infection confined to a single anatomical system or site. The opposite of focal disease is widespread, multi-system infection, which is called systemic disease.

003.0	Salmonella gastroenteritis — *gastrointestinal infection*
003.1	Salmonella septicemia — *bloodstream infection*
003.20	Unspecified localized salmonella infection — *unknown localized site*
003.21	Salmonella meningitis — *infection of membranes of brain/spinal cord*
003.22	Salmonella pneumonia — *infection of lungs*
003.23	Salmonella arthritis — *infection of joint*
003.24	Salmonella osteomyelitis — *infection of bone*
003.29	Other localized salmonella infections — *other localized site*
003.8	Other specified salmonella infections — *other salmonella infection*
003.9	Unspecified salmonella infection — *unspecified salmonella infection*

004 SHIGELLOSIS

Shigellosis is a bacterium that causes an acute infection of the bowel with fever, irritability, drowsiness, anorexia, nausea, vomiting, diarrhea, abdominal pain, and distension. Blood, pus, and mucus are found in the stool. Ingestion of food contaminated by feces of infected individuals is the most common source of infection. Incubation period is one to four days.

There are four species in the Shigella genus and they differ according to their biochemical reactions. All cause dysentery in humans and some primates.

Suspected Shigella carrier is reported with V02.3.

004.0	Shigella dysenteriae — *subgroup A, severe dysenteria; type 1 can be fatal in children; Schmitz bacillus, Bacillus dysenteriae or Bacterium dysenteriae*
004.1	Shigella flexneri — *subgroup B; S. paradysenteriae and Flexner's bacillus*
004.2	Shigella boydii — *subgroup C; tropical locales, causing severe diarrhea*
004.3	Shigella sonnei — *subgroup D, milder dysentery; Sonne-Duval bacillus or Bacterium sonnei.*
004.8	Other specified shigella infections — *other than A,B,C,D*
004.9	Unspecified shigellosis — *unknown Shigella infection*

005 OTHER FOOD POISONING (BACTERIAL)

Food poisoning as reported with 005 reports the ingestion of bacteria that leads to gastrointestinal infection.

Staphylococcal enterotoxin is a common cause of food poisoning that can occur when an infected food handler introduces the staph into egg, milk, or meat products. The infection multiplies in the protein-rich media. An acute bout of diarrhea and vomiting usually occurs within a few hours of ingestion, and resolves within several hours. Hypovolemia poses the greatest risk to the elderly, the young, and the immunosuppressed, but this form of food poisoning rarely is fatal.

Clostridium botulinum is a neurotoxic bacterium and ingestion of contaminated food leads to optic neurology symptoms including diplopia, loss of accommodation, or blepharoptosis. Gastrointestinal symptoms including vomiting and diarrhea may precede neurological symptoms. No fever is present. Improperly canned food is the most common source of botulism. With treatment, the mortality rate of botulism is still significant although at less than 10 percent.

C. perfringens is commonly found in soil, air, and water. When the bacterium contaminates meat, it forms spores that cause mild gastroenteritis in type A or severe, life-threatening gastroenteritis in type C. Both are reported with 005.2.

Japan has the highest incidence of food poisoning by *Vibrio parahaemolyticus*, caused by the ingestion of undercooked or raw fish.

Food poisoning by *Vibrio vulnificus* is the result of eating raw seafood. Resulting gastroenteritis can be severe and may be fatal to persons with liver disease.

Bacillus cereus (005.89) is commonly found in soil, milk, and other dried food, such as cereals, herbs, and spices. Meat pies, fried rice and puddings are frequently implicated in outbreaks.

005.0	Staphylococcal food poisoning — *Staphylococcal toxemia due to food*
005.1	Botulism — *Clostridium botulinum*
005.2	Food poisoning due to Clostridium perfringens (C. welchii) — *enteritis necroticans*
005.3	Food poisoning due to other Clostridia — *other or unknown*
005.4	Food poisoning due to Vibrio parahaemolyticus — *from fish; common to Japan*
005.81	Food poisoning due to Vibrio vulnificus — *severe enteritis from seafood; may progress to septicemia*
005.89	Other bacterial food poisoning — *Bacillus cereus*
005.9	Unspecified food poisoning

006 AMEBIASIS

There are 50 million annual cases of amebiasis worldwide, with 40,000 to 50,000 deaths attributed to amebiasis annually.

Amebiasis is most common in tropical areas where crowded living conditions and poor sanitation exist. Africa, Latin America, Southeast Asia, and India have significant health problems associated with amebiasis. In amebiasis, protozoa can live in the large intestine without causing symptoms; or it can invade the colon wall causing colitis, acute dysentery, or chronic diarrhea. The infection may spread through the blood to the liver, and rarely, to the lungs, brain, or other organs.

Transmission occurs through ingestion of feces in contaminated food or water, use of human feces as fertilizer, or person-to-person contact. Malnutrition and alcoholism predispose a person to more severe disease, as does immunosuppression. Recent travel to a tropical region is a risk factor. In the United States, immunosuppressed populations, people living in institutions, people with disabilities, and male homosexuals are considered higher risk groups, although the infection rate in the United States is low at less than 1 percent.

Codes in the rubric 006 are used to report infection or ulceration due to *Entamoeba histolytica*. If the ameba is other than *Entamoeba histolytica*, report 007.8 instead. Meningoencephalitis due to *Naegleria gruber* is reported with 136.2. Suspected carrier of amebic disease is reported with V02.2.

✔5th   Needs fifth-digit   **OK**   Valid three-digit code

006.0	Acute amebic dysentery without mention of abscess — *sudden, severe dysentery*
006.1	Chronic intestinal amebiasis without mention of abscess — *persistent dysentery*
006.2	Amebic nondysenteric colitis — *inflamed colon but no dysentery*
006.3	Amebic liver abscess — *liver infection*
006.4	Amebic lung abscess — *lung with or without liver infection*
006.5	Amebic brain abscess — *brain with or without lung and/or liver*
006.6	Amebic skin ulceration — *cutaneous amebiasis*
006.8	Amebic infection of other sites — *including seminal vesicle, bladder, appendix or other site infection, ameboma*
006.9	Unspecified amebiasis — *unknown or unspecified*

007 OTHER PROTOZOAL INTESTINAL DISEASES

Giardia lamblia is the most common intestinal parasite in the United States and is classified to this rubric. Giardiasis is an infection of the lumen of the small intestine, spread by contaminated food and water or by direct contact. Commonly, contaminated water from lakes or streams is a source of the disease. Most cases are asymptomatic, but those with symptoms experience diarrhea, nausea, lassitude, anorexia, and weight loss.

Cryptosporidiosis is usually transmitted person-to-person and the symptoms are mild and self-limited in a healthy population. However, cryptosporidiosis is frequently seen as an opportunistic infection in the acquired immune deficiency syndrome (AIDS), causing profound dehydration and electrolyte imbalances. There is no specific antibiotic therapy for cryptosporidiosis. Treatment consists of rehydration and electrolyte management. In the case of an AIDS patient with cryptosporidiosis and volume depletion, report the AIDS first (042), followed by cryptosporidiosis (007.4) and volume depletion (276.5).

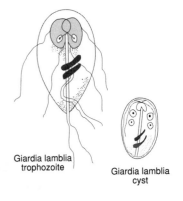

Giardia lamblia
trophozoite

Giardia lamblia
cyst

007.0	Balantidiasis — *Balantidium coli infection*
007.1	Giardiasis — *Giardia lamblia, lambliasis infection*
007.2	Coccidiosis — *Isospora belli, Isospora hominis infection*
007.3	Intestinal trichomoniasis — *Trichomonas infection*
007.4	Cryptosporidiosis — *Cryptosporidium infection is self-limiting in immunocompetent cattle workers, debilitating in immunosuppressed patients*
007.5	Cyclosporiasis — *dysentery from Cyclospora infection*
007.8	Other specified protozoal intestinal diseases — *including chilomastigiasis, craigiasis*
007.9	Unspecified protozoal intestinal disease — *unknown*

008 INTESTINAL INFECTIONS DUE TO OTHER ORGANISMS

Intestinal infections caused by *E. coli* are covered in the 008 rubric. The infections are classified by the degree of penetration into intestinal tissue. Infections or food poisoning caused by other agents are reported with codes in the 005 rubric.

Congenital *E. coli* is coded to 771.8, generalized *E. coli* (septicemia) to 038.42, and *E. coli* in conditions classified elsewhere to 041.4 (code first the disease then the bacterial agent).

Gastroenteritis and enteritis due to a specified virus is coded to 008.61-008.69. Use 008.69 to report a specified virus when it is not elsewhere classified or 088.8 to report the infection when it is not elsewhere classified or otherwise specified.

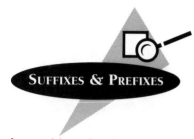

SUFFIXES & PREFIXES

colo-: pertaining to the colon

entero-: pertaining to the intestines

gastro-: pertaining to the stomach

-hemorrhagic: bleeding

-invasive: penetrating

-itis: inflammation

-pathogenic: causing disease

-toxogenic: producing a toxin

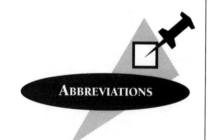

ABBREVIATIONS

Clostridium difficile: *C. difficile*

Staphylococcus: Staph

008.00	Intestinal infection due to unspecified E. coli — *not otherwise specified*
008.01	Intestinal infection due to enteropathogenic E. coli — *inflammation of intestines*
008.02	Intestinal infection due to enterotoxigenic E. coli — *toxic reaction in intestinal mucosa, causing voluminous watery secretions*
008.03	Intestinal infection due to enteroinvasive E. coli — *infection penetrates intestinal mucosa*
008.04	Intestinal infection due to enterohemorrhagic E. coli — *infection penetrates intestinal mucosa, causing ulceration and bleeding*
008.09	Intestinal infection due to other intestinal E. coli infections
008.1	Intestinal infection due to Arizona group of paracolon bacilli — *Arizona (bacillus)*
008.2	Intestinal infection due to aerobacter aerogenes — *Enterobacter aerogenes*
008.3	Intestinal infections due to proteus (mirabilis) (morganii) — *Morganella morganii, Salmonella morganii*
008.41	Intestinal infections due to staphylococcus
008.42	Intestinal infections due to pseudomonas
008.43	Intestinal infections due to campylobacter
008.44	Intestinal infections due to yersinia enterocolitica
008.45	Intestinal infections due to clostridium difficile
008.46	Intestinal infections due to other anerobes
008.47	Intestinal infections due to other gram-negative bacteria
008.49	Intestinal infection due to other organisms
008.5	Intestinal infection due to unspecified bacterial enteritis
008.61	Intestinal infection, enteritis due to rotavirus
008.62	Intestinal infection, enteritis due to adenovirus
008.63	Intestinal infection, enteritis due to Norwalk virus
008.64	Intestinal infection, enteritis due to other small round viruses (SRVs)
008.65	Intestinal infection, enteritis due to calcivirus
008.66	Intestinal infection, enteritis due to astrovirus
008.67	Intestinal infection, enteritis due to enterovirus not elsewhere classified
008.69	Intestinal infection, enteritis due to other viral enteritis
008.8	Intestinal infection due to other organism, NEC

009 ILL-DEFINED INTESTINAL INFECTIONS

Use this series of codes only when more specific information in not available. If the source of infection is known, use an infective enteritis code from the 001-008 series. Noninfective colitis, enteritis, or gastroenteritis is reported with codes in the 555-558 series, and diarrhea due to noninfectious causes is reported with 787.91. Allergic diarrhea is reported with 558.3; nervous diarrhea with 306.4.

Colitis is the inflammation of the colon, while enteritis is the inflammation of the intestine, especially small intestine. Gastroenteritis is inflammation of the mucous membranes of the stomach and intestines. Diarrhea describes copious, loose bowels without evidence of infection or inflammation of the gastrointestinal tract.

009.0	Infectious colitis, enteritis, and gastroenteritis — *known to be infectious*
009.1	Colitis, enteritis, and gastroenteritis of presumed infectious origin — *presumed to be infectious*
009.2	Infectious diarrhea — *known to be infectious*
009.3	Diarrhea of presumed infectious origin — (Use aditional code for associated: 711.1; 372.33) — *presumed to be infectious*

↙5th Needs fifth-digit   **OK** Valid three-digit code

010-018 Tuberculosis

Tuberculosis (TB) is a bacterial infection that usually attacks the lungs, but which may also affect other organs. The disease is caused by *Mycobacterium tuberculosis*. TB is transmitted by inhaling air droplets exhaled by an infected person, or sometimes, the infection is absorbed through the skin. Medical technicians handling TB specimens may contract the disease through skin wounds. TB has also been reported in people who have received tattoos or circumcisions in nonsterile conditions.

Symptoms of TB include coughing, chest pain, shortness of breath, loss of appetite, weight loss, fever, chills, and fatigue. Children and people with weakened immune systems are the most susceptible to TB.

A person may become infected with TB bacteria and not develop the disease. An immune system may destroy the bacteria completely. Only 5 percent to 10 percent of people infected with TB actually become sick.

Some tuberculosis codes are found in other sections of ICD-9. Congenital tuberculosis is reported with 771.2, and the late effects of tuberculosis are reported with codes in the 137 series. If an asymptomatic person tests positive for TB, report 795.5. Report exposure to TB without further information on tests or infection status with V01.1, and report the need for a BCG inoculation against TB with V03.2. Do not report personal history of tuberculosis (V12.01) in patients with active disease.

010 PRIMARY TUBERCULOUS INFECTION

Primary TB is the stage of the disease absent of any noticeable symptoms. The disease is not contagious in the early stage. Macrophages, immune cells that detect and destroy foreign matter, ingest the TB bacteria and transport them to the lymph nodes where they may be inhibited, destroyed, or may multiply.

010.0 ✒5th Primary tuberculous complex — *first infection, lung*
010.1 ✒5th Tuberculous pleurisy in primary progressive tuberculosis — *first infection, lung and lung lining*
010.8 ✒5th Other primary progressive tuberculosis infection — *primary site other than pulmonary*
010.9 ✒5th Primary tuberculous infection, unspecified — *unknown primary tuberculosis*

011 PULMONARY TUBERCULOSIS

If the bacteria multiply, active primary tuberculosis will develop along with typical symptoms of TB: coughing, night sweats, weight loss, and fever. A chest x-ray typically shows shadows or fluid collection between the lung and its lining.

If the bacteria are suppressed but not destroyed, they will be contained in a mass known as a granuloma or tubercle: a wall of immune cells around inactive bacteria to protect the body from infection. As long as the immune system remains strong, the TB bacteria remain walled off and inactive. The tubercle gradually collects calcium deposits to form a Ghon focus.

Initial tubercles in the lung usually heal, leaving permanent scars that appear as shadows in chest x-rays. At this primary stage of TB, the disease does not progress, but bacteria may

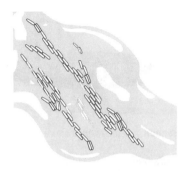

Mycobacterium tuberculosis is the cause of almost all cases of TB in the U.S. Multiplying organisms often appear as parallel bundles of rods, known as cording. Infection commonly is by inhalation of droplets containing TB

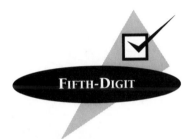

FIFTH-DIGIT

The following fifth-digit subclassification is for use with categories 010-018:

0 unspecified

1 bacteriological or histological examination not done

2 bacteriological or histological examination unknown (at present)

3 tubercle bacilli found (in sputum) by microscopy

4 tubercle bacilli not found (in sputum) by microscopy, but found by bacterial culture

5 tubercle bacilli not found by bacteriological examination, but tuberculosis confirmed histologically

6 tubercle bacilli not found by bacteriological or histological examination but tuberculosis confirmed by other methods (inoculation of animals)

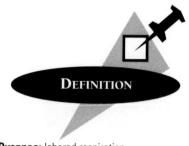

DEFINITION

Dyspnea: labored respiration

Ghon's foci: calcified nodules in the lower or middle lung field.

Hemoptysis: blood in sputum

Simon's foci: nodular scars in the apices of the lung, evidence of TB that progressed in the primary stage and may seed later disease.

remain dormant in the body for many years. If the immune system becomes weakened, the tubercle opens, releases the bacteria, and the infection may develop into secondary TB.

011.0 ✓5th Tuberculosis of lung, infiltrative — *clusters of TB bacilli in lung*
011.1 ✓5th Tuberculosis of lung, nodular — *infiltration of TB leads to formation of nodules*
011.2 ✓5th Tuberculosis of lung with cavitation — *further infiltration of TB leads to cavities*
011.3 ✓5th Tuberculosis of bronchus — *clusters of TB bacilli in bronchial tissue*
011.4 ✓5th Tuberculous fibrosis of lung — *TB cells in lungs surrounded by fibrous tissue*
011.5 ✓5th Tuberculous bronchiectasis — *TB causes bronchial dilation and cough*
011.6 ✓5th Tuberculous pneumonia (any form) — *TB causes inflammatory reaction of lung*
011.7 ✓5th Tuberculous pneumothorax — *TB causes spontaneous rupture of lung tissue*
011.8 ✓5th Other specified pulmonary tuberculosis — *not elsewhere classified*
011.9 ✓5th Unspecified pulmonary tuberculosis — *unknown type*

012 OTHER RESPIRATORY TUBERCULOSIS

Rubric 012 is used to report tuberculosis of respiratory sites other than the lung without lung involvement, such as the pleura, intrathoracic lymph nodes, trachea or bronchus alone, larynx (including the glottis), and the mediastinum, nasopharynx, nose or sinus.

Tuberculosis of other respiratory sites, such as the nose can be due to a primary or secondary infection with tuberculosis mycobacerium.

A pleural effusion occurs after the initial infection. The result of a release of a small amount of tuberculoprotein within the lung into the plural space causing an inflammatory response and a resulting accumlation of fluid.

At the time of the initial infection hilar, and mediastinal lymph nodes become seeded with bacilli, other lymph nodes may also become involved. The infection may progress to clinical significance, may become active at a late date, or may never become active.

012.0 ✓5th Tuberculous pleurisy — *inflammation of lung lining*
012.1 ✓5th Tuberculosis of intrathoracic lymph nodes — *hilar, mediastinal, tracheobronchial lymph infection*
012.2 ✓5th Isolated tracheal or bronchial tuberculosis — *without lung involvement*
012.3 ✓5th Tuberculous laryngitis — *infection of glottis*
012.8 ✓5th Other specified respiratory tuberculosis — *mediastinum, nasopharynx, nose, or sinus infection, other*

013 TUBERCULOSIS OF MENINGES AND CENTRAL NERVOUS SYSTEM

Nearly all TB in the United States originates as a pulmonary disease, though before pasteurization, infection commonly occurred at other anatomical sites with the ingestion of contaminated milk or milk products. Today in the United States, sites other than the lung are considered secondary to pulmonary infection.

013.0 ✓5th Tuberculous meningitis — *infection of cerebral or spinal meninges*
013.1 ✓5th Tuberculoma of meninges — *enlarged tubercle in lining or brain or spinal cord*
013.2 ✓5th Tuberculoma of brain — *enlarged tubercle in brain*
013.3 ✓5th Tuberculous abscess of brain — *abscess of brain*
013.4 ✓5th Tuberculoma of spinal cord — *enlarged tubercle in spinal cord*
013.5 ✓5th Tuberculous abscess of spinal cord — *abscess of spinal cord*
013.6 ✓5th Tuberculous encephalitis or myelitis — *inflammation of brain or spinal cord*

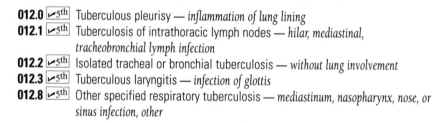

✓5th   Needs fifth-digit   **OK**   Valid three-digit code

013.8 ✔5th Other specified tuberculosis of central nervous system — *other CNS site*
013.9 ✔5th Unspecified tuberculosis of central nervous system — *unknown CNS site*

014 TUBERCULOSIS OF INTESTINES, PERITONEUM, AND MESENTERIC GLANDS

Infection of the intestinal tract by the tuberculin bacillus can occur through the blood, through swallowing the organisms from the pulmonary tract, or through penetration of the intestinal layers from granuloma or from other infected sites.

Wide-spread intra-abdominal infection may result in peritonitis which may present in an exudative form with ascites, or a fibrotic form with slight to no ascites but with intraperitoneal adhesions. Peritoneal tuberculous is often associated with a concomitant pleural effusion.

014.0 ✔5th Tuberculous pertonitis — *inflammation of the lining of the abdomen*
014.8 ✔5th Tuberculosis of intestines, peritoneum, and mesentric glands, other — *anus, intestine, rectum, retroperitoneal lymph nodes, mesenteric glands, other*

015 TUBERCULOSIS OF BONES AND JOINTS

Tuberculosis of the bone or joints is usually limited to cases in which the primary TB occurs during childhood. Sometimes, the symptoms do not present themselves for years. In joint disease, arthritis is present. In bone infection, bone may be destroyed. In Pott's disease, the patient may be asymptomatic until deformity occurs or vertebrae collapse.

When coding tuberculosis of bones or joints, report the TB code first, followed by codes that best describe the manifestation, such as arthropathy (subclassification 711.4), necrosis or osteitis (730.8), or synovitis/tenosynovitis (727.01). In Pott's disease, also report any curvature of spine (737.43) or spondylitis (720.81).

015.0 ✔5th Tuberculosis of vertebral column — *Pott's disease, sacrum, spine, vertebra, lordosis, scoliosis, intervertebral*
015.1 ✔5th Tuberculosis of hip — *joint or bone infection*
015.2 ✔5th Tuberculosis of knee — *joint or bone infection*
015.5 ✔5th Tuberculosis of limb bones — *long bones, hands, feet, wrist, ankle, dactylitis*
015.6 ✔5th Tuberculosis of mastoid — *mastoiditis*
015.7 ✔5th Tuberculosis of other specified bone — *jaw, bony pelvis, shoulder blade, other bone*
015.8 ✔5th Tuberculosis of other specified joint — *wrist, ankle, sacroiliac, shoulder, other joint*
015.9 ✔5th Tuberculosis of unspecified bones and joints — *cartilage, ganglion, rheumatism, other synovitis or tenosynovitis*

016 TUBERCULOSIS OF GENITOURINARY SYSTEM

When coding tuberculosis of the genitourinary system, report the TB code first, followed by codes that best described the manifestation, such as nephropathy (583.81), prostatitis (601.4), or pyelitis (590.81).

016.0 ✔5th Tuberculosis of kidney — *renal, perinephritic*
016.1 ✔5th Tuberculosis of bladder — *cystitis*
016.2 ✔5th Tuberculosis of ureter — *ureter only*
016.3 ✔5th Tuberculosis of other urinary organs — *urethra*
016.4 ✔5th Tuberculosis of epididymis — *epididymis only*

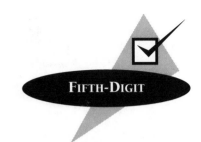

FIFTH-DIGIT

The following fifth-digit subclassification is for use with categories 010-018:

0 unspecified

1 bacteriological or histological examination not done

2 bacteriological or histological examination unknown (at present)

3 tubercle bacilli found (in sputum) by microscopy

4 tubercle bacilli not found (in sputum) by microscopy, but found by bacterial culture

5 tubercle bacilli not found by bacteriological examination, but tuberculosis confirmed histologically

6 tubercle bacilli not found by bacteriological or histological examination but tuberculosis confirmed by other methods (inoculation of animals)

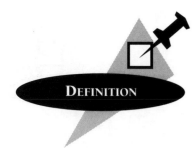

DEFINITION

Erythema nodosum: an inflammatory, allergic reaction to infection, presenting as painful nodules on the shin. Seen most often in TB or sarcoidosis.

Hemoptysis: blood in the sputum.

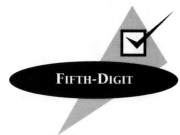

FIFTH-DIGIT

The following fifth-digit subclassification is for use with categories 010-018:

0 unspecified

1 bacteriological or histological examination not done

2 bacteriological or histological examination unknown (at present)

3 tubercle bacilli found (in sputum) by microscopy

4 tubercle bacilli not found (in sputum) by microscopy, but found by bacterial culture

5 tubercle bacilli not found by bacteriological examination, but tuberculosis confirmed histologically

6 tubercle bacilli not found by bacteriological or histological examination but tuberculosis confirmed by other methods (inoculation of animals)

016.5 ✓5th Tuberculosis of other male genital organs — *bulbourethral gland, Cowper's gland, penis, prepuce, prostate, scrotum, spermatic cord, testis*
016.6 ✓5th Tuberculous oophoritis and salpingitis — *fallopian tube, ovary*
016.7 ✓5th Tuberculosis of other female genital organs — *broad ligament, cervix, endometrium, placenta, uterus*
016.9 ✓5th Genitourinary tuberculosis, unspecified — *unknown genitourinary site*

017 TUBERCULOSIS OF OTHER ORGANS

When coding tuberculosis of other organs, report the TB code first, followed by codes that best described the manifestation, such as episcleritis (379.09), myocarditis (422.0), or interstitial keratitis (370.59).

017.0 ✓5th Tuberculosis of skin and subcutaneous cellular tissue — *cellulitis, colliquativa, cutis, scrofuloderma*
017.1 ✓5th Erythema nodosum with hypersensitivity reaction in tuberculosis — *Bazin's disease, erythema induratum, tuberculosis indurativa*
017.2 ✓5th Tuberculosis of peripheral lymph nodes — *axilla, cervical, neck*
017.3 ✓5th Tuberculosis of eye — *conjunctiva, globe, iris, lacrimal apparatus, retina*
017.4 ✓5th Tuberculosis of ear — *inner ear, middle ear; excludes mastoid*
017.5 ✓5th Tuberculosis of thyroid gland — *thyroid*
017.6 ✓5th Tuberculosis of adrenal glands — *bronze (Addison's) disease, adrenal gland*
017.7 ✓5th Tuberculosis of spleen — *spleen*
017.8 ✓5th Tuberculosis of esophagus — *esophagus*
017.9 ✓5th Tuberculosis of other specified organs — *artery, breast, buccal cavity, endocardium, muscle, palate, parotid, parathyroid, pericardium, perineum, pituitary, thymus, stomach, vein*

018 MILIARY TUBERCULOSIS

Tuberculosis bacilli may be seeded to distant organs through the lymphatic or vascular system. Miliary tuberculosis is named for the pale, disseminated lesions that resemble millet seeds. Miliary tuberculosis is most commonly seen in bone marrow, eye, lymph nodes, liver, spleen, kidney, adrenal gland, prostate, seminal vesicle, fallopian tube, endometrium, or meninges. Affected organs may eventually develop progressive, isolated organ infection.

018.0 ✓5th Acute miliary tuberculosis — *sudden, severe onset*
018.8 ✓5th Other specified miliary tuberculosis — *other*
018.9 ✓5th Unspecified miliary tuberculosis — *unknown*

020-027 Zoonotic Bacterial Diseases

020 PLAGUE

Plague, an acute infection caused by the bacillus *Yersinia pestis*, occurs in three forms among people: bubonic plague, pneumonic plague, and septicemic plague. All three varieties have been called "black death" because in untreated cases, respiratory failure precedes death by several hours, and during this time, the hypoxic victim's skin may turn deep purple. Plague responds well to modern antibiotics. In the United States, sporadic infections are seen primarily in the Southwest.

Bubonic plague is transmitted by the bite of insects that are normally rodent parasites. The most important of these insects is the rat flea *Xenopsylla cheopis*. Bubonic plague is characterized by buboes: enlarged, inflamed lymph nodes, in the groin, armpit, or neck. Other symptoms include headache, fever, nausea, vomiting, and aching joints. Untreated, bubonic plague's fatality rate is 30 percent to 75 percent.

✓5th Needs fifth-digit   **OK** Valid three-digit code

Septicemic plague may be initiated by direct contact of contaminated hands, food, or objects with the mucous membranes of the nose or throat. Untreated, pneumonic plague's fatality rate is 95 percent; septicemic, nearly 100. In treated cases, the fatality drops to 10 percent or less.

Pneumonic plague is characterized by lung infection and, as a primary infection, is often transmitted by inhaling bacteria-carrying air droplets exhaled by an infected person. Secondary pneumonic plague begins as another form of plague before infecting the lungs.

Prophylactic inoculation against plague is reported with V03.3.

020.0	Bubonic plague — *most common, with swollen lymph glands*
020.1	Cellulocutaneous plague — *inflammation and necrosis of the skin*
020.2	Septicemic plague — *infection in bloodstream*
020.3	Primary pneumonic plague — *plague infects lung first*
020.4	Secondary pneumonic plague — *infection spreads to lung*
020.5	Pneumonic plague, unspecified
020.8	Other specified types of plague
020.9	Unspecified plague

021 TULAREMIA

A sudden fever, chill, headache, myalgia, and fatigue characterize tularemia.

It is a fairly uncommon disease, seen in the United States most commonly in Oklahoma, Missouri, and Alaska. The infective agent, *Francisella tularensis,* enters the body through a tick bite or by direct contact with the skin. The bacillus can penetrate unbroken skin, and can therefore be transmitted by handling tainted meat or cleaning wild game, usually rodents such as squirrels or rabbits.

Tularemia responds well to antibiotic treatment and, with treatment, death is rare. Without treatment, mortality of tularemia is about 5 percent. Once infected, the patient develops immunity.

Tularemia codes are selected on the basis of site of initial infection: skin, lung, gastrointestinal system, eye, or other site. To report prophylactic vaccination against tularemia, see V03.4.

021.0	Ulceroglandular tularemia — *lesion at cutaneous site of bacillus penetration*
021.1	Enteric tularemia — *intestinal infection*
021.2	Pulmonary tularemia — *infection of lung and/or bronchus*
021.3	Oculoglandular tularemia — *conjunctival infection with possible spread to cornea, lacrimal systems*
021.8	Other specified tularemia — *glandular or other*
021.9	Unspecified tularemia — *site unknown*

022 ANTHRAX

Anthrax is a caused by *Bacillus anthracis.* Anthrax is rare in the United States, but is seen occasionally in animals in agricultural regions including Texas, Louisiana, Mississippi, Oklahoma, and South Dakota. Human infection in the United States is usually due to an occupational exposure to animal products imported from other countries where anthrax is more common.

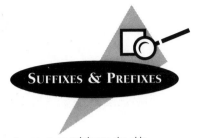

SUFFIXES & PREFIXES

-cutaneous: pertaining to the skin

pneumo-: pertaining to the lung

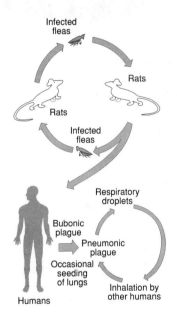

Infected fleas

Rats

Rats

Infected fleas

Respiratory droplets

Bubonic plague

Pneumonic plague

Occasional seeding of lungs

Inhalation by other humans

Humans

Anthrax infection can occur in three forms: cutaneous (skin), inhalation, and gastrointestinal. Symptoms vary according to the form of infection, but usually occur within seven days.

In most cases, the anthrax bacterium enters a cut or abrasion on the skin. This is called cutaneous anthrax. Skin infection begins as a raised itchy bump that resembles an insect bite. The bump develops into a vesicle and, from there, a painless ulcer, usually 1 centimeter to 3 centimeters in diameter, within 48 hours. Lymph glands in the adjacent area may swell. About 20 percent of untreated cases of cutaneous anthrax will result in death. However, death is rare with drug therapy.

Pulmonary anthrax is caused by inhalation of the anthrax bacterium. It presents like cold symptoms and progresses. Untreated, pulmonary anthrax has a high mortality rate.

The intestinal form of anthrax is rare, and may follow the consumption of contaminated meat. Intestinal anthrax is characterized by an acute gastroenteritis progressing into septicemia.

In pneumonia, report the anthrax infection first, followed by the manifestation of the disease, anthrax pneumonia (484.5).

DEFINITION

Anthrax: an infection of *Bacillus anthracis* classified by route of infection.

022.0	Cutaneous anthrax —	*infection through superficial wound*
022.1	Pulmonary anthrax —	*infection in lungs*
022.2	Gastrointestinal anthrax —	*acute gastrointestinal infection*
022.3	Anthrax septicemia —	*infection in bloodstream*
022.8	Other specified manifestations of anthrax —	*other site of infection*
022.9	Unspecified anthrax —	*unknown site of infection*

023 BRUCELLOSIS

Brucellosis is also known as "undulant fever" or "Bangs disease" and is a systemic infection caused by exposure to any of several brucella species. The species are specific to the type of animal usually infected: sheep/goats, cattle, swine, or dogs.

The infection enters the body through a break in the skin. Onset of symptoms can be within three days to 30 days. Symptoms of brucellosis infection in humans include fever, night sweats, fatigue, anorexia, weight loss, headache, and arthralgia. In animals, the primary sign of infection is abortion in females and epididymitis in males.

Worldwide, brucellosis remains a major source of disease in humans and domesticated animals. B. abortus is the most common form in the United States.

023.0	Brucella melitensis —	*contact infected sheep/goats*
023.1	Brucella abortus —	*contact infected cattle*
023.2	Brucella suis —	*contact infected swine*
023.3	Brucella canis —	*contact infected dogs*
023.8	Other brucellosis —	*more than one source*
023.9	Burcellosis, unspecified —	*unknown animal contact*

024 GLANDERS OK

Glanders is an equine disease communicable to man and caused by *Burkholderia mallei* (formerly *Pseudomonas mallei*). Nearly all cases of glanders in the United States occur among people who are professionally or recreationally exposed to horses, although glanders

✔5th   Needs fifth-digit   **OK**   Valid three-digit code

can be transmitted from human to human and in the laboratory. Glanders cases have not appeared in the United States since the 1940s. Outbreaks do occur in South America, Asia, African, and the Middle East. Symptoms of glanders include headache, chills, fever, and vomiting.

025 MELIOIDOSIS **OK**

Also known as Whitmore's disease or pseudoglanders, melioidosis is a rare infection caused by *Pseudomonas pseudomallei*. Most cases are limited to Asia. The disease is acquired through exposure to contaminated soil or water to a break in the skin. Symptoms range from a skin lesion at the site of infection, to pneumonia or septicemia. Patients with melioidosis may suffer relapses years after the initial infection has resolved.

026 RAT-BITE FEVER

Rat-bite fever begins with a rat bite, scratch, or ingestion of contaminated food or water. While the initial wound may heal promptly, it usually becomes swollen and painful again within a few weeks of the bite. At that time, regional lymph nodes may swell and there may be chills, fever, and a skin rash. Periods of relapse may subside and recur. Code selection is based on the type of infection: *Spirillum minus* or *Streptobacillus moniliformis*.

026.0 Spirillary fever — *Spirillum minus infection, Sodoku*
026.1 Streptobacillary fever — *Streptobacillus moniliformis infection, Haverhill fever*
026.9 Unspecified rat-bite fever — *unknown*

027 OTHER ZOONOTIC BACTERIAL DISEASE

Use this rubric to report zoonotic bacterial disease not described earlier in the chapter. In all cases, code the zoonotic bacterial disease first, followed by manifestations of the infection, as in the case of listeriosis with meningitis (320.7). Report congenital listeriosis infection with 771.2.

027.0 Listeriosis — *infection by Listeria monocytogenes*
027.1 Erysipelothrix infection — *infection by Erysipelothrix insidiosa*
027.2 Pasteurellosis — *infection by Pasteurella multocida (P. septica)*
027.8 Other specified zoonotic bacterial diseases — *Yersinia septica, others*
027.9 Unspecified zoonotic bacterial disease — *unknown*

030-041 Other Bacterial Diseases

030 LEPROSY

Mycobacterium leprae causes leprosy. Leprosy, also known as Hansen's disease, can be treated effectively with several drugs. If left untreated, the disease can result in severe disfigurement, especially of the feet, hands, and face. It is rarely fatal.

Ninety percent of the 900,000 leprosy cases worldwide occur in just 16 nations, and India and Brazil have the highest numbers of cases. Only 7,000 registered cases of leprosy currently exist in the United States. Most of these patients are immigrants who acquired the disease in their home countries.

Leprosy has two main forms: tuberculoid and lepromatous. In tuberculoid leprosy, skin lesions are few and small, with few bacteria present. Lepromatous leprosy, is a more severe disease, with symptomatic widespread lesions and significant bacteria.

Leprosy is not easily transmitted, but likely is transmitted person-to-person through nasal droplets released from an infected person. Less than 5 percent of people who are infected with *Mycobacterium leprae* actually develop leprosy. For most, the immune system fights off infection. Immunosuppressed patients are no more likely to develop leprosy and research has not discovered what, if anything, predisposes a person to the disease.

Treating leprosy using multidrug therapy can halt the progression of the disease, though there are side effects. Inflammation develops in patients when leprosy bacteria are killed and erythema nodosum leprosum (ENL) is a risk in patients during drug therapy. The painful skin sores characteristic of ENL are thought to be a result of abnormal immune reactions to the killed bacteria. ENL is reported with 695.2.

When coding leprosy, report the leprosy code, and identify any manifestations in addition to the leprosy, such as infective and deformity-creating dermatitis of the eyelid (373.4) or corneal lesion (371.89).

030.0	Lepromatous leprosy (type L) — *widespread lesions and bacteria*
030.1	Tuberculoid leprosy (type T) — *small lesions, few bacteria*
030.2	Indeterminate leprosy (group I) — *uncharacteristic, early manifestation*
030.3	Borderline leprosy (group B) — *transitional; neither tuberculoid or lepromatous; dimorphous*
030.8	Other specified leprosy — *not elsewhere classified*
030.9	Unspecified leprosy — *unknown type*

031 DISEASES DUE TO OTHER MYCOBACTERIA

Mycobacteria cause leprosy and tuberculosis. In this rubric, other mycobacterial diseases are classified by site of infection.

Mycobacterium avium-intracellulare (MAC) affects up to 40 percent of human immunodeficiency virus (HIV)-infected people in the United States, while the disseminated form of the disease (DMAC) affects 15 percent to 24 percent of AIDS patients and other people with severely impaired immune systems. Severe anemia, fever, night sweats, anorexia, and diarrhea characterize DMAC. It is a significant cause of AIDS morbidity. When coding these cases, sequence the code for AIDS (042) first, followed by the code for MAC or DMAC (031.2).

031.0	Pulmonary diseases due to other mycobacteria — *lung infection; Battey disease, avium, intracellulare, kansasii, fortuitum, xenopi*
031.1	Cutaneous diseases due to other mycobacteria — *skin infection; Buruli ulcer; marinum (M. balnei)*
031.2	Disseminated diseases due to other mycobacteria — *more than one site; DMAC, MAC*
031.8	Other specified diseases due to other mycobacteria — *not elsewhere classified; kasongo, kakerifu*
031.9	Unspecified diseases due to mycobacteria — *unknown or atypical*

032 DIPHTHERIA

An acute, contagious disease, diphtheria is one of the childhood diseases that common immunizations protect against. (The D in DPT is for the diphtheria vaccine). The infective agent is *Corynebacterium diphtheriae*.

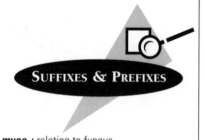

SUFFIXES & PREFIXES

myco-: relating to fungus

Diphtheria usually presents with sore throat, with its hallmark fibrous membrane most commonly seen on the tonsil or nasopharynx. This membrane can combine with pharyngeal edema to obstruct breathing. However, diphtheria can attack other organs rather than presenting as a sore throat, and the codes in this rubric are therefore classified by site of infection.

Report suspected carrier of diphtheria with V02.4 and report prophylactic vaccination against diphtheria with V03.5 (diptheria alone). Vaccinations for diphtheria in combination with other diseases are in the V06 series of codes.

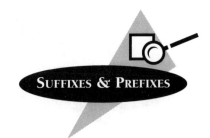

SUFFIXES & PREFIXES

032.0	Faucial diphtheria — *tonsillar*
032.1	Nasopharyngeal diphtheria — *deep, soft tissue of nose and pharynx*
032.2	Anterior nasal diphtheria — *superficial, soft tissue of the nose*
032.3	Laryngeal diphtheria — *larynx*
032.81	Conjunctival diphtheria — *conjunctiva*
032.82	Diphtheritic myocarditis — *wall of the heart*
032.83	Diphtheritic peritonitis — *abdominal membrane lining*
032.84	Diphtheritic cystitis — *bladder*
032.85	Cutaneous diphtheria — *skin*
032.89	Other specified diphtheria — *neurological or other complication*

-pharyngo-: pharynx

laryngo-: larynx

naso-: nose

033 WHOOPING COUGH

An acute, contagious disease, whooping cough is one of the childhood diseases that common immunizations protect against. The P in DPT is for the pertussis (whooping cough) vaccine.

The infective agent in whopping cough is *Bordetella pertussis*. A milder disease clinically indistinguishable from *B. pertussis* is caused by *B. parapertussis*. *B. bronchiseptica* also creates symptoms of whooping cough.

The course of whopping cough is approximately six weeks and has three stages: catarrhal (nocturnal cough, sneezing, and lacrimation); paroxysmal (thick mucus, choking spells); and convalescence, when the severity of the symptoms diminishes. Mortality for the most severe form of whopping cough, pertussis, is about 2 percent in children under a year old.

Report any pneumonia concurrent to whooping cough separately with 484.3. Prophylactic vaccination is reported with V03.6 (pertussis alone) or with a code from the V06 series for pertussis vaccination in combination with other prophylactic vaccinations.

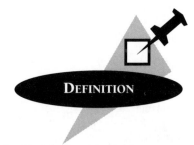

DEFINITION

Cystitis: infection of the bladder.

Myocarditis: infections of the wall of the heart.

Peritonitis: infection of the abdominal membrane lining.

033.0	Whooping cough due to Bordetella pertussis (P. pertussis) — *B. pertussis*
033.1	Whooping cough due to Bordetella parapertussis (B. parapertussis) — *B. parapertussis*
033.8	Whooping cough due to other specified organism — *B. bronchiseptica*
033.9	Whooping cough, unspecified organism — *unknown organism*

034 STREPTOCOCCAL SORE THROAT AND SCARLET FEVER

Strep throat is a common pharyngeal infection presenting with a red, sore throat and fever. Strep throat responds readily to antibiotic treatment. Without antibiotics, strep throat can progress into scarlet fever, typified by a red blush to the skin of the chest and abdomen, that blanches under pressure. Streptococcal infections can progress to endocarditis, pneumonias, and septicemias.

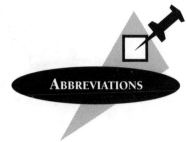

Streptococcal: strep

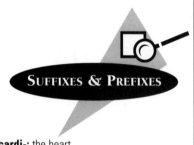

cardi-: the heart

encephalo-: the brain

endo-: within

mening-: membranes of the brain and spinal cord

myo-: muscle

peri-: around, lining

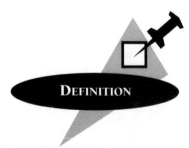

Risus sardonicus: tonic facial muscles create an artificial smile and raised eyebrow, characteristic of lockjaw

Trismus: lack of jaw mobility seen in lockjaw

Suspected carrier of streptococcus is reported with V02.51 for Group B and V02.52 for other strains of streptococcus.

034.0	Streptococcal sore throat — *simple strep throat*	
034.1	Scarlet fever — *red rash spreading from trunk*	

035 ERYSIPELAS `OK`

Formerly called St Anthony's fire, erysipelas is a hot, bright red, superficial cellulitis, involving dermal lymphatics that is usually caused by a streptococcal infection. If the erysipelas infection is of the external ear, report the erysipelas first, and the site of infection with 380.13. For erysipelas as a maternal complication of childbirth, see rubric 670.

036 MENINGOCOCCAL INFECTION

Neisseria meningitidis is a common cause of meningitis. Called also meningococcus, the bacteria may invade the spinal cord, brain, heart, joints, optic nerve, or bloodstream. A pink or petechial rash may accompany the disease. Although the bacterium is found in the nasopharynx of 5 percent of the population, only a fraction of carriers ever develop the disease. It is seen most commonly in infants or in epidemics among persons who live in close quarters (barracks, schools). Prophylactic meningococcal vaccination is administered during epidemics and is reported with V03.89. Suspected carrier of meningitis is reported with V02.59.

036.0	Meningococcal meningitis — *infection of membranes lining brain or spinal cord*
036.1	Meningococcal encephalitis — *infection of brain*
036.2	Meningococcemia — *invasion of bloodstream*
036.3	Waterhouse-Friderichsen syndrome, meningococcal — *vascular collapse and shock*
036.40	Meningococcal carditis, unspecified — *site of heart infection unknown*
036.41	Meningococcal pericarditis — *infection of lining of heart*
036.42	Meningococcal endocarditis — *infection within heart cavities*
036.43	Meningococcal myocarditis — *infection of muscle of heart*
036.81	Meningococcal optic neuritis — *infection of optic nerve*
036.82	Meningococcal arthropathy — *infection of joint*
036.89	Other specified meningococcal infections — *other specific site of infection*
036.9	Unspecified meningococcal infection — *unknown site of infection*

037 TETANUS `OK`

Tetanus is an infection by *Clostridium tetani*, and is commonly called "lockjaw" because of the tonic spasms that occur in voluntary muscles. *C. tetani* is found in soil and animal feces, and infection may result from insignificant or deep wounds. The infected patient may have difficulty swallowing, speaking, or respiration as a result of the tonic spasms caused by the infection.

In the United States, the highest number of tetanus cases is seen among intravenous drug abusers and in burn victims or as a complication of abortion or pregnancy. See the index of ICD-9 for entries relating to tetanus occurring as a result of abortion or childbirth.

Tetanus has a high mortality rate and is one of the diseases that common childhood immunizations protect against. (The T in DPT is for tetanus vaccine). Report prophylactic vaccination for tetanus with V03.7. If tetanus immunization occurs in conjunction with other immunizations, see the V06 series of immunization codes.

✔5th Needs fifth-digit   `OK` Valid three-digit code

038 SEPTICEMIA

Septicemia is the invasion of the bloodstream that results in multisystemic infection. Codes in this series are classified according to the infective bacterial agent.

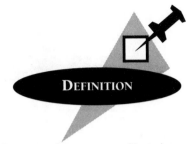

Septicemia, also called septic syndrome or sepsis, occurs when a localized infection (a urinary tract infection, operative wound infection, or infected tooth) metastasizes and the bacterium is spread throughout the body. The disease is acute, and symptoms may include shaking chills, fever, abdominal pain, vomiting, and diarrhea. Septicemia treatments include antibiotic therapy, drainage of any abscess, or reoperation.

Gram-negative: a category of bacteria.

Septicemia: infection that invades the bloodstream and becomes systemic.

"Sepsis" can be an ambiguous term in the medical record and care should be taken in coding to differentiate generalized sepsis represented in this code rubric from other bacterial infections. For example, one physician may document urosepsis, meaning a general sepsis originating as a urinary tract infection, while another physician may document urosepsis, meaning urine contaminated with bacteria. The former would be reported with a code from this rubric, while the latter would be reported with 599.0.

The incidence of septicemia in staphylococcal infection is related to the organism identified. As many as 90 percent of staphylococcal aureus infection cases are true sepsis, while less than 50 percent of non-aureus staphylococcus cases are true sepsis.

When septicemia is iatrogenic, arising from a complication of an implanted device or other medical intervention, the complication code should be reported first, followed by the appropriate septicemia code.

For septicemia associated with pregnancy, childbirth, or abortion, see the index of ICD-9-CM. Shigella septicemia is reported with 004.9. Septicemia from anthrax is reported with 022.3, and from salmonella, 003.1. For gonococcal septicemia, see 098.89, and for herpetic septicemia, see 054.5. Postoperative septicemia is reported with 998.59.

038.0	Streptococcal septicemia — *other than Streptococcus pneumoniae*
038.10	Unspecified staphylococcal septicemia — *unknown staphylococcus*
038.11	Staphylococcus aureus septicemia — *also called S. pyogenes*
038.19	Other staphylococcal septicemia
038.2	Pneumococcal septicemia — *septicemia from bacteria common to pneumonia*
038.3	Septicemia due to anaerobes — *due to bacteroides*
038.40	Septicemia due to unspecified gram-negative organism — *not otherwise specified*
038.41	Septicemia due to hemophilus influenzae (H. influenzae) — *also called Pfeiffer's bacillus*
038.42	Septicemia due to Escherichia coli (E. coli) — *also called colon bacillus and Escherich's bacillus*
038.43	Septicemia due to pseudomonas — *family Pseudomonadaceae*
038.44	Septicemia due to serratia — *family Enterobacteriaceae*
038.49	Other septicemia due to gram-negative organism — *including Proteus vulgaris*
038.8	Other specified septicemia — *not elsewhere classified*
038.9	Unspecified septicemia — *disseminated, unknown cause*

039 ACTINOMYCOTIC INFECTIONS

Infections by *Actinomyces israeli* are classified in this rubric according to site, at which multiple, communicating abscesses often form granulated tissue. The disease is most

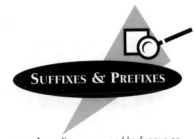

-mycosis: a disease caused by fungus or yeast

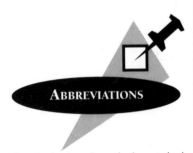

ABBREVIATIONS

TSS: toxic shock syndrome is characterized by high fever, diarrhea, skin rash, and shock and often associated with the use of tampons. Usually caused by *Staphylococcus aureus.*

commonly seen in adult males and is slowly progressive, although it is sometime seen as a local complication of intrauterine device (IUD) placement in women.

039.0	Cutaneous actinomycotic infection — *superficial skin infection*	
039.1	Pulmonary actinomycotic infection — *lung involvement with chest pain, fever, cough*	
039.2	Abdominal actinomycotic infection — *intestinal involvement with anorexia, pain, fever, vomiting and irregular bowels*	
039.3	Cervicofacial actinomycotic infection — *"lumpy jaw" in oral mucosa or neck*	
039.4	Madura foot — *deep foot infection following penetrating injury*	
039.8	Actinomycotic infection of other specified sites — *site not elsewhere classified, multiple sites, or generalized*	
039.9	Actinomycotic infection of unspecified site — *unknown site*	

040 OTHER BACTERIAL DISEASES

Gas gangrene is the result of infection by the *Clostridium bacteria*, usually at the site of injury or a recent surgical wound. It is an acute condition, with red, extremely painful tissue swelling in quick progression to surrounding areas. Involved tissue is destroyed. Gas gangrene has a high mortality rate. Clostridia species of bacteria produce many toxins that cause tissue death and systemic symptoms, including sweating, fever, and shock. Untreated, gas gangrene can lead to renal failure, coma, and death. Treatments include wound debridement, amputation, antibiotics, and hyperbaric oxygen treatment. Gas gangrene associated with abortion, pregnancy, or labor and delivery should be reported with codes from that section of ICD-9. Check the ICD-9 index for more information. Also check the ICD-9 index for a complex list of gangrene diagnoses other than gas gangrene.

Whipple's disease primarily effects middle-aged men and presents as chronic diarrhea, anemia, arthralgia, and abdominal pain. Whipple's disease is incorrectly classified in ICD-9 as an infective disease, because little was known about the disease when ICD-9-CM was developed in the 1970s. In fact, it is an intestinal malabsorption disorder. In ICD-10-CM, Whipple's disease is correctly classified to the Digestive System chapter under a rubric for nutritional malabsorption disorders. Even though it is incorrectly classified as an infection, Whipple's disease is still correctly reported as 040.2 in ICD-9.

040.0	Gas gangrene — *clostridial myonecrosis, malignant edema*	
040.1	Rhinoscleroma — *Klebsiella rhinoscleromatis infection of nose, nasopharynx*	
040.2	Whipple's disease — *intestinal lipodystrophy*	
040.3	Necrobacillosis — *Fusobacterium necrophorum abscess or necrosis*	
040.81	Tropical pyomyositis — *including Bungpagga*	
040.89	Other specified bacterial diseases — *not elsewhere classified, including toxic shock syndrome*	

041 BACTERIAL INFECTION IN CONDITIONS CLASSIFIED ELSEWHERE AND OF UNSPECIFIED SITE

This rubric of ICD-9 provides supplemental codes to identify bacterial agents in diseases classified elsewhere. They usually are sequenced after the disease manifestation. When coding a disease caused by an infectious organism, report the disease first, followed by the code that identifies the infectious agent. For example, urinary tract infection due to *E. coli* is sequenced as 599.0, then 041.4. Codes in this rubric can also be used to classify bacterial infections of unspecified nature or site.

✓5th Needs fifth-digit   **OK** Valid three-digit code

041.00 Unspecified streptococcus infection in conditions classified elsewhere and of unspecified site

041.01 Streptococcus infection in conditions classified elsewhere and of unspecified site, group A

041.02 Streptococcus infection in conditions classified elsewhere and of unspecified site, group B

041.03 Streptococcus infection in conditions classified elsewhere and of unspecified site, group C

041.04 Streptococcus infection in conditions classified elsewhere and of unspecified site, group D

041.05 Streptococcus infection in conditions classified elsewhere and of unspecified site, group G

041.09 Other streptococcus infection in conditions classified elsewhere and of unspecified site

041.10 Unspecified staphylococcus infection in conditions classified elsewhere and of unspecified site

041.11 Staphylococcus aureus infection in conditions classified elsewhere and of unspecified site

041.19 Other staphylococcus infection in conditions classified elsewhere and of unspecified site

041.2 Pneumococcus infection in conditions classified elsewhere and of unspecified site

041.3 Friedländer's bacillus infection in conditions classified elsewhere and of unspecified site — *Klebsiella pneumoniae infection*

041.4 Escherichia coli (E. coli) infection in conditions classified elsewhere and of unspecified site

041.5 Hemophilus influenzae (H. influenzae) infection in conditions classified elsewhere and of unspecified site

041.6 Proteus (mirabilis) (morganii) infection in conditions classified elsewhere and of unspecified site

041.7 Pseudomonas infection in conditions classified elsewhere and of unspecified site

041.81 Mycoplasma infection in conditions classified elsewhere and of unspecified site

041.82 Bacillus fragilis infection in conditions classified elsewhere and of unspecified site

041.83 Clostridium perfringens infection in conditions classified elsewhere and of unspecified site

041.84 Infection due to other anaerobes in conditions classified elsewhere and of unspecified site — *gram negative anaerobes, bacteroides (fragilis)*

041.85 Infection due to other gram-negative organisms in conditions classified elsewhere and of unspecified site — *Aerobacter aerogenes, Mima polymorpha, Serratia*

041.86 Helicobacter pylori (H. pylori) infection — *associated with peptic ulcers*

041.89 Infection due to other specified bacteria in conditions classified elsewhere and of unspecified site — *not elsewhere classified*

041.9 Bacterial infection, unspecified, in conditions classified elsewhere and of unspecified site

042 Human Immunodeficiency Virus (HIV) Infection

042 HUMAN IMMUNODEFICIENCY VIRUS [HIV] DISEASE OK

HIV is divided into two categories, HIV I and HIV II. HIV I is seen worldwide; HIV II is limited to Africa and other countries and is seldom seen in the United States. HIV I has far-

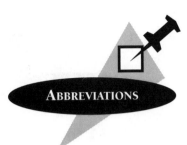

ABBREVIATIONS

MRSA: methicillin-resistant *Staphylococcus aureus*, an infection seen in hospitalized patients by a staph organism resistant to antibiotics like nafcillin, oxacillin, and all cephalosporins.

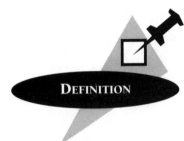

DEFINITION

Fomite: an object that may serve as an agent of transmission of an infection, as it is able to harbor pathogenic microorganisms; for example, a telephone or a hand towel.

Nosocomial: hospital acquired. A nosocomial infection is iatrogenic, or caused by medical care, in this case, in a hospital environment. Common nosocomial infections include those caused by *Enterobacter, Klebsiella, Serratia, Pseudomonas, Proteus, Acinetobacter,* or *Candida.*

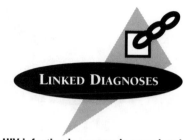

LINKED DIAGNOSES

HIV infection is commonly associated with the following conditions:

Candidiasis

Cryptococcosis outside of lung

Cryptosporidial diarrhea

Disseminated histoplasmosis

Kaposi's sarcoma

Pneumocystis carinii pneumonia

Toxoplasmic encephalitis

ranging health effects and manifestations. This code is reserved for patients with active HIV I infections, or AIDS. HIV II cases are reported with 079.53.

HIV I is a blood-borne virus in that it is transmitted through body fluids containing blood or plasma. Transmission of HIV I can occur sexually or non-sexually through the exchange of body fluids infected with a high concentration of the virus, mainly blood, semen, or vaginal/cervical secretions.

In HIV I, the body's immune system is attacked, reducing its ability to protect itself against a variety of illnesses. Over time, the infected person becomes more susceptible to opportunistic infections or cancers that attack the body and can cause death. AIDS related complex (ARC) includes general lymphadenopathy, anorexia, fever, malaise, diarrhea, anemia, oral hairy leukoplakia, and oral candidiasis. If the patient is being treated for AIDS or an AIDS-related illness, the code for HIV I infection (042) should be sequenced first, followed by codes for manifestations of HIV I infection. If the patient is being treated for an illness unrelated to AIDS, for example, an injury, AIDS would be reported secondarily to the injury.

While 042 is used to report HIV I in patients that have HIV I related illnesses, V08 reports patients who have tested positive for HIV I but who remain asymptomatic. When HIV test results are inconclusive, 795.71 reports nonspecific serologic evidence of HIV.

If the patient is pregnant and has an HIV positive history, use a code from the series 647.6, followed by the appropriate HIV code for infection or positive test. Maternal antibodies can falsely cause a newborn to test positive for HIV. Infants testing positive should be reported with 795.71 unless they exhibit active infections of AIDS. By 18 months, the maternal antibodies will dissipate, and another HIV test will reveal whether the asymptomatic child is truly HIV positive.

Take care not to use 042 in cases of "rule-out" or "suspected" AIDS, as this diagnosis can create a flag in the patient's data files that could interfere with ability to obtain life or health insurance.

045-049 Poliomyelitis and Other Non-arthropod-borne Viral Disease of Central Nervous System

045 ACUTE POLIOMYELITIS

Poliomyelitis is an infectious viral disease of the central nervous system that sometimes results in paralysis. The World Health Organization (WHO) declared the Western Hemisphere polio-free in 1994. Today, polio is most prevalent in areas of Africa, the Middle East and South Asia.

Three types of poliovirus have been identified: the Brunhilde (type 1), Lansing (type 2), and Leon (type 3) strains. Immunity to one strain does not provide protection against the other two. Type 1 causes 85 percent of paralytic infection, type 2 causes 5 percent, and type 3 causes 10 percent.

Polio enters the body through the digestive tract and spreads along nerve cells to affect various parts of the central nervous system. The incubation period ranges from four days to 35 days. Symptoms include fatigue, headache, fever, vomiting, constipation, and stiffness of

5th   Needs fifth-digit   **OK**   Valid three-digit code

the neck. Polio infection can cause permanent paralysis. However, nonparalytic cases far outnumber paralytic cases of polio. No drug has proven effective against polio infection, so treatment is symptomatic.

A third of patients who recover from poliomyelitis develop post-polio syndrome (PPS) 30 years to 40 years later. PPS causes fatigue, muscle weakness, and muscle and joint pain. Late effects of polio, including PPS, deformities, or paralysis in non-active disease, are reported with 138. Sequence first the manifestation, for example, progressive muscular atrophy (335.21), then report the late effect. Congenital polio is reported with 771.2. Do not report personal history of poliomyelitis (V12.02) in patients with active disease.

Exposure to poliovirus is reported with V01.2, and prophylactic vaccination is reported with V04.0. Routine immunization is largely responsible for the eradication of poliomyelitis in the United States.

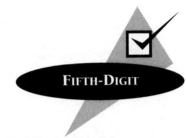

FIFTH-DIGIT

The following fifth-digit subclassification is for use with category 045:

0 poliovirus, unspecified type - unknown

1 poliovirus type 1 - Brunhilde

2 poliovirus type 2 - Lansing

3 poliovirus type 3 - Leon

045.0 ✓5th Acute paralytic poliomyelitis specified as bulbar — *infection at site where brain merges with spinal cord*

045.1 ✓5th Acute poliomyelitis with other paralysis — *infection of peripheral or spinal nerves*

045.2 ✓5th Acute nonparalytic poliomyelitis — *pain, stiffness, or paresthesia without paralysis*

045.9 ✓5th Acute unspecified poliomyelitis — *unknown type*

046 SLOW VIRUS INFECTION OF CENTRAL NERVOUS SYSTEM

Jakob-Creutzfeldt disease is a progressive, fatal disease causing dementia and seizures in adults. Transmission occurs from contaminated humans or human cadavers, although 10 percent of cases are familial in origin. Jakob-Creutzfeldt disease is related to mad cow disease, another form of spongiform encephalopathy with European outbreaks.

Kuru is limited exclusively to New Guinea natives, where the disease has nearly been eradicated. The disease is linked to cannibalism and Fore tribal rituals.

Subacute sclerosing panencephalitis (SSPE) is a rare, progressive, and grave disorder, occurring months or years following measles or measles vaccination, and usually before age 20. Mental faculties are diminished, seizures occur, and the patient deteriorates until death, usually within three years.

All slow virus infections in this rubric may present with manifestations that should be reported in addition to the infection source. Dementia should be reported with 294.11, with behavioral disturbance, or 294.10, without behavioral disturbance.

046.0 Kuru — *New Guinea-based neural disease*

046.1 Jakob-Creutzfeldt disease — *spongiform encephalopathy similar to "mad cow" disease*

046.2 Subacute sclerosing panencephalitis — *Dawson's, Van Bogaert's, Bodechtel-Guttmann disease*

046.3 Progressive multifocal leukoencephalopathy — *cerebral cortex infection in immunosuppressed*

046.8 Other specified slow virus infection of central nervous system — *not elsewhere classified*

046.9 Unspecified slow virus infection of central nervous system — *unknown slow virus infection of CNS*

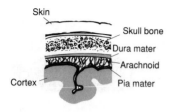

Skin
Skull bone
Dura mater
Arachnoid
Cortex
Pia mater

The meninges constitute the three layers that cover the brain and spinal cord: the dura mater, pia mater, and arachnoid

047 MENINGITIS DUE TO ENTEROVIRUS

Meningitis is the inflammation of the membranes surrounding the brain or spinal cord, in this case, due to an aseptic, abacterial, or a viral enterovirus infection not included in other rubrics in this section of ICD-9.

Viral infections must be differentiated from bacterial and other infections. Typically, a viral infection of the central nervous system is suspected by default, when a culture fails to grow bacteria. A virus may be isolated in spinal fluid or other tissues, but viruses causing aseptic meningitis are identified in less than half of all cases.

Coxsackie virus causes symptoms resembling polio, but without paralysis. It is most commonly seen in children during warm months.

ECHO virus is an acronym for enteric cytopathic human orphan virus and is also most prevalent during warm months.

047.0	Meningitis due to coxsackie virus — *Coxsackievirus*
047.1	Meningitis due to ECHO virus — *echovirus*
047.8	Other specified viral meningitis — *not elsewhere classified*
047.9	Unspecified viral meningitis — *unknown type*

048 OTHER ENTEROVIRUS DISEASES OF CENTRAL NERVOUS SYSTEM `OK`

This rubric represents all enterovirus disease of the central nervous system not elsewhere classified. Among these is Boston exanthem, a mild illness with a rash and fever caused by echovirus 16. It is named after an epidemic that occurred in Boston, Mass.

049 OTHER NON-ARTHROPOD-BORNE VIRAL DISEASES OF CENTRAL NERVOUS SYSTEM

Late effects of viral encephalitis are reported with 139.0.

049.0	Lymphocytic choriomeningitis — *Arenavirus*
049.1	Meningitis due to adenovirus — *Adenovirus*
049.8	Other specified non-arthropod-borne viral diseases of central nervous system — *not elsewhere classified*
049.9	Unspecified non-arthropod-borne viral disease of central nervous system — *unknown type*

050-057 Viral Diseases Accompanied by Exanthem

050 SMALLPOX

Smallpox was a highly contagious human disease caused by the virus variolae. There are two strains: variolae major, which had severe symptoms and high mortality of 20 percent to 40 percent, and variolae minor, which had less severe symptoms and a lower mortality of less than 1 percent. The virus has been eliminated from the modern human population. Some virus remains in government laboratory storage, and WHO still retains a classification for the disease in ICD-9 and ICD-10.

In the unlikely event a patient experiences exposure to the smallpox virus, report V01.3 and call the Centers for Disease Control. Prophylactic vaccination against smallpox is reported with V04.1.

ᐦ5th Needs fifth-digit   `OK` Valid three-digit code

050.0	Variola major — *severe form*
050.1	Alastrim — *mild form*
050.2	Modified smallpox — *reinfection form*
050.9	Unspecified smallpox — *unknown type*

051 COWPOX AND PARAVACCINIA

Cowpox is also called vaccinia because it is closely related to variola, the causative virus of smallpox, and infection by cowpox renders the patient immune to smallpox. Cowpox infection is due to Poxvirus bovis infection from milking cattle, and is much milder than smallpox, with hard lesions and low fever. Vaccinia as a result of inoculation is reported with 999.0, not with 051.1.

051.0	Cowpox — *vaccinia from cattle*
051.1	Pseudocowpox — *paravaccinia infection*
051.2	Contagious pustular dermatitis — *Poxvirus from sheep or goats*
051.9	Unspecified paravaccinia — *unknown paravaccinia infection*

052 CHICKENPOX

Varicella zoster virus causes chickenpox and herpes zoster. Chickenpox is the initial, acute phase of the disease, and herpes zoster is a reactivation of the virus in a latent stage.

Chickenpox is highly contagious and usually mild, but it may be severe in infants, adults, or the immunosuppressed. More than 95 percent of Americans have been infected by chickenpox by the time they reach adulthood. In the United States, 4 million people are infected with chickenpox each year. Chickenpox has a characteristic itchy rash, which then forms blisters that dry into scabs. An infected person may have anywhere from only a few or more than 500 lesions.

An adult bout of chickenpox is more likely to have complications than a childhood infection. These complications may occur when the *Varicella zoster* virus inflames the brain, lung, or other organ, or when infection is accompanied by manifestations of high fever, or when the patient is immunosuppressed. Secondary infections are also considered complications. If the complication to chickenpox cannot be described in the codes presented in this rubric, report a code from rubric 052 first, and codes describing the complications or manifestations secondarily, as in the case of myocarditis (422.0) or arthritis (711.50-711.59).

Inoculation against chickenpox is reported with V05.4.

052.0	Postvaricella encephalitis — *with inflammation of brain*
052.1	Varicella (hemorrhagic) pneumonitis — *with lung infection*
052.7	Chickenpox with other specified complications — *complications not listed above*
052.8	Chickenpox with unspecified complication — *unknown complication*
052.9	Varicella without mention of complication — *no complications mentioned*

053 HERPES ZOSTER

Varicella zoster virus causes chickenpox and herpes zoster. Chickenpox is the initial, acute phase of the disease, and herpes zoster is a reactivation of the virus in a latent stage. Herpes zoster is often referred to as shingles or zona. In herpes zoster, the virus causes unilateral eruptions and painful neuralgia along a nerve path. The disease is classified according to site.

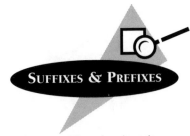

SUFFIXES & PREFIXES

pseudo-: resembling, often deceptive

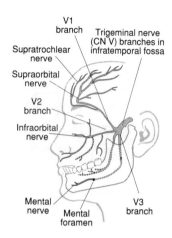

V1
branch

Trigeminal nerve
(CN V) branches in
infratemporal fossa

Supratrochlear
nerve

Supraorbital
nerve

V2
branch

Infraorbital
nerve

Mental
nerve

Mental
foramen

V3
branch

Trigeminal neuralgia,
also known as tic douloureaux,
is a severe facial pain brought
on by mere touch in an area
of one of the divisions of the
trigeminal nerve, usually
along the V2 branch

053.0	Herpes zoster with meningitis — *inflammation of brain and/or spinal cord*
053.10	Herpes zoster with unspecified nervous system complication — *unknown nervous system complication*
053.11	Geniculate herpes zoster — *affecting facial nerve*
053.12	Postherpetic trigeminal neuralgia — *causing oral or nasal pain*
053.13	Postherpetic polyneuropathy — *multiple nerve involvement*
053.19	Other herpes zoster with nervous system complications
053.20	Herpes zoster dermatitis of eyelid — *unilateral, eyelid*
053.21	Herpes zoster keratoconjunctivitis — *unilateral in cornea and conjunctiva*
053.22	Herpes zoster iridocyclitis — *unilateral in iris and ciliary body*
053.29	Other ophthalmic herpes zoster complications — *other eye complication*
053.71	Otitis externa due to herpes zoster
053.79	Other specified herpes zoster complications
053.8	Unspecified herpes zoster complication
053.9	Herpes zoster without mention of complication

054 HERPES SIMPLEX

Herpes simplex is an infection of the herpes simplex virus (HSV), including HSV-1 and HSV-2. The infection causes multiple clusters of fluid-filled, inflamed blisters on the skin or mucous membranes and is usually transmitted by direct contact. HSV-1 is commonly seen about the mouth, lips, and conjunctiva. HSV-2 usually affects genitals and is often transmitted through sexual contact. However, either type of HSV can occur in either site.

The virus can remain dormant and be reactivated by emotional stress, fever, or photosensitivity. Typically, the virus is localized, and code selection is based on the anatomy affected. Herpes simplex infections of the lips or mouth are considered the most benign form of the disease and are reported as "uncomplicated," with 054.9. Systemic manifestations can occur, especially in infants and in the immunosuppressed.

This rubric excludes congenital herpes simplex, which is reported with 771.2.

054.0	Eczema herpeticum — *invading pre-existing skin inflammation*
054.10	Unspecified genital herpes — *unknown site*
054.11	Herpetic vulvovaginitis — *vulva and vagina*
054.12	Herpetic ulceration of vulva — *vulva*
054.13	Herpetic infection of penis — *penis*
054.19	Other genital herpes — *other specified site*
054.2	Herpetic gingivostomatitis — *oral mucosa*
054.3	Herpetic meningoencephalitis — *inflammation of brain and spinal cord*
054.40	Unspecified ophthalmic complication herpes simplex — *unknown eye complication*
054.41	Herpes simplex dermatitis of eyelid — *inflammation and lesions on lid*
054.42	Dendritic keratitis — *inflammation and ulcers of cornea*
054.43	Herpes simplex disciform keratitis — *inflammation and edema of cornea*
054.44	Herpes simplex iridocyclitis — *inflammation of iris and ciliary body*
054.49	Herpes simplex with other ophthalmic complications — *eye complication not elsewhere classified*
054.5	Herpetic septicemia — *herpes simplex disseminated through bloodstream*
054.6	Herpetic whitlow — *painful herpes lesion on fingertip; "herpetic felon"*
054.71	Visceral herpes simplex — *infection of thoracic or abdominal organ*
054.72	Herpes simplex meningitis — *inflammation of lining of brain or spinal cord*
054.73	Herpes simplex otitis externa — *inflammation and lesions of external ear*

✔5th   Needs fifth-digit   **OK**   Valid three-digit code

054.79   Other specified herpes simplex complications — *complication not elsewhere classified*

054.8   Unspecified herpes simplex complication — *unknown complications*

054.9   Herpes simplex without mention of complication — *uncomplicated "fever blister"*

055 MEASLES

Measles is an acute infection caused by paramyxovirus and presents with a hacking cough, rash, and fevers. German measles (rubella) is a different infection, reported with codes from the 056 rubric.

Measles are usually transmitted from person to person via airborne respiratory droplets. Pharyngitis is common. Koplik's spots are white, grainy spots that can occur in the buccal mucosa and are an early symptom of measles.

In the United States, measles outbreaks have been greatly reduced by government immunization programs. Measles has a low mortality rate in healthy individuals, and if the disease follows a normal course with high fever, Koplik's spots, generalized rash, and cough, report 055.9.

Patients with measles are susceptible to streptococcal infection, worsening of TB, or reactivation of an inactive mycobacterial infection. Sequence the measles code first, followed by codes for the secondary infection.

Measles are classified according to complication. In most cases, the complication occurs after the symptoms of the measles have diminished. Pneumonia as a complication is most common in infants.

Prophylactic vaccination against measles is reported with V04.2 as a separate inoculation, or V06.4 for measles-mumps-rubella (MMR) inoculation.

055.0   Postmeasles encephalitis — *brain infection*

055.1   Postmeasles pneumonia — *lung infection*

055.2   Postmeasles otitis media — *middle ear infection*

055.71   Measles keratoconjunctivitis — *inflammation of cornea and conjunctiva*

055.79   Other specified measles complications — *complication not elsewhere classified*

055.8   Unspecified measles complication — *unknown complication*

055.9   Measles without mention of complication — *typical course of rash, fever, and cough*

056 RUBELLA

Rubella is also called German measles or three-day measles. It is a highly contagious virus, but the symptoms are mild and short-lived in most people. Symptoms include malaise, arthralgia, rash, headache, and fever. Rubella during pregnancy, however, can result in abortion, stillbirth, or in congenital defects. Because of its highly contagious nature and affect upon the fetus, rubella is considered a serious health threat.

Rubella codes are selected according to complication. If the infection runs its normal course, report rubella without complication with 056.9. Consult the index to report rubella during pregnancy.

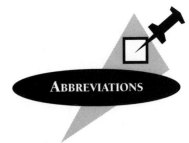

ABBREVIATIONS

AMS: atypical measles syndrome, most commonly seen in young adults

MIG: measles immune globulin

SSPE: subacute sclerosing panencephalitis, often associated with measles

This rubric excludes congential rubella, which is reported with 771.0. Exposure to rubella is reported with V01.4 Prophylactic vaccination against rubella is reported with V04.3 as a separate inoculation or V06.4 for measles-mumps-rubella (MMR) inoculation.

056.00	Unspecified rubella neurological complication — *unknown nervous complication*
056.01	Encephalomyelitis due to rubella — *inflammation of brain and spinal cord*
056.09	Other neurological rubella complications — *nervous complication not elsewhere classified*
056.71	Arthritis due to rubella — *inflammation of joint*
056.79	Rubella with other specified complications — *complication not elsewhere classified, not nervous system*
056.8	Unspecified rubella complications — *unknown complication*
056.9	Rubella without mention of complication — *typical course of rash and fever*

057 OTHER VIRAL EXANTHEMATA

This rubric captures rash-causing viruses that are not specifically outlined in rubrics 050-056. Report 057.0 for fifth disease, also called Sticker's disease. Report 057.8 for any of the following: Dukes (-Filatow) disease, exanthema subitum or sixth disease, fourth disease, parascarlatina, pseudoscarlatina, roseola infantum, and Zahorsky's disease.

057.0	Erythema infectiosum (fifth disease) — *contagious rash, livid on cheeks*
057.8	Other specified viral exanthemata — *including fourth disease, sixth disease, roseola infantum, others*
057.9	Unspecified viral exanthem — *unknown viral exanthemata*

060-066 Arthropod-borne Viral Diseases

Insects are the vectors that carry the diseases classified to this section of ICD-9. Early attempts to classify these diseases were made along geographic lines and according to the insect believed to be the vector. An arbovirus is a common shortened name for arthropod-borne virus.

Mosquitoes are the most common vector, or transmitting agent, for arboviruses. The bite of mosquito often transmits the disease from bird to mosquito. The bite of mosquito to man transmits the disease to man. In equine disease, the mosquitoes transmit disease to horses, or from horses to man. Seldom is the disease carried from man to mosquito to man.

060 YELLOW FEVER

Yellow fever is transmitted from mosquito to man. In cities, the bite of an *Aedes aegypti* mosquito causes the infection; in the jungle (sylvan), *Haemagogus* and other forest canopy mosquitoes acquire the virus from jungle primates and transmit the virus to man. In the United States, cases of yellow fever are usually limited to people who have been abroad. Yellow fever is most commonly seen in central Africa, South America, and Central America.

Yellow fever causes high fever, headache, jaundice, and hemorrhage. The pulse is slow. Mortality rate can be as high as 10 percent.

Prophylactic inoculation against yellow fever is reported with V04.4.

DEFINITION

Exanthemata: an eruption.

Faget's sign: slowed pulse occurring with high fever, as seen in yellow fever.

060.0	Sylvatic yellow fever — *origin in jungle or woods; usually transmitted animal to man, by mosquito*
060.1	Urban yellow fever — *origin in city or town; usually transmitted man to man, by mosquito*
060.9	Unspecified yellow fever — *unknown*

061 DENGUE OK

Dengue is transmitted to man by the bite of the *Aedes* mosquito. The disease is endemic throughout tropical and subtropical regions, and is usually seen in the United States only when people come to this country already infected with the virus.

Dengue causes chills, headache, backache and prostration. Joint and leg aches and onset of high fever are rapid.

This rubric excludes hemorrhagic fever caused by dengue, which is reported with 065.4.

062 MOSQUITO-BORNE VIRAL ENCEPHALITIS

These diseases cause central nervous system symptoms like tremors, convulsion, coma and confusion, as well as headache, vomiting, and fever. Geographic differences are significant among the varieties. Japanese encephalitis is seen in the Far East. Eastern equine encephalitis (EEE) is most common in the Atlantic and Gulf Coast states, upper New York and western Michigan. Western equine encephalitis (WEE) is seen in areas west of the Mississippi. St. Louis encephalitis is most common in the United States and Caribbean. Australian encephalitis is usually limited to New Guinea and Australia, and California encephalitis.

Report Venezuelan equine encephalitis with 066.2.

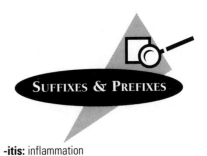

SUFFIXES & PREFIXES

-itis: inflammation

encephalo-: pertaining to the brain

062.0	Japanese encephalitis — *Flavivirus; Japanese B*
062.1	Western equine encephalitis — *Alphavirus; WEE*
062.2	Eastern equine encephalitis — *Alphavirus; EEE*
062.3	St. Louis encephalitis — *Flavivirus; in United States*
062.4	Australian encephalitis — *Flavivirus; in Australia*
062.5	California virus encephalitis
062.8	Other specified mosquito-borne viral encephalitis — *including Ilheus virus*
062.9	Unspecified mosquito-borne viral encephalitis — *unknown*

063 TICK-BORNE ENCEPHALITIS

In tick-borne encephalitis, a tick is the vector instead of a mosquito. Included in this rubric are diseases limited to Russia, Central Europe, and Great Britain. Only the Powassan encephalitis, reported with 063.8, is commonly found in North America, both in New York and in Canada. Any other variety is likely to be found among travelers.

063.0	Russian spring-summer (taiga) encephalitis — *Russia, central Europe*
063.1	Louping ill — *British Isles*
063.2	Central European encephalitis — *central Europe*
063.8	Other specified tick-borne viral encephalitis — *including Langat and Powassan (New York)*
063.9	Unspecified tick-borne viral encephalitis

064 VIRAL ENCEPHALITIS TRANSMITTED BY OTHER AND UNSPECIFIED ARTHROPODS OK

Report viral encephalitis not otherwise specified, unknown vector, with 049.9, reserving this code for encephalitis caused by an unidentified arbovirus.

065 ARTHROPOD-BORNE HEMORRHAGIC FEVER

This rubric specifies a hemorrhagic fever. If hemorrhage is not a component, seek other codes. For example, hemorrhagic dengue fever is reported with 065.4, as is hemorrhagic Chikungunya fever. For Chikungunya fever without mention of hemorrhage, report 066.3; for dengue fever without mention of hemorrhage, report 061. In all cases, with or without hemorrhage, yellow fever is reported with 060.0-060.9.

Hemorrhagic fever is not endemic to the United States. Codes in this category may apply to infections obtained while abroad, primarily in Russia and Asia.

065.0	Crimean hemorrhagic fever (CHF Congo virus) — *Crimea and Russian Don and Volga river valleys*
065.1	Omsk hemorrhagic fever — *Siberia*
065.2	Kyasanur Forest disease — *India*
065.3	Other tick-borne hemorrhagic fever — *other*
065.4	Mosquito-borne hemorrhagic fever — *Dengue hemorrhagic; Chikungunya hemorrhagic*
065.8	Other specified arthropod-borne hemorrhagic fever — *including mite-borne hemorrhagic*
065.9	Unspecified arthropod-borne hemorrhagic fever — *unknown hemorrhagic arbovirus*

066 OTHER ARTHROPOD-BORNE VIRAL DISEASES

This rubric captures arbovirus infections not classified as hemorrhagic, as causing encephalitis, and not the specific infections of yellow fever or dengue. Colorado tick fever, reported with 066.1, is the arbovirus in this section that would be likely to be seen in the United States, and causes fever, malaise, headaches, and myalgia. This is a different infection than Rocky Mountain spotted fever, a rickettsioses infection that causes a petechial rash in addition to fever, malaise, headache, and myalgia. Rocky Mountain spotted fever is reported with 082.0.

066.0	Phlebotomus fever — *sandfly-borne; Asia, Mideast, South America*
066.1	Tick-borne fever — *American mountain; Colorado*
066.2	Venezuelan equine fever
066.3	Other mosquito-borne fever — *Bunyamwera; O'nyong-nyong; Rift valley*
066.8	Other specified arthropod-borne viral diseases — *including Chandipura and Piry fever*
066.9	Unspecified arthropod-borne viral disease — *unknown arbovirus*

070-079 Other Diseases Due to Viruses and Chlamydiae

This rubric covers a broad spectrum of infection not elsewhere classified.

070 VIRAL HEPATITIS

Hepatitis is an inflammation or infection of the liver. ICD-9 differentiates all hepatitis into two categories: viral and nonviral. Further, hepatitis caused by specific viruses like Epstein-Barr or cytomegaloviruses are considered separately, and do not fall into the general

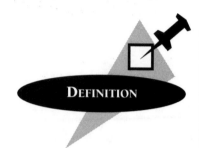

DEFINITION

Arbovirus: arthropod-borne virus. An arbovirus uses an insect, usually a mosquito but also tick or sandfly, as a vector to transmit disease from animal to man.

Arthropod: refers to insects.

✎5th   Needs fifth-digit   OK   Valid three-digit code

accepted usage of the phrase "viral hepatitis." Viral hepatitis is considered to be hepatitis caused by the hepatitis virus and this rubric covers acute and chronic stages of that disease.

Symptoms of hepatitis range from flu-like illness to liver failure and death. Initially, nausea and malaise are common. Later in the course of the disease, jaundice and an enlarged liver are common.

Hepatitis A (HAV) is spread through fecal contamination or by eating contaminated, raw shellfish and is considered to be a milder form of hepatitis. Exposure to hepatitis B (HBV) is limited to direct contact with contaminated blood or blood products, or through sexual congress. HB is the source of many chronic liver ailments. The hepatitis C virus (HCV) causes 80 percent of hepatitis cases resulting from blood transfusions, and also is associated with more chronic and severe liver ailments. The hepatitis E virus (HEV) is associated with fecal contamination and is a milder form of the disease.

For chronic viral hepatitis with an acute exacerbation, two codes should be reported to describe each condition: the chronic and the acute.

Nonviral hepatitis is classified to rubric 571 in the Digestive System chapter. Other infectious hepatitis is reported with codes from the 573 rubric. Report cytomegalic inclusion virus hepatitis with 573.1 and 078.5; hepatitis due to mononucleosis with 075 with 573.1, and due to Coxsackie virus with 074.8 with 573.1. Suspected carrier of viral hepatitis is reported with codes from the V02.6 rubric. Prophylactic inoculation against viral hepatitis is reported with V05.3.

070.0	Viral hepatitis A with hepatic coma
070.1	Viral hepatitis A without mention of hepatic coma
070.2 ✔5th	Viral hepatitis B with hepatic coma
070.3 ✔5th	Viral hepatitis B without mention of hepatic coma
070.41	Acute or unspecified hepatitis C with hepatic coma
070.42	Hepatitis delta without mention of active hepatitis B disease with hepatic coma
070.43	Hepatitis E with hepatic coma
070.44	Chronic hepatitis C with hepatic coma
070.49	Other specified viral hepatitis with hepatic coma
070.51	Acute or unspecified hepatitis C without mention of hepatic coma
070.52	Hepatitis delta without mention of active hepatitis B disease or hepatic coma
070.53	Hepatitis E without mention of hepatic coma
070.54	Chronic hepatitis C without mention of hepatic coma
070.59	Other specified viral hepatitis without mention of hepatic coma
070.6	Unspecified viral hepatitis with hepatic coma
070.9	Unspecified viral hepatitis without mention of hepatic coma

071 RABIES OK

This code is used to report active rabies infection, not simple exposure to rabies. Rabies, or hydrophobia, is an acute infectious disease caused by a neurotropic virus found in the saliva of rabid mammals. Canine vaccination has nearly eliminated canine rabies in the United States and cases of wild animal bites are rare. Rabies causes restlessness, fever, excessive salivation, and painful laryngeal spasms.

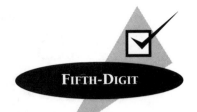

FIFTH-DIGIT

The following fifth-digit subclassification is for use with categories 070.2 and 070.3:

0 acute or unspecified, without mention of hepatitis delta

1 acute or unspecified, with hepatitis delta

2 chronic, without mention of hepatitis delta

3 chronic, with hepatitis delta

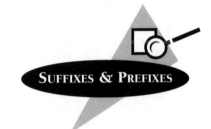

SUFFIXES & PREFIXES

Hepat: pertaining to the liver

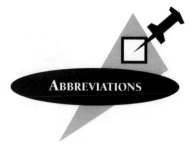

ARS: anti-rabies serum

HDCV: human diploid cell rabies vaccine

RIG: rabies immune globulin

RVA: rabies vaccine, absorbed

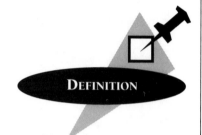

DEFINITION

Mumps: contagious and infectious disease caused by *Paramyxovirus*. Symptoms are fever, inflammation and swelling of the parotid gland.

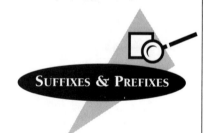

SUFFIXES & PREFIXES

encephal-: pertaining to the brain

mening-: pertaining to the lining of the brain and/or spinal cord

orch-: pertaining to the testis

pancreat-: pertaining to the pancreas, an endocrine and exocrine gland in the abdomen

Exposure to rabies is usually treated successfully with immediate local wound cleansing and administration of rabies immune globulin. If a person has been exposed to rabies, but infection status is unknown or an infection has not developed, report V01.5. To report inoculation against rabies, whether following exposure or as a prophylactic measure for high-risk individuals like wildlife handlers, report V04.5.

If the patient develops rabies, the diagnosis is no longer an imminent death sentence. Supportive treatment of respiratory system, circulatory system, and central nervous system complications can result in positive outcome for the symptomatic rabies patient. Rabies is often described as urban or sylvan, depending on the source of infection. Whether the vector is from the city or the wilderness, rabies infection is reported with 071.

072 MUMPS

Mumps presents as an acute infection of the salivary glands, usually the parotids, caused by *Paramyxovirus*. Inhaling respiratory droplets from an infected person can spread the disease. Most cases occur in children two years or older. Mumps causes painful swelling of the salivary glands, pain upon chewing, and high fever. Complications may occur, especially in adults. Code selection for mumps is determined by complication. In cases that follow the normal uncomplicated course of swollen parotid glands and high fever, report 072.9.

Prophylactic vaccination against mumps is reported with V04.6 as a separate inoculation or V06.4 for measles-mumps-rubella (MMR) inoculation.

072.0	Mumps orchitis — *inflammation of testis*
072.1	Mumps meningitis — *inflammation of lining of brain and/or spinal cord*
072.2	Mumps encephalitis — *inflammation of brain*
072.3	Mumps pancreatitis — *inflammation of pancreas*
072.71	Mumps hepatitis — *inflammation of liver*
072.72	Mumps polyneuropathy — *inflammation of nerves*
072.79	Mumps with other specified complications — *specified inflammation not elsewhere classified*
072.8	Unspecified mumps complication — *complication not elsewhere classified*
072.9	Mumps without mention of complication — *normal course of mumps*

073 ORNITHOSIS

Ornithosis is also called psittacosis. The disease is caused by *Chlamydia psittaci* and transmitted most commonly by parrots, parakeets, or lovebirds, but sometimes by domestic birds like pigeons, turkeys or canaries, or by some seabirds. Infection usually occurs when dust or droppings are inhaled by man, or rarely, by a bird bite. Ornithosis can also be transmitted from man to man, but this is very rare.

Symptoms include fever, malaise, and cough, in the case of lung infection. Ornithosis has a 30 percent mortality rate without treatment, but responds well to antibiotics. Code selection for ornithosis is a based on site of infection. Report any significant symptoms, like cough or shortness of breath, secondarily.

073.0	Ornithosis with pneumonia — *pulmonary infection*
073.7	Ornithosis with other specified complications — *complication not elsewhere classified*

✔5th Needs fifth-digit   **OK** Valid three-digit code

| 073.8 | Ornithosis with unspecified complication — *complication not specified* |
| 073.9 | Unspecified ornithosis — *no complications* |

074 SPECIFIC DISEASES DUE TO COXSACKIE VIRUS

Coxsackie virus commonly causes infection in summer and fall, and is transmitted man-to-man via oral secretions, feces, or blood. Herpangina is an acute infection of *Coxsackie* virus, causing throat lesions, fever and vomiting, generally seen in children during the summer months. Epidemic pleurodynia is a *Coxsackie* infection causing severe paroxysmal pain in the chest and fever, usually limited to young adults and children. It is also called Bornholm disease or devil's grip.

Coxsackie carditis is infection of the heart. Code selection is based on whether the infection occurs in the outer lining of the heart, the heart cavities, or the heart muscle. In infants, a *Coxsackie* infection of the heart muscle can be life threatening, but this infection can occur at any age.

Hand, foot, and mouth disease is a *Coxsackie* infection of the hands, feet, and oral mucosa, most commonly seen in preschool children. It is usually a mild infection.

Report *Coxsackie* meningitis with 047.0 and Coxsackie enteritis with 008.67. Coxsackie virus infection of the nervous system, not elsewhere classified, is reported with 048.

074.0	Herpangina — *vesicular pharyngitis; typically children in summer*
074.1	Epidemic pleurodynia — *chest pain with fever; typically children and young adults*
074.20	Coxsackie carditis, unspecified — *inflammation of heart unspecified*
074.21	Coxsackie pericarditis — *inflammation of outer lining of heart*
074.22	Coxsackie endocarditis — *inflammation of within the heart cavities*
074.23	Coxsackie myocarditis — *inflammation of muscle of heart*
074.3	Hand, foot, and mouth disease — *lesions on hands, feet, and mouth; typically preschoolers*
074.8	Other specified diseases due to Coxsackievirus — *including acute lymphonodular pharyngitis*

075 INFECTIOUS MONONUCLEOSIS **OK**

Infectious mononucleosis is an active infection by the Epstein-Barr virus, causing fever, sore throat, enlarged lymph glands spleen, and fatigue. It is most commonly seen in teens and young adults, and runs a mild course in most cases.

In mononucleosis with hepatitis, report 075 and 573.1.

076 TRACHOMA

Trachoma is caused by infection with the organism *Chlamydia trachomatis*. It begins slowly as a mild conjunctivitis that develops into a severe onset infection. The initial stage lasts several weeks and is followed by a chronic stage in which the lids remain swollen, and the cornea becomes eroded, scarred, and vascularized. The lids develop contractures and may turn outward, pulling away form the eye. Eventually, the eyelashes turn in, rubbing on the cornea at the front of the eye. The scarring on the cornea leads to severe vision loss and blindness, usually when people are 40 years to 50 years old.

Report late effects of trachoma with 139.1. Code the sequelae first, as in vision loss (369.00-369.9), followed by 139.1.

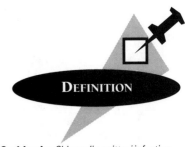

DEFINITION

Ornithosis: *Chlamydia psittaci* infection often transmitted from birds to humans.

Trachoma: a contagious form of conjunctivitis.

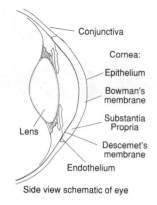

Side view schematic of eye

Labels:
- Conjunctiva
- Cornea:
  - Epithelium
  - Bowman's membrane
  - Substantia Propria
  - Descemet's membrane
  - Endothelium
- Lens

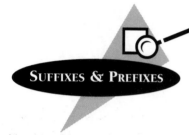

SUFFIXES & PREFIXES

adeno-: pertaining to a gland

conjunctiv-: pertaining to the conjunctiva of the eye

kerat-: pertaining to the cornea

076.0	Initial stage trachoma — *mild inflammation of conjunctiva with pain*	
076.1	Active stage trachoma — *acute inflammation of conjunctiva with pain*	
076.9	Unspecified trachoma — *stage unknown*	

077 OTHER DISEASES OF CONJUNCTIVA DUE TO VIRUSES AND CHLAMYDIAE

Other diseases and infections of the conjunctiva can be found in the Nervous System chapter under rubrics 372 and 373, as well as under specific infective agents, for example, herpes zoster keratoconjunctivitis (053.21) or trachoma (076.0-076.9).

Codes in this rubric are organized by infective agent and symptoms. Inclusion conjunctivitis is caused by *Chlamydia trachomatis* and adenovirus type B causes epidemic keratoconjunctivitis and pharyngoconjunctival fever.

077.0	Inclusion conjunctivitis — *due to Chlamydia trachomatis*
077.1	Epidemic keratoconjunctivitis — *shipyard eye; due to adenovirus type B*
077.2	Pharyngoconjunctival fever — *due to adenovirus type B*
077.3	Other adenoviral conjunctivitis — *acute adenoviral follicular conjunctivitis*
077.4	Epidemic hemorrhagic conjunctivitis
077.8	Other viral conjunctivitis — *including Newcastle conjunctivitis*
077.98	Unspecified diseases of conjunctiva due to Chlamydiae
077.99	Unspecified diseases of conjunctiva due to viruses — *unknown virus*

078 OTHER DISEASES DUE TO VIRUSES AND CHLAMYDIAE

This rubric addresses specific viral and chlamydial diseases not specified elsewhere.

More than 50 types of human papilloma viruses (HPV) cause plantar and genital warts in humans. These infections may be asymptomatic or produce warts or mucosal lesions.

Commonly, human papilloma virus causes viral warts. They may be documented as condyloma, verruca, or verruca vulgaris and are reported with 078.10. Viral warts caused by condylomata acuminata are sexually transmitted genital warts, distinct from other viral warts in that they are associated with cervical dysplasia and carcinoma of the cervix, penis and vulva. They are reported with 078.11. Condyloma acuminatum are commonly called genital warts on the patient record but, unless condyloma acuminatum is noted, the patient record only supports use of a nonspecific code, 078.19, for genital warts, not otherwise specified.

Cytomegaloviral disease (CMV) is a human salivary gland virus and member of the herpes group. It affects only humans, and can range in symptoms from being a benign and asymptomatic infection to causing significant impairment or death in infants and the immunosuppressed. In symptomatic cases, fatigue, lymphadenopathy, and low fever may be present.

CMV is a most common and serious organ transplant infection complication. If CMV infection follows transplant, assign a code from category 996.8 to identify the transplanted organ, and 078.5 to report the infection. When appropriate, an additional code is used to identify the manifestation of CMV infection, as in hepatitis (573.1) or pneumonia (484.1). For congenital cytomegaloviral infection, report 771.1.

078.0	Molluscum contagiosum — *poxvirus causing small bumps on skin or conjunctiva*
078.10	Unspecified viral warts — *horny skin wars; human papilloma virus*
078.11	Condyloma acuminatum — *clusters of lesions on genitalia; STD*

✔5th Needs fifth-digit   **OK** Valid three-digit code

078.19	Other specified viral warts — *including Verruca plantaris, Verruca plana; fig wart*
078.2	Sweating fever — *sweating disease; miliary fever*
078.3	Cat-scratch disease — *mild and benign lymphoreticulosis*
078.4	Foot and mouth disease — *aphthous fever; ulcers on mouth, legs and feet*
078.5	Cytomegaloviral disease — *CMV*
078.6	Hemorrhagic nephrosonephritis — *Russia and Korea*
078.7	Arenaviral hemorrhagic fever — *Argentina and Bolivia*
078.81	Epidemic vertigo — *dizziness*
078.82	Epidemic vomiting syndrome — *winter vomiting disease*
078.88	Other specified diseases due to Chlamydiae — *not elsewhere classified*
078.89	Other specified diseases due to viruses — *including Marburg disease, Lassa fever; green monkey disease, pseudorabies, tanapox, and Aujeszky's disease*

079 VIRAL AND CHLAMYDIAL INFECTION IN CONDITIONS CLASSIFIED ELSEWHERE AND OF UNSPECIFIED SITE

HIV II, generally not seen in the United States, is on the rise elsewhere in the world. Report HIV II with 079.53 and HIV I with 042.

Respiratory syncytial virus (RSV) is a common cause of respiratory disease in winter in the United States. Infants are most vulnerable to the disease. Each year, RSV causes 4,500 U.S. deaths and 90,000 hospitalizations. For some respiratory infections, report the infection first and RSV as the infective agent secondarily, as in tracheobronchitis due to RSV, with 466.0 and 079.6. Some respiratory infection codes identify RSV as the infective agent, so only one code is necessary. Bronchiolitis due to RSV is reported with a single code, 466.11, and pneumonia due to RSV is reported with a single code, 480.1.

Hantavirus is an arbovirus that causes severe respiratory distress in its victims. The mortality rate for Hantavirus is about 50 percent, with treatment. Most commonly transmitted to humans when they inhale dust from feces of infected mice, most cases are seen in the Four Corners area of the United States. Report 079.81 secondarily to pneumonia or other infection code from the Respiratory System chapter of ICD-9; Hantavirus should not be reported as a primary or principal diagnosis.

079.0	Adenovirus infection in conditions classified elsewhere and of unspecified site
079.1	ECHO virus infection in conditions classified elsewhere and of unspecified site
079.2	Coxsackievirus infection in conditions classified elsewhere and of unspecified site
079.3	Rhinovirus infection in conditions classified elsewhere and of unspecified site
079.4	Human papilloma virus in conditions classified elsewhere and of unspecified site
079.50	Unspecified retrovirus in conditions classified elsewhere and of unspecified site
079.51	Human t-cell lymphotrophic virus, type I (HTLV-I), in conditions classified elsewhere and of unspecified site
079.52	Human t-cell lymphotrophic virus, type II (HTLV-II), in conditions classified elsewhere and of unspecified site
079.53	Human immunodeficiency virus, type 2 (HIV 2), in conditions classified elsewhere and of unspecified site

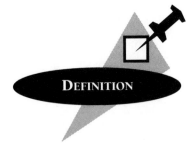

DEFINITION

Condyloma acuminatum: a wart-like lesion on the external genitalia. Also referred to as genital warts.

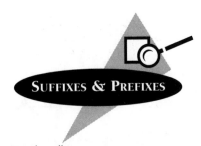

SUFFIXES & PREFIXES

cyte-: the cell

megalo-: large

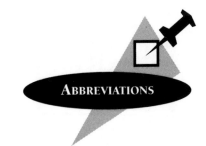

ABBREVIATIONS

CMV: cytomegalovirus

HTLV: human T-cell lymphotrophic virus. Type I has been known to cause adult T cell lymphoma, myelopathy and spastic paraparesis. Type II is spread by sexual contact, transfusion, and IV drug use.

RSV: respiratory syncytial virus, a virus that can cause severe bronchitis and bronchopneumonia in children

079.59	Other specified retrovirus, in conditions classified elsewhere and of unspecified site
079.6	Respiratory syncytial virus (RSV)
079.81	Hantavirus infection
079.88	Other specified chlamydial infection, in conditions classified elsewhere and of unspecified site
079.89	Other specified viral infection, in conditions classified elsewhere and of unspecified site
079.98	Unspecified chlamydial infection, in conditions classified elsewhere and of unspecified site
079.99	Unspecified viral infection, in conditions classified elsewhere and of unspecified site

080-088 Rickettsioses and Other Arthropod-borne Diseases

Rickettsial diseases are usually perpetuated by a cycle from animal to insect vector to man. The illnesses are sudden in onset and include fever, myalgia, malaise, headache, and, sometimes, rash. In some cases, rickettsioses produce a localized ulcer or lesion at the site of the insect bite.

080 LOUSE-BORNE (EPIDEMIC) TYPHUS OK

Rickettsia prowazekii transmitted by feces from the human body louse (*Pediculus humanus*), through a break in the skin, often from scratching, or by entry of the louse droppings into mucus membranes. Epidemic typhus causes headache, rash, and high fever, and is most dangerous to people older than 50. Report 080 for primary typhus infection.

081 OTHER TYPHUS

Other varieties of typhus are classified by infective agent and by vector. Brill's disease is a reoccurrence of epidemic typhus (080) and is reported with 081.1.

081.0	Murine (endemic) typhus — *Rickettsia typi (mooseri); rat flea*
081.1	Brill's disease — *Rickettsia prowazekii recurrence*
081.2	Scrub typhus — *Rickettsia tsutsugamushi; chigger*
081.9	Unspecified typhus — *unknown*

082 TICK-BORNE RICKETTSIOSES

These diseases typically begin with a tick bite in which a lesion develops at the site of the bite. This may be called an eschar, or, in boutonneuse fever, a tache noire. Lymphadenopathy, low fever, and a rash usually follow.

Rocky Mountain spotted fever is endemic to the United States and is a spotted fever reported with 082.0. Colorado tick fever, reported with 066.1, is a different infection than Rocky Mountain spotted fever, which causes a petechial rash in addition to fever, malaise, headache, and myalgia. Rocky Mountain spotted fever is reported with 082.0.

Boutonneuse fever, caused by *Rickettsioses conorii*, occurs in Africa, India, Europe, the Mideast, and near the Caspian, Black, and Mediterranean seas. Normally, boutonneuse fever, Queensland tick typhus, and North Asian tick fever are seen in the United States only among travelers who return with an infection.

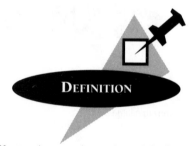

DEFINITION

Vector: the agent that carries an infection from one host to another, as in a mosquito transferring disease from man to man, or a flea transferring disease from rodent to man.

⌐5th Needs fifth-digit **OK** Valid three-digit code

Ehrlichiosis is likely caused by various *Ehrlichia* species and code selection is based on the species. Infection resembles Rocky Mountain spotted fever, without a rash, and illness may extend for weeks or months. The infection responds to antibiotics.

082.0	Spotted fevers — *Rocky Mountain spotted fever*
082.1	Boutonneuse fever — *Africa, India, Mediterranean*
082.2	North Asian tick fever — *Siberia*
082.3	Queensland tick typhus — *Australia*
082.40	Ehrlichiosis, unspecified — *unknown type*
082.41	Ehrlichiosis chafeensis [E. chafeensis]
082.49	Other ehrlichiosis — *other than E. chaffeensis*
082.8	Other specified tick-borne rickettsioses
082.9	Unspecified tick-borne rickettsiosis

083 OTHER RICKETTSIOSES

These specific varieties of rickettsioses infection do not fall into the previous rubric classifications. Report 083.9 for an infection known to be rickettsioses, but of unknown type and unknown vector.

083.0	Q fever — *Coxiella burnetii*
083.1	Trench fever — *Quintan, Wolhynian, Werner-His fever*
083.2	Rickettsialpox — *Rickettsia akari; mite*
083.8	Other specified rickettsioses — *not elsewhere classified*
083.9	Unspecified rickettsiosis — *unknown*

084 MALARIA

Malaria is a mosquito-borne protozoan infection endemic to the tropics. It is transmitted man to mosquito to man and has largely been eradicated in the United States through insecticide programs and drugs. Most cases of malaria in the United States are seen in people who have traveled abroad. Sometimes, these infected travelers may even spawn a stateside epidemic of malaria. Rarely, malaria may be transmitted through a blood transfusion or shared needle.

Malaria causes malaise and headache with intermittent fever and chill. Jaundice usually develops. Some varieties, most notably Blackwater fever, can cause more serious complications including hemolysis.

Malaria is coded according to species of *Plasmodium*: *P. falciparum, P. malariae, P. ovale, P. vivax,* or mixed species. A code is also provided in this rubric for therapeutically induced malaria (084.7), regardless of species. Do not report personal history of malaria (V12.03) in patients with active disease.

084.0	Falciparum malaria (malignant tertian) — *Plasmodium falciparum*
084.1	Vivax malaria (benign tertian) — *Plasmodium vivax*
084.2	Quartan malaria — *Plasmodium malariae*
084.3	Ovale malaria — *Plasmodium ovale*
084.4	Other malaria — *monkey malaria*
084.5	Mixed malaria — *more than one parasite*
084.6	Unspecified malaria — *unknown*
084.7	Induced malaria — *therapeutically induced*
084.8	Blackwater fever — *Plasmodium falciparum; with hemoglobinuria*
084.9	Other pernicious complications of malaria — *including algid and cerebral malaria*

085 LEISHMANIASIS

Leishmaniasis is an infection by *Leishmania*, a genus of parasitic protozoa, usually seen in developing nations and rare in the United States, though seen in parts of South America. The focus of infection and the infective agent are variables that create a broad spectrum of disease associated with leishmaniasis.

085.0	Visceral leishmaniasis (kala-azar) — *L. donovani; systemic; in Far East, USSR, Africa, Mediterranean, South and Central America*
085.1	Cutaneous leishmaniasis, urban — *L tropica minor; dry/ulcerating lesions; boils*
085.2	Cutaneous leishmaniasis, Asian desert — *L. tropica major; wet/necrotizing skin lesions*
085.3	Cutaneous leishmaniasis, Ethiopian — *L. ethiopica; widespread skin lesions*
085.4	Cutaneous leishmaniasis, American — *L mexicana; L. tegumentaria diffusa; skin lesions*
085.5	Mucocutaneous leishmaniasis, (American) — *L. braziliensis; called espundia, uta, chiclero ulcer*
085.9	Unspecified leishmaniasis — *unknown Leishmaniasis species*

086 TRYPANOSOMIASIS

Trypanosomiasis is caused by protozoa *Trypanosoma* and causes chronic disease with symptoms including fever, lymphadenopathy, headache, and edema. Complications can affect the central nervous system and major organs and can be fatal. International travelers may return to the United States with a trypanosomiasis infection, but the protozoa is endemic only in Africa and South America, so it is seldom seen in North America.

Report the trypanosomiasis code first, followed by any manifestation codes that may apply, for example, encephalitis (323.2), meningitis (321.3). However, cardiomyopathy from Chagas' disease requires only 086.0, and other specific forms of Chagas' disease are reported with 078.88.

086.0	Chagas' disease with heart involvement — *Trypanosoma cruzi; heart involvement*
086.1	Chagas' disease with other organ involvement — *Trypanosoma cruzi; other organ involvement*
086.2	Chagas' disease without mention of organ involvement — *Trypanosoma cruzi; no organ infection*
086.3	Gambian trypanosomiasis — *Trypanosoma gambiense*
086.4	Rhodesian trypanosomiasis — *Trypanosoma rhodesiense*
086.5	African trypanosomiasis, unspecified — *sleeping sickness*
086.9	Unspecified trypanosomiasis — *unknown trypanosomiasis*

087 RELAPSING FEVER

Relapsing fever is an infection caused by **Borrelia** and the symptoms are episodic and may include fever and arthralgia. Code selection is based on the vector. Report 087.9 if the vector is unknown.

087.0	Louse-borne relapsing fever — *lice as vector*
087.1	Tick-borne relapsing fever — *tick as vector*
087.9	Unspecified relapsing fever — *unknown vector*

✔5th Needs fifth-digit   **OK** Valid three-digit code

088 OTHER ARTHROPOD-BORNE DISEASES

This category identifies arthropod-borne diseases not elsewhere classified.

Bartonellosis is in infection of *Bartonella bacilliformis*, transmitted by sandflies in the Andes Mountains of South America. Cases in the United States are rare.

Babesiosis identifies a group of tick-borne diseases infected with the *Babesia* protozoa. Rare in humans, it causes fever, chills, anemia, splenomegaly, and muscle pain. People with a history of splenectomy have a high mortality rate for babesiosis. In others, it resolves within weeks.

Lyme disease is caused by the bite of a tick infected with *Borrelia burgdorferi* and causes joint disorders, skin lesions, and flu-like symptoms. It is endemic to most parts of the United States as well as in Russia, Australia, and the Far East.

088.0	Bartonellosis — *Bartonella bacilliformis; sandflies; Andes*
088.81	Lyme disease — *Borrelia burgdorferi; ticks, United States*
088.82	Babesiosis — *Babesia; ticks*
088.89	Other specified arthropod-borne diseases — *not elsewhere classified*
088.9	Unspecified arthropod-borne disease — *unknown*

090-099 Syphilis and Other Venereal Diseases

It is estimated that 400,000 people seek treatment for syphilis in the United States each year. Syphilis is caused by the spirochete *Treponema pallidum*. The disease is divided into four categories: congenital syphilis, and the three stages of acquired syphilis: early syphilis, a contagious stage with mild symptoms; latent syphilis, asymptomatic and infectious; and the late or tertiary stage, with significant symptoms but not contagious. Infection is transmitted by an infected mother to her fetus or by sexual contact. Rare instances of infection from kissing or close bodily contact have been documented, as the spirochete enters the body through the mucous membranes or skin. Syphilis responds to antibiotic treatment.

The disease can manifest itself in any stage, and may be asymptomatic for years. Usually, the first symptoms are lymphadenopathy and a localized chancre. However, the variety of manifestations can make clinical recognition of syphilis difficult.

Syphilis codes are classified as congenital, early, or latent. The disease is further classified according to its manifestations.

Report exposure to syphilis with V01.6, and carrier of syphilis with V02.8.

090 CONGENITAL SYPHILIS

Up to 80 percent of syphilitic mothers pass the infection to their fetus. Symptoms do not develop in most neonates, so diagnosis in the hospital nursery is usually the result of tests performed on the infant because of the mother's medical history.

Early congenital syphilis may manifest itself within two years of birth with a rash on the patient's palms and soles, swollen lymph glands, an enlarged spleen, and/or characteristic syphilitic chancres near mucous membranes. Other symptoms may include osteochondritis, epiphysitis, periostitis, chronic coryza, or choroiditis. Syphilis is confirmed with serologic

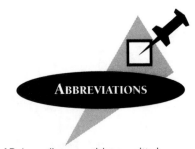

ABBREVIATIONS

LD: Lyme disease, a tick-transmitted, inflammatory disease that causes skin lesions, and abnormalities in the joints, nerves and heart.

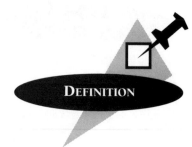

Alopecia areata: bald patches that may be a symptom of syphilis.

Condyloma lata: papules in the mucosal junctions and moist areas of the skin, associated with syphilis.

Gumma: chronic granulomatous reaction to syphilis.

Rhagades: fissured lesions around the mouth, associated with syphilis.

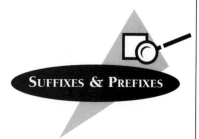

uvea-: uveal tract which includes the iris, ciliary body, and choroid

tests. Early symptomatic syphilis is sometimes called Wegner's disease. If neurological manifestations are present, use codes from the 090.4 series of codes rather than 090.0.

Latent early congenital syphilis has no clinical manifestations and is diagnosed through serologic testing within the first two years of life. If a test of spinal fluid is positive for syphilis, the disease is not considered latent, even if the patient does not show symptoms. Instead, the condition is reported as congenital syphilitic meningitis (090.42).

090.0	Early congenital syphilis, symptomatic — *from birth to two years old, symptoms*
090.1	Early congenital syphilis, latent — *from birth to two years old, no symptoms*
090.2	Unspecified early congenital syphilis — *from birth to two years, symptoms unknown*
090.3	Syphilitic interstitial keratitis — *congenital corneal infection*
090.40	Unspecified juvenile neurosyphilis — *unknown site of infection*
090.41	Congenital syphilitic encephalitis — *infection of brain*
090.42	Congenital syphilitic meningitis — *infection of the lining of the brain or spinal cord*
090.49	Other juvenile neurosyphilis — *not elsewhere classified*
090.5	Other late congenital syphilis, symptomatic — *older than two years with symptoms*
090.6	Late congenital syphilis, latent — *older than two years, no symptoms*
090.7	Late congenital syphilis, unspecified — *older than two years, symptoms unknown*
090.9	Congenital syphilis, unspecified — *unknown age in child with unknown symptoms*

091 EARLY SYPHILIS, SYMPTOMATIC

Generally, early syphilis is the period from initial infection and the first two years of the disease. Early syphilis can be further divided into primary or secondary syphilis. In primary syphilis, a painless chancre appears at the site of infection and regional swelling of lymph nodes occurs as the spirochetes invade the lymphatic system. The lymphadenopathy is sometimes called bubo. In secondary syphilis, the infection spreads to secondary sites. Codes in this section are selected based on whether the infection is primary or secondary and, then, by anatomic site.

If early syphilis has complications involving the heart or nervous system, report codes in the 093 or 094 rubrics instead.

091.0	Genital syphilis (primary) — *genital lesion in new case of syphilis*
091.1	Primary anal syphilis — *anal lesion in new case of syphilis*
091.2	Other primary syphilis — *lesion in new case of syphilis, not genital or anal*
091.3	Secondary syphilis of skin or mucous membranes — *secondary lesions within two years of initial infection*
091.4	Adenopathy due to secondary syphilis — *secondary lymph gland inflammation within two years of initial infection*
091.50	Early syphilis, syphilitic uveitis, unspecified — *secondary inflammation of uvea in eye within two years of initial infection*
091.51	Early syphilis, syphilitic chorioretinitis (secondary) — *secondary inflammation of retina and choroid of eye within two years of initial infection*
091.52	Early syphilis, syphilitic iridocyclitis (secondary) — *secondary inflammation of iris and ciliary body of eye within two years of initial infection*

↙5th Needs fifth-digit   **OK** Valid three-digit code

091.61 Early syphilis, secondary syphilitic periostitis — *secondary inflammation of outer layers of bone within two years of initial infection*

091.62 Early syphilis, secondary syphilitic hepatitis — *secondary inflammation of liver within two years of initial infection*

091.69 Early syphilis, secondary syphilis of other viscera — *secondary inflammation of other abdominal organs within two years of initial infection*

091.7 Early syphilis, secondary syphilis, relapse — *return of symptoms after asymptomatic period within two years of initial infection*

091.81 Early syphilis, acute syphilitic meningitis (secondary) — *sudden, severe inflammation of lining of the brain or spinal cord within two years of initial infection*

091.82 Early syphilis, syphilitic alopecia — *secondary loss of hair of within two years of initial infection*

091.89 Early syphilis, other forms of secondary syphilis — *other secondary manifestation within two years of initial infection*

091.9 Early syphilis, unspecified secondary syphilis

092 EARLY SYPHILIS, LATENT

Latent early syphilis has no clinical manifestations and is diagnosed through serologic testing within the first two years of infection. If a test of spinal fluid is positive for syphilis, the disease is not considered latent, even if the patient does not show symptoms. Instead, the condition is reported with a code from the 094 rubric for neurosyphilis.

092.0 Early syphilis, latent, serological relapse after treatment — *other than congenital; results positive-negative-positive within first two years*

092.9 Early syphilis, latent, unspecified — *other than congenital; within first two years, no symptoms*

093 CARDIOVASCULAR SYPHILIS

This rubric is reserved for any syphilitic infection of the cardiovascular system, except congenital infection, which is reported with 090.5 instead. Select the code based on anatomic site of infection. Clinical diagnosis is based on echocardiography (ECG) and serologic test for syphilis. Syphilis infection within the heart may lead to congestive heart failure, which is reported in addition to syphilis with 428.0. Often, cardiovascular complications occur in tandem with neurosyphilis and, in these cases, report codes from both the 093 and 094 rubrics.

093.0 Aneurysm of aorta, specified as syphilitic — *dilation of syphilitic aorta*

093.1 Syphilitic aortitis — *inflammation of main artery leading from heart*

093.20 Unspecified syphilitic endocarditis of valve — *inflammation of unknown heart valve*

093.21 Syphilitic endocarditis, mitral valve — *inflammation of mitral valve*

093.22 Syphilitic endocarditis, aortic valve — *inflammation of aortic valve*

093.23 Syphilitic endocarditis, tricuspid valve — *inflammation of tricuspid valve*

093.24 Syphilitic endocarditis, pulmonary valve — *inflammation of pulmonary value*

093.81 Syphilitic pericarditis — *inflammation of outer lining of heart*

093.82 Syphilitic myocarditis — *inflammation of muscle of heart*

093.89 Other specified cardiovascular syphilis — *other inflammation of heart, including Babinski-Vaquez syndrome*

094 NEUROSYPHILIS

In neurosyphilis, spirochetes infect the nerves, spinal cord, or brain. Codes in this rubric are organized by anatomy and severity. Tabes dorsalis is a progressive degeneration of

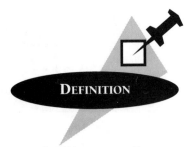

DEFINITION

Latent: to be hidden or not manifest.

Periostitis: inflammation of outer layers of bone.

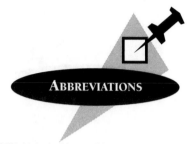

BFP: biologic false positive

FTA-ABS: fluorescent treponemal antibody absorption

HATTS: hemagglutination treponemal tests for syphilis

MHA-TP: microhemagglutination assay for antibodies to *T. pallidum*

RPR: rapid plasma reagin.

STS: serologic tests for syphilis.

VDRL: Veneral Disease Research Laboratory.

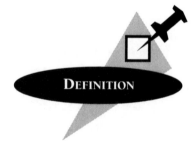

DEFINITION

Tabes dorsalis: progressive degeneration of the nerves associated with long-term syphilis.

nerves and general paresis describes progressive degeneration of brain. Both conditions are considered the most severe and systemic forms of neurosyphilis.

Most symptomatic neurosyphilis is a form of late syphilis, meaning the patient has been infected for more than two years. Any presence of infection in the spinal fluid is considered a form a neurosyphilis, even if the patient is otherwise asymptomatic. Asymptomatic neurosyphilis can be an early or late form of the disease, and is reported with 094.3.

Disorders including dementia and some forms of arthropathy are associated with some forms of neurosyphilis and should be reported in addition to the neurosyphilis code.

094.0	Tabes dorsalis — *progressive degeneration of nerves in long-term syphilis*
094.1	General paresis — *degeneration of brain in long-term syphilis*
094.2	Syphilitic meningitis — *inflammation of lining of the brain and/or spinal cord*
094.3	Asymptomatic neurosyphilis — *positive spinal fluid, but no symptoms*
094.81	Syphilitic encephalitis — *inflammation of the brain in neurosyphilis*
094.82	Syphilitic Parkinsonism — *tremors, decreased motor function, muscular rigidity*
094.83	Syphilitic disseminated retinochoroiditis — *inflammation of retina and choroid*
094.84	Syphilitic optic atrophy — *degeneration of the eye and its nerves*
094.85	Syphilitic retrobulbar neuritis — *inflammation of the posterior optic nerve*
094.86	Syphilitic acoustic neuritis — *inflammation of acoustic nerve*
094.87	Syphilitic ruptured cerebral aneurysm — *rupture of blood vessel in brain*
094.89	Other specified neurosyphilis — *including Argyll Robertson's syndrome, erosion of spine, Heubner's disease*
094.9	Unspecified neurosyphilis

095 OTHER FORMS OF LATE SYPHILIS, WITH SYMPTOMS

This rubric covers symptomatic syphilitic infections of more than two years organized by site of secondary infection. Cardiovascular syphilis (093) and neurosyphilis (094) are excluded from this rubric.

095.0	Syphilitic episcleritis — *inflammation of external surface of sclera*
095.1	Syphilis of lung — *pulmonary infection*
095.2	Syphilitic peritonitis — *inflammation of the abdominal membrane lining*
095.3	Syphilis of liver — *hepatic infection*
095.4	Syphilis of kidney — *inflammation of one or both kidneys*
095.5	Syphilis of bone — *infection of bone*
095.6	Syphilis of muscle — *myositis from syphilis*
095.7	Syphilis of synovium, tendon, and bursa — *Verneuil's disease, bursitis, synovitis*
095.8	Other specified forms of late symptomatic syphilis
095.9	Unspecified late symptomatic syphilis

096 LATE SYPHILIS, LATENT **OK**

In latent late syphilis, a positive serologic test has indicated the patient has the disease, but there are no symptoms after an infection of two or more years. The spinal fluid is clear. For asymptomatic late syphilis with infected spinal fluid, 094.3 is reported instead.

097 OTHER AND UNSPECIFIED SYPHILIS

This rubric contains nonspecific codes for use in cases when the timetable of syphilitic infection or the specific site of secondary infection is unknown. These codes are not to be used for patients under two years of age. See the codes in rubric 090 for congenital and juvenile syphilis.

📐5th Needs fifth-digit   **OK** Valid three-digit code

097.0   Unspecified late syphilis — *after first two years, unknown symptoms*
097.1   Unspecified latent syphilis
097.9   Unspecified syphilis — *unknown acquired syphilis*

098 GONOCOCCAL INFECTIONS

Gonorrhea is an acute infection caused by *Neisseria gonorrhoeae*, usually transmitted sexually. Women are often asymptomatic, while men tend to develop urinary symptoms from gonococcus rather quickly. Diagnosis is based on bacteriologic examination of discharge or urine. Gonorrhea responds to antibiotic treatment, though several courses may be required to eradicate the disease.

Gonococcal infection is classified by site. In the most common site of infection, the genitourinary system, a further distinction is made between chronic and acute cases. Report chronic infection codes when the infection has continued for two months or longer. If the patient is infected with a penicillin-resistant form of gonorrhea, report V09.0 Infection with microorganisms resistant to penicillins, in addition to the code for chronic gonorrhea. Chlamydial infections frequently occur with gonorrhea and should be reported in addition to the gonorrhea code, with *Chlamydia* codes from the 099 rubric.

Report exposure to gonorrhea with V01.6, and carrier of gonorrhea with V02.7.

098.0   Gonococcal infection (acute) of lower genitourinary tract — *sudden onset; bartholinitis, urethritis, vulvovaginitis*
098.10   Gonococcal infection (acute) of upper genitourinary tract, site unspecified — *sudden onset; upper genitourinary tract site unknown*
098.11   Gonococcal cystitis (acute) — *sudden onset; bladder*
098.12   Gonococcal prostatitis (acute) — *sudden onset; prostate*
098.13   Gonococcal epididymo-orchitis (acute) — *sudden onset; epididymis, testis*
098.14   Gonococcal seminal vesiculitis (acute) — *sudden onset; seminal vesicle*
098.15   Gonococcal cervicitis (acute) — *sudden onset; cervix*
098.16   Gonococcal endometritis (acute) — *sudden onset; uterus*
098.17   Gonococcal salpingitis, specified as acute — *sudden onset; fallopian tubes*
098.19   Other gonococcal infections (acute) of upper genitourinary tract — *sudden onset; upper genitourinary tract not elsewhere classified*
098.2   Gonococcal infections, chronic, of lower genitourinary tract — *persistent infection; bartholinitis, urethritis, vulvovaginitis*
098.30   Chronic gonococcal infection of upper genitourinary tract, site unspecified — *persistent infection, upper genitourinary tract site unknown*
098.31   Gonococcal cystitis, chronic — *persistent infection; bladder*
098.32   Gonococcal prostatitis, chronic — *persistent infection; prostate*
098.33   Gonococcal epididymo-orchitis, chronic — *persistent infection; epididymis, testis*
098.34   Gonococcal seminal vesiculitis, chronic — *persistent infection; seminal vesicle*
098.35   Gonococcal cervicitis, chronic — *persistent infection; cervix*
098.36   Gonococcal endometritis, chronic — *persistent infection; uterus*
098.37   Gonococcal salpingitis (chronic) — *persistent infection; fallopian tubes*
098.39   Other chronic gonococcal infections of upper genitourinary tract — *persistent infection; upper genitourinary tract not elsewhere classified*
098.40   Gonococcal conjunctivitis (neonatorum) — *infection of conjunctiva at birth*
098.41   Gonococcal iridocyclitis — *inflammation of iris and ciliary body*
098.42   Gonococcal endophthalmia — *inflammation and infection of the contents of the eyeball*
098.43   Gonococcal keratitis — *inflammation and infection of cornea*

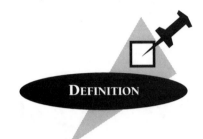

DEFINITION

Epididymo-orchitis: inflammation of the testes and epididymis.

Prostatitis: inflammation of the prostate.

Salpingitis: inflammation of the fallopian tube.

Enophthalmia: inflammation and infection of the tissues of the eyeball.

Neonatorum: newborn period.

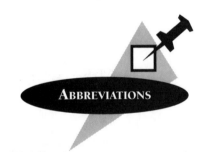

ABBREVIATIONS

GU: genitourinary

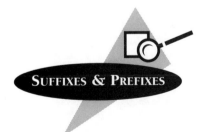

SUFFIXES & PREFIXES

-cycl-: the ciliary body of the eye

irid-: the iris of the eye

098.49	Other gonococcal infection of eye — *other infection of eye due to gonorrhea*
098.50	Gonococcal arthritis — *inflammation of joint*
098.51	Gonococcal synovitis and tenosynovitis — *inflammation of viscid fluid of joint, causing pain and swelling*
098.52	Gonococcal bursitis — *inflammation of sac-like cavities in joint*
098.53	Gonococcal spondylitis — *inflammation of vertebrae*
098.59	Other gonococcal infection of joint — *gonococcal rheumatism; other joint inflammation not elsewhere classified*
098.6	Gonococcal infection of pharynx — *inflammation of pharynx*
098.7	Gonococcal infection of anus and rectum — *proctitis*
098.81	Gonococcal keratosis (blennorrhagica) — *skin lesions*
098.82	Gonococcal meningitis — *inflammation of the lining of the brain or spinal cord*
098.83	Gonococcal pericarditis — *inflammation of the outer lining of the heart*
098.84	Gonococcal endocarditis — *inflammation of the tissues lining the cavities of the heart*
098.85	Other gonococcal heart disease — *heart inflammation, not elsewhere classified*
098.86	Gonococcal peritonitis
098.89	Gonococcal infection of other specified sites — *other infection, not elsewhere classified*

099 OTHER VENEREAL DISEASES

This category identifies sexually transmitted diseases not elsewhere classified.

Chancroid is a localized infection by *Hemophilus ducreyi*, causing genital ulcers and infecting the inguinal lymph nodes. Care must be taken to distinguish chancroid infection from herpes simplex infection. This diagnosis made via cultures or microscopic examination.

The most common sexually transmitted disease in the United States is chlamydial infection and its most common manifestation is urethritis. At least 50 percent of nongonococcal urethritis cases in the United States are due to *Chlamydia*. In the past, chlamydial urethritis was reported generically as NGU. As a result, a specific code for NGU due to chlamydial infection falls under rubric 099.4 Other nongonococcal urethritis, rather than under 099.5 Other veneral diseases due to *Chlamydia trachomatis*. Codes in the 099.5 rubric exclude urethral infection.

In cases of genitourinary infection, other than urethra and due to *Chlamydia trachomatis*, an additional code may be required to specify the site of genitourinary infection. For example, sequence 099.54 *Chlamydia trachomatis infection of other genitourinary site* first, and 614.9 *Unspecified inflammatory disease of female pelvic organs and tissues*, second, to report pelvic inflammatory disease due to *Chlamydia*.

Trachoma, a chlamydial infection of the eye, is not venereal and is reported in the rubric 076.

For Reiter's disease (099.3) use a second code to report manifestations of the infection, such as conjunctivitis (372.33).

099.0	Chancroid — *STD of Haemophilus ducreyi; skin lesions*
099.1	Lymphogranuloma venereum — *STD of Chlamydia trachomatis; skin lesions*
099.2	Granuloma inguinale — *STD of Calymmatobacterium granulomatis; anogenital skin ulcers*
099.3	Reiter's disease — *STD of unknown etiology; urethritis, conjunctivitis*

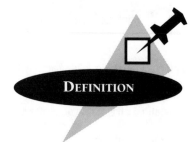

DEFINITION

Chancroid: sexually transmitted infection that causes chancre sores at the site of infection.

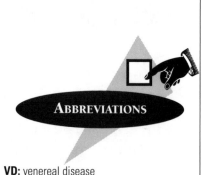

ABBREVIATIONS

VD: venereal disease

↵5th Needs fifth-digit   **OK** Valid three-digit code

099.40	Unspecified nongonococcal urethritis (NGU) — *STD, nonspecific NGU*
099.41	Nongonococcal urethritis (NGU) due to Chlamydia trachomatis — *STD, NGU from Chlamydia trachomatis*
099.49	Nongonococcal urethritis (NGU) due to other specified organism — *STD, NGU from other specified source not elsewhere classified*
099.50	Chlamydia trachomatis infection of unspecified site — *STD, unknown site*
099.51	Chlamydia trachomatis infection of pharynx — *STD, throat*
099.52	Chlamydia trachomatis infection of anus and rectum — *STD, proctitis*
099.53	Chlamydia trachomatis infection of lower genitourinary sites — *STD, excluding urethra*
099.54	Chlamydia trachomatis infection of other genitourinary sites — *STD, including pelvic inflammatory disease, testis*
099.55	Chlamydia trachomatis infection of unspecified genitourinary site — *STD, unknown site*
099.56	Chlamydia trachomatis infection of peritoneum — *STD, including perihepatitis*
099.59	Chlamydia trachomatis infection of other specified site — *STD, specified site not elsewhere classified*
099.8	Other specified venereal diseases — *STD, other disease, not elsewhere classified*
099.9	Unspecified venereal disease — *STD, unknown*

100-104 Other Spirochetal Diseases

These spirochetal diseases are not classified as sexually transmitted diseases because they are transmitted from person to person through general body contact.

100 LEPTOSPIROSIS

Leptospirosis is an infection due to any serotype of *Leptospira*. Dogs and rats are the most common carriers of leptospirosis and, in the United States, the most common source of infection is swimming in contaminated water. The infection usually enters the host through mucous membranes or injured skin. Less than 100 cases are reported in the United States annually.

100.0	Leptospirosis icterohemorrhagica — *Weil's, Mathieu's, Wassilieff's disease*
100.81	Leptospiral meningitis (aseptic) — *inflammation of membranes of brain and spinal cord*
100.89	Other specified leptospiral infections — *including Fort Bragg fever; swamp fever*
100.9	Unspecified leptospirosis — *unknown*

101 VINCENT'S ANGINA

Vincent's angina is an infection of the oral mucosa causing painful bleeding, salivation, edema, and breath odor, caused by fusiform bacillus and a spirochete.

102 YAWS

Yaws is an infection by *Treponema pallidum* subspecies pertenue causing lesions of the skin, bone, and soft tissue. Upon infection, a lesion develops at the site and the yaws spirochete enters the body. This lesion is called the "mother yaw." Yaws is endemic to equatorial countries with high humidity, so cases in the United States are limited to travelers.

| 102.0 | Initial lesions of yaws — *initial, mother yaw* |
| 102.1 | Multiple papillomata and wet crab yaws due to yaws — *butter, plantar, palmar yaws* |

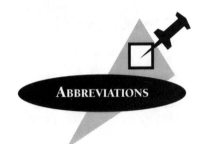

ABBREVIATIONS

ANUG: acute necrotizing ulcerative gingivitis, also known as trench mouth, Vincent's angina, or Fusospirochetosis

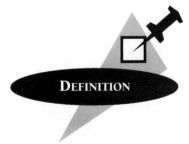

DEFINITION

Vincent's angina: an infection causing ulcers on the tonsils and pharynx.

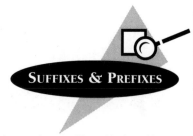

SUFFIXES & PREFIXES

-keratosis: an epidermal lesion with an overgrowth of skin

hyper-: above, more than, over

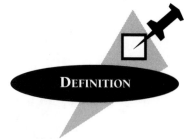

DEFINITION

Nonvenereal: not sexually transmitted

Pinta: *Treponema carateum* infection causing blue, red, white, or purple skin spots.

102.2	Other early skin lesions due to yaws — *cutaneous, less than five years since onset*	
102.3	Hyperkeratosis due to yaws — *overgrowth of skin on palms and bottoms of feet*	
102.4	Gummata and ulcers due to yaws — *rubbery lesions and dead skin*	
102.5	Gangosa due to yaws — *massive, mutilating lesions of nose and oral cavity*	
102.6	Bone and joint lesions due to yaws — *goundou, bone gumma, osteitis*	
102.7	Other manifestations due to yaws — *mucosal, juxta-articular nodules*	
102.8	Latent yaws — *asymptomatic with positive test*	
102.9	Unspecified yaws — *including parangi*	

103 PINTA

Pinta is an infection by *Treponema pallidum* subspecies *carateum* confined to the skin and causing progressive lesions. Pinta is confined to the Indians of Mexico, and Central and South America, so causes in the United States is limited to travelers.

103.0	Primary lesions of pinta — *first stage, early disease*
103.1	Intermediate lesions of pinta — *pigmented lesions, mid-disease*
103.2	Late lesions of pinta — *vitiligo, late in disease*
103.3	Mixed lesions of pinta
103.9	Unspecified pinta

104 OTHER SPIROCHETAL INFECTION

Nonvenereal endemic syphilis is an infection of *Treponema pallidum* subspecies *endemicum* found in the eastern Mediterranean region and Africa. It initially causes skin lesions that may progress to soft tissue and bone lesions.

104.0	Nonvenereal endemic syphilis — *lesions on skin and mucosa, not from STD*
104.8	Other specified spirochetal infections — *including bronchospirochetosis, Castellani's bronchitis*
104.9	Unspecified spirochetal infection — *unknown*

110-118 Mycoses

These diseases are usually considered chronic and may be present for years before a diagnosis is made. Seldom are the symptoms acute, except with immunocompromised hosts. In the immunocompromised host, also report the health problem that causes the immune deficiency. Clinical manifestations of mycoses can be fever, anorexia, malaise, or depression. Many of the infections are geographically limited; each has a typical clinical course.

110 DERMATOPHYTOSIS

Dermatophytoses are superficial fungal infections of the skin. Ringworm, though no worm is present, and athlete's foot are common names for the disease. Dermatophytosis is classified according to the site of the lesion. This rubric includes infections by species of *Epidermophyton, Microsporum,* and *Trichophyton tinea.*

110.0	Dermatophytosis of scalp and beard — *kerion, sycosis, black dot tinea of scalp*
110.1	Dermatophytosis of nail — *onychomycosis, tinea unguium*
110.2	Dermatophytosis of hand — *tinea manuum*
110.3	Dermatophytosis of groin and perianal area — *Dhobie itch, tinea cruris, Baerensprung's disease*
110.4	Dermatophytosis of foot — *athlete's foot; tinea pedis*
110.5	Dermatophytosis of the body — *herpes circinatus; tinea imbricata*

✓5th Needs fifth-digit   **OK** Valid three-digit code

110.6 Deep seated dermatophytosis — *Majocchi's granuloma*
110.8 Dermatophytosis of other specified sites — *not elsewhere classified*
110.9 Dermatophytosis of unspecified site — *unknown site*

111 DERMATOMYCOSIS, OTHER AND UNSPECIFIED

These superficial fungal infections of the skin are fungal infections other than ringworm, not elsewhere classified, or have an unknown fungal infectious agent.

111.0 Pityriasis versicolor — *Malassezia (Pityrosporum) furfur; tinea flava, tinea versicolor*
111.1 Tinea nigra — *Cladosporium infection; pityriasis nigra*
111.2 Tinea blanca — *Trichosporon (beigelii) cutaneum; white piedra, Beigel's morbus*
111.3 Black piedra — *Piedraia hortae infection*
111.8 Other specified dermatomycoses — *including acladiosis and chromotrichomycosis*
111.9 Unspecified dermatomycosis — *unknown*

112 CANDIDIASIS

Candidiasis is a yeast infection caused by *Candida* (usually *C. albicans* but also *C. tropicalis*, *C. parapsilosis*). Topical infections are quite common in the United States and are found in simple cases of diaper rash and vulvovaginal infection. However, *Candida* is an opportunistic illness and significant, systemic infection is seen among the immunosuppressed. Candidiasis involving the respiratory system is considered a clinically defining disease of AIDS. The code for HIV (AIDS) infection (042) should be sequenced first, followed by codes for manifestations of HIV infection. Thrush is considered a clinically significant form of *Candida* infection in adults, as it may be an indicator of AIDS. Thrush, an oral infection, is considered benign in children.

112.0 Candidiasis of mouth — *thrush*
112.1 Candidiasis of vulva and vagina — *vaginal yeast infection*
112.2 Candidiasis of other urogenital sites — *other than vulva and vagina*
112.3 Candidiasis of skin and nails — *intertrigo, onychia, perionyxis*
112.4 Candidiasis of lung — *pneumonia*
112.5 Disseminated candidiasis — *grave, systemic infection associated with immunosuppression*
112.81 Candidal endocarditis — *infection of lining of cavities of heart*
112.82 Candidal otitis externa — *infection of outer ear*
112.83 Candidal meningitis — *infection of lining of brain or spinal cord*
112.84 Candidiasis of the esophagus — *infection in throat*
112.85 Candidiasis of the intestine — *infection in intestines*
112.89 Other candidiasis of other specified sites — *including bronchomoniliasis*
112.9 Candidiasis of unspecified site — *unknown site*

114 COCCIDIOIDOMYCOSIS

Coccidioidomycosis is a fungal disease caused by *Coccidioidomycosis immitis* and common to the Southwestern United States. It is acquired by inhaling contaminated dust. The primary infection is an acute respiratory infection. Progressive disease may infect organs, bones, or nervous system. A disseminating form of coccidioidomycosis is considered a clinically defining disease for AIDS.

Coccidioidomycosis infection is classified by site of infection, and by its primary or progressive form.

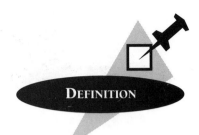

DEFINITION

Dermatomycosis: an infection of the skin, hair, or nails.

Dermatophytosis: an infection of the skin, hair, or nails.

Kerion: a large, soft lesion of the scalp due to a superficial fungal infection (dermatomycosis) of the hair follicles.

Perleche: candidiasis of the corners of the mouth.

Pityriasis: a scaly eruption on the skin.

Thrush: oral candidiasis.

Tinea: also referred to as ringworm, a fungal infection of the skin, hair, or nails.

Yeast infection: common name for vaginal or vulvovaginal infection by *Candida albicans*.

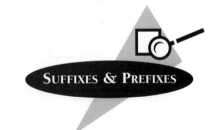

SUFFIXES & PREFIXES

-iasis: a condition or state

candida-: a type of yeast-like fungus

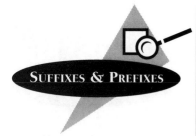

SUFFIXES & PREFIXES

extra-: without, outside of

-mycosis: a disease caused by yeast or fungus

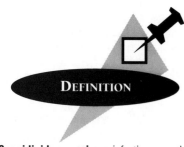

DEFINITION

Coccidioidomycosis: an infection caused by the inhalation of dust containing *Coccidioides immitis.*

Histoplasmosis: an infection caused by inhalation of fungal spores. The infection starts in the lungs and can manifest in the meninges of the brain, heart, peritoneum, and adrenals.

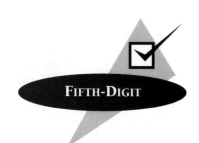

FIFTH-DIGIT

The following fifth-digit subclassification is for use with category 115:

0 without mention of manifestation

1 meningitis

2 retinitis

3 pericarditis

4 endocarditis

5 pneumonia

9 other

114.0	Primary coccidioidomycosis (pulmonary) — *acute, self-limiting lung infection*
114.1	Primary extrapulmonary coccidioidomycosis — *other acute, self-limited infection*
114.2	Coccidioidal meningitis — *infection of the lining of the brain or spinal cord*
114.3	Other forms of progressive coccidioidomycosis — *including disseminated infection*
114.4	Chronic pulmonary coccidioidomycosis — *persisting infection of lung*
114.5	Unspecified pulmonary coccidioidomycosis — *lung infection, unknown whether chronic or acute*
114.9	Unspecified coccidioidomycosis — *unknown infection, or Posada-Wernicke disease*

115 HISTOPLASMOSIS

Histoplasmosis is a fungal disease caused by *Histoplasma capsulatum* in the United States or *Histoplasma duboisii* in Africa. Pulmonary infection and lesion characterize the disease. The disseminating form of histoplasmosis is considered a clinically defining disease for AIDS.

H. capsulatum is common to the eastern and Midwestern United States. It is also called small form histoplasmosis, while the African variety is called large form.

Histoplasmosis is classified according to American (small) or African (large) and by site of infection. Histoplasmosis can present with significant symptoms, including cough, or shortness of breath. Also report any significant symptoms secondarily.

115.0	5th	Histoplasma capsulatum — *small form seen in United States*
115.1	5th	Histoplasma duboisii — *large form seen in Africa*
115.9	5th	Unspecified Histoplasmosis — *unknown form*

116 BLASTOMYCOTIC INFECTION

Blastomycosis is a fungal infection common to North American and Africa. Paracoccidioidomycosis is confined to South America. Lobomycosis is an infection by *Loboa loboi,* uncultured yeast that causes keloidal blastomycosis.

116.0	Blastomycosis — *Blastomyces (Ajellomyces) dermatitidis; Chicago disease*
116.1	Paracoccidioidomycosis — *Paracoccidioides (Blastomyces) brasiliensis; South American form*
116.2	Lobomycosis — *Loboa (Blastomyces) loboi; keloidal form*

117 OTHER MYCOSES

The fungus aspergillosis is commonly found in decaying leaves, stored grain, or bird droppings. It can cause three types of lung disease: as a colonization or aspergilloma in a healed site of previous lung disease (as in tuberculosis or lung abscess); as an invasive infection of the lung parenchyma that may spread via the blood stream to other parts of the body; or as an allergic reaction in people with asthma, cystic fibrosis, or whom are immunosuppressed. In the case of aspergillosis pneumonia, assign codes 117.3 for aspergillosis infection and 484.6 for the pneumonia. For allergic bronchopulmonary aspergillosis (ABA), report 518.6, along with an appropriate asthma code from the 493.9 series.

Mycotic mycetomas are infections by various genera and species of *Ascomycetes* and *Deuteromycetes,* such as *Acremonium (Cephalosporium) falciforme, Neotestudina rosatii, Madurella grisea, Madurella mycetomi, Pyrenochaeta romeroi,* and *Zopfii (Leptosphaeria) senagalensis.* Report actinomycotic mycetomas with codes from the 039 rubric.

5th   Needs fifth-digit   **OK**   Valid three-digit code

Cryptococcosis is an infection by *Cryptococcus neoformans*. It is a clinically defining infection of AIDS. The primary infection is respiratory and can be followed by infections in organs, bones, or the nervous system. Cryptococcosis is sometimes called European blastomycosis or torulosis, after its former name, Torula histolytica.

117.0	Rhinosporidiosis — *Rhinosporidium loboi*
117.1	Sporotrichosis — *Sporothrix (Sporotrichum) schenckii*
117.2	Chromoblastomycosis — *Cladosporium carrionii Fonsecaea compactum, Fonsecaea pedrosoi, Phialophora verrucosa*
117.3	Aspergillosis — *A. fumigatus, A. flavus, A. terreus groups*
117.4	Mycotic mycetomas — *various Ascomycetes and Deuteromycetes; Madura foot*
117.5	Cryptococcosis — *Cryptococcus neoformans; Busse-Buschke's disease*
117.6	Allescheriosis (Petriellidosis) — *Allescheria (Petriellidium) boydii*
117.7	Zygomycosis (Phycomycosis or Mucormycosis) — *various Absidia, Basidiobolus, Conidiobolus, Cunninghamella, Entomophthora, Mucor, Rhizopus, Saksenaea*
117.8	Infection by dematiacious fungi (Phaehyphomycosis) — *various fungi including Cladosporium trichoides (bantianum), Dreschlera hawaiiensis, Phialophora gougerotii, Phialophora jeanselmei*
117.9	Other and unspecified mycoses — *unknown pneumomycosis*

118 OPPORTUNISTIC MYCOSES OK

Use this code to report infection of skin, subcutaneous tissues, or organs by a wide variety of fungi generally considered to be pathogenic to compromised hosts only. Among the opportunistic mycoses would be the species of *Alternaria, Dreschlera*, and *Fusarium*. These infections are most likely to occur in patients after radiation therapy or during therapy with corticosteroids or immunosuppressants. People with AIDS, Hodgkin's lymphoma, or diabetes are susceptible to opportunistic mycoses.

120-129 Helminthiases

Helminthiases are diseases caused by worms. Worms are soft-bodied invertebrates and the infections can arise in a variety of ways, from person-to-person contact, contact with infested water, or ingestion of larvae in undercooked meat. Most helminthiasis infections occur in underdeveloped countries.

Infection by intestinal parasites is rarely life threatening, especially when the victim is in good health and proper treatment is instituted. Instead, discomfort and inconvenience are the more likely problems caused by intestinal parasites. However, helminthiasis is a significant problem in underdeveloped countries since these infections rob their hosts of essential nutrients. They often cause local irritation throughout the gastrointestinal tract. Diagnosis of intestinal parasites is usually done by analysis of stool specimens.

Worm infestations in ICD-9 are initially classified by type of worms: flukes, tapeworms, nematodes, and hookworms.

120 SCHISTOSOMIASIS (BILHARZIASIS)

Schistosomiasis, also known as bilharzia or blood fluke, is a water-borne parasitic disease carried by water snails. It is the major health risk in the rural areas of Central China and Egypt and continues to rank high in other developing countries. The main forms of

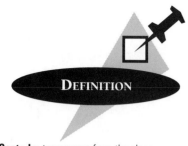

DEFINITION

Cestode: tapeworms from the class *Cestoidea*.

Echinococcosis: infection caused by larval forms of tapeworms of the genus *Echinococcus*.

Schistosomiasis: infection caused by *Schistosoma*, a genus of flukes of trematode parasites.

Trematode: a fluke from the class *Trematoda*.

schistosomiasis are caused by five species, and classification of infection is based on the species. The disease is contracted through contact with infested water.

The eggs of the schistosomes in the excreta of an infected host open on contact with water and release a parasite, the miracidium, which seeks a fresh water snail. Once it has found its snail host, the miracidium produces thousands of new parasites (cercariae). The snail excretes the cercariae into the surrounding water. They penetrate the skin, continuing the biological cycle once they have made their way to the victim's blood vessels as worms

In intestinal schistosomiasis, the worms reside in the blood vessels lining the intestine. In urinary schistosomiasis, they live in the blood vessels of the bladder. Only about a half of the eggs are excreted in the feces (intestinal schistosomiasis) or in the urine (urinary schistosomiasis). The rest remain in the host, damaging other vital organs. It is the eggs and not the worms that cause damage.

120.0	Schistosomiasis due to schistosoma haematobium — *urinary schistosomiasis; S. haematobium*
120.1	Schistosomiasis due to schistosoma mansoni — *intestinal schistosomiasis; S. mansoni*
120.2	Schistosomiasis due to schistosoma japonicum — *intestinal schistosomiasis; S. japonicum*
120.3	Cutaneous schistosomiasis — *S. dermatitis*
120.8	Other specified schistosomiasis — *S, bovis; S intercalatum; S. mattheei; S. spindale. S chestermani*
120.9	Unspecified schistosomiasis — *unknown schistosomiasis*

121 OTHER TREMATODE INFECTIONS
Trematodes other than bilharziasis are classified in this rubric. Most are very uncommon in the United States.

121.0	Opisthorchiasis — *Opisthorchis; cat liver fluke*
121.1	Clonorchiasis — *Clonorchis sinensis; oriental liver fluke*
121.2	Paragonimiasis — *Paragonimus; oriental lung fluke*
121.3	Fascioliasis — *Fasciola; sheep liver fluke*
121.4	Fasciolopsiasis — *Fasciolopsis (buski); intestinal fluke*
121.5	Metagonimiasis — *Metagonimus yokogawai*
121.6	Heterophyiasis — *Heterophyes*
121.8	Other specified trematode infections — *other trematode including Dicrocoelium dendriticum, Echinostoma ilocanum; Gastrodiscoides homines*
121.9	Unspecified trematode infection — *unknown fluke disease*

122 ECHINOCOCCOSIS
Echinococcosis is an infection by the tapeworm *Echinococcus*. Diseases are classified according to serotype: *E. granulosus* or *E. multilocularis* and by site of infection. Other tapeworm infestations are reported with codes from the 123 rubric.

122.0	Echinococcus granulosus infection of liver — *tapeworm*
122.1	Echinococcus granulosus infection of lung — *tapeworm*
122.2	Echinococcus granulosus infection of thyroid — *tapeworm*
122.3	Other echinococcus granulosus infection — *not elsewhere classified*
122.4	Unspecified echinococcus granulosus infection — *unknown site*
122.5	Echinococcus multilocularis infection of liver — *tapeworm*
122.6	Other echinococcus multilocularis infection — *not elsewhere classified*

✎5th Needs fifth-digit   **OK** Valid three-digit code

122.7	Unspecified echinococcus multilocularis infection — *unknown site*
122.8	Unspecified echinococcus of liver — *unknown type, of liver*
122.9	Other and unspecified echinococcosis — *unknown type, other than liver*

123 OTHER CESTODE INFECTION

Tapeworms other than *Echinococcus* are reported under this rubric.

123.0	Taenia solium infection, intestinal form — *adult pork tapeworm*
123.1	Cysticercosis — *larval pork tapeworm*
123.2	Taenia saginata infection — *Taenia saginata; beef tapeworm*
123.3	Taeniasis, unspecified — *unknown Taeniasis infection*
123.4	Diphyllobothriasis, intestinal — *adult fish tapeworm*
123.5	Sparganosis (larval diphyllobothriasis) — *larval fish tapeworm*
123.6	Hymenolepiasis — *rat tapeworm*
123.8	Other specified cestode infection — *dog tapeworm*
123.9	Unspecified cestode infection — *unknown*

124 TRICHINOSIS OK

Trichinosis is an infection by the roundworm, *Trichinella spiralis*, smallest of the parasitic nematodes. *Trichinella* is found in the muscle of bear and pig and, generally, infection occurs when undercooked meat is eaten. Infection is rare but not unknown in the United States. Patients may be asymptomatic or may have gastrointestinal symptoms, muscle pains, fever, and periorbital edema. Trichinosis is also known as trichinellosis and trichiniasis.

125 FILARIAL INFECTION AND DRACONTIASIS

Worms in the *Filaria* or *Dracunculus* family cause diseases in this rubric. Most are uncommon in the United States. Many of the filarial infections cause congestion in the lymphatic system that can lead to other manifestations, including elephantiasis or chyluria.

In dracontiasis, a threadlike worm up to 120 centimeters long inhabits the subcutaneous and muscle tissues of man. Dracontiasis is limited to Africa, India, and Arabia.

125.0	Bancroftian filariasis — *Wuchereria bancrofti*
125.1	Malayan filariasis — *Brugia (Wuchereria) malayi*
125.2	Loiasis — *African eyeworm; Loa loa*
125.3	Onchocerciasis — *Onchocerca volvulus*
125.4	Dipetalonemiasis — *Acanthocheilonema perstans; Caribbean, Central and South America*
125.5	Mansonella ozzardi infection — *Filariasis ozzardi*
125.6	Other specified filariasis — *Acanthocheilonema streptocerca, Dipetalonema streptocerca*
125.7	Dracontiasis — *Guinea worm; Africa, India, Asia; subcutaneous worm up to 120 cm*
125.9	Unspecified filariasis — *unknown variety*

126 ANCYLOSTOMIASIS AND NECATORIASIS

Rubric 126 classifies varieties of hookworm infection. Several infective agents, the most common being *Ancylostoma duodenale* and *Necator americanus*, can cause hookworm. Symptoms include gastrointestinal pain and anemia, though many patients are asymptomatic. *A. duodenale* is common in the Far East and the Mediterranean. *N. americanus* is more common in tropical areas. Currently, incidence of hookworm is very rare in the United States, though the incidence is thought to be as high as one in four people worldwide.

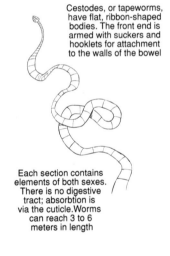

Cestodes, or tapeworms, have flat, ribbon-shaped bodies. The front end is armed with suckers and hooklets for attachment to the walls of the bowel

Each section contains elements of both sexes. There is no digestive tract; absorbtion is via the cuticle. Worms can reach 3 to 6 meters in length

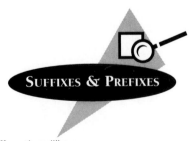

SUFFIXES & PREFIXES

filar-: threadlike

Hookworm is classified according to the infective agent. In symptomatic infection, eggs from the patient's stool can be examined to identify the type of hookworm.

126.0	Ancylostomiasis and necatoriasis due to ancylostoma duodenale — *hookworm*
126.1	Ancylostomiasis and necatoriasis due to necator americanus — *hookworm*
126.2	Ancylostomiasis and necatoriasis due to ancylostoma braziliense — *hookworm*
126.3	Ancylostomiasis and necatoriasis due to ancylostoma ceylanicum — *hookworm*
126.8	Ancylostomiasis and necatoriasis due to other specified ancylostoma — *hookworm not elsewhere classified*
126.9	Unspecified ancylostomiasis and necatoriasis — *unknown hookworm*

127 OTHER INTESTINAL HELMINTHIASIS

Ascariasis is infection by *Ascaris lumbricoides* and may cause gastrointestinal or pulmonary symptoms. It is seen worldwide.

Strongyloidiasis is threadworm infection, endemic to the tropics that may cause gastric pain, vomiting, and diarrhea.

127.0	Ascariasis — *Ascaris lumbricoides; roundworm*
127.1	Anisakiasis — *larval infection*
127.2	Strongyloidiasis — *Strongyloides stercoralis*
127.3	Trichuriasis — *Trichuris trichiura; whipworm*
127.4	Enterobiasis — *Enterobius vermicularis; pinworm or threadworm*
127.5	Capillariasis — *Capillaria philippinensis*
127.6	Trichostrongyliasis — *Trichostrongylus species*
127.7	Other specified intestinal helminthiasis — *Oesophagostomum apiostomum*
127.8	Mixed intestinal helminthiasis — *not elsewhere classified*
127.9	Unspecified intestinal helminthiasis — *unknown*

128 OTHER AND UNSPECIFIED HELMINTHIASIS

Toxocariasis is an invasion of the viscera by *Toxocara canis* or *Toxocara cati*, which normally cause diseases confined to dogs and cats. Symptoms are fever, cough, or skin rash and some patients experience recurring pneumonias. Most cases are seen in the very young or very old. Report any significant symptoms or manifestations in addition to the toxocariasis.

128.0	Toxocariasis — *visceral larva migrans syndrome*
128.1	Gnathostomiasis — *Gnathostoma spinigerum*
128.8	Other specified helminthiasis — *not elsewhere classified*
128.9	Unspecified helminth infection — *unknown*

129 INTESTINAL PARASITISM, UNSPECIFIED `OK`

Use this code only if the disease is known to be parasitic and the parasite is unknown. If the parasite is known, use the appropriate "not elsewhere classified" code from other rubrics in this section.

130-136 Other Infectious and Parasitic Diseases

The diseases in this section of ICD-9 are a mixed bag of infections or parasites. Single-cell organisms, amebae, protozoa, mites and lice, fly larvae, or parasites of unknown etiology may cause the infections. As the last subclassification for infectious and parasitic diseases in this chapter, this section provides a hodgepodge of significant diseases that are reorganized or reclassified under ICD-10. In ICD-10, toxoplasmosis is reclassified with other protozoal diseases and trichomoniasis is reclassified with other sexually transmitted diseases. All infestations are given their own subclassification. Sarcoidosis is no longer considered an infectious disease and in ICD-10 is reclassified as a disease of the immune system and moved to another chapter entirely.

130 TOXOPLASMOSIS

Toxoplasmosis is caused by a single-celled parasite, *Toxoplasma gondii*. It is found throughout the world. Millions of people in the United States are infected with the Toxoplasma parasite, but very few have symptoms because the immune system usually keeps the parasite from causing illness.

Toxoplasmosis is an opportunistic disease and a danger to the unborn and to the immunocompromised patient. Congenital toxoplasmosis is classified to the Congenital Anomalies chapter of ICD-9, with 771.2, and toxoplasmosis in pregnancy is classified to the Pregnancy and Childbirth chapter, with a code from the rubric 655.4.

Toxoplasmosis is classified according to site or system infected. If multiple sites or systems are infection, report 130.8 *Multisystem disseminated toxoplasmosis*. In the case of AIDS, the code for HIV infection (042) should be sequenced first, followed by codes for toxoplasmosis infection. Any functional disturbance (visual or mental disorder, for example) may be reported secondarily.

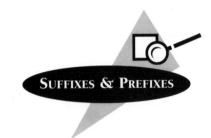

SUFFIXES & PREFIXES

-encephal-: the brain

chorio-: the choroid plexus of the eye

hepa-: the liver

mening-: the meninges of the brain

myocard-: the muscle of the heart

pneuma-: pertaining to the lung

130.0	Meningoencephalitis due to toxoplasmosis — *inflammation of brain and its lining*
130.1	Conjunctivitis due to toxoplasmosis — *inflammation of the mucous lining of the eye*
130.2	Chorioretinitis due to toxoplasmosis — *infection of the posterior lining of the eye*
130.3	Myocarditis due to toxoplasmosis — *inflammation of the lining of the heart*
130.4	Pneumonitis due to toxoplasmosis — *inflammation of the lungs*
130.5	Hepatitis due to toxoplasmosis — *inflammation of the liver*
130.7	Toxoplasmosis of other specified sites — *not elsewhere classified*
130.8	Multisystemic disseminated toxoplasmosis — *multiple organ systems; seen in the immunocompromised patient*
130.9	Unspecified toxoplasmosis — *unknown*

131 TRICHOMONIASIS

Trichomonas vaginalis is parasitic flagellated protozoa infestation that is usually sexually transmitted, although transmission by other routes, such as moist, soiled washcloths, has been documented. Most people infected with trichomoniasis are asymptomatic, and most infections are in the genitourinary system. Symptomatic infections are characterized by a white discharge from the genital tract and itching. Complications of infection can be vaginitis, urethritis, enlargement of the prostate, or epididymitis.

This rubric classifies only trichomoniasis from *T. vaginalis*. Intestinal trichomoniasis may be caused by any of several other forms of *Trichomonas*, and is reported with 007.3.

131.00	Unspecified urogenital trichomoniasis — *STD with infection of urinary or reproductive organs*
131.01	Trichomonal vulvovaginitis — *STD with infection of vulva or vagina*
131.02	Trichomonal urethritis — *STD with infection of urethra*

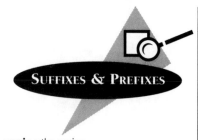

-vagin-: the vagina

prostat-: the prostate

ureth-: the urethra

vulvo-: the vulva

131.03	Trichomonal prostatitis — *STD with infection of prostate*	
131.09	Other urogenital trichomoniasis — *STD infection at genitourinary site not elsewhere classified*	
131.8	Trichomoniasis of other specified sites — *infection, not genitourinary or intestinal, site not elsewhere classified*	
131.9	Unspecified trichomoniasis — *unknown*	

132 PEDICULOSIS AND PHTHIRUS INFESTATION

This rubric classifies lice infestations. Lice suck the blood of the host and cause severe itching and loss of sleep. Louse saliva or feces irritate some sensitive hosts, increasing the chance of secondary infection from excessive scratching.

Head lice are *Pediculus capitis*, and they live mainly on the scalp and neck hairs of their human host. Head lice are mainly acquired by direct head-to-head contact with an infested person's hair, but may be transferred with shared combs, hats, and other hair accessories. Infestation is seen most often in children and in whites more frequently than other ethnic groups. Most commonly, epidemics are seen among school children. Head lice do not transmit infectious agents from person to person.

Body lice are *Pediculus humanus* and are closely related to head lice, but are less frequently encountered in the United States. Body lice feed on the body, though may be discovered on the scalp and facial hair. They usually remain on clothing near the skin and generally deposit their eggs on or near the seams of garments. Body lice are acquired mainly through direct contact with an infested person or clothing and bedding, and are most commonly found on individuals who infrequently change or wash their clothes. Body lice serve as vectors of certain human pathogens including louse-borne typhus, louse-borne relapsing fever, and trench fever.

Pubic or crab lice are *Phthirus pubis* and have a short crab-like body easily distinguished from that of head and body lice. Pubic lice are most frequently found among the pubic hairs of the infested person, but may also be found elsewhere on the body. The infestation by pubic lice is termed 'phthiriasis.' Pubic lice are acquired mainly through sexual contact or by sharing a bed with an infested person. Public lice do not transmit infectious agents from person to person.

132.0	Pediculus capitis (head louse) — *nits, head lice*	
132.1	Pediculus corporis (body louse) — *body lice; may be vector to other disease*	
132.2	Phthirus pubis (pubic louse) — *crabs; usually sexually transmitted*	
132.3	Mixed pediculosis and phthirus infestation — *infestation of more than one category above*	
132.9	Unspecified pediculosis — *unknown infestation by lice*	

133 ACARIASIS

Acariasis is a mite infestation. Acarid infestation is classified according to the type of mite. Scabies is caused by *Sarcoptes scabiei*; all other known mites would be classified to 133.8, and unknown infestation would be classified to 133.9.

Scabies causes intense itching and sometimes, secondary infection. Report any significant secondary manifestations.

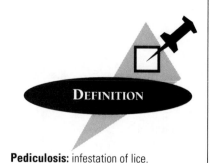

DEFINITION

Pediculosis: infestation of lice.

133.0   Scabies — *Sarcoptes scabiei*
133.8   Other acariasis — *chiggers and other mites, not elsewhere classified*
133.9   Unspecified acariasis — *unknown mite*

134 OTHER INFESTATION

Myiasis is an infestation by fly larvae (maggots), and is most commonly seen in wound or ulcer sites. Myiasis is usually cutaneous, but is also found in nasal mucosa or in the intestines. Hirudiniasis is an infestation of mucous membranes or skin by leeches. While clinical myiasis and hirudiniasis are occasionally pursued as therapeutic interventions, these codes refer to nonclinical infestations.

134.0   Myiasis — *Dermatobia (hominis); maggot infestation*
134.1   Other arthropod infestation — *sand fleas or other infestations not elsewhere classified*
134.2   Hirudiniasis — *leech infestation*
134.8   Other specified infestations — *not elsewhere classified*
134.9   Unspecified infestation — *unknown*

135 SARCOIDOSIS OK

Sarcoidosis is a disease of unknown etiology that has many presentations. It can have an acute onset and rapid resolution, or it can come upon the patient slowly, and become an increasingly debilitating chronic condition. Also called sarcoid, the disorder is characterized by epithelioid tubercles in organs and tissues.

Incidence of sarcoid in the United States exceeds that of tuberculosis. Common symptoms include hilar adenopathy, shortness of breath, weight loss, arthralgia, night sweats, and erythema nodosum. The symptoms will vary according to the organs that are affected by sarcoidosis, though nearly all cases show decreased pulmonary function and mediastinal (hilar) adenopathy. Patients with chronic infection frequently have skin lesions. Tissue biopsy is the best method of diagnosing sarcoidosis.

Manifestations of sarcoidosis are reported in addition to the infection. These may include cardiac involvement (425.8), pulmonary involvement (517.8), joint involvement (713.7), or erythema nodosum (695.2). Multiple codes may be required to complete the clinical picture. Report 135 *Sarcoidosis* first, and the manifestations or symptoms of the infection in descending order of severity.

136 OTHER AND UNSPECIFIED INFECTIOUS AND PARASITIC DISEASES

Most of the diseases in this category are "other," not "unspecified." They are listed here by default. There may be no room remaining in the rubric to which they would normally be classified.

Ainhum is an African disease, seen primarily in black males and causing stricture at a distal joint of a digit on the foot or hand. The stricture is progressive, leading to spontaneous amputation. Another name for the disease is dactylolysis spontanea.

Behcet's syndrome is a disease of unknown etiology causing inflammation and lesions of the mucous membrane, joints, and gastrointestinal and nervous systems. It is most common in men in their third decade in Japan and Mediterranean countries.

Free-living amoeba, *Naegleria*, can cause a grave form of meningoencephalitis. The infection is acquired by swimming in infected lakes.

Pneumocystosis is an infection of *Pneumocystis carinii fungus*, causing pneumonia in immunocompromised patients. It is the leading cause of death among AIDS patients. Patients with intact immune systems are not affected by pneumocystosis.

Psorospermosis is an infection by *P. haeckeli*, water-borne microscopic organism. Sarcosporidiosis is an infection by *Sarcocystis* causing muscle cysts and intestinal inflammation.

If the source of infection is found no where else in ICD-9 and a thorough search of the index does not give better direction, report 136.8 for candiru infestation, microsporidiosis, or an infectious disease not yet classified to ICD-9. If the source of infection remains undiagnosed, report 136.9.

136.0	Ainhum — *African; stricture causes loss of digit*	
136.1	Behcet's syndrome — *unknown etiology; inflammation and lesions*	
136.2	Specific infections by free-living amebae — *ameba causing meningoencephalitis*	
136.3	Pneumocystosis — *Pneumocystis carinii; fungus infection seen in the immunocompromised patient*	
136.4	Psorospermiasis — *Psorospermic infection*	
136.5	Sarcosporidiosis — *Sarcocystis infection; muscle cysts*	
136.8	Other specified infectious and parasitic diseases — *not elsewhere classified, includes candiru infestation, microsporidiosis*	
136.9	Unspecified infectious and parasitic diseases — *unknown*	

137-139 Late Effects of Infectious and Parasitic Diseases

A late effect is a residual effect of a condition that is no longer acute or an illness that has resolved. There is no time frame associated with a late effect; it can be reported at any time after the condition has resolved. Two codes are required to report late effects: one code for residual condition and the second code for the cause of the late effect. Never report the acute condition that caused the late effect with a late effect code.

137 LATE EFFECTS OF TUBERCULOSIS

This category is used to indicate conditions classifiable to 010-018 as the cause of the late effects, which are classified elsewhere. The conditions are reported first, with the late effect code being reported secondarily. Late effects include sequelae, or complications due to old or inactive TB. When using late effect codes from this category, there should be no evidence of active disease.

137.0	Late effects of respiratory or unspecified tuberculosis — *sequelae*
137.1	Late effects of central nervous system tuberculosis — *sequelae*
137.2	Late effects of genitourinary tuberculosis — *sequelae*
137.3	Late effects of tuberculosis of bones and joints — *sequelae*
137.4	Late effects of tuberculosis of other specified organs — *sequelae*

138 LATE EFFECTS OF ACUTE POLIOMYELITIS **OK**

This category is used to indicate conditions classifiable to 045 as the cause of the late effects, which are classified elsewhere. The conditions are reported first, with the late effect code being reported secondarily. Late effects include sequelae, or complications due to old or inactive polio. When using late effect codes from this category, there should be no evidence of active disease.

139 LATE EFFECTS OF OTHER INFECTIOUS AND PARASITIC DISEASES

This category is to be used to indicate conditions classifiable to 001-009, 020-041, or 046-136 as the cause of the late effects, which are classified elsewhere. The conditions are reported first, with the late effect code being reported secondarily. Late effects include sequelae, or complications due to old or inactive infection. When using late effects codes from this category, there should be no evidence of active infection.

139.0	Late effects of viral encephalitis — *sequelae*
139.1	Late effects of trachoma — *sequelae*
139.8	Late effects of other and unspecified infectious and parasitic diseases — *sequelae*

Chapter 2

140-239
Neoplasms

Neoplasms in ICD-9 are classified as malignant, carcinoma in situ, uncertain, unknown, or benign. In most cases, anatomic location of the neoplasm is specified in code selection.

In malignancy, the neoplasm invades surrounding tissue or sheds cells that seed malignancies in other body sites. Malignant neoplasms are therefore classified as primary, for the original site, or secondary, a seeded site. Classifications within malignant neoplasms also specify certain malignancies as leukemias, Kaposi's sarcoma, melanoma, lymphomas and carcinoma in situ. Interestingly, in ICD-10-CM, in situ cancers are divided into two categories: carcinoma in situ and melanoma in situ.

A benign neoplasm may grow, but does not invade, and so remains a circumscribed lesion. Uncertain behavior is undetermined and unspecified behavior is unknown.

Because of the nature of malignancy, this chapter classifies anatomy differently than other chapters of ICD-9. In this chapter, malignancies are often classified according to contiguous anatomic site rather than by distinct organ system. Therefore, body parts that in other chapters may be classified separately are grouped together here. For example, soft tissue malignancies, whether blood vessels, tendons, or nerves, are classified under a single rubric for connective and soft tissue.

All neoplasms are classified to this chapter, whether or not they are functionally active. A functionally active neoplasm is a growth that performs functions ascribed to surrounding tissue, as in a thyroid tumor that secretes thyroxine and causes hyperthyroidism in the patient. An additional code from Chapter 3 may be reported to identify functional activity associated with any neoplasm, for example, catecholamine-producing malignant pheochromocytoma of adrenal, 194.0 for neoplasm and 255.6 for adrenal hypofunction; basophil adenoma of pituitary with Cushing's syndrome, 227.3 for neoplasm and 255.0 for Cushing's syndrome.

The index of ICD-9 provides a complex and complete table of neoplasms for easy code lookup. The index is organized alphabetically by anatomy. Find the anatomical site, and the table will identify the codes for primary, secondary, and carcinoma in situ, as well as the codes for benign, uncertain, and unspecified behaviors. After looking up the anatomical site and finding the appropriate code, refer to the tabular section of ICD-9 to see appropriate includes and excludes notes and instructions for use of that code. Kaposi's sarcoma is excluded from the index and can be found in the alphabetized index under Kaposi's.

Morphology of Neoplasms

The World Health Organization has published an adaptation of the International Classification of Diseases for oncology (ICD-O). It contains a coded nomenclature for the morphology of neoplasms, which is reproduced here for those who wish to use it in conjunction with Chapter 2 of the International Classification of Diseases, 9th Revision, Clinical Modification.

The morphology code numbers consist of five digits; the first four identify the histological type of the neoplasm and the fifth indicates its behavior. The one-digit behavior code is as follows:

/0 Benign

/1 Uncertain whether benign or malignant
   Borderline malignancy

/2 Carcinoma in situ
   Intraepithelial
   Noninfiltrating
   Noninvasive

/3 Malignant, primary site

/6 Malignant, metastatic site
   Secondary site

/9 Malignant, uncertain whether primary or metastatic site

In the nomenclature below, the morphology code numbers include the behavior code appropriate to the histological type of neoplasm, but this behavior code should be changed if other reported information makes this necessary. For example, "chordoma (M9370/3)" is assumed to be malignant; the term "benign chordoma" should be coded M9370/0. Similarly, "superficial spreading adenocarcinoma (M8143/3)" described as "noninvasive" should be coded M8143/2 and "melanoma (M8720/3)" described as "secondary" should be coded M8720/6.

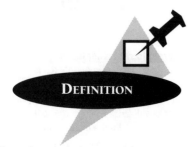

Commissure: the juncture of the upper and lower lip.

Vermilion border: the exposed, pigmented, fleshy margin of the lip.

ICD-Oncology Classification

The ICD-Oncology identifying the morphology of neoplasms is provided in the margins of this chapter for easy access. These are published by the World Health Organization (WHO) and consist of five digits. The first four identify the histological type of neoplasm and the fifth digit indicates its behavior as benign (/0); uncertain (/1); carcinoma in situ (/2); malignant, primary (/3); malignant, secondary (/6); or malignant uncertain (/9). These M codes are listed in the right-hand margins of Chapter 2 for quick reference, and are used in reporting malignancies to the national cancer registry. In many cases, the index to ICD-9 can help in M code selections, which are based on morphology and histology rather than anatomic site.

PERSONAL HISTORY OF MALIGNANT NEOPLASM

Codes from the V10 rubric describe personal history of malignant neoplasm, but these codes should never be assigned to patients who have active or recurring disease or are still receiving treatment for their malignancy, except when that disease is secondary. When a previously excised malignant neoplasm recurs at the same site, it is still considered a primary malignancy of that site. If the malignant neoplasm recurs at a different site, it is reported as a secondary malignant neoplasm and an additional code to identify a history of the malignancy of the primary site is reported from the V10 rubric.

Furthermore, when assigning a personal history code, the site should reflect the site of the primary malignant neoplasm, not a metastatic site. Rubric V10 reports only the primary malignancy. There is no method for reporting a history of malignancy in a secondary site.

SEQUENCING ISSUES

The main rule for sequencing malignancies and their manifestations is to sequence first the reason for the encounter.

In cases of a metastasized malignancy, if a secondary malignancy causes a functional problem, sequence the codes as follows: (1) the functional problem; (2) the secondary malignant neoplasm causing the problem; and (3) the site of the original, metastasized neoplasm (primary site). For example, if a patient with prostate cancer comes to the physician with acute abdominal pain and is found to have a blocked bowel, the result of a secondary malignancy in the ileum, the following codes would be reported in this sequence:

560.89	Other intestinal obstruction without mention of hernia
197.4	Secondary malignant neoplasm of small intestine, including duodenum
185	Malignant neoplasm of the prostate

If the patient is being treated for a condition unrelated to the neoplasm, report the reason for treatment first, followed by the neoplasm, if it could affect the course of care. For example, if a patient with breast cancer fractures her hip, the fracture would be sequenced first, followed by the code for the cancer. However, if the patient's breast neoplasm is known to be benign, only the hip fracture would be reported, since the neoplasm would not affect care, unless the benign neoplasm were discovered in the course of care for the hip fracture. In that case, it would be reported as a secondary diagnosis.

If a patient is seen solely for chemotherapy or radiotherapy, either on an inpatient or outpatient basis, V58.1 *Encounter or admission for chemotherapy* or V58.0 *Encounter or*

5th   Needs fifth-digit   **OK**   Valid three-digit code

admission for radiotherapy should be sequenced first, and the code for the malignancy reported secondarily. If the patient receives other care related to the malignancy at the time of the therapy, the therapy would not be sequenced first, but secondary to the malignant neoplasm code.

Codes from the signs and symptoms chapter of ICD-9 should never be sequenced first when reporting malignancies. If manifestations cannot be specified with other codes, report the malignancy first, followed by any appropriate signs or symptoms.

140-149 Malignant Neoplasm of Lip, Oral Cavity, and Pharynx

This section of ICD-9 classifies malignancies of the mouth and throat. The pharynx (throat) is a tube that begins at the internal nares, behind the nasal cavity, and ends at the larynx. While malignant neoplasms of the pharynx are classified in this subsection of ICD -9, malignant neoplasms of the larynx are found in the respiratory section, under rubric 161.

140 MALIGNANT NEOPLASM OF LIP

The lips, or labia, are highly mobile structures that surround the mouth opening. They contain skeletal muscles; primary is orbicularis oris, the sphincter muscle that encircles the mouth and lies between the outer skin (integument) and the mucous membranes of the lips. The labial glands, which are similar to salivary glands, lie between the muscle and mucous membrane tissues. The lips also have many sensory nerves, and abundant capillary vessels that produce the normal reddish color. The external margin of the lips, the vermilion border, marks the boundary between the skin of the face and the mucous membrane that lines the alimentary canal of the digestive system.

Anatomically, the lips are divided into two distinct segments. The vermilion border is the pigmented, fleshy, outer lip, and may be described in the medical record as the lipstick area or external lip. The interior aspect is the second segment. Lined in buccal mucosa, the interior aspect may be described as the mucosa, buccal aspect, or frenulum. The commissure of the lip is the juncture of the upper and lower lips, whether at the vermilion border or interior aspect. Malignant neoplasms of the lip are classified according to upper, lower, or commissure of lip; and whether it is vermilion border or buccal aspect. For overlapping sites, report 140.8 *Other sites of lip*.

140.0	Malignant neoplasm of upper lip, vermilion border — *pigmented, fleshy margin up upper lip*
140.1	Malignant neoplasm of lower lip, vermilion border — *pigmented, fleshy margin of lower lip*
140.3	Malignant neoplasm of upper lip, inner aspect — *mucous membrane lined, inner margin, upper lip*
140.4	Malignant neoplasm of lower lip, inner aspect — *mucous membrane lined, inner margin, lower lip*
140.5	Malignant neoplasm of lip, inner aspect, unspecified as to upper or lower — *mucous membrane lined inner margin, unknown lip*
140.6	Malignant neoplasm of commissure of lip — *juncture of upper and lower lip*
140.8	Malignant neoplasm of other sites of lip — *contiguous or overlapping sites*
140.9	Malignant neoplasm of lip, vermilion border, unspecified as to upper or lower — *pigmented, fleshy margin, unknown lip*

The following table shows the correspondence between the morphology code and the different sections of Chapter 2:

Morphology Code	ICD-9-CM Chapter 2	Histology/ Behavior
Any	0 210-229	Benign neoplasms
M8000-M8004	1 239	Neoplasms of unspecified nature
M8010+	1 235-238	Neoplasms of uncertain behavior
Any	2 230-234	Carcinoma in situ
Any	3 140-195 200-208	Malignant neoplasms, stated or presumed to be primary
Any	6 196-198	Malignant neoplasms, stated or presumed to be secondary

The ICD-O behavior digit /9 is inapplicable in an ICD context, since all malignant neoplasms are presumed to be primary (/3) or secondary (/6) according to other information on the medical record.

Only the first-listed term of the full ICD-O morphology nomenclature appears against each code number in the list below. The ICD-9-CM Alphabetical Index (Volume 2), however, includes all the ICD-O synonyms as well as a number of other morphological names still likely to be encountered on medical records but omitted from ICD-O as outdated or otherwise undesirable.

A coding difficulty sometimes arises where a morphological diagnosis contains two qualifying adjectives that have different code numbers. An example is "transitional cell epidermoid carcinoma." "Transitional cell carcinoma NOS" is M8120/3 and "epidermoid carcinoma

141 MALIGNANT NEOPLASM OF TONGUE

The tongue is a strong muscle that is attached to the floor of the mouth within the curve of the jawbone. It is anchored to muscles at the rear of the mouth, which attach to the base of the skull and to the hyoid bone. The underside of the tongue is attached to the floor of the mouth by membranes. These form a distinct vertical fold in the centerline, called the frenulum linguae. The tongue contains mucous, serous, and lymph glands. The lymph glands at the back of the tongue form the lingual tonsils.

The surface of the tongue is covered with the lingual membrane, a specialized tissue with a variety of papillae protruding from it. These papillae nodules produce the characteristic rough surface of the tongue. Between the papillae are the taste buds, the sensory nerve organs that provide the sensations of flavor. The muscle fibers of the tongue are also heavily supplied with nerves, to provide for manipulation and safe placement of food in the mouth and between the teeth for chewing. The tongue also aids in swallowing and in the formation of sounds of speech.

Malignant neoplasms of the tongue are classified according to site. If multiple or contiguous sites on the tongue are involved, report 141.8 *Other sites of tongue*. For secondary malignant neoplasm of tongue, report 198.89 and for carcinoma in situ, report 239.0.

141.0	Malignant neoplasm of base of tongue — *fixed, dorsal base*
141.1	Malignant neoplasm of dorsal surface of tongue — *dorsal surface, anterior two-thirds*
141.2	Malignant neoplasm of tip and lateral border of tongue — *tip and front edge*
141.3	Malignant neoplasm of ventral surface of tongue — *anterior two-thirds; frenulum linguae*
141.4	Malignant neoplasm of anterior two-thirds of tongue, part unspecified — *mobile part of tongue NOS*
141.5	Malignant neoplasm of junctional zone of tongue — *border of tongue at junction*
141.6	Malignant neoplasm of lingual tonsil — *lymphoid tissue of tongue*
141.8	Malignant neoplasm of other sites of tongue — *contiguous or overlapping sites*
141.9	Malignant neoplasm of tongue, unspecified site — *unknown*

142 MALIGNANT NEOPLASM OF MAJOR SALIVARY GLANDS

These codes report malignant neoplasms of major salivary glands, but not of surrounding tissues. Salivary glands secrete saliva to aid in mastication and to keep the mouth moist. The major salivary glands are the parotid, sublingual, and submandibular glands.

The parotid is the most common site of salivary gland tumor, and mucoepidermoid carcinoma is the most common type of parotid cancer.

Symptoms of parotid tumor include pain, enlargement of nodule, and sometimes facial nerve paralysis or lymphadenopathy.

Some types of salivary gland tumors classified as malignant are the following carcinomas: mucoepidermoid; adenoid cystic; epithelial-myoepithelial; primary squamous cell; biphasic malignancy; ex-pleomorphic adenoma; malignant onocytoma; clear cell; or acinic cell.

Do not use these codes to report cancers in minor salivary glands. The minor salivary glands are distributed in the lips, palate, uvula, tongue, peritonsillar area, and cheek. Report

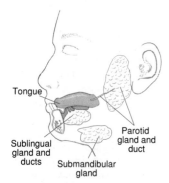

Tongue

Sublingual gland and ducts

Submandibular gland

Parotid gland and duct

The parotid gland is a common site for malignant lesions. Occurrence is several times the frequency of other major salivary glands

↳5th Needs fifth-digit   **OK** Valid three-digit code

malignant neoplasms of minor salivary glands with codes specific to the anatomical site in which they are located.

142.0 Malignant neoplasm of parotid gland — *salivary gland in cheek, in front of ear*

142.1 Malignant neoplasm of submandibular gland — *salivary gland at base of mandible*

142.2 Malignant neoplasm of sublingual gland — *salivary gland at base of tongue*

142.8 Malignant neoplasm of other major salivary glands — *contiguous or overlapping sites*

142.9 Malignant neoplasm of salivary gland, unspecified — *unknown*

143 MALIGNANT NEOPLASM OF GUM

More than 95 percent of cancers of the oral cavity are squamous cell carcinomas, found most commonly in males, aged 50-70, with a history of tobacco and alcohol use. For malignant neoplasms of contiguous or overlapping sites of the gum, report 143.8 *Other sites of gum.*

143.0 Malignant neoplasm of upper gum — *gingiva, alveolar mucosa, interdental papillae*

143.1 Malignant neoplasm of lower gum — *gingiva, alveolar mucosa, interdental papillae*

143.8 Malignant neoplasm of other sites of gum — *contiguous or overlapping upper and lower sites*

143.9 Malignant neoplasm of gum, unspecified site — *unknown*

144 MALIGNANT NEOPLASM OF FLOOR OF MOUTH

More than 95 percent of cancers of the oral cavity are squamous cell carcinomas, found most commonly in males, aged 50-70, with a history of tobacco and alcohol use. Cancers of the floor of the mouth have a higher incidence of lymph node involvement than do cancers of the lip, palate, or buccal mucosa, which explains their classification separately in ICD-9 from other parts of the inside of the mouth.

For malignant neoplasms of contiguous or overlapping sites of the parts of mouth, report 144.8 *Other specified parts of mouth.*

144.0 Malignant neoplasm of anterior portion of floor of mouth — *anterior to premolar-canine juncture*

144.1 Malignant neoplasm of lateral portion of floor of mouth — *on the side*

144.8 Malignant neoplasm of other sites of floor of mouth — *overlapping site*

144.9 Malignant neoplasm of floor of mouth, part unspecified — *unknown*

145 MALIGNANT NEOPLASM OF OTHER AND UNSPECIFIED PARTS OF MOUTH

More than 95 percent of cancers of the oral cavity are squamous cell carcinomas, found most commonly in males, aged 50-70, with a history of tobacco and alcohol use.

The vestibule of the mouth is the part of the oral cavity inside the cheeks and lips and outside the dentoalveolar structures (the teeth and gums). It includes the mucosal and submucosal tissue of the lips and cheeks, and the labial and buccal frenulum, or frenum, the connecting folds of membrane that support and restrain the lips and cheeks. Secretions from the salivary glands lubricate the vestibule.

Do not use this rubric for reporting the floor of the mouth (144), lips (140), or nasopharyngeal surface of soft palate (147).

NOS" is M8070/3. In such circumstances, the higher number (M8120/3 in this example) should be used, as it is usually more specific.

Coded Nomenclature for Morphology of Neoplasms

M800 Neoplasms NOS

M8000/0 Neoplasm, benign

M8000/1 Neoplasm, uncertain whether benign or malignant

M8000/3 Neoplasm, malignant

M8000/6 Neoplasm, metastatic

M8000/9 Neoplasm, malignant, uncertain whether primary or metastatic

M8001/0 Tumor cells, benign

M8001/1 Tumor cells, uncertain whether benign or malignant

M8001/3 Tumor cells, malignant

M8002/3 Malignant tumor, small cell type

M8003/3 Malignant tumor, giant cell type

M8004/3 Malignant tumor, fusiform cell type

M801-M804 Epithelial neoplasms NOS

M8010/0 Epithelial tumor, benign

M8010/2 Carcinoma in situ NOS

M8010/3 Carcinoma NOS

M8010/6 Carcinoma, metastatic NOS

M8010/9 Carcinomatosis

M8011/0 Epithelioma, benign

M8011/3 Epithelioma, malignant

M8012/3 Large cell carcinoma NOS

M8020/3 Carcinoma, undifferentiated type NOS

M8021/3 Carcinoma, anaplastic type NOS

M8022/3 Pleomorphic carcinoma

M8030/3 Giant cell and spindle cell carcinoma

M8031/3 Giant cell carcinoma

M8032/3 Spindle cell carcinoma

M8033/3 Pseudosarcomatous carcinoma

M8034/3 Polygonal cell carcinoma

M8035/3 Spheroidal cell carcinoma

M8040/1 Tumorlet

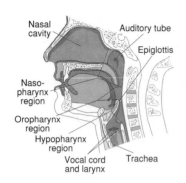

Nasal cavity
Auditory tube
Epiglottis
Naso-pharynx region
Oropharynx region
Hypopharynx region
Vocal cord and larynx
Trachea

145.0	Malignant neoplasm of cheek mucosa — *buccal mucosa, inner aspect cheek*
145.1	Malignant neoplasm of vestibule of mouth — *buccal sulcus; labial sulcus*
145.2	Malignant neoplasm of hard palate — *anterior, rigid*
145.3	Malignant neoplasm of soft palate — *posterior, soft*
145.4	Malignant neoplasm of uvula
145.5	Malignant neoplasm of palate, unspecified
145.6	Malignant neoplasm of retromolar area
145.8	Malignant neoplasm of other specified parts of mouth — *overlapping sites*
145.9	Malignant neoplasm of mouth, unspecified site — *unknown*

146 MALIGNANT NEOPLASM OF OROPHARYNX

The part of the pharynx that lies posterior to the oral cavity is called the oropharynx. It extends from its upper part at the soft palate down to its lower part that ends at the level of the hyoid bone. The lingual and palatine tonsils are located in the oropharynx. Most oropharyngeal tumors are squamous carcinomas, many with deep infiltrations.

Take care to determine the type of oropharyngeal tissue in which the tumor lies. Some tumors of the parapharyngeal space are actually major salivary gland tumors, or carotid body tumors, and should be reported as such. Minor salivary tumors at this site, however, are reported with codes in this rubric.

Oropharyngeal tumors drain bilaterally to lymph nodes, and the incidence of nodal involvement in oropharyngeal malignancy is 70 percent.

146.0	Malignant neoplasm of tonsil — *faucial, palatine*
146.1	Malignant neoplasm of tonsillar fossa — *sinus tonsillaris*
146.2	Malignant neoplasm of tonsillar pillars (anterior) (posterior) — *faucial pillar, palatoglossal arch*
146.3	Malignant neoplasm of vallecula — *Anterior and medial surface of pharyngoepiglottic fold*
146.4	Malignant neoplasm of anterior aspect of epiglottis — *glossoepiglottic fold, epiglottis*
146.5	Malignant neoplasm of junctional region of oropharynx — *junction of free margin of epiglottis, aryepiglottic fold, and pharyngoepiglottic fold*
146.6	Malignant neoplasm of lateral wall of oropharynx — *on the side of the throat*
146.7	Malignant neoplasm of posterior wall of oropharynx — *on the back of the throat*
146.8	Malignant neoplasm of other specified sites of oropharynx — *contiguous or overlapping sites; brachial cleft*
146.9	Malignant neoplasm of oropharynx, unspecified site — *unknown*

147 MALIGNANT NEOPLASM OF NASOPHARYNX

The part of the pharynx that lies behind (posterior) the nasal cavity is called the nasopharynx. The nasopharynx extends from behind the nasal cavity to the soft palate. There are two openings from the nasopharynx to the nose (internal nares) and two openings to the ears (Eustachian tubes). The adenoids (pharyngeal tonsil) are located on the posterior wall of the nasopharynx. The most common tumor of the nasopharynx is squamous cell carcinoma. Lymph node metastases occur in 80 percent of patients with nasopharyngeal cancer.

147.0	Malignant neoplasm of superior wall of nasopharynx — *roof of nasopharynx*
147.1	Malignant neoplasm of posterior wall of nasopharynx — *adenoid; pharyngeal tonsil*

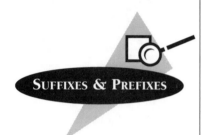

SUFFIXES & PREFIXES

hypo-: below, less than, under

naso-: pertaining to the nose

oro-: pertaining to the mouth

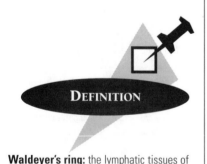

DEFINITION

Waldeyer's ring: the lymphatic tissues of the lingual, pharyngeal, and palatine tonsils.

✔5th   Needs fifth-digit   **OK**   Valid three-digit code

147.2	Malignant neoplasm of lateral wall of nasopharynx — *pharyngeal recess; fossa of Rosenmüller; opening of auditory tube*
147.3	Malignant neoplasm of anterior wall of nasopharynx — *floor of nasopharynx; posterior margin of nasal septum; nasopharyngeal surface of soft palate*
147.8	Malignant neoplasm of other specified sites of nasopharynx — *contiguous or overlapping sites*
147.9	Malignant neoplasm of nasopharynx, unspecified site — *unknown*

148 MALIGNANT NEOPLASM OF HYPOPHARYNX

The lowest part of the pharynx is called the laryngopharynx or hypopharynx. It extends from the hyoid bone and ends at a point where it breaks into two parts, the esophagus and larynx, by blending in with them. More than 95 percent of hypopharyngeal cancers are squamous carcinoma, and the most common site is the periform sinus, which occur on either side of the larynx. These account for 60 percent of hypopharyngeal cancers. Lymphatic involvement is seen in about 70 percent of hypopharyngeal malignancy.

148.0	Malignant neoplasm of postcricoid region of hypopharynx
148.1	Malignant neoplasm of pyriform sinus — *pyriform fossa*
148.2	Malignant neoplasm of aryepiglottic fold, hypopharyngeal aspect
148.3	Malignant neoplasm of posterior hypopharyngeal wall — *aryepiglottic fold NOS; interarytenoid fold NOS*
148.8	Malignant neoplasm of other specified sites of hypopharynx — *overlapping sites*
148.9	Malignant neoplasm of hypopharynx, unspecified site — *unknown*

149 MALIGNANT NEOPLASM OF OTHER AND ILL-DEFINED SITES WITHIN THE LIP, ORAL CAVITY AND PHARYNX

This rubric captures malignant neoplasms in the pharynx and oral cavity that have less specific anatomic boundaries. Waldeyer's ring includes the lymphatic tissues of the lingual, pharyngeal, and palatine tonsils. Report 149.8 if the malignancy is not limited to one of the specific structures, but has invaded contiguous or overlapping structures.

149.0	Malignant neoplasm of pharynx, unspecified — *unknown part*
149.1	Malignant neoplasm of Waldeyer's ring — *lymphatic tissues of the lingual, pharyngeal, and palatine tonsils*
149.8	Malignant neoplasm of other sites within the lip and oral cavity — *point of origin cannot be assigned to any one of the categories 140-148*
149.9	Malignant neoplasm of ill-defined sites of lip and oral cavity — *unknown*

150-159 Malignant Neoplasm of Digestive Organs and Peritoneum

This subsection of ICD-9 classifies malignancies of the body parts that carry food through the digestive system where nutrients are absorbed, to the anus where the waste is excreted. These body parts include the esophagus, stomach, intestines, and anus.

Structures that support the digestive process from outside this continuous tube are also included in this system: gall bladder, pancreas, and liver. These organs provide secretions that are critical to food absorption and use by the body.

The digestive system is a group of organs that breaks down and changes food chemically for absorption as simple, soluble substances by blood, lymph systems, and body tissues. The digestive system begins in the mouth, continues in the pharynx and esophagus, the stomach, the small and large intestines, the rectum, and the anus.

M8041/3	Small cell carcinoma NOS
M8042/3	Oat cell carcinoma
M8043/3	Small cell carcinoma, fusiform cell type

M805-M808 Papillary and squamous cell neoplasms

M8050/0	Papilloma NOS (except Papilloma of urinary bladder M8120/1)
M8050/2	Papillary carcinoma in situ
M8050/3	Papillary carcinoma NOS
M8051/0	Verrucous papilloma
M8051/3	Verrucous carcinoma NOS
M8052/0	Squamous cell papilloma
M8052/3	Papillary squamous cell carcinoma
M8053/0	Inverted papilloma
M8060/0	Papillomatosis NOS
M8070/2	Squamous cell carcinoma in situ NOS
M8070/3	Squamous cell carcinoma NOS
M8070/6	Squamous cell carcinoma, metastatic NOS
M8071/3	Squamous cell carcinoma, keratinizing type NOS
M8072/3	Squamous cell carcinoma, large cell, nonkeratinizing type
M8073/3	Squamous cell carcinoma, small cell, nonkeratinizing type
M8074/3	Squamous cell carcinoma, spindle cell type
M8075/3	Adenoid squamous cell carcinoma
M8076/2	Squamous cell carcinoma in situ with questionable stromal invasion
M8076/3	Squamous cell carcinoma, microinvasive
M8080/2	Queyrat's erythroplasia
M8081/2	Bowen's disease
M8082/3	Lymphoepithelial carcinoma

M809-M811 Basal cell neoplasms

M8090/1	Basal cell tumor
M8090/3	Basal cell carcinoma NOS
M8091/3	Multicentric basal cell carcinoma
M8092/3	Basal cell carcinoma, morphea type

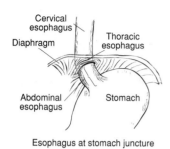

Cervical esophagus
Diaphragm
Thoracic esophagus
Abdominal esophagus
Stomach

Esophagus at stomach juncture

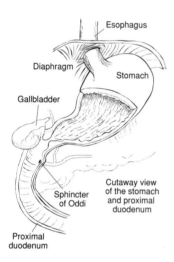

Esophagus
Diaphragm
Stomach
Gallbladder
Sphincter of Oddi
Cutaway view of the stomach and proximal duodenum
Proximal duodenum

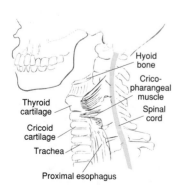

Hyoid bone
Crico-pharangeal muscle
Thyroid cartilage
Spinal cord
Cricoid cartilage
Trachea
Proximal esophagus

Digestion involves mechanical and chemical processes. Mechanical actions include chewing in the mouth, churning action in the stomach, and intestinal peristaltic action. These mechanical forces move the food through the digestive tract and mix it with secretions containing enzymes which accomplish three chemical reactions: the conversion of carbohydrates to simple sugars, the breakdown of proteins into amino acids, and the conversion of fats into fatty acids and glycerol.

The stomach churns and mixes the food with hydrochloric acid and enzymes and gradually releases materials into the upper small intestine (the duodenum) through the pyloric sphincter.

The majority of the digestive process occurs in the small intestine where most foods are hydrolysed and absorbed. The products of digestion are actively or passively transported through the wall of the small intestine and assimilated into the body. The stomach and the large intestine (colon) can also absorb water, alcohol, certain salts and crystalloids, and some drugs. Water-soluble digestive products (minerals, amino acids, and carbohydrates) are transferred into the blood system and transported to the liver. Many fats, resynthesized in the intestinal wall, are picked up by the lymphatic system and enter the blood stream through the vena caval system, bypassing the liver.

Remaining undigested matter is passed into the large intestine (the colon) where water is extracted. This solid mass (the stool) is propelled into the rectum, where it is held until excreted through the anus.

150 MALIGNANT NEOPLASM OF ESOPHAGUS

The esophagus is the alimentary canal connecting the pharynx to the stomach. Symptoms of carcinoma of the esophagus include difficulty swallowing, weight loss, coughing, and pain. Hoarseness is often seen.

Carcinoma of the esophagus is more common among men and has been linked in the United States to heavy use of alcohol and tobacco. A majority of these cancers are squamous cell or adenocarcinoma. Anatomically, 20 percent occur in the upper third of the esophagus; 30 percent in the mid-esophagus; and 50 percent in the lower esophagus.

Adenocarcinoma is more common in the lower esophagus, while squamous cell carcinoma is common in the mid to the upper esophagus.

Cancers in this rubric are classified by site, with one exception. According to ICD-9 exclusion notes, if squamous cell carcinoma is present at the distal end of the esophagus (the cardia), report 150.5 *Malignant neoplasm of lower third of esophagus*. However, if adenocarcinoma is present in the distal end of the esophagus (the cardia), report 151.0 *Malignant neoplasm of cardia*.

If the malignancy is of contiguous and overlapping sites, report 150.8 *Malignant neoplasm of other specified part of esophagus*.

150.0	Malignant neoplasm of cervical esophagus — *above the diaphragm*
150.1	Malignant neoplasm of thoracic esophagus — *within the diaphragm*
150.2	Malignant neoplasm of abdominal esophagus — *below the diaphragm*
150.3	Malignant neoplasm of upper third of esophagus — *proximal third*
150.4	Malignant neoplasm of middle third of esophagus — *mid*

✓5th   Needs fifth-digit   **OK**   Valid three-digit code

150.5	Malignant neoplasm of lower third of esophagus — *distal third*
150.8	Malignant neoplasm of other specified part of esophagus — *contiguous or overlapping sites of esophagus whose point of origin cannot be determined*
150.9	Malignant neoplasm of esophagus, unspecified site — *unknown*

151 MALIGNANT NEOPLASM OF STOMACH

The stomach has four functions: to act as a reservoir for food; to mix food; to begin the digestive process; and to allow the absorption of some substances.

The stomach begins at the portal between the esophagus and the stomach - the cardia. It ends at the portal to duodenum — the pylorus. In between is the corpus, or the body of the stomach. The corpus is divided into the upper portion, the fundus, which is served by the oxyntic gland, and the lower portion or the antrum, served by the pyloric gland and the large midportion, the body). There are no clear demarcations between the segments of the corpus. The lesser and greater curvatures of the stomach refer to the short and long walls of the organ.

Stomach cancer is rarely found before age 40 and is twice as common in men as in women. The most common types of stomach cancers are ulcerating carcinomas, polypoid carcinomas, superficial spreading carcinomas, linitis plastica, and advanced carcinoma.

Cancers in this rubric are classified by site, with one exception. According to ICD-9 exclusion notes, if squamous cell carcinoma is present at the distal end of the esophagus (the cardia), report 150.5 *Malignant neoplasm of lower third of esophagus*. However, if adenocarcinoma is present in the distal end of the esophagus (the cardia), report 151.0 *Malignant neoplasm of cardia*.

If the malignancy is of contiguous and overlapping sites, report 151.8 *Malignant neoplasm of other specified sites of stomach*.

151.0	Malignant neoplasm of cardia — *cardiac orifice; cardio-esophageal junction*
151.1	Malignant neoplasm of pylorus — *pre-pylorus, pyloric canal*
151.2	Malignant neoplasm of pyloric antrum — *lower portion of the stomach preceding the pylorus; antrum of stomach*
151.3	Malignant neoplasm of fundus of stomach — *upper portion of the stomach proceeding from the cardia*
151.4	Malignant neoplasm of body of stomach — *central segment*
151.5	Malignant neoplasm of lesser curvature of stomach, unspecified — *not classifiable to 151.1-151.4*
151.6	Malignant neoplasm of greater curvature of stomach, unspecified — *not classifiable to 151.0-151.4*
151.8	Malignant neoplasm of other specified sites of stomach — *anterior wall, posterior wall, contiguous or overlapping parts*
151.9	Malignant neoplasm of stomach, unspecified site — *unknown, including carcinoma ventriculi, gastric cancer, Brinton's disease*

152 MALIGNANT NEOPLASM OF SMALL INTESTINE, INCLUDING DUODENUM

The small intestine, often called the small bowel, is the portion of the alimentary canal from the pylorus to the cecum and is divided into the upper two-fifths, the jejunum, and the balance (the ilium). There is no demarcation between the two portions of small bowel, but, generally, the jejunum resides to the left side of the peritoneum and the ileum resides to the right and into the pelvis. The duodenum lies between the pylorus valve at the exit of the

M8093/3	Basal cell carcinoma, fibroepithelial type
M8094/3	Basosquamous carcinoma
M8095/3	Metatypical carcinoma
M8096/0	Intraepidermal epithelioma of Jadassohn
M8100/0	Trichoepithelioma
M8101/0	Trichofolliculoma
M8102/0	Tricholemmoma
M8110/0	Pilomatrixoma

M812-M813 Transitional cell papillomas and carcinomas

M8120/0	Transitional cell papilloma NOS
M8120/1	Urothelial papilloma
M8120/2	Transitional cell carcinoma in situ
M8120/3	Transitional cell carcinoma NOS
M8121/0	Schneiderian papilloma
M8121/1	Transitional cell papilloma, inverted type
M8121/3	Schneiderian carcinoma
M8122/3	Transitional cell carcinoma, spindle cell type
M8123/3	Basaloid carcinoma
M8124/3	Cloacogenic carcinoma
M8130/3	Papillary transitional cell carcinoma

M814-M838 Adenomas and adenocarcinomas

M8140/0	Adenoma NOS
M8140/1	Bronchial adenoma NOS
M8140/2	Adenocarcinoma in situ
M8140/3	Adenocarcinoma NOS
M8140/6	Adenocarcinoma, metastatic NOS
M8141/3	Scirrhous adenocarcinoma
M8142/3	Linitis plastica
M8143/3	Superficial spreading adenocarcinoma
M8144/3	Adenocarcinoma, intestinal type
M8145/3	Carcinoma, diffuse type
M8146/0	Monomorphic adenoma
M8147/0	Basal cell adenoma
M8150/0	Islet cell adenoma
M8150/3	Islet cell carcinoma
M8151/0	Insulinoma NOS

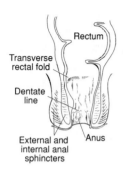

stomach, and the jejunum. The most common form of small intestine malignancy is adenocarcinoma in the proximal jejunum.

The small intestine is a common site for melanoma metastases, and these should be classified as secondary cancers rather than with the 152 rubric.

Cancer of the small bowel is classified by site. If the malignancy is of contiguous or overlapping sites, report 152.8 *Malignant neoplasm of other specified sites of small intestine*. Cancer of the ileocecal valve is reported with 153.4 *Malignant neoplasm of the cecum*.

152.0	Malignant neoplasm of duodenum — *small intestine immediate to the pylorus*
152.1	Malignant neoplasm of jejunum — *middle portion of the small intestine*
152.2	Malignant neoplasm of ileum — *distal small intestine that connects to the large intestine*
152.3	Malignant neoplasm of Meckel's diverticulum — *abnormal pouch near the terminal part of the ilium near the ileocecal juncture*
152.8	Malignant neoplasm of other specified sites of small intestine — *duodenojejunal junction; contiguous or overlapping sites*
152.9	Malignant neoplasm of small intestine, unspecified site — *unknown*

153 MALIGNANT NEOPLASM OF COLON

The large intestine, or colon, extends from the end of the ileum to the rectum. The rectum, however, is excluded from rubric 153 and classified in 154. The right colon consists of the cecum, ascending colon, hepatic flexure, and proximal transverse colon. The left colon consists of the distal transverse colon, the splenic flexure, the descending colon, sigmoid colon, and rectosigmoid colon.

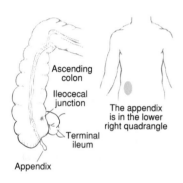

Colon cancer is the second to lung cancer as the most common form of cancer in the United States. About 150,000 new cases are diagnosed and 60,000 deaths occur each year. Adenocarcinoma is the most common form of colon cancer.

If the malignancy is causing obstruction or other manifestation, report the manifestation first, and the neoplasm secondarily.

153.0	Malignant neoplasm of hepatic flexure — *juncture of the ascending and transverse colons*
153.1	Malignant neoplasm of transverse colon — *middle portion of the large intestines, between the hepatic and splenic flexures*
153.2	Malignant neoplasm of descending colon — *between the splenic flexure and the sigmoid colon; left colon*
153.3	Malignant neoplasm of sigmoid colon — *S-shaped colon between the descending colon and the rectum*
153.4	Malignant neoplasm of cecum — *pouch at the beginning of the large intestine, including ileocecal valve*
153.5	Malignant neoplasm of appendix — *attached to the cecum*
153.6	Malignant neoplasm of ascending colon — *first portion of the large intestine between the cecum and the hepatic flexure; right colon*
153.7	Malignant neoplasm of splenic flexure — *bend between the transverse and descending colons*
153.8	Malignant neoplasm of other specified sites of large intestine — *not elsewhere classified or contiguous or overlapping sites*
153.9	Malignant neoplasm of colon, unspecified site — *unknown*

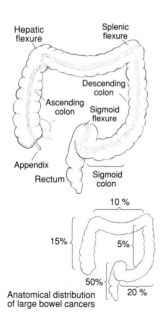

Anatomical distribution of large bowel cancers

⤶5th   Needs fifth-digit   **OK**   Valid three-digit code

154 MALIGNANT NEOPLASM OF RECTUM, RECTOSIGMOID JUNCTION, AND ANUS

The rectum begins at the rectosigmoid junction and ends at the anus. The rectum and rectosigmoid junctions are the most common sites for cancer in the colon, accounting for more than 30 percent of cases. In these cancers, the most common symptoms are rectal bleeding with bowel movement and pain upon defecation (tenesmus).

Diseases in this rubric are classified according to site. Report 154.8 *Malignant neoplasm of other specified sites* if the malignancy is of contiguous or overlapping sites. If the malignancy is causing bleeding, obstruction or other manifestation, report the manifestation first, and the malignancy secondarily.

154.0	Malignant neoplasm of rectosigmoid junction — *colon with rectum; rectosigmoid (colon)*
154.1	Malignant neoplasm of rectum — *rectal ampulla*
154.2	Malignant neoplasm of anal canal — *including anal sphincter*
154.3	Malignant neoplasm of anus, unspecified site — *unknown*
154.8	Malignant neoplasm of other sites of rectum, rectosigmoid junction, and anus — *including anorectum, cloacogenic zone, contiguous or overlapping sites*

155 MALIGNANT NEOPLASM OF LIVER AND INTRAHEPATIC BILE DUCTS

Primary liver cancer is uncommon in the United States; however, the liver is a common site for metastases, and would be reported with 197.7 Secondary malignant neoplasm of the mediastinum. About 80 percent of primary liver cancers are hepatomas.

For cancers of the hepatic duct, report 156.1 *Malignant neoplasm of extrahepatic bile ducts.*

155.0	Malignant neoplasm of liver, primary — *including all lobes; hepatoblastoma, liver carcinoma*
155.1	Malignant neoplasm of intrahepatic bile ducts — *including canaliculi biliferi, interlobular bile ducts; intrahepatic biliary passages, gall duct; intrahepatic bile ducts*
155.2	Malignant neoplasm of liver, not specified as primary or secondary — *unknown whether a metastasis*

156 MALIGNANT NEOPLASM OF GALLBLADDER AND EXTRAHEPATIC BILE DUCTS

Gallbladder cancer is uncommon and usually seen only in the elderly. Bile duct tumors are somewhat more common, but still usually limited to older patients. Most of these cancers are adenocarcinomas. Disease is classified according to site. If the malignancy is of contiguous and overlapping sites, report 156.8 *Other specified sites of gallbladder and extrahepatic bile ducts.*

156.0	Malignant neoplasm of gallbladder — *gallbladder*
156.1	Malignant neoplasm of extrahepatic bile ducts — *including biliary, common bile, cystic, hepatic duct; sphincter of Oddi*
156.2	Malignant neoplasm of ampulla of Vater — *area of dilation at the juncture of common bile and pancreatic ducts near their opening into the lumen of the duodenum*

M8151/3	Insulinoma, malignant
M8152/0	Glucagonoma NOS
M8152/3	Glucagonoma, malignant
M8153/1	Gastrinoma NOS
M8153/3	Gastrinoma, malignant
M8154/3	Mixed islet cell and exocrine adenocarcinoma
M8160/0	Bile duct adenoma
M8160/3	Cholangiocarcinoma
M8161/0	Bile duct cystadenoma
M8161/3	Bile duct cystadenocarcinoma
M8170/0	Liver cell adenoma
M8170/3	Hepatocellular carcinoma NOS
M8180/0	Hepatocholangioma, benign
M8180/3	Combined hepatocellular carcinoma and cholangiocarcinoma
M8190/0	Trabecular adenoma
M8190/3	Trabecular adenocarcinoma
M8191/0	Embryonal adenoma
M8200/0	Eccrine dermal cylindroma
M8200/3	Adenoid cystic carcinoma
M8201/3	Cribriform carcinoma
M8210/0	Adenomatous polyp NOS
M8210/3	Adenocarcinoma in adenomatous polyp
M8211/0	Tubular adenoma NOS
M8211/3	Tubular adenocarcinoma
M8220/0	Adenomatous polyposis coli
M8220/3	Adenocarcinoma in adenomatous polyposis coli
M8221/0	Multiple adenomatous polyps
M8230/3	Solid carcinoma NOS
M8231/3	Carcinoma simplex
M8240/1	Carcinoid tumor NOS
M8240/3	Carcinoid tumor, malignant
M8241/1	Carcinoid tumor, argentaffin NOS
M8241/3	Carcinoid tumor, argentaffin, malignant
M8242/1	Carcinoid tumor, nonargentaffin NOS
M8242/3	Carcinoid tumor, nonargentaffin, malignant
M8243/3	Mucocarcinoid tumor, malignant

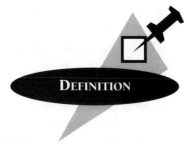

Peritoneum: the sac or lining of the abdomen

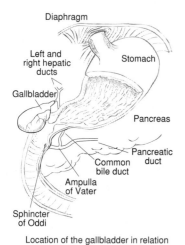

Location of the gallbladder in relation to select surrounding structures

retro-: behind, backward

156.8   Malignant neoplasm of other specified sites of gallbladder and extrahepatic bile ducts — *not elsewhere classified or of contiguous or overlapping sites*

156.9   Malignant neoplasm of biliary tract, part unspecified site — *unknown or involving both intrahepatic and extrahepatic bile ducts*

157 MALIGNANT NEOPLASM OF PANCREAS

The pancreas is a slender organ lying behind the stomach in the abdomen. The head of the pancreas is curved near the duodenum; the body is the main portion, and the tail is the portion that abuts the spleen. There are no clear demarcations between the parts of the pancreas.

The pancreas produces pancreatic juice, enzymes that assist in digestion. It also creates insulin, which regulates blood glucose levels.

Pancreatic cancer is one of the leading causes of cancer in the United States, after lung cancer and colon cancer. It is most common in people aged 50-70. Symptoms include weight loss, jaundice, and abdominal or back pain. Pancreatic cancer is most common in the head of the gland, with 66 percent of malignancies occurring there. Ductal adenocarcinoma is the most common type of malignancy in pancreatic cancer.

If the cancer is in the islets of Langerhans, insulin regulation could be affected. Any functional activity resulting from the malignancy should be separately reported. If the cancer occurs in overlapping or contiguous portions of the pancreas, report 157.8 *Other specified sites of pancreas.*

157.0   Malignant neoplasm of head of pancreas — *including Bard-Pic's syndrome*
157.1   Malignant neoplasm of body of pancreas — *main portion*
157.2   Malignant neoplasm of tail of pancreas — *tail*
157.3   Malignant neoplasm of pancreatic duct — *including Santorini, Wirsung ducts*
157.4   Malignant neoplasm of islets of Langerhans — *structures in the pancreas that produce insulin, somatostatin, or glucagon*
157.8   Malignant neoplasm of other specified sites of pancreas — *including ectopic tissue, contiguous or overlapping sites*
157.9   Malignant neoplasm of pancreas, part unspecified — *unknown*

158 MALIGNANT NEOPLASM OF RETROPERITONEUM AND PERITONEUM

The retroperitoneum is the space behind the peritoneum and in front of the spine. The peritoneum is the membrane that holds the abdominal organs. A majority of peritoneal malignancies are secondary, with the exception of peritoneal mesothelioma, a rare cancer arising in the mesodermal lining of the peritoneum. Retroperitoneal tumors are usually of mesodermal tissue.

If the malignancy spans both the peritoneum and retroperitoneum, ICD-9 instructs us to report this condition with 158.8 *Malignant neoplasm of specified parts of peritoneum.*

158.0   Malignant neoplasm of retroperitoneum — *including periadrenal, perirenal, perinephric, retrocecal tissues*
158.8   Malignant neoplasm of specified parts of peritoneum — *including Douglas cul-de-sac, mesentery; mesocolon; omentum; peritoneum; rectouterine pouch; or contiguous or sites*
158.9   Malignant neoplasm of peritoneum, unspecified — *unknown*

↙5th   Needs fifth-digit   **OK**   Valid three-digit code

159 MALIGNANT NEOPLASM OF OTHER AND ILL-DEFINED SITES WITHIN THE DIGESTIVE ORGANS AND PERITONEUM

This rubric is reserved for nonspecific malignancies of digestive sites and the peritoneum. When a digestive malignancy has progressed so that the point of origin cannot be assigned to a specific code in rubrics 150-158, report 159.8 *Malignant neoplasm of other and ill-defined sites of digestive system and intra-abdominal organs.*

159.0   Malignant neoplasm of intestinal tract, part unspecified — *not elsewhere specified*

159.1   Malignant neoplasm of spleen, not elsewhere classified — *angiosarcoma, fibrosarcoma of spleen*

159.8   Malignant neoplasm of other sites of digestive system and intra-abdominal organs — *point of origin cannot be assigned to any one of the categories 150-158*

159.9   Malignant neoplasm of ill-defined sites of digestive organs and peritoneum — *generalized "alimentary canal," "gastrointestinal tract"*

160-165 Malignant Neoplasm of Respiratory and Intrathoracic Organs

The respiratory system can be divided into two main sections: the upper and the lower respiratory tracts. The upper respiratory tract is located outside the thorax (the chest cavity), and is composed of the nose, the pharynx (nasopharynx, oropharynx, and hypopharynx. Malignant neoplasms of this upper portion of respiratory anatomy are classified in 140-149, as part of the oral cavity. This subsection includes the larynx, and the lower respiratory tract contained within the thorax and consisting of the trachea, bronchial tree, and the lungs, and pleura. Also classified to this subsection because of their anatomic locations are malignant neoplasms of the heart, thymus and mediastinum. However, great vessels are classified to 171.4.

The respiratory system functions as follows: air enters the body through the nose, where it is warmed, filtered and humidified as it passes through the nasal cavity. The air passes into the pharynx and from the pharynx into the trachea (the "windpipe"). The epiglottis in the pharynx prevents food from entering the trachea. The upper part of the trachea contains the three parts of the larynx and the vocal chords. At its base, the trachea divides into the left and right primary bronchi. Each bronchus divides into smaller branches known as segmental bronchi. These divide into tiny bronchioles that terminate in the microscopic ducts and alveoli sacs of the lungs where gas exchange takes place.

The lungs are large, paired organs in the thorax. The right lung has three lobes. The left lung cavity contains two lobes and encloses the heart. Thin sheets of epithelium (the pleura) separate the inside of the chest cavity from the outer surface of the lungs and the heart.

The respiratory system functions as an air distributor and gas exchanger, to supply oxygen and remove carbon monoxide from the body's cells. All parts of the respiratory system, except the microscopic alveoli of the lungs, function as air distributors. Only the alveoli sacks and ducts serve as gas exchangers. In addition to air distribution and gas exchange, the respiratory system and its structures provide for such functions as yawning, sneezing, coughing, hiccups, sound production (including speech), and the sense of smell (olfaction). The respiratory system also assists in homeostasis (regulation of pH in the body).

Malignancies in this section are classified according to anatomic site. If malignancies are found in multiple sites within an anatomic system, a code for "other sites" is in most cases

M8244/3	Composite carcinoid
M8250/1	Pulmonary adenomatosis
M8250/3	Bronchiolo-alveolar adenocarcinoma
M8251/0	Alveolar adenoma
M8251/3	Alveolar adenocarcinoma
M8260/0	Papillary adenoma NOS
M8260/3	Papillary adenocarcinoma NOS
M8261/1	Villous adenoma NOS
M8261/3	Adenocarcinoma in villous adenoma
M8262/3	Villous adenocarcinoma
M8263/0	Tubulovillous adenoma
M8270/0	Chromophobe adenoma
M8270/3	Chromophobe carcinoma
M8280/0	Acidophil adenoma
M8280/3	Acidophil carcinoma
M8281/0	Mixed acidophil-basophil adenoma
M8281/3	Mixed acidophil-basophil carcinoma
M8290/0	Oxyphilic adenoma
M8290/3	Oxyphilic adenocarcinoma
M8300/0	Basophil adenoma
M8300/3	Basophil carcinoma
M8310/0	Clear cell adenoma
M8310/3	Clear cell adenocarcinoma NOS
M8311/1	Hypernephroid tumor
M8312/3	Renal cell carcinoma
M8313/0	Clear cell adenofibroma
M8320/3	Granular cell carcinoma
M8321/0	Chief cell adenoma
M8322/0	Water-clear cell adenoma
M8322/3	Water-clear cell adenocarcinoma
M8323/0	Mixed cell adenoma
M8323/3	Mixed cell adenocarcinoma
M8324/0	Lipoadenoma
M8330/0	Follicular adenoma
M8330/3	Follicular adenocarcinoma NOS
M8331/3	Follicular adenocarcinoma, well differentiated type
M8332/3	Follicular adenocarcinoma, trabecular type
M8333/0	Microfollicular adenoma

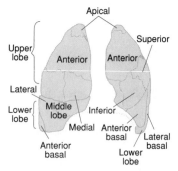

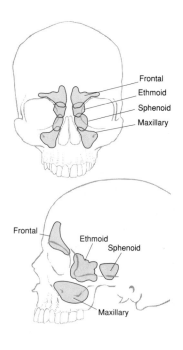

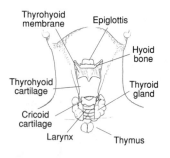

Anterior view of lungs. The left lung is divided into superior and inferior lobes. The right lung has three segments. The subdivisions are defined by the areas served by bronchial divisions

appropriate to report multiple sites. If the malignancy results in functional abnormalities, report the malignancy first, followed by the functional problem. For nonspecific or multiple thoracic or intrathoracic malignancies, report 195.1 *Malignant neoplasm of the thorax*. If the malignancy is carcinoma in situ, report with codes from the 231 rubric instead. If respiratory or thoracic malignancies are secondary, see codes in the 196-199 rubrics.

160 MALIGNANT NEOPLASM OF NASAL CAVITIES, MIDDLE EAR, AND ACCESSORY SINUSES

The nasal cavity opens into the vestibule that is just inside of the nostrils and continues to the respiratory area where bone in three shelves (formed by the nasal cavity) called the superior, middle, and inferior nasal turbinates (nasal conchae) are located. The turbinates come close to the nasal septum and subdivide the nasal cavity into passageways.

160.0	Malignant neoplasm of nasal cavities — *including nasal cartilage, septum, conchae, fossa, mucosa, internal nose*
160.1	Malignant neoplasm of auditory tube, middle ear, and mastoid air cells — *including eustachian tube, inner ear, middle ear, antrum tympanicum, tympanic cavity*
160.2	Malignant neoplasm of maxillary sinus — *sinus behind cheekbones; including maxillary antrum and Highmore antrum*
160.3	Malignant neoplasm of ethmoidal sinus — *sinus between the eyes on either side of the nose*
160.4	Malignant neoplasm of frontal sinus — *sinus above the eyes*
160.5	Malignant neoplasm of sphenoidal sinus — *sinus behind the eyes on either side of the nose*
160.8	Malignant neoplasm of other sites of nasal cavities, middle ear, and accessory sinuses — *contiguous or overlapping sites of nasal cavities, middle and inner ear, and accessory sinuses*
160.9	Malignant neoplasm of site of nasal cavities, middle ear, and accessory sinus, unspecified site — *unknown*

161 MALIGNANT NEOPLASM OF LARYNX

The larynx has several functions: speech, protection of the airways, respiration, and fixation of the chest. It is commonly called the "voicebox." Most laryngeal malignancies are squamous cell carcinomas and 90 percent of laryngeal cancers occur in males. Hoarseness and throat pain are common symptoms. Malignant neoplasms of the larynx are classified according to site. If the malignancy spans two sites of the larynx, ICD-9 instructs us to report this condition with 161.8 Malignant neoplasm of specified sites of larynx. Do not use codes in this rubric to report malignancies of the epiglottis (146.4), or hypopharynx (rubric 148).

161.0	Malignant neoplasm of glottis — *true vocal cord including intrinsic larynx, commissure*
161.1	Malignant neoplasm of supraglottis — *false vocal cord including aryepiglottic fold, epiglottis, extrinsic larynx, ventricular bands*
161.2	Malignant neoplasm of subglottis — *larynx below the vocal cords and above the trachea*
161.3	Malignant neoplasm of laryngeal cartilages — *including arytenoid, cricoid, cuneiform, thyroid cartilage*
161.8	Malignant neoplasm of other specified sites of larynx — *contiguous or overlapping sites of larynx whose point of origin cannot be determined*
161.9	Malignant neoplasm of larynx, unspecified site — *unknown*

✔5th Needs fifth-digit   **OK** Valid three-digit code

162 MALIGNANT NEOPLASM OF TRACHEA, BRONCHUS, AND LUNG

Lung cancer is the most common cancer in the United States, with more than 150,000 cases diagnosed and more than 100,000 dying from the disease annually. Malignant tumors of the lung may be squamous cell, adenocarcinoma, small cell, large cell, adenosquamous, carcinoid, or bronchial gland carcinoma. Lung cancer is considered one of the most lethal forms of cancer, with only 20 percent of patients surviving one year after diagnosis. Symptoms include wheezing, pneumonia, and pain, as well as symptoms from metastatic sites of disease. The most common site of metastatic lung cancer is the liver, but brain, kidney, and adrenal gland are also common sites. Lung cancer is classified according to the lobe of the lung. Report 162.8 if the cancer invades contiguous or overlapping sites in the lung or bronchus if the point of origin cannot be determined.

162.0   Malignant neoplasm of trachea — *in the breathing tube anterior to the esophagus and extending from the larynx to the right and left bronchi.*

162.2   Malignant neoplasm of main bronchus — *including carina and hilus of lung*

162.3   Malignant neoplasm of upper lobe, bronchus, or lung — *including Cuiffini-Pancoase syndrome, Hare's syndrome, Tobias' syndrome*

162.4   Malignant neoplasm of middle lobe, bronchus, or lung — *Middle lobe, bronchus or lung*

162.5   Malignant neoplasm of lower lobe, bronchus, or lung — *Lower lobe, bronchus or lung*

162.8   Malignant neoplasm of other parts of bronchus or lung — *contiguous or overlapping sites of bronchus or lung whose point of origin cannot be determined*

162.9   Malignant neoplasm of bronchus and lung, unspecified site — *unknown*

163 MALIGNANT NEOPLASM OF PLEURA

The pleura line the lung and localized mesothelioma. Diffuse malignant mesothelioma is the most common form of pleural malignancy. Cancers of the pleura are classified according to site. The parietal pleura are the outer lining of the lung, and the visceral pleura are the inner lining. Report 163.8 if the malignancy is overlapping or in contiguous parts of the pleura.

163.0   Malignant neoplasm of parietal pleura — *outer lining of the lung*

163.1   Malignant neoplasm of visceral pleura — *inner lining of the lung.*

163.8   Malignant neoplasm of other specified sites of pleura — *contiguous or overlapping sites of pleura whose point of origin cannot be determined*

163.9   Malignant neoplasm of pleura, unspecified site — *unknown*

164 MALIGNANT NEOPLASM OF THYMUS, HEART, AND MEDIASTINUM

The thymus is a bilateral, lymph-rich organ that produces T lymphocytes that circulate throughout the body to provide an immune function. The organ is anterior to the heart, in the upper mediastinum and is a common site for neoplasms. The most common type of thymoma is epithelial, accounting for 45 percent of cases. Since some lymphomas and Hodgkin's granulomas arise in thymus tissue, check documentation to be sure of appropriate use of codes from this rubric.

The mediastinum is the compartment between the sternum and lungs/ heart (anterior), and the spine and lungs/heart (posterior). Because of the general nature of the mediastinum in anatomical descriptions, care should be taken that a more specific site isn't overlooked when coding malignant neoplasm of the mediastinum. The thymus (164.0) and parathyroid (194.1) reside in the mediastinum, but are reported with more specific codes, as are neurogenic tumors in the mediastinum (classify to nerve).

M8334/0	Macrofollicular adenoma
M8340/3	Papillary and follicular adenocarcinoma
M8350/3	Nonencapsulated sclerosing carcinoma
M8360/1	Multiple endocrine adenomas
M8361/1	Juxtaglomerular tumor
M8370/0	Adrenal cortical adenoma NOS
M8370/3	Adrenal cortical carcinoma
M8371/0	Adrenal cortical adenoma, compact cell type
M8372/0	Adrenal cortical adenoma, heavily pigmented variant
M8373/0	Adrenal cortical adenoma, clear cell type
M8374/0	Adrenal cortical adenoma, glomerulosa cell type
M8375/0	Adrenal cortical adenoma, mixed cell type
M8380/0	Endometrioid adenoma NOS
M8380/1	Endometrioid adenoma, borderline malignancy
M8380/3	Endometrioid carcinoma
M8381/0	Endometrioid adenofibroma NOS
M8381/1	Endometrioid adenofibroma, borderline malignancy
M8381/3	Endometrioid adenofibroma, malignant

M839-M842 Adnexal and skin appendage neoplasms

M8390/0	Skin appendage adenoma
M8390/3	Skin appendage carcinoma
M8400/0	Sweat gland adenoma
M8400/1	Sweat gland tumor NOS
M8400/3	Sweat gland adenocarcinoma
M8401/0	Apocrine adenoma
M8401/3	Apocrine adenocarcinoma
M8402/0	Eccrine acrospiroma
M8403/0	Eccrine spiradenoma
M8404/0	Hidrocystoma
M8405/0	Papillary hydradenoma
M8406/0	Papillary syringadenoma
M8407/0	Syringoma NOS
M8410/0	Sebaceous adenoma
M8410/3	Sebaceous adenocarcinoma

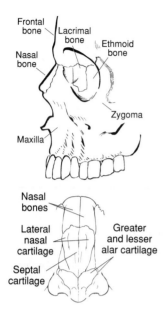

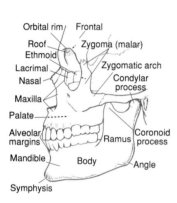

The heart is the muscle responsible for circulation of blood throughout the body. It is divided into four cavities, the right and left atria and the right and left ventricles. The left atrium receives oxygenated blood from the lung, and passes it along to the left ventricle, which pushes the blood through the circulatory system to nourish the body's cells. The right atrium receives the blood that has completed its circuit through the body. From the right atrium, the blood is circulated to the right ventricle, which pumps it back into the lungs for reoxygenation. Four major valves separate the chambers and prevent backflow of blood. The valves consist of flaps called cusps; the ends of the cusps between the atria and ventricles extend into the ventricles where they are connected to the papillary muscles by fibrous cords called the chordae tendineae.

Malignant neoplasms of the heart are rarely seen as primary neoplasms. When primary cancer of the heart occurs, it occurs most commonly in children. The most common cardiac malignancy is cardiac sarcoma, accounting for 30 percent of the cases. Complications from cardiac cancer can be grave and include heart failure, hemorrhagic pericardial effusion with tamponade, and arrhythmia. A primary cancer of the heart is also prone to metastases to the spine and other major organs.

Report malignant neoplasms of the great vessels with 171.4 *Malignant neoplasm of the thorax.* If the malignancy is overlapping or in contiguous parts of the heart and mediastinum, report 164.8 *Malignant neoplasm of other specified site.*

164.0	Malignant neoplasm of thymus — *lymphoid and endocrine organ behind the sternum*
164.1	Malignant neoplasm of heart — *including endocardium, epicardium, myocardium and pericardium*
164.2	Malignant neoplasm of anterior mediastinum — *soft and connective tissue between the lungs, in the cavity between the heart and the sternum*
164.3	Malignant neoplasm of posterior mediastinum — *soft and connective tissue between the lungs, in the cavity between the heart and the spinal column*
164.8	Malignant neoplasm of other parts of mediastinum — *contiguous or overlapping sites of thymus, heart, and mediastinum*
164.9	Malignant neoplasm of mediastinum, part unspecified — *unknown*

165 MALIGNANT NEOPLASM OF OTHER AND ILL-DEFINED SITES WITHIN THE RESPIRATORY SYSTEM AND INTRATHORACIC ORGANS

This rubric is reserved for nonspecific malignancies of respiratory and intrathoracic organs. When a respiratory malignancy has progressed to a point that it cannot be assigned to a specific code in rubrics 160-164, report 165.8 *Malignant neoplasm of other and ill-defined sites of respiratory system and intra-thoracic organs.*

165.0	Malignant neoplasm of upper respiratory tract, part unspecified — *the respiratory organs above the diaphragm*
165.8	Malignant neoplasm of other sites within the respiratory system and intrathoracic organs — *point of origin cannot be assigned to any one of the categories 160-164*
165.9	Malignant neoplasm of ill-defined sites within the respiratory system — *respiratory tract not otherwise specified*

170-176 Malignant Neoplasm of Bone, Connective Tissue, Skin, and Breast

Codes in this section of ICD-9 refer to malignancies in the bone, connective tissue, skin, and breast.

170 MALIGNANT NEOPLASM OF BONE AND ARTICULAR CARTILAGE

Primary malignancies of the bone are uncommon compared to the incidence of metastases to the bone. For metastasized cancers, see 198.5 *Secondary malignant neoplasm of the bone and bone marrow*. Malignancies of the bone are classified in ICD-9 according to anatomic site and type of bone (long or short). Cartilage and periosteum malignancies are classified to the appropriate bone code. Cartilage malignancies are classified to the 171 rubric, as connective tissue.

Multiple myeloma is the most common bone malignancy, occurring usually in older adults. Osteosarcoma is most commonly seen in children and young adults. Pain, swelling, limit to range of motion, or pathological fracture are common symptoms.

170.0 Malignant neoplasm of bones of skull and face, except mandible — *including ethmoid, frontal, turbinate, malar, occipital, orbital, zygomatic, sphenoid, temporal*

170.1 Malignant neoplasm of mandible — *inferior maxilla, lower jaw bone*

170.2 Malignant neoplasm of vertebral column, excluding sacrum and coccyx — *meaning bony spine, vertebra*

170.3 Malignant neoplasm of ribs, sternum, and clavicle — *including costal cartilage, costovertebral joint, xiphoid process*

170.4 Malignant neoplasm of scapula and long bones of upper limb — *including acromion, radius, ulna, humerus*

170.5 Malignant neoplasm of short bones of upper limb — *including bones of hand and wrist; carpal, cuneiform, scaphoid, semilunar of lunate, navicular, phalanges, unciform, trapezoid, pisiform*

170.6 Malignant neoplasm of pelvic bones, sacrum, and coccyx — *including coccygeal vertebra, ilium, ischium, pubic bone, sacral vertebra*

170.7 Malignant neoplasm of long bones of lower limb — *including femur, fibula, tibia*

170.8 Malignant neoplasm of short bones of lower limb — *including bones of knee, foot and ankle; astragalus talus, calcaneus, cuboid, navicular of knee, patella, phalanges, tarsal, metatarsal*

170.9 Malignant neoplasm of bone and articular cartilage, site unspecified — *unknown*

171 MALIGNANT NEOPLASM OF CONNECTIVE AND OTHER SOFT TISSUE

Malignant neoplasms of the connective tissue and other soft tissue are classified according to site rather than specific type of tissue. These codes can be used to classify malignant neoplasms of blood vessels, bursa, fascia, fat, ligament (except uterine), muscle, peripheral, sympathetic, and parasympathetic nerves, synovia, or tendons.

Cartilage is a type of dense connective tissue (hyaline, elastic, and fibrocartilage) that is found in joints. Hyaline cartilage is located at joints over the ends of long bones; fibrocartilage is found at other body sites, such as the pubic symphysis, intervertebral discs, menisci of the knee, and the point where the hip bones fuse anteriorly.

M8420/0 Ceruminous adenoma

M8420/3 Ceruminous adenocarcinoma

M843 Mucoepidermoid neoplasms

M8430/1 Mucoepidermoid tumor

M8430/3 Mucoepidermoid carcinoma

M844-M849 Cystic, mucinous, and serous neoplasms

M8440/0 Cystadenoma NOS

M8440/3 Cystadenocarcinoma NOS

M8441/0 Serous cystadenoma NOS

M8441/1 Serous cystadenoma, borderline malignancy

M8441/3 Serous cystadenocarcinoma NOS

M8450/0 Papillary cystadenoma NOS

M8450/1 Papillary cystadenoma, borderline malignancy

M8450/3 Papillary cystadenocarcinoma NOS

M8460/0 Papillary serous cystadenoma NOS

M8460/1 Papillary serous cystadenoma, borderline malignancy

M8460/3 Papillary serous cystadenocarcinoma

M8461/0 Serous surface papilloma NOS

M8461/1 Serous surface papilloma, borderline malignancy

M8461/3 Serous surface papillary carcinoma

M8470/0 Mucinous cystadenoma NOS

M8470/1 Mucinous cystadenoma, borderline malignancy

M8470/3 Mucinous cystadenocarcinoma NOS

M8471/0 Papillary mucinous cystadenoma NOS

M8471/1 Papillary mucinous cystadenoma, borderline malignancy

M8471/3 Papillary mucinous cystadenocarcinoma

M8480/0 Mucinous adenoma

M8480/3 Mucinous adenocarcinoma

M8480/6 Pseudomyxoma peritonei

M8481/3 Mucin-producing adenocarcinoma

M8490/3 Signet ring cell carcinoma

Soft tissue generally includes the deep fascia, muscles, tendons, and ligaments. Deep fascia lies beneath the second layer of subcutaneous tissue (hypodermis) of the integumentary system. Deep fascia in the musculoskeletal system lines extremities and holds together groups of muscles. There are three types of muscle tissue: skeletal, cardiac, and visceral. Muscle tissue consists of specialized cells that allow contraction to produce voluntary or involuntary movement of body parts.

Tendons are fibrous cords that vary in length. They are found at the ends of muscles and connecting muscles to bones. Ligaments are bands of fibrous tissue that connect two or more bones or cartilage.

If the malignant neoplasm is of contiguous or overlapping soft tissue sites and the point of origin cannot be determined, report 171.8.

171.0	Malignant neoplasm of connective and other soft tissue of head, face, and neck — *including blood vessel, fascia, fat, muscle, cartilage of eye and ear, ligament, and peripheral, sympathetic, and parasympathetic nerve and ganglia*
171.2	Malignant neoplasm of connective and other soft tissue of upper limb, including shoulder — *including blood vessel, fascia, fat, muscle, ligament, and peripheral, sympathetic, and parasympathetic nerve and ganglia*
171.3	Malignant neoplasm of connective and other soft tissue of lower limb, including hip — *including blood vessel, fascia, fat, muscle, ligament, and peripheral, sympathetic, and parasympathetic nerve and ganglia*
171.4	Malignant neoplasm of connective and other soft tissue of thorax — *including blood vessel, fascia, fat, muscle, ligament, and peripheral, sympathetic, and parasympathetic nerve and ganglia*
171.5	Malignant neoplasm of connective and other soft tissue of abdomen — *including blood vessel, fascia, fat, muscle, ligament, and peripheral, sympathetic, and parasympathetic nerve and ganglia*
171.6	Malignant neoplasm of connective and other soft tissue of pelvis — *including blood vessel, fascia, fat, muscle, ligament, and peripheral, sympathetic, and parasympathetic nerve and ganglia*
171.7	Malignant neoplasm of connective and other soft tissue of trunk, unspecified site — *including blood vessel, fascia, fat, muscle, ligament, and peripheral, sympathetic, and parasympathetic nerve and ganglia*
171.8	Malignant neoplasm of other specified sites of connective and other soft tissue — *contiguous or overlapping sites of connective tissue whose point of origin cannot be determined*
171.9	Malignant neoplasm of connective and other soft tissue, site unspecified — *site unknown*

172 MALIGNANT MELANOMA OF SKIN

The integumentary system is a diverse and complex organ forming the boundary and barrier between the internal environment of the body and the outside world. Although quite thin, the skin (or cutaneous membrane) is the largest human organ, usually 12 to 20 square feet in area and comprising 12 percent of the total body weight. The depth of the skin varies from 0.5 mm in thin areas such as the eyelids to 5.0 mm or more at its thickest over the back.

There are three integrated layers in the skin: the thinner outer layer (epidermis), the dense connective layer (dermis), and the loose subcutis or subcutaneous layer (also called the hypodermis or superficial fascia) which is composed of fat and areolar tissue.

⌐5th   Needs fifth-digit   **OK**   Valid three-digit code

The epidermis consists of three distinct cell types: keratinocytes that provide structure, melanocytes that contribute color and filter ultraviolet light, and Langerhans cells that contribute to the immune response. These cells form up to five strata over the dermal epidermal junction or basement membrane. Beneath the epidermal junction lies the dermis, composed of a papillary and a reticular layer. The dermis is rich in skin receptor nerves, blood vessels, and in sweat glands. It provides attachment for smooth and skeletal muscle fibers and the hair follicles. The lipocyte cells of the subcutis, joined to the bottom of the dermis, produce lipids for the subcutaneous tissue to make the fatty, insulating layer that cushions the body against shocks and provides an energy source.

Melanomas are skin cancers that are usually pigmented but otherwise vary in size and presentation. They are among the most invasive of the cancers. Change is the hallmark of melanoma; adjacent tissue is usually transformed. The most common type of melanoma is superficial spreading melanoma, accounting for 65 percent of all melanomas. They are most common on women's legs, or men's trunks. Other types of melanoma include nodular, with dark papules or plaques, and solar lentigo, arising as a flat tan macule on areas of skin that have had long-term sun exposure, especially on the hands and forehead.

Melanoma begins as a skin cancer, but aggressively metastasizes to other systems or organs. These secondary sites are not classified in ICD-9 as melanomas, but as secondary malignant neoplasms, classified by site in rubrics 196-199.

Do not report personal history of malignant melanoma of skin (V10.83) in patients with a recurrence; instead, report the active disease. The personal history code is reserved for patients who have completed treatment and are without recurrence of melanoma.

172.0	Malignant melanoma of skin of lip — *skin only, outer aspect only*
172.1	Malignant melanoma of skin of eyelid, including canthus — *skin of eyelid*
172.2	Malignant melanoma of skin of ear and external auditory canal — *including auricle, external canal, tragus, helix, pinna, concha, pinna*
172.3	Malignant melanoma of skin of other and unspecified parts of face — *including external cheek and nose, chin but not neck, forehead, but not scalp*
172.4	Malignant melanoma of skin of scalp and neck — *but not chin or forehead*
172.5	Malignant melanoma of skin of trunk, except scrotum — *including axilla, breast, buttock, groin, perianal skin, perineum, umbilicus*
172.6	Malignant melanoma of skin of upper limb, including shoulder — *shoulder, arm, and hand*
172.7	Malignant melanoma of skin of lower limb, including hip — *hip, leg, and foot*
172.8	Malignant melanoma of other specified sites of skin — *contiguous or overlapping sites of skin*
172.9	Melanoma of skin, site unspecified — *unknown*

173 OTHER MALIGNANT NEOPLASM OF SKIN

Skin cancers other than melanoma may be basal cell or squamous cell carcinomas. No distinction is made between basal and squamous cells in ICD-9 classification. Basal cell carcinoma is usually small, shiny, and firm, but may also be crusty and ulcerous. A squamous cell carcinoma is often more pigmented, but it, too, is highly variable in appearance.

Skin cancers in this rubric are classified according to location. For melanoma, see codes in rubric 172; for Kaposi's sarcoma, see rubric 176. Cancers of the skin of the genitalia are reported with genitalia codes, 184.0-184.9 and 187.1-187.9.

M8490/6	Metastatic signet ring cell carcinoma

M850-M854 Ductal, lobular, and medullary neoplasms

M8500/2	Intraductal carcinoma, noninfiltrating NOS
M8500/3	Infiltrating duct carcinoma
M8501/2	Comedocarcinoma, noninfiltrating
M8501/3	Comedocarcinoma NOS
M8502/3	Juvenile carcinoma of the breast
M8503/0	Intraductal papilloma
M8503/2	Noninfiltrating intraductal papillary adenocarcinoma
M8504/0	Intracystic papillary adenoma
M8504/2	Noninfiltrating intracystic carcinoma
M8505/0	Intraductal papillomatosis NOS
M8506/0	Subareolar duct papillomatosis
M8510/3	Medullary carcinoma NOS
M8511/3	Medullary carcinoma with amyloid stroma
M8512/3	Medullary carcinoma with lymphoid stroma
M8520/2	Lobular carcinoma in situ
M8520/3	Lobular carcinoma NOS
M8521/3	Infiltrating ductular carcinoma
M8530/3	Inflammatory carcinoma
M8540/3	Paget's disease, mammary
M8541/3	Paget's disease and infiltrating duct carcinoma of breast
M8542/3	Paget's disease, extramammary (except Paget's disease of bone)

M855 Acinar cell neoplasms

M8550/0	Acinar cell adenoma
M8550/1	Acinar cell tumor
M8550/3	Acinar cell carcinoma

M856-M858 Complex epithelial neoplasms

M8560/3	Adenosquamous carcinoma
M8561/0	Adenolymphoma
M8570/3	Adenocarcinoma with squamous metaplasia
M8571/3	Adenocarcinoma with cartilaginous and osseous

173.0	Other malignant neoplasm of skin of lip — *skin only, outer aspect only*
173.1	Other malignant neoplasm of skin of eyelid, including canthus — *skin of eyelid*
173.2	Other malignant neoplasm of skin of ear and external auditory canal — *including auricle, external canal, tragus, helix, pinna, concha, pinna*
173.3	Other malignant neoplasm of skin of other and unspecified parts of face — *including external cheek and nose, chin but not neck, forehead, but not scalp*
173.4	Other malignant neoplasm of scalp and skin of neck — *but not chin or forehead*
173.5	Other malignant neoplasm of skin of trunk, except scrotum — *including axilla, breast, buttock, groin, perianal skin, perineum, umbilicus*
173.6	Other malignant neoplasm of skin of upper limb, including shoulder — *shoulder, arm and hand*
173.7	Other malignant neoplasm of skin of lower limb, including hip — *Ship, leg and foot*
173.8	Other malignant neoplasm of other specified sites of skin — *contiguous or overlapping sites of skin*
173.9	Other malignant neoplasm of skin, site unspecified — *unknown*

174 MALIGNANT NEOPLASM OF FEMALE BREAST

The female breasts are located in the subcutaneous tissue of the front thorax, forming elevations. The mammary glands, accessory organs of the female reproductive system, are contained within these elevations. Each breast contains 15 to 20 lobes of glandular tissue consisting of smaller lobuli of alveoli (secreting cells) and ducts. The smaller ducts unite into a single milk-carrying duct for each lobe and these converge toward the nipple. The glandular tissue is contained within dense connective tissue that attaches to the pectoral muscle, and with suspensory ligaments that extend from the skin to the pectoral muscle to provide support. The nipple is located near the tip of each breast surrounded by a circular area of pigmented and irregular surfaced skin called the areola.

The function of the mammary gland is lactation — secretion of colostrum and subsequently milk for the nourishment of newborn infants. Successful lactation relies on pre- and post-natal production of hormones including progesterone, estrogen, prolactin, and oxytocin.

Malignant neoplasms of the female breast are classified according to site. The upper, outer quadrant of the breast is the most likely site for a malignancy; a full 50 percent of breast disease occurs in this quadrant. This is followed by 18 percent in the nipple; 15 percent in the upper, inner quadrant; 6 percent in the lower, inner quadrant; and 1 percent in the lower, outer quadrant. The remaining percentage (10 percent) is distributed in the axillary tail and in multiple sites.

If a malignancy is found in several sites of the breast, report 174.8 *Other specified sites of female breast*, which includes multiple sites. Do not code each site separately. If the malignancy is in the skin of the breast, report 172.5 (melanoma) or 173.5 (other skin malignancy).

174.0	Malignant neoplasm of nipple and areola of female breast — *female only*
174.1	Malignant neoplasm of central portion of female breast — *female only*
174.2	Malignant neoplasm of upper-inner quadrant of female breast — *female only*
174.3	Malignant neoplasm of lower-inner quadrant of female breast — *female only*
174.4	Malignant neoplasm of upper-outer quadrant of female breast — *female only*

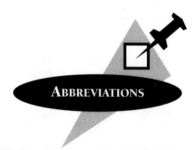

ABBREVIATIONS

KS: Kaposi's sarcoma, also called Multiple Idiopathic Hemorrhagic Sarcoma, is a neoplasm characterized by vascular skin lesions.

✔5th Needs fifth-digit   **OK** Valid three-digit code

174.5	Malignant neoplasm of lower-outer quadrant of female breast — *female only*
174.6	Malignant neoplasm of axillary tail of female breast — *female only*
174.8	Malignant neoplasm of other specified sites of female breast — *female only; including ectopic sites or overlapping sites*
174.9	Malignant neoplasm of breast (female), unspecified site — *female only; unknown site*

175 MALIGNANT NEOPLASM OF MALE BREAST

Malignant neoplasms of the male breast are classified by site: both nipple and areola or other. If the malignancy is in the skin of the breast, report 172.5 (melanoma) or 173.5 (other skin malignancy) instead. Breast cancer in men occurs at only 1 percent of the rate it occurs in women.

175.0	Malignant neoplasm of nipple and areola of male breast — *male only*
175.9	Malignant neoplasm of other and unspecified sites of male breast — *male only; including ectopic sites*

176 KAPOSI'S SARCOMA

Kaposi's sarcoma is a malignancy characterized by numerous vascular skin tumors. Kaposi's sarcoma was once found only rarely, in aging men, usually of Italian or Jewish decent. Today, incidence is common in the United States, as a manifestation of Acquired Immune Deficiency Syndrome (AIDS).

A diagnosis of Kaposi's sarcoma of the skin is significant because it is often the first clinical manifestation of AIDS in a Human Immunodeficiency Virus (HIV) positive patient, though Kaposi's sarcoma itself is rarely a cause of death. Disseminated Kaposi's sarcoma can involve lymph nodes, viscera, and the gastrointestinal tract.

Kaposi's syndrome is classified according to site of lesion. More than one code may be required to describe disseminated sarcoma, and Kaposi's is never reported with secondary neoplasm codes.

Do not reference the table of neoplasms to assign codes for Kaposi's sarcoma; Kaposi's sarcoma codes are omitted from the table. Instead, refer to Kaposi's sarcoma in the index of ICD-9 where a complete indexing is provided.

176.0	Kaposi's sarcoma of skin — *any site*
176.1	Kaposi's sarcoma of soft tissue — *including aponeurosis, bursa, blood vessel, connective tissue, fat, fascia, ligament, muscle*
176.2	Kaposi's sarcoma of palate — *hard or soft*
176.3	Kaposi's sarcoma of gastrointestinal sites — *stomach, intestine, anus, liver, spleen, pancreas*
176.4	Kaposi's sarcoma of lung — *any site*
176.5	Kaposi's sarcoma of lymph nodes — *any site, but excluding lymphatic channels*
176.8	Kaposi's sarcoma of other specified sites — *including external genitalia, scrotum, vulva, and oral cavity not elsewhere specified*
176.9	Kaposi's sarcoma of unspecified site — *viscera not otherwise specified, or unknown*

	metaplasia
M8572/3	Adenocarcinoma with spindle cell metaplasia
M8573/3	Adenocarcinoma with apocrine metaplasia
M8580/0	Thymoma, benign
M8580/3	Thymoma, malignant

M859-M867 Specialized gonadal neoplasms

M8590/1	Sex cord-stromal tumor
M8600/0	Thecoma NOS
M8600/3	Theca cell carcinoma
M8610/0	Luteoma NOS
M8620/1	Granulosa cell tumor NOS
M8620/3	Granulosa cell tumor, malignant
M8621/1	Granulosa cell-theca cell tumor
M8630/0	Androblastoma, benign
M8630/1	Androblastoma NOS
M8630/3	Androblastoma, malignant
M8631/0	Sertoli-Leydig cell tumor
M8632/1	Gynandroblastoma
M8640/0	Tubular androblastoma NOS
M8640/3	Sertoli cell carcinoma
M8641/0	Tubular androblastoma with lipid storage
M8650/0	Leydig cell tumor, benign
M8650/1	Leydig cell tumor NOS
M8650/3	Leydig cell tumor, malignant
M8660/0	Hilar cell tumor
M8670/0	Lipid cell tumor of ovary
M8671/0	Adrenal rest tumor

M868-M871 Paragangliomas and glomus tumors

M8680/1	Paraganglioma NOS
M8680/3	Paraganglioma, malignant
M8681/1	Sympathetic paraganglioma
M8682/1	Parasympathetic paraganglioma
M8690/1	Glomus jugulare tumor
M8691/1	Aortic body tumor
M8692/1	Carotid body tumor
M8693/1	Extra-adrenal paraganglioma NOS
M8693/3	Extra-adrenal paraganglioma, malignant
M8700/0	Pheochromocytoma NOS

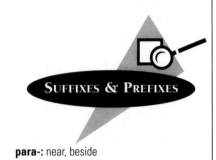

SUFFIXES & PREFIXES

para-: near, beside

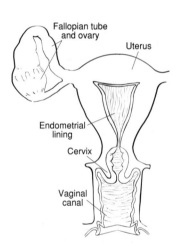

Fallopian tube and ovary

Uterus

Endometrial lining

Cervix

Vaginal canal

179-189 Malignant Neoplasm of Genitourinary Organs

Codes in this subsection of ICD-9 are classified according to site of malignant neoplasm in the female or male reproductive system or in the urinary system.

179 MALIGNANT NEOPLASM OF UTERUS, PART UNSPECIFIED **OK**

Use this valid three-digit code to report a malignant neoplasm of the uterus when the specific location is unknown. Use a more specific code whenever possible, as this code is nonspecific and its use may cause reimbursement delays. Use 182.8 *Malignant neoplasm of other specified sites of body of uterus* when the neoplasm is of contiguous or overlapping sites of the uterus.

180 MALIGNANT NEOPLASM OF CERVIX UTERI

Cancer of the cervix uteri ay be asymptomatic or may cause vaginal discharge, pain, or postcoital bleeding. Most cervical cancers are squamous cell cancers.

Cervical cancer is classified as of the endocervix, the mucous membrane lining the canal of the cervix; or exocervix, the squamous epithelium of the cervix. Report other specified site, 180.8, if the malignancy is of the cervical stump following hysterectomy; of the squamocolumnar junction of the cervix, or of the malignancy is of contiguous or overlapping sites of the endocervix and exocervix.

180.0	Malignant neoplasm of endocervix — *cervical canal opening into uterus*
180.1	Malignant neoplasm of exocervix — *cervical canal opening into vagina*
180.8	Malignant neoplasm of other specified sites of cervix — *including cervical stump, squamocolumnar junction of cervix, or contiguous or overlapping sites*
180.9	Malignant neoplasm of cervix uteri, unspecified site — *unknown*

181 MALIGNANT NEOPLASM OF PLACENTA **OK**

The placenta is an organ of pregnancy, operating as an exchange point for waste from the fetus and nourishment from the mother. In rare cases, an anomalous placenta may develop when no viable fetus exists, as in the case of hydatidiform mole. Use this valid three-digit code to report choriocarcinoma, also called chorioepithelioma. Hydatidiform mole or pregnancy precedes choriocarcinoma. It is an epithelial malignancy that metastasizes rapidly.

Do not use this code to report a hydatidiform mole (630), malignant hydatidiform mole (236.1), or chorioadenoma (236.1).

182 MALIGNANT NEOPLASM OF BODY OF UTERUS

The uterus is the muscular female organ where the fetus develops until delivery. Normally only three inches long and the shape of a pear, the uterus expands greatly during pregnancy.

Malignant neoplasms of the body of the uterus are classified according to site: the body of the uterus, including the fundus and endometrium; and the isthmus of the uterus, the narrow, distal portion of the uterus between the main body and the cervix. Endometrial carcinoma is a common malignancy that affects primarily postmenopausal women. Symptoms include postmenopausal bleeding, though symptoms may not be present until metastases become symptomatic. Endometrial carcinoma is reported with 182.0 *Malignant neoplasm of the corpus uteri, except isthmus.*

Report 182.8 *Malignant neoplasm of other specified site of body of uterus* if the malignancy is of contiguous or overlapping sites of the uterus. See codes in the 183 rubric to report cancer of the uterine ligaments.

182.0   Malignant neoplasm of corpus uteri, except isthmus — *including cornu, endometrium, myometrium, fundus*

182.1   Malignant neoplasm of isthmus — *narrow portion of the uterus between the cervix and the main body of the uterus.*

182.8   Malignant neoplasm of other specified sites of body of uterus — *including contiguous or overlapping sites*

183 MALIGNANT NEOPLASM OF OVARY AND OTHER UTERINE ADNEXA

The ovary is the female gonad and produces the ova. The organs are situated on either side of the uterus and lie near bilateral fallopian tubes, which carry the ova from the ovary to the uterus. Ligaments secure the female reproductive organs in the abdominal cavity.

Ovarian malignancies often present as an abdominal mass. Common types of ovarian malignancies include mucinous cystadenocarcinoma and endometrioid carcinoma. Other ovarian cancers are hormone producing and include Sertoli-Leydig cell tumors, adrenal cell rest tumors, granulosa-theca cell tumors. Use an additional code to report any functional activity associated with the ovarian malignancy. If the ovarian malignancy is bilateral, it is usually metastasized disease, rather than a primary malignancy.

This rubric excludes Douglas' cul-de-sac, reported with 158.8. If the malignancy is of contiguous or overlapping sites of ovary and uterine adnexa, report 183.8 *Malignant neoplasm of other specified sites of uterine adnexa.*

183.0   Malignant neoplasm of ovary — (Use additional code to identify any functional activity) — *female gonad*

183.2   Malignant neoplasm of fallopian tube — *oviduct, uterine tube*

183.3   Malignant neoplasm of broad ligament of uterus — *fold of peritoneum extending from the side of the uterus to the wall of the pelvis; mesovarium, parovarian region*

183.4   Malignant neoplasm of parametrium of uterus — *connective tissue between the uterus and the broad ligament; uterosacral ligament*

183.5   Malignant neoplasm of round ligament of uterus — *ligament between the uterus and the wall of the pelvis*

183.8   Malignant neoplasm of other specified sites of uterine adnexa — *including tubo-ovarian, utero-ovarian, or contiguous or overlapping sites of ovary and other uterine adnexa*

183.9   Malignant neoplasm of uterine adnexa, unspecified site — *unknown*

184 MALIGNANT NEOPLASM OF OTHER AND UNSPECIFIED FEMALE GENITAL ORGANS

Malignancies of external female genitalia and the vagina are classified to this rubric. If the malignancy affects both labia majora and labia minor, report 184.8 for contiguous or overlapping sites, rather than 184.4 for unspecified vulva.

M8700/3	Pheochromocytoma, malignant
M8710/3	Glomangiosarcoma
M8711/0	Glomus tumor
M8712/0	Glomangioma
M872-M879 Nevi and melanomas	
M8720/0	Pigmented nevus NOS
M8720/3	Malignant melanoma NOS
M8721/3	Nodular melanoma
M8722/0	Balloon cell nevus
M8722/3	Balloon cell melanoma
M8723/0	Halo nevus
M8724/0	Fibrous papule of the nose
M8725/0	Neuronevus
M8726/0	Magnocellular nevus
M8730/0	Nonpigmented nevus
M8730/3	Amelanotic melanoma
M8740/0	Junctional nevus
M8740/3	Malignant melanoma in junctional nevus
M8741/2	Precancerous melanosis NOS
M8741/3	Malignant melanoma in precancerous melanosis
M8742/2	Hutchinson's melanotic freckle
M8742/3	Malignant melanoma in Hutchinson's melanotic freckle
M8743/3	Superficial spreading melanoma
M8750/0	Intradermal nevus
M8760/0	Compound nevus
M8761/1	Giant pigmented nevus
M8761/3	Malignant melanoma in giant pigmented nevus
M8770/0	Epithelioid and spindle cell nevus
M8771/3	Epithelioid cell melanoma
M8772/3	Spindle cell melanoma NOS
M8773/3	Spindle cell melanoma, type A
M8774/3	Spindle cell melanoma, type B
M8775/3	Mixed epithelioid and spindle cell melanoma
M8780/0	Blue nevus NOS
M8780/3	Blue nevus, malignant
M8790/0	Cellular blue nevus

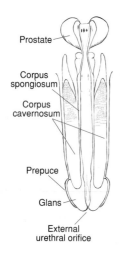

Prostate

Corpus
spongiosum

Corpus
cavernosum

Prepuce

Glans

External
urethral orifice

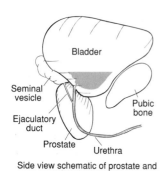

Bladder

Seminal
vesicle

Ejaculatory
duct

Prostate

Urethra

Pubic
bone

Side view schematic of prostate and
related structures

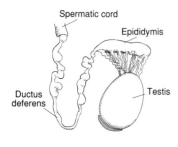

Spermatic cord

Epididymis

Ductus
deferens

Testis

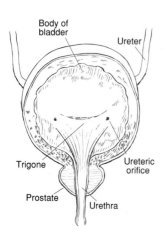

Body of
bladder

Ureter

Trigone

Ureteric
orifice

Prostate

Urethra

184.0 Malignant neoplasm of vagina — *including Gartner's duct, vaginal vault*

184.1 Malignant neoplasm of labia majora — *outer fold of skin and fat on either side of the vagina, including Bartholin's gland*

184.2 Malignant neoplasm of labia minora — *inner fold of skin between the labia major and the vagina*

184.3 Malignant neoplasm of clitoris — *clitoris*

184.4 Malignant neoplasm of vulva, unspecified site — *specific site in vulva unknown*

184.8 Malignant neoplasm of other specified sites of female genital organs — *Mullerian duct; contiguous or overlapping sites of female genital organs*

184.9 Malignant neoplasm of female genital organ, site unspecified — *unknown*

185 MALIGNANT NEOPLASM OF PROSTATE **OK**

The prostate is a singular, walnut-sized gland in the male. It surrounds the neck of the bladder and its ducts empty into the prostatic portion of the urethra. The prostate contributes fluid that helps to liquefy semen.

Adenocarcinoma of the prostate is the most common form of cancer in males older than 50 in the United States. Symptoms are uncommon until late in the disease course, when ureteral obstruction when hematuria may occur.

For cancer of the seminal vesicles, see 187.8 *Malignant neoplasm of other specified sites of male genital organs.*

186 MALIGNANT NEOPLASM OF TESTIS

The testes are a pair of male gonads found in the scrotum and produce spermatozoa for fertilization. Leydig cells in the testes produce testosterone.

Most testicular masses are malignant and testicular cancer is more common among males with a history of undescended testes, even if the condition has been corrected surgically. Testicular tumors rarely cause functional problems. If functional problems occur, however, use an additional code to report it.

186.0 Malignant neoplasm of undescended testis — (Use additional code to identify any functional activity) — *ectopic, retained*

186.9 Malignant neoplasm of other and unspecified testis — (Use additional code to identify any functional activity) — *descended, scrotal*

187 MALIGNANT NEOPLASM OF PENIS AND OTHER MALE GENITAL ORGANS

The penis has two functions in males: sexual and excretory. The urethra may convey semen, or urine. The tip of the penis is called the glans penis, and is covered in mucous membrane. The prepuce, or foreskin, is a fold of skin at the juncture where the body of the penis meets the glans penis; this extra skin is removed in circumcision. The corpora cavernosa are twin cylinders that extend the length of the organ called the body of the penis. Cancer of the penis usually occurs in uncircumcised males and human papillomavirus infection has been linked to penile cancer rates.

Report 187.8 *Malignant neoplasm of male genital organs* if the malignancy is of contiguous or overlapping sites of the penis or other male reproductive organs.

187.1 Malignant neoplasm of prepuce — *foreskin*

187.2 Malignant neoplasm of glans penis — *head, distal end*

✔5th Needs fifth-digit   **OK** Valid three-digit code

187.3 Malignant neoplasm of body of penis — *including corpus cavernosum, shaft*

187.4 Malignant neoplasm of penis, part unspecified — *including skin of penis not otherwise specified*

187.5 Malignant neoplasm of epididymis — *tube in which sperm is stored*

187.6 Malignant neoplasm of spermatic cord — *tube that carries sperm to the ejaculatory duct; vas deferens*

187.7 Malignant neoplasm of scrotum — *pouch of skin and muscle, but not the contents (testes)*

187.8 Malignant neoplasm of other specified sites of male genital organs — *including seminal vesicle, Mullerian duct, tunica vaginalis, and contiguous or overlapping sites of penis and other male genital organs*

187.9 Malignant neoplasm of male genital organ, site unspecified — *unknown*

188 MALIGNANT NEOPLASM OF BLADDER

The bladder lies in front (anterior) of the rectum in men and in front (anterior) of the vagina in women. As the bladder fills with urine, impulses from both voluntary and involuntary nerves signal that the bladder is full. When full, the bladder releases the urine it has stored through urination (voiding) via a tube called the urethra that connects the bladder floor to the outside of the body. Internal and external urinary muscle sphincters control the urine flow and stops the urine.

Malignant neoplasms of the bladder are classified by site. The dome of the bladder is the ceiling and the trigone is the triangular lower portion of the bladder bounded by the ureteral and urethral openings. Symptoms of malignant neoplasm of the bladder include hematuria, urinary urgency or frequency, or secondary infection at the tumor site. Pain or urinary retention may be present.

Males are twice as likely to develop bladder cancers as are females, and more than 90 percent of these cancers are transitional cell carcinomas. The most common site for cancer in the bladder is in the trigone.

If the malignancy is of contiguous and overlapping sites and the point of origin cannot be determined, report 188.8 *Malignant neoplasm of other specified sites of bladder.*

188.0 Malignant neoplasm of trigone of urinary bladder — *lower portion of the bladder, bounded by a triangle created by the points at which the urethra and two ureters attach to the bladder*

188.1 Malignant neoplasm of dome of urinary bladder — *top wall of the bladder*

188.2 Malignant neoplasm of lateral wall of urinary bladder — *side wall of the bladder*

188.3 Malignant neoplasm of anterior wall of urinary bladder — *front wall of the bladder*

188.4 Malignant neoplasm of posterior wall of urinary bladder — *back wall of the bladder*

188.5 Malignant neoplasm of bladder neck — *internal urethral orifice*

188.6 Malignant neoplasm of ureteric orifice — *bladder surrounding the ureter's opening*

188.7 Malignant neoplasm of urachus — *remnant of the fetal urinary tract*

188.8 Malignant neoplasm of other specified sites of bladder — *contiguous or overlapping sites of bladder*

188.9 Malignant neoplasm of bladder, part unspecified — *unknown*

M880 Soft tissue tumors and sarcomas NOS

M8800/0	Soft tissue tumor, benign
M8800/3	Sarcoma NOS
M8800/9	Sarcomatosis NOS
M8801/3	Spindle cell sarcoma
M8802/3	Giant cell sarcoma (except of bone M9250/3)
M8803/3	Small cell sarcoma
M8804/3	Epithelioid cell sarcoma

M881-M883 Fibromatous neoplasms

M8810/0	Fibroma NOS
M8810/3	Fibrosarcoma NOS
M8811/0	Fibromyxoma
M8811/3	Fibromyxosarcoma
M8812/0	Periosteal fibroma
M8812/3	Periosteal fibrosarcoma
M8813/0	Fascial fibroma
M8813/3	Fascial fibrosarcoma
M8814/3	Infantile fibrosarcoma
M8820/0	Elastofibroma
M8821/1	Aggressive fibromatosis
M8822/1	Abdominal fibromatosis
M8823/1	Desmoplastic fibroma
M8830/0	Fibrous histiocytoma NOS
M8830/1	Atypical fibrous histiocytoma
M8830/3	Fibrous histiocytoma, malignant
M8831/0	Fibroxanthoma NOS
M8831/1	Atypical fibroxanthoma
M8831/3	Fibroxanthoma, malignant
M8832/0	Dermatofibroma NOS
M8832/1	Dermatofibroma protuberans
M8832/3	Dermatofibrosarcoma NOS

M884 Myxomatous neoplasms

M8840/0	Myxoma NOS
M8840/3	Myxosarcoma

M885-M888 Lipomatous neoplasms

M8850/0	Lipoma NOS
M8850/3	Liposarcoma NOS
M8851/0	Fibrolipoma
M8851/3	Liposarcoma, well differentiated type
M8852/0	Fibromyxolipoma
M8852/3	Myxoid liposarcoma
M8853/3	Round cell liposarcoma
M8854/3	Pleomorphic liposarcoma

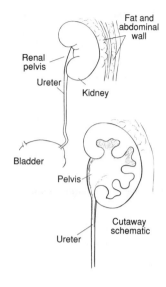

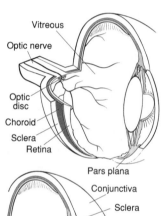

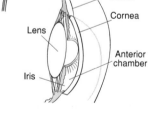

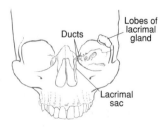

189 MALIGNANT NEOPLASM OF KIDNEY AND OTHER UNSPECIFIED URINARY ORGANS

The kidneys are paired organs between the parietal peritoneum and the posterior abdominal wall (retroperitoneal). They are located in the area of the last thoracic vertebrae to the third lumbar vertebrae.

Think of the kidneys as the body's blood filter. Items no longer needed are removed from the blood by the filter (kidneys) and eliminated in the form of urine, and elements needed are put back into the blood to be used by the cells and tissues of the body. Some of the blood the heart outputs with each cardiac cycle is sent to the kidneys to be filtered via two renal arteries (one to each kidney). In the kidneys the renal arteries drain into other small arteries, then into even smaller arterioles and capillary networks called glomerulus where filtration takes place. Once the blood has been filtered and cleaned in the kidneys, it goes through venous capillaries that change into small veins called venules. Venules drain into larger veins that finally drain into the renal veins. The renal veins return the blood that has been filtered to the heart via the inferior vena cava.

Cup-like projections in each of the kidneys, called the renal calyces, drain the urine. Urine that has collected in the renal pelvis is transported via a process called peristalsis to storage in the bladder. The ureters enter the bladder (one at each side) at its base (top) and deposit the urine they carry into the bladder. Each ureter includes a valve that prevents urine that has been placed into the bladder from backing up into the ureters and the renal pelvis.

Wilms' tumor is nephroblastoma, a childhood malignancy of the kidney and reported with 189.0. The tumor begins in utero and may be asymptomatic for years, though it is usually diagnosed before age 5.

189.0	Malignant neoplasm of kidney, except pelvis — *parenchyma, Wilms' tumor*
189.1	Malignant neoplasm of renal pelvis — *portal of the kidney from which the ureters collect urine; renal calyces, rreteropelvic junction*
189.2	Malignant neoplasm of ureter — *one of a pair of tubes that transport urine from the kidneys to the bladder*
189.3	Malignant neoplasm of urethra — *tube that eliminates urine from the bladder, and in males, serves as a genital duct*
189.4	Malignant neoplasm of paraurethral glands — *glands and ducts of the urethra*
189.8	Malignant neoplasm of other specified sites of urinary organs — *contiguous or overlapping sites of kidney and other urinary organs*
189.9	Malignant neoplasm of urinary organ, site unspecified — *unknown*

190-195 Malignant Neoplasm of Other and Unspecified Sites

Anatomical sites that don't fall under other rubrics are classified here for malignant neoplasms. Cancers of the eye, the brain, the central nervous system, and glands, as well as undefined locations are reported in this section of ICD-9.

Secondary malignant neoplasms are also reported in this section. Secondary malignancies are sites to which the primary cancer has spread. They are usually classified by anatomical site.

190 MALIGNANT NEOPLASM OF EYE

The eye is the organ of sight and has a complex physiology. The eyeball rests in fatty tissue in the bony orbit of the skull where it is protected from jarring actions. A malignant

▶5th   Needs fifth-digit   **OK**   Valid three-digit code

neoplasm of the orbit lies in these fatty and other tissues between the eyeball and the skull. The eyeball can be divided into several segments: the anterior segment, which includes the lens and all tissue anterior to the lens in the eyeball; and the posterior segment, which includes everything in the eyeball that is situated behind the lens. The eye is basically a fluid-filled ball. Intraocular pressure in the anterior segment of the eye is maintained through the flow of aqueous humor, or tears. The lacrimal system provides these tears and is also an agent in their disposal. Tears are produced in the lacrimal glands, located bilaterally behind the eyebrow, and the lacrimal ducts carry the tears to the eye or away from the eye to the nose. Pressure in the posterior segment of the eye is maintained by gel-like vitreous humor.

A thin, vascular, mucous membrane covers the inner eyelids and the white outer shell of the eye (sclera). This membrane is called the conjunctiva. The cornea is the bulging "window" through which we see, and the retina is the light-sensitive "viewing screen" at the back of the eye. The choroid is a vascular layer of the inside of the eyeball.

A congenital cancer that is usually detected before age 2, retinoblastoma is reported with 190.5 *Malignant neoplasm of retina*. Retinoblastoma is a malignancy of the retina and occurs bilaterally in 25 percent of patients with the disease.

If the malignant neoplasm is of the skin of the eyelid, it should be reported with codes for malignant neoplasm of the skin (172.1, 173.1). A malignancy of the optic nerve is reported with 192.0 *Malignant neoplasm of cranial nerves*, and of the orbital bone, 170.0 *Malignant neoplasm of skull and face, except mandible*. If the malignant neoplasm is of contiguous or overlapping parts of the eye, report 190.8 *Malignant neoplasm of other specified sites of eye*.

190.0	Malignant neoplasm of eyeball, except conjunctiva, cornea, retina, and choroid — *including ciliary body, sclera, lens, iris, uveal tract*
190.1	Malignant neoplasm of orbit — *tissue between the sclera of the eyeball and the orbital bone; retrobulbar tissue, extraocular muscle*
190.2	Malignant neoplasm of lacrimal gland — *tear-producing gland located behind the eyebrow; excludes lacrimal duct, sac*
190.3	Malignant neoplasm of conjunctiva — *mucous membrane lining the anterior eyeball and the inner aspect of the eyelid*
190.4	Malignant neoplasm of cornea — *clear dome that covers the anterior segment of the eye*
190.5	Malignant neoplasm of retina — *light-sensitive lining of the posterior segment of the eye*
190.6	Malignant neoplasm of choroid — *vascular layer of the globe of the eye*
190.7	Malignant neoplasm of lacrimal duct — *passage that carries tears to the eye and nose; lacrimal sac, nasolacrimal duct.*
190.8	Malignant neoplasm of other specified sites of eye — *contiguous or overlapping sites of eye*
190.9	Malignant neoplasm of eye, part unspecified — *unknown*

191 MALIGNANT NEOPLASM OF BRAIN

All brain tumors are "malignant" in that they may lead to death as they compromise the circulation of fluids in the brain through compression of obstruction. However, neoplasms classified to this rubric must also be of a metastasizing nature: a true malignancy. The incidences of benign and malignant neoplasms of the brain are about the same at 50 percent.

M8855/3	Mixed type liposarcoma
M8856/0	Intramuscular lipoma
M8857/0	Spindle cell lipoma
M8860/0	Angiomyolipoma
M8860/3	Angiomyoliposarcoma
M8861/0	Angiolipoma NOS
M8861/1	Angiolipoma, infiltrating
M8870/0	Myelolipoma
M8880/0	Hibernoma
M8881/0	Lipoblastomatosis

M889-M892 Myomatous neoplasms

M8890/0	Leiomyoma NOS
M8890/1	Intravascular leiomyomatosis
M8890/3	Leiomyosarcoma NOS
M8891/1	Epithelioid leiomyoma
M8891/3	Epithelioid leiomyosarcoma
M8892/1	Cellular leiomyoma
M8893/0	Bizarre leiomyoma
M8894/0	Angiomyoma
M8894/3	Angiomyosarcoma
M8895/0	Myoma
M8895/3	Myosarcoma
M8900/0	Rhabdomyoma NOS
M8900/3	Rhabdomyosarcoma NOS
M8901/3	Pleomorphic rhabdomyosarcoma
M8902/3	Mixed type rhabdomyosarcoma
M8903/0	Fetal rhabdomyoma
M8904/0	Adult rhabdomyoma
M8910/3	Embryonal rhabdomyosarcoma
M8920/3	Alveolar rhabdomyosarcoma

M893-M899 Complex mixed and stromal neoplasms

M8930/3	Endometrial stromal sarcoma
M8931/1	Endolymphatic stromal myosis
M8932/0	Adenomyoma
M8940/0	Pleomorphic adenoma
M8940/3	Mixed tumor, malignant NOS
M8950/3	Mullerian mixed tumor
M8951/3	Mesodermal mixed tumor
M8960/1	Mesoblastic nephroma
M8960/3	Nephroblastoma NOS
M8961/3	Epithelial nephroblastoma
M8962/3	Mesenchymal

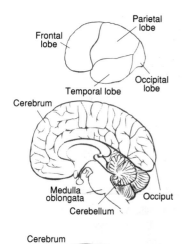

Frontal lobe
Parietal lobe
Occipital lobe
Temporal lobe
Cerebrum
Medulla oblongata
Occiput
Cerebellum

Cerebrum
Tentorium
Medulla
Cerebellum
Posterior fossa compartment (subtentorial)

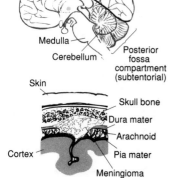

Skin
Skull bone
Dura mater
Arachnoid
Cortex
Pia mater
Meningioma

The tentorium is a dural sheath that divides the cranial cavity and supports the occipital lobes

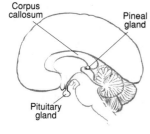

Corpus callosum
Pineal gland
Pituitary gland

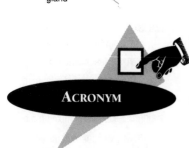

ACRONYM

MEN-II: multiple endocrine neoplasia, type II, also called Sipple's syndrome, is comprised of medullary carcinoma of the thyroid, pheochromocytoma, and hyperparathroidism.

Symptoms of a neoplasm of the brain include headache, seizures, personality changes, impaired mental or physical functions, or in children, an enlarged head. Use an additional code to report any manifestations associated with the malignancy.

Malignant neoplasms of the brain are classified according to location. Symptoms usually correspond to site. Malignant neoplasms of contiguous or overlapping sites in the brain are reported with 191.8. Do not use codes in this rubric to report cancers of the cranial nerves (192.0), of the retrobulbar area (190.1), or of the pituitary gland (194.3).

191.0	Malignant neoplasm of cerebrum, except lobes and ventricles — *including basal ganglia, globus pallidus; cerebral cortex; hypothalamus; corpus striatum; thalamus, cerebrum, internal capsule*
191.1	Malignant neoplasm of frontal lobe of brain — *frontal lobe*
191.2	Malignant neoplasm of temporal lobe of brain — *including hippocampus, uncus*
191.3	Malignant neoplasm of parietal lobe of brain — *parietal lobe*
191.4	Malignant neoplasm of occipital lobe of brain — *occipital lobe*
191.5	Malignant neoplasm of ventricles of brain — *including choroid plexus, floor of ventricle*
191.6	Malignant neoplasm of cerebellum NOS — *including cerebellopontine angle*
191.7	Malignant neoplasm of brain stem — *including cerebral peduncle, midbrain, medulla oblongata, pons, stem*
191.8	Malignant neoplasm of other parts of brain — *including corpus callosum, tapetum, and contiguous or overlapping sites of brain*
191.9	Malignant neoplasm of brain, unspecified site — *unknown*

192 MALIGNANT NEOPLASM OF OTHER AND UNSPECIFIED PARTS OF NERVOUS SYSTEM

Malignant neoplasms of the spine, meninges, cranial nerves, or sites unknown in the nervous system are classified in this rubric. Primary malignancies arising at these sites are much more rare than malignancies of the brain.

Report 192.8 *Malignant neoplasm of other specified sites of nervous system* if the neoplasm is of overlapping or contiguous sites of the nervous system. Peripheral, sympathetic or parasympathetic nerve malignancies are classified in rubric 171.

192.0	Malignant neoplasm of cranial nerves — *including olfactory bulb*
192.1	Malignant neoplasm of cerebral meninges — *including dura mater, falx, meninges, tentorium*
192.2	Malignant neoplasm of spinal cord — *including cauda equina*
192.3	Malignant neoplasm of spinal meninges — *lining of the spinal cord*
192.8	Malignant neoplasm of other specified sites of nervous system — *contiguous or overlapping sites of other parts of nervous system*
192.9	Malignant neoplasm of nervous system, part unspecified — *unknown*

193 MALIGNANT NEOPLASM OF THYROID GLAND **OK**

The thyroid gland is located just below the cricoid cartilage near the larynx and its purpose is to secrete thyroxine and triiodothyronine. Thyroxine and triiodothyronine increase the rate of cell metabolism.

Papillary adenocarcinoma accounts for 85 percent of thyroid cancers, and usually appears in young adults. Though the only symptom of thyroid cancer may be a palpable node, some patients with thyroid cancer present with symptoms of hyporthyroidism or

✓5th Needs fifth-digit   **OK** Valid three-digit code

hyperthyroidism. Use an additional code to report any functional activity associated with the malignancy.

194 MALIGNANT NEOPLASM OF OTHER ENDOCRINE GLANDS AND RELATED STRUCTURES

The parathyroid glands come in pairs — the superior and inferior pair — that are embedded in the posterior thyroid. The adrenal glands are situated above each kidney, and the pituitary gland is located in the sella turcica of the sphenoid bone. The pineal gland, located at the base of the corpus callosum, secretes melatonin; the carotid body, located in the fork of the carotid artery, monitors blood oxygen. The aortic body at the aortic arch and right subclavian artery regulates reflex respiration.

Malignancies of the endocrine glands can create functional activities in those glands. For example, adrenal tumors can cause virilizing or feminizing symptoms. Pituitary cancers can cause gigantism, Cushing's disease, amenorrhea or galactorrhea, or acromegaly. Report these functional activities in addition to the cancer.

Neuroblastoma is a common tumor of childhood that may affect the adrenal gland, retroperitoneum, central nervous system, or thoracic cavity. Usually seen in children under age 5, neuroblastomas present with a complex of symptoms according to the site of malignancy. A majority of the neuroblastomas arise in the adrenal gland. The ICD-9 index identifies 194.0 *Malignant neoplasm of adrenal gland* as the code for neuroblastoma for unspecified site. However, if a site other than adrenal gland is specified, consult the Neoplasm Table in ICD-9 for the correct code as classified by site.

194.0	Malignant neoplasm of adrenal gland — (Use additional code to identify any functional activity) — *including cortex, medulla, suprarenal gland*
194.1	Malignant neoplasm of parathyroid gland — (Use additional code to identify any functional activity) — *including superior and inferior*
194.3	Malignant neoplasm of pituitary gland and craniopharyngeal duct — (Use additional code to identify any functional activity) — *including craniobuccal pouch, Rathke's pouch, hypophysis, sella turcica*
194.4	Malignant neoplasm of pineal gland — (Use additional code to identify any functional activity) — *located at the base of the corpus callosum*
194.5	Malignant neoplasm of carotid body — (Use additional code to identify any functional activity) — *located at the fork in the carotid artery*
194.6	Malignant neoplasm of aortic body and other paraganglia — (Use additional code to identify any functional activity) — *located at aortic arch and right subclavian artery; including coccygeal body, para-aortic body, glomus jugulare*
194.8	Malignant neoplasm of other endocrine glands and related structures — (Use additional code to identify any functional activity) — *if the sites of multiple involvements are known, they should be coded separately.*
194.9	Malignant neoplasm of endocrine gland, site unspecified — (Use additional code to identify any functional activity) — *unknown*

195 MALIGNANT NEOPLASM OF OTHER AND ILL-DEFINED SITES

Use this rubric only as a last resort when the specific site of primary cancer cannot be identified or when the primary cancer has grown to invade two anatomic areas that would normally be reported with two codes and the point of origin cannot be determined.

	nephroblastoma
M8970/3	Hepatoblastoma
M8980/3	Carcinosarcoma NOS
M8981/3	Carcinosarcoma, embryonal type
M8982/0	Myoepithelioma
M8990/0	Mesenchymoma, benign
M8990/1	Mesenchymoma NOS
M8990/3	Mesenchymoma, malignant
M8991/3	Embryonal sarcoma

M900-M903 Fibroepithelial neoplasms

M9000/0	Brenner tumor NOS
M9000/1	Brenner tumor, borderline malignancy
M9000/3	Brenner tumor, malignant
M9010/0	Fibroadenoma NOS
M9011/0	Intracanalicular fibroadenoma NOS
M9012/0	Pericanalicular fibroadenoma
M9013/0	Adenofibroma NOS
M9014/0	Serous adenofibroma
M9015/0	Mucinous adenofibroma
M9020/0	Cellular intracanalicular fibroadenoma
M9020/1	Cystosarcoma phyllodes NOS
M9020/3	Cystosarcoma phyllodes, malignant
M9030/0	Juvenile fibroadenoma

M904 Synovial neoplasms

M9040/0	Synovioma, benign
M9040/3	Synovial sarcoma NOS
M9041/3	Synovial sarcoma, spindle cell type
M9042/3	Synovial sarcoma, epithelioid cell type
M9043/3	Synovial sarcoma, biphasic type
M9044/3	Clear cell sarcoma of tendons and aponeuroses

M905 Mesothelial neoplasms

M9050/0	Mesothelioma, benign
M9050/3	Mesothelioma, malignant
M9051/0	Fibrous mesothelioma, benign
M9051/3	Fibrous mesothelioma, malignant
M9052/0	Epithelioid mesothelioma, benign
M9052/3	Epithelioid mesothelioma,

195.0 Malignant neoplasm of head, face, and neck — *including cheek, jaw, nose, supraclavicular region*

195.1 Malignant neoplasm of thorax — *including axilla, chest wall, or intrathoracic region*

195.2 Malignant neoplasm of abdomen — *intrabdominal*

195.3 Malignant neoplasm of pelvis — *including groin; sacrococcygeal, inguinal, or presacral regions; rectovaginal or rectovesical septums; or overlapping sites*

195.4 Malignant neoplasm of upper limb — *including shoulder, arm, or hand*

195.5 Malignant neoplasm of lower limb — *including hip, leg. or foot*

195.8 Malignant neoplasm of other specified sites — *not elsewhere classified, including back and flank*

196-199 Secondary and Unspecified Malignant Neoplasms

All cancers shed cells into the patient's circulation. When these cells adhere to the vascular endothelium and begin to multiply into new tumors, the cancer is said to have metastasized. The new cancers are considered secondary malignancies, the primary malignancy being the "mother" site.

When a cancer recurs at the site of the original malignancy, it is still considered a primary malignancy and should not be reported with secondary malignancy codes. If the cancer recurs at a different site, these codes are appropriate, along with an additional code from the V10 rubric to identify a history of the malignancy of the primary site.

The secondary malignancy is sequenced first in coding if the patient is receiving treatment solely for the secondary malignancy. Otherwise, the code for the secondary site follows the code for the primary malignancy site.

196 SECONDARY AND UNSPECIFIED MALIGNANT NEOPLASM OF LYMPH NODES

Secondary malignancies are classified according to site in this rubric. Metastases of cancers to lymphatic sites are fairly common since lymphatic fluid circulates the body and is filtered in the lymph nodes. The primary cancer may near the affected lymph tissue or distant from it.

196.0 Secondary and unspecified malignant neoplasm of lymph nodes of head, face, and neck — *including cervicofacial, supraclavicular*

196.1 Secondary and unspecified malignant neoplasm of intrathoracic lymph nodes — *including bronchopulmonary, mediastinal, intercostal, tracheobronchial, intrathoracic, Virchow's*

196.2 Secondary and unspecified malignant neoplasm of intra-abdominal lymph nodes — *including aortic, intestinal, retroperitoneal, mesenteric,*

196.3 Secondary and unspecified malignant neoplasm of lymph nodes of axilla and upper limb — *including axillary, brachial, infraclavicular, epitrochlea, pectoral*

196.5 Secondary and unspecified malignant neoplasm of lymph nodes of inguinal region and lower limb — *including Cloquet, femoral, popliteal, groin, Rosenmueller's, tibial*

196.6 Secondary and unspecified malignant neoplasm of intrapelvic lymph nodes — *including hypogastric, obturator, iliac, parametrial*

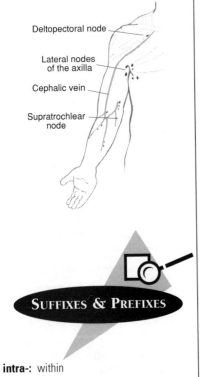

Deltopectoral node

Lateral nodes of the axilla

Cephalic vein

Supratrochlear node

SUFFIXES & PREFIXES

intra-: within

5th Needs fifth-digit   **OK** Valid three-digit code

196.8 Secondary and unspecified malignant neoplasm of lymph nodes of multiple sites — *including lymphatic channel or vessel not elsewhere classified*

196.9 Secondary and unspecified malignant neoplasm of lymph nodes, site unspecified — *unknown*

197 SECONDARY MALIGNANT NEOPLASM OF RESPIRATORY AND DIGESTIVE SYSTEMS

Secondary malignancies are classified according to site in this rubric. Report metastases to lymph nodes with codes from the rubric 196.

197.0 Secondary malignant neoplasm of lung — *including bronchus*

197.1 Secondary malignant neoplasm of mediastinum — *soft tissue between sternum and the spinal column, between the lungs*

197.2 Secondary malignant neoplasm of pleura — *lining of the lung*

197.3 Secondary malignant neoplasm of other respiratory organs — *including trachea*

197.4 Secondary malignant neoplasm of small intestine including duodenum — *duodenum, ilium, jejunum*

197.5 Secondary malignant neoplasm of large intestine and rectum — *colon, rectum*

197.6 Secondary malignant neoplasm of retroperitoneum and peritoneum — *mesentery, mesocolon, omentum, retroperitoneal tissue*

197.7 Secondary malignant neoplasm of liver — *liver, specified as secondary*

197.8 Secondary malignant neoplasm of other digestive organs and spleen — *including spleen, pancreas, gall bladder/duct, ampulla of Vater, sphincter of Oddi*

198 SECONDARY MALIGNANT NEOPLASM OF OTHER SPECIFIED SITES

Secondary malignancies are classified according to site in this rubric. Report metastases to lymph nodes with codes from the rubric 196.

198.0 Secondary malignant neoplasm of kidney — *including parenchyma, calyx, hilus, pelvis*

198.1 Secondary malignant neoplasm of other urinary organs — *including bladder, ureter, urethra, prostate utricle*

198.2 Secondary malignant neoplasm of skin — *including skin of breast and except genital*

198.3 Secondary malignant neoplasm of brain and spinal cord — *brain and spinal cord nerve root*

198.4 Secondary malignant neoplasm of other parts of nervous system — *including meninges, parasympathetic, sympathetic, peripheral nerves and ganglia*

198.5 Secondary malignant neoplasm of bone and bone marrow — *bone and associated cartilage or marrow*

198.6 Secondary malignant neoplasm of ovary — *female gonad*

198.7 Secondary malignant neoplasm of adrenal gland — *including suprarenal gland*

198.81 Secondary malignant neoplasm of breast — *male or female*

198.82 Secondary malignant neoplasm of genital organs — *including Mullerian duct, oviduct, cervical stump, endometrial stroma*

198.89 Secondary malignant neoplasm of other specified sites — *including pharynx, tongue, thyroid, salivary pituitary, connective tissue*

malignant

M9053/0 Mesothelioma, biphasic type, benign

M9053/3 Mesothelioma, biphasic type, malignant

M9054/0 Adenomatoid tumor NOS

M906-M909 Germ cell neoplasms

M9060/3 Dysgerminoma

M9061/3 Seminoma NOS

M9062/3 Seminoma, anaplastic type

M9063/3 Spermatocytic seminoma

M9064/3 Germinoma

M9070/3 Embryonal carcinoma NOS

M9071/3 Endodermal sinus tumor

M9072/3 Polyembryoma

M9073/1 Gonadoblastoma

M9080/0 Teratoma, benign

M9080/1 Teratoma NOS

M9080/3 Teratoma, malignant NOS

M9081/3 Teratocarcinoma

M9082/3 Malignant teratoma, undifferentiated type

M9083/3 Malignant teratoma, intermediate type

M9084/0 Dermoid cyst

M9084/3 Dermoid cyst with malignant transformation

M9090/0 Struma ovarii NOS

M9090/3 Struma ovarii, malignant

M9091/1 Strumal carcinoid

M910 Trophoblastic neoplasms

M9100/0 Hydatidiform mole NOS

M9100/1 Invasive hydatidiform mole

M9100/3 Choriocarcinoma

M9101/3 Choriocarcinoma combined with teratoma

M9102/3 Malignant teratoma, trophoblastic

M911 Mesonephromas

M9110/0 Mesonephroma, benign

M9110/1 Mesonephric tumor

M9110/3 Mesonephroma, malignant

M9111/1 Endosalpingioma

M912-M916 Blood vessel tumors

M9120/0 Hemangioma NOS

M9120/3 Hemangiosarcoma

M9121/0 Cavernous hemangioma

M9122/0 Venous hemangioma

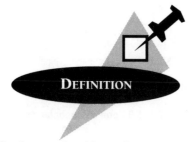

DEFINITION

Carcinomatosis: widespread dissemination of carcinoma in several sites.

Disseminated: widely scattered.

Generalized: involving the whole organ.

Hodgkin's
granuloma: granular, inflammatory lesions in the lymph nodes

paragranuloma: a neoplasm resembling, but different than a granuloma

sarcoma: a neoplasm in the connective tissue

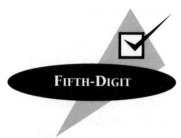

FIFTH-DIGIT

The following fifth-digit subclassification is for use with categories 200-202:

0 unspecified site, extranodal and solid organ sites

1 lymph nodes of head, face, and neck

2 intrathoracic lymph nodes

3 intra-abdominal lymph nodes

4 lymph nodes of axilla and upper limb

5 lymph nodes of inguinal region and lower limb

6 intrapelvic lymph nodes

7 spleen

8 lymph nodes of multiple sites

199 MALIGNANT NEOPLASM WITHOUT SPECIFICATION OF SITE

Secondary malignancies in this rubric are general, though they do have some specific uses. Up to 7 percent of cancer patients are diagnosed with a secondary malignancy for which the primary site cannot be found (e.g., UPO (unknown primary origin)). In these cases, report the secondary malignancy first, followed by 199.1 *Malignant neoplasm of unspecified site* to report the unknown primary site. In cases where laboratory results indicate metastases to an unknown site, report the secondary malignancy with the same code, 199.1. In ICD-10, separate codes have been created to report secondary and primary malignant neoplasms of unknown sites.

199.0 Disseminated malignant neoplasm — *carcinomatosis, multiple in unspecified site*

199.1 Other malignant neoplasm of unspecified site — *unspecified primary or secondary site; Eaton-Lambert syndrome*

200-208 Malignant Neoplasm of Lymphatic and Hematopoietic Tissue

Malignant neoplasms of the lymphatic and hematopoietic tissues are considered primary neoplasms and do not spread to secondary sites. The malignant cells circulate to other areas through the lymphatic or blood systems.

Cancers of the lymphatic sytem are called lymphomas and they are more common after age 50. They occur most frequently in the groin (inguinal), neck (cervical), and armpit (axillary) nodes.

Some of the types of neoplasms that are included in this section are lymphosarcomas, Hodgkin's disease, lymphomas, malignant histyocytosis, multiple myeloma, myeloid leukemia, acute leukemia, and chronic leukemia. These diseases are classified by type, by site, and in some cases, by status of remission or chronic or acute phase.

Do not use codes in this series to report secondary or unspecified lymph node malignancies, secondary bone marrow malignancies, or spleen cancer.

If the encounter is solely for the purpose of chemotherapy, the V code for chemotherapy (V58.1) should be sequenced first, and the malignancy sequenced secondarily.

200 LYMPHOSARCOMA AND RETICULOSARCOMA

Lymphosarcoma is a form on non-Hodgkin's lymphoma in which the cells are either a small or large lymphocyte.

Reticulosarcoma (200.1) along with reticulum cell carcoma and histiocytic sarcoma is a form of non-Hodgkin's lymphoma derived from the histiocyte, a macrophage present in connective tissue.

Burkitt's tumor or lymphoma is a form of non-Hodgkin's lymphoma characterized by an undifferentiated B-cell tumor. There are two variants: endemic (African) and sporadic. The endemic variant is associated with Epstein-Barr virus infection and has a variable diagnosis. The sporadic variant has a very poor prognosis. Jaw and orbital involvement is typical in endemic Burkitt's lymphoma and abdominal disease predominates in sporadic Burkitt's lymphoma.

✔5th   Needs fifth-digit   **OK**   Valid three-digit code

200.0 ✔5th Reticulosarcoma — *reticulum cell sarcoma; pleomorphic cell type*
200.1 ✔5th Lymphosarcoma — *lymphoblastoma, prolymphocytic*
200.2 ✔5th Burkitt's tumor or lymphoma — *malignant lymphoma*
200.8 ✔5th Other named variants of lymphosarcoma and reticulosarcoma — *mixed cell type; reticulolymphosarcoma; lymphoplasmacytoid*

201 HODGKIN'S DISEASE

Hodgkin's disease is the most common type of lymphoma, and most commonly affects young and middle-aged adults. Hodgkin's disease is a painless, progressive replacement of lymph nodes, spleen, and other lymphatic tissue with tumor tissue consisting of atypical histiocytes together with lymphocytes, eosinophils, plasma cells and fibrous tissue. In Hodgkin's lymphoma, Reed-Sternberg cells are present.

201.0 ✔5th Hodgkin's paragranuloma
201.1 ✔5th Hodgkin's granuloma
201.2 ✔5th Hodgkin's sarcoma
201.4 ✔5th Hodgkin's disease, lymphocytic-histiocytic predominance
201.5 ✔5th Hodgkin's disease, nodular sclerosis — *cellular phase*
201.6 ✔5th Hodgkin's disease, mixed cellularity — *mixed cellularity*
201.7 ✔5th Hodgkin's disease, lymphocytic depletion — *lymphocytic depletion; diffuse fibrosis;reticular type*
201.9 ✔5th Hodgkin's disease, unspecified type — *Paltauf-Sternberg disease*

202 OTHER MALIGNANT NEOPLASMS OF LYMPHOID AND HISTIOCYTIC TISSUE

Nodular lymphoma is a non-Hodgkin's lymphoma in which lymphoma cells are clustered into identifiable nodules or follicles, and malignant histiocytosis presents with progressive, abnormal histiocytes in the blood. Mycosis fungoides is an uncommon, chronic T cell lymphoma affecting the skin and sometimes internal organs, usually in patients 50 years or older. T cell lymphoma often appears as a rash and goes undiagnosed for a period. Sezary disease is an extension of mucosis fungoides that affects the blood. Leukemic reticuloendotheliosis is a chronic leukemia with preponderance of large, mononuclear cells with hairy appearance in the marrow, spleen, liver, and blood. In Letterer-Siwe disease, reticuloendotheliosis occurs in early childhood and presents with skin eruptions, anemia, and enlarged liver, spleen, and lymph nodes.

202.0 ✔5th Nodular lymphoma — *Brill-Symmers disease; lymphosarcoma; reticulosarcoma*
202.1 ✔5th Mycosis fungoides — *cutaneous T-cell lymphoma*
202.2 ✔5th Sezary's disease — *mycosis fungoides infecting blood*
202.3 ✔5th Malignant histiocytosis — *histiocytic medullary reticulosis; malignant reticuloendotheliosis/reticulosis*
202.4 ✔5th Leukemic reticuloendotheliosis — *hairy cell leukemia*
202.5 ✔5th Letterer-Siwe disease — *acute differentiated progressive histiocytosis; histiocytosis X; infantile reticuloendotheliosis*
202.6 ✔5th Malignant mast cell tumors — *mast cell sarcoma; mastocytoma;; mastocytosis*
202.8 ✔5th Other malignant lymphomas — *NOS, diffuse*
202.9 ✔5th Other and unspecified malignant neoplasms of lymphoid and histiocytic tissue — *including malignant neoplasm of bone marrow NOS*

203 MULTIPLE MYELOMA AND IMMUNOPROLIFERATIVE NEOPLASMS

Multiple myeloma is an uncontrolled proliferation of plasma cells and results in a number of organ dysfunctions and symptoms of bone pain or fracture, renal failure, infection, anemia, hypercalcemia, as well as clotting, neurologic, or vascular abnormalities. When a patient with multiple myelomas develops a complication from the disease, the complication

M9123/0	Racemose hemangioma
M9124/3	Kupffer cell sarcoma
M9130/0	Hemangioendothelioma, benign
M9130/1	Hemangioendothelioma NOS
M9130/3	Hemangioendothelioma, malignant
M9131/0	Capillary hemangioma
M9132/0	Intramuscular hemangioma
M9140/3	Kaposi's sarcoma
M9141/0	Angiokeratoma
M9142/0	Verrucous keratotic hemangioma
M9150/0	Hemangiopericytoma, benign
M9150/1	Hemangiopericytoma NOS
M9150/3	Hemangiopericytoma, malignant
M9160/0	Angiofibroma NOS
M9161/1	Hemangioblastoma

M917 Lymphatic vessel tumors

M9170/0	Lymphangioma NOS
M9170/3	Lymphangiosarcoma
M9171/0	Capillary lymphangioma
M9172/0	Cavernous lymphangioma
M9173/0	Cystic lymphangioma
M9174/0	Lymphangiomyoma
M9174/1	Lymphangiomyomatosis
M9175/0	Hemolymphangioma

M918-M920 Osteomas and osteosarcomas

M9180/0	Osteoma NOS
M9180/3	Osteosarcoma NOS
M9181/3	Chondroblastic osteosarcoma
M9182/3	Fibroblastic osteosarcoma
M9183/3	Telangiectatic osteosarcoma
M9184/3	Osteosarcoma in Paget's disease of bone
M9190/3	Juxtacortical osteosarcoma
M9191/0	Osteoid osteoma NOS
M9200/0	Osteoblastoma

M921-M924 Chondromatous neoplasms

M9210/0	Osteochondroma
M9210/1	Osteochondromatosis NOS
M9220/0	Chondroma NOS
M9220/1	Chondromatosis NOS
M9220/3	Chondrosarcoma NOS

is generally sequenced first, followed by the myeloma. For example, if a patient with multiple myeloma sustains a stress fracture of the femur, the codes would be sequenced:

733.14 Pathologic fracture of the neck of femur
203.00 Multiple myeloma without mention of remission

Multiple myeloma is often described as metastatic to the bone, but because this is part of the disease, the bone metastases should not be reported separately as a secondary malignant neoplasm.

203.0 ✔5th Multiple myeloma — *Kahler's disease; myelomatosis*
203.1 ✔5th Plasma cell leukemia — *plasmacytic leukemia*
203.8 ✔5th Other immunoproliferative neoplasms — *other immunoproliferative neoplasms*

204 LYMPHOID LEUKEMIA

Lymphoid leukemia is a malignant proliferation of immature lymphocytes called lymphoblasts. The acute condition is common in children and fatal if untreated. The chronic conditions is a generalized, progressive form of lymphocytic leukemia predominantly affecting men over the age of 50. It is the least malignant form of leukemia.

204.0 ✔5th Acute lymphoid leukemia — *lymphoblastic, usually in childhood*
204.1 ✔5th Chronic lymphoid leukemia — *lymphoblastic, more mature, usually in middle/old age*
204.2 ✔5th Subacute lymphoid leukemia — *subacute*
204.8 ✔5th Other lymphoid leukemia — *aleukemic leukemia*
204.9 ✔5th Unspecified lymphoid leukemia — *unknown*

205 MYELOID LEUKEMIA

Myeloid leukemia is a rapid and malignant proliferation of immature myelocytes called myeloblasts. The acute condition is common in children and fatal if untreated. The chronic condition is a fatal disease characterized by abnormal proliferation of premature granulocytes called myeloblasts, promyelocytes, metamyelocytes, and myelocytes, in bone marrow, peripheral blood, and body tissues.

When a patient has an acute exacerbation of chronic myelogenous leukemia with blastic transformation, assign 205.10 *Chronic myeloid leukemia, without mention of remission* since the acute/blastic exacerbation is included in the code for chronic leukemia. The "acute" designation in this rubric is reserved for acute promyelocytic leukemia.

205.0 ✔5th Acute myeloid leukemia — *acute promyelocytic; differentiated cell populations*
205.1 ✔5th Chronic myeloid leukemia — *more granulocytic cells; usually in young adults, eosinophilic/neutrophilic*
205.2 ✔5th Subacute myeloid leukemia — *subacute*
205.3 ✔5th Myeloid sarcoma — *chloroma, granulocytic carcoma, green malignancy airising from bone marrow*
205.8 ✔5th Other myeloid leukemia — *aleukemic*
205.9 ✔5th Unspecified myeloid leukemia — *unknown*

206 MONOCYTIC LEUKEMIA

When a patient has an acute exacerbation of chronic monocytic leukemia, assign 206.10 Chronic monocytic leukemia, without mention of remission since the acute exacerbation is included in the code for chronic leukemia. The "acute" designation in this rubric is

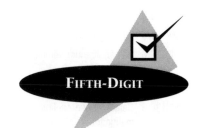

FIFTH-DIGIT

The following fifth-digit subclassification is for use with categories 203, 204, 205, 206, 207, and 208:

0 without mention of remission

1 in remission

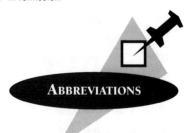

ABBREVIATIONS

ALL: acute lymphocytic leukemia, lymphoblastic leukemia with undifferentiated cell populations

AML: acute myelogenous leukemia, myeloid leukemia with undifferentiated cell populations

CLL: chronic lymphocytic leukemia, lymphoblastic leukemia with more mature lymphocytes in the blood, bone marrow, and lymphoid organs

CML: chronic myelogenous leukemia, myeloid leukemia with more granulocytic cells of all stages in the blood, bone marrow, liver, and spleen

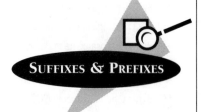

SUFFIXES & PREFIXES

-blastic: an immature cell

-cytic: cell

-genous: originating, producing

-oid: resembling

lymph-: a fluid in the lymphatic system

✔5th Needs fifth-digit　　**OK** Valid three-digit code

reserved for an uncommon form of myelogenous leukemia with monocytes as predominant cells.

206.0 ✓5th Acute monocytic leukemia — *uncommon; monocytes as predominant cells*
206.1 ✓5th Chronic monocytic leukemia — *chronic*
206.2 ✓5th Subacute monocytic leukemia — *subacute*
206.8 ✓5th Other monocytic leukemia — *aleukemic*
206.9 ✓5th Unspecified monocytic leukemia — *unknown, including Schilling-type*

207 OTHER SPECIFIED LEUKEMIA

This rubric is reserved for several leukemias that do not classify to the other rubrics. Leukemias of unspecified cell types are classified to rubric 208.

207.0 ✓5th Acute erythremia and erythroleukemia — *acute erythremic myelosis; Di Guglielmo's disease; erythremic myelosis*
207.1 ✓5th Chronic erythremia — *including Heilmeyer-Schöner disease*
207.2 ✓5th Megakaryocytic leukemia — *megakaryocytic myelosis; thrombocytic leukemia*
207.8 ✓5th Other specified leukemia — *including lymphosarcoma cell leukemia*

208 LEUKEMIA OF UNSPECIFIED CELL TYPE

Use these leukemia codes when documentation does not provide sufficient information or when the patient's specific diagnosis has not yet been established although leukemia is certain.

208.0 ✓5th Acute leukemia of unspecified cell type — *acute leukemia NOS; stem cell leukemia; blast cell leukemia*
208.1 ✓5th Chronic leukemia of unspecified cell type — *not otherwise specified*
208.2 ✓5th Subacute leukemia of unspecified cell type — *not otherwise specified*
208.8 ✓5th Other leukemia of unspecified cell type — *other leukemia of unspecified cell type*
208.9 ✓5th Unspecified leukemia — *unknown; Bennett's disease*

210-212 Benign Neoplasms of Digestive and Respiratory System and Intrathoracic Organs

Benign neoplasms are tumors characterized by dividing cells that adhere to each other, so that the mass remains a circumscribed lesion. Benign neoplasms are classified according to site. Many cysts and embryonic cysts are excluded from this classification.

Benign neoplasms of the digestive system are classified by site in these rubrics. The margin of the anus is excluded from this rubric and would be reported with 216.5 *Benign neoplasm of skin of trunk, except scrotum.*

210 BENIGN NEOPLASM OF LIP, ORAL CAVITY, AND PHARYNX

Neoplasms are classified by site in this rubric. Excluded from this rubric are cysts, ranulas, and radicular cysts.

210.0 Benign neoplasm of lip — *frenulum labii, inner aspect, mucosa*
210.1 Benign neoplasm of tongue — *including lingual tonsil*
210.2 Benign neoplasm of major salivary glands — *parotid, sublingual, submandibular; Warthin's tumor*
210.3 Benign neoplasm of floor of mouth — *floor of mouth*
210.4 Benign neoplasm of other and unspecified parts of mouth — *including gingiva, oral mucosa, palate, uvula, labial commissure*

M9221/0 Juxtacortical chondroma
M9221/3 Juxtacortical chondrosarcoma
M9230/0 Chondroblastoma NOS
M9230/3 Chondroblastoma, malignant
M9240/3 Mesenchymal chondrosarcoma
M9241/0 Chondromyxoid fibroma

M925 Giant cell tumors
M9250/1 Giant cell tumor of bone NOS
M9250/3 Giant cell tumor of bone, malignant
M9251/1 Giant cell tumor of soft parts NOS
M9251/3 Malignant giant cell tumor of soft parts

M926 Miscellaneous bone tumors
M9260/3 Ewing's sarcoma
M9261/3 Adamantinoma of long bones
M9262/0 Ossifying fibroma

M927-M934 Odontogenic tumors
M9270/0 Odontogenic tumor, benign
M9270/1 Odontogenic tumor NOS
M9270/3 Odontogenic tumor, malignant
M9271/0 Dentinoma
M9272/0 Cementoma NOS
M9273/0 Cementoblastoma, benign
M9274/0 Cementifying fibroma
M9275/0 Gigantiform cementoma
M9280/0 Odontoma NOS
M9281/0 Compound odontoma
M9282/0 Complex odontoma
M9290/0 Ameloblastic fibro-odontoma
M9290/3 Ameloblastic odontosarcoma
M9300/0 Adenomatoid odontogenic tumor
M9301/0 Calcifying odontogenic cyst
M9310/0 Ameloblastoma NOS
M9310/3 Ameloblastoma, malignant
M9311/0 Odontoameloblastoma
M9312/0 Squamous odontogenic tumor
M9320/0 Odontogenic myxoma
M9321/0 Odontogenic fibroma NOS
M9330/0 Ameloblastic fibroma
M9330/3 Ameloblastic fibrosarcoma

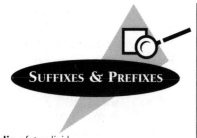

-lip-: fat or lipid

-oma: a tumor or neoplasm

angio-: pertaining to blood or lymph vessels

fibro-: fiber

myelo-: bone marrow, spinal cord, or the sheath of nerve fibers

myxo-: mucous

210.5	Benign neoplasm of tonsil — *faucial, palatine*
210.6	Benign neoplasm of other parts of oropharynx — *including mesopharynx, tonsillar fossa/pillars, vallecula, brachial cleft, anterior epiglottis*
210.7	Benign neoplasm of nasopharynx — *including adenoid, pharyngeal tonsil, posterior nasal septum, choana*
210.8	Benign neoplasm of hypopharynx — *including arytenoid fold, pyriform fossa, postcricoid region, laryngopharynx*
210.9	Benign neoplasm of pharynx, unspecified — *site specified only a "throat"*

211 BENIGN NEOPLASM OF OTHER PARTS OF DIGESTIVE SYSTEM

Neoplasms are classified by site in this rubric.

211.0	Benign neoplasm of esophagus — *esophagus*
211.1	Benign neoplasm of stomach — *cardia, body, fundus, pylorus*
211.2	Benign neoplasm of duodenum, jejunum, and ileum — *small intestine*
211.3	Benign neoplasm of colon — *large intestine, appendix, cecum, ileocecal valve, Cronkhite-Canada syndrome*
211.4	Benign neoplasm of rectum and anal canal — *anal canal, sphincter, rectosigmoid junction*
211.5	Benign neoplasm of liver and biliary passages — *ampulla of Vater, gallbladder, sphincter of Oddi, hepatic or cystic or common bile duct*
211.6	Benign neoplasm of pancreas, except islets of Langerhans — *head, tail, or body, except insulin-producing cells*
211.7	Benign neoplasm of islets of Langerhans — (Use additional code to identify any functional activity) — *insulin producing cells*
211.8	Benign neoplasm of retroperitoneum and peritoneum — *mesentery, mesoappendix, mesocolon, omentum, retroperitoneal tissue*
211.9	Benign neoplasm of other and unspecified site of the digestive system — *including spleen and generalized sites*

212 BENIGN NEOPLASM OF RESPIRATORY AND INTRATHORACIC ORGANS

Neoplasms are classified by site in this rubric. Classify thoracic or intrathoracic benign neoplasms, not otherwise specified to 229.8.

212.0	Benign neoplasm of nasal cavities, middle ear, and accessory sinuses — *including sinus, eustachian tube, septum, nasal cartilage*
212.1	Benign neoplasm of larynx — *vocal cords including laryngeal cartilage, suprahyoid epiglottis, glottis*
212.2	Benign neoplasm of trachea
212.3	Benign neoplasm of bronchus and lung — *including carina, hilus*
212.4	Benign neoplasm of pleura — *membrane surrounding lung*
212.5	Benign neoplasm of mediastinum — *thoracic soft tissue not elsewhere classified*
212.6	Benign neoplasm of thymus — *lymphoid tissue in upper, anterior mediastinum*
212.7	Benign neoplasm of heart — *including myocardium, pericardium, endocardium*
212.8	Benign neoplasm of other specified sites of respiratory and intrathoracic organs — *not elsewhere classified*
212.9	Benign neoplasm of respiratory and intrathoracic organs, site unspecified — *unknown*

213-215 Benign Neoplasms of Bone, Connective, and Soft Tissues

Neoplasms are classified by type (benign or lipoma) and by site in this rubric.

213 BENIGN NEOPLASM OF BONE AND ARTICULAR CARTILAGE

Bone and cartilage are not differentiated in this rubric. Code selection is based on anatomic site. Benign neoplasms for some cartilage sites are classified elsewhere: ear, eyelid, nose (212.0), larynx (212.1), synovia (215.0-215.9), and exostosis NOS (726.91).

213.0 Benign neoplasm of bones of skull and face — *including cranial bone, turbinates, orbit, patella*

213.1 Benign neoplasm of lower jaw bone — *including mandible*

213.2 Benign neoplasm of vertebral column, excluding sacrum and coccyx — *including intervertebral cartilage or disc*

213.3 Benign neoplasm of ribs, sternum, and clavicle — *including xiphoid process, costal cartilage*

213.4 Benign neoplasm of scapula and long bones of upper limb — *including long bones, upper extremity*

213.5 Benign neoplasm of short bones of upper limb — *including short bones, upper extremity*

213.6 Benign neoplasm of pelvic bones, sacrum, and coccyx — *including acetabulum, cuboid*

213.7 Benign neoplasm of long bones of lower limb — *including long bones, lower extremity*

213.8 Benign neoplasm of short bones of lower limb — *including short bones, lower extremity*

213.9 Benign neoplasm of bone and articular cartilage, site unspecified — *unknown*

214 LIPOMA

A lipoma is a soft nodule of fat that can occur subcutaneously or in any organ system. Treatment is not usually required, unless the lipoma is causing discomfort or compression. Other words used to describe lipomas are angiolipoma, fibrolipoma, hibernoma, myelolipoma, and myxolipoma. Lipomas are classified by site.

214.0 Lipoma of skin and subcutaneous tissue of face — *also called angiolipoma, fibrolipoma, hibernoma, or myelolipoma*

214.1 Lipoma of other skin and subcutaneous tissue — *excluding face*

214.2 Lipoma of intrathoracic organs — *including intrathoracic, mediastinum, thymus*

214.3 Lipoma of intra-abdominal organs — *including peritoneum, retroperitoneum, stomach, kidney*

214.4 Lipoma of spermatic cord — *also called angiolipoma, fibrolipoma, hibernoma, or myelolipoma*

214.8 Lipoma of other specified sites — *not elsewhere classified, including muscle*

214.9 Lipoma of unspecified site — *unknown*

215 OTHER BENIGN NEOPLASM OF CONNECTIVE AND OTHER SOFT TISSUE

Soft tissue includes blood vessel, bursa, fascia, ligament, muscle, peripheral, sympathetic, or parasympathetic nerve and ganglia, synovia, and tendon. Classify benign neoplasm of cartilage to rubric 212 or 213, and of breast to 217. Classify connective tissue of internal organs to the appropriate organ, except for hemangioma, or lipoma.

M9340/0 Calcifying epithelial odontogenic tumor

M935-M937 Miscellaneous tumors

M9350/1 Craniopharyngioma

M9360/1 Pinealoma

M9361/1 Pineocytoma

M9362/3 Pineoblastoma

M9363/0 Melanotic neuroectodermal tumor

M9370/3 Chordoma

M938-M948 Gliomas

M9380/3 Glioma, malignant

M9381/3 Gliomatosis cerebri

M9382/3 Mixed glioma

M9383/1 Subependymal glioma

M9384/1 Subependymal giant cell astrocytoma

M9390/0 Choroid plexus papilloma NOS

M9390/3 Choroid plexus papilloma, malignant

M9391/3 Ependymoma NOS

M9392/3 Ependymoma, anaplastic type

M9393/1 Papillary ependymoma

M9394/1 Myxopapillary ependymoma

M9400/3 Astrocytoma NOS

M9401/3 Astrocytoma, anaplastic type

M9410/3 Protoplasmic astrocytoma

M9411/3 Gemistocytic astrocytoma

M9420/3 Fibrillary astrocytoma

M9421/3 Pilocytic astrocytoma

M9422/3 Spongioblastoma NOS

M9423/3 Spongioblastoma polare

M9430/3 Astroblastoma

M9440/3 Glioblastoma NOS

M9441/3 Giant cell glioblastoma

M9442/3 Glioblastoma with sarcomatous component

M9443/3 Primitive polar spongioblastoma

M9450/3 Oligodendroglioma NOS

M9451/3 Oligodendroglioma, anaplastic type

M9460/3 Oligodendroblastoma

M9470/3 Medulloblastoma NOS

M9471/3 Desmoplastic medulloblastoma

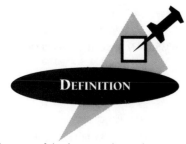

DEFINITION

Intramural: benign, smooth muscle tumor within the wall of the uterus.

Submucous: benign, smooth muscle tumor beneath the lining of the uterus.

Subserous: benign, smooth muscle tumor beneath the serous membrane of the uterus.

Uterine leiomyoma: also referred to as fibroids.

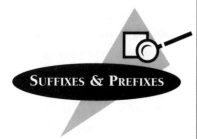

SUFFIXES & PREFIXES

-cyst-: a sac

dermato-: pertaining to the skin

fibro-: fiber

hydro-: water or hydrogen

syring-: tube-shaped

215.0 Other benign neoplasm of connective and other soft tissue of head, face, and neck — *including blood vessel, bursa, fascia, ligament, muscle, or peripheral, sympathetic, and parasympathetic nerve*

215.2 Other benign neoplasm of connective and other soft tissue of upper limb, including shoulder — *including blood vessel, bursa, fascia, ligament, muscle, or peripheral, sympathetic, and parasympathetic nerve*

215.3 Other benign neoplasm of connective and other soft tissue of lower limb, including hip — *including blood vessel, bursa, fascia, ligament, muscle, or peripheral, sympathetic, and parasympathetic nerve*

215.4 Other benign neoplasm of connective and other soft tissue of thorax — *including blood vessel, bursa, fascia, ligament, muscle, or sympathetic and parasympathetic nerve*

215.5 Other benign neoplasm of connective and other soft tissue of abdomen — *including blood vessel, bursa, fascia, ligament, muscle, or sympathetic and parasympathetic nerve*

215.6 Other benign neoplasm of connective and other soft tissue of pelvis — *including blood vessel, bursa, fascia, ligament, muscle, or sympathetic and parasympathetic nerve*

215.7 Other benign neoplasm of connective and other soft tissue of trunk, unspecified — *including blood vessel, bursa, fascia, ligament, muscle, or sympathetic and parasympathetic nerve*

215.8 Other benign neoplasm of connective and other soft tissue of other specified sites — *not elsewhere classified*

215.9 Other benign neoplasm of connective and other soft tissue of unspecified site — *unknown*

216-217 Benign Neoplasms of Integumentary System

216 BENIGN NEOPLASM OF SKIN
Codes in this rubric report such benign neoplasms as blue nevus, dermatofibroma, hydrocystoma, pigmented nevus, syringoadenoma, and syringoma.

216.0 Benign neoplasm of skin of lip — *including blue nevus, pigmented nevus, dermatofibroma, syringoadenoma, hydrocystoma*

216.1 Benign neoplasm of eyelid, including canthus — *including blue nevus, pigmented nevus, dermatofibroma, syringoadenoma, hydrocystoma*

216.2 Benign neoplasm of ear and external auditory canal — *including blue nevus, pigmented nevus, dermatofibroma, syringoadenoma, hydrocystoma*

216.3 Benign neoplasm of skin of other and unspecified parts of face — *including blue nevus, pigmented nevus, dermatofibroma, syringoadenoma, hydrocystoma*

216.4 Benign neoplasm of scalp and skin of neck — *including blue nevus, pigmented nevus, dermatofibroma, syringoadenoma, hydrocystoma*

216.5 Benign neoplasm of skin of trunk, except scrotum — *including blue nevus, pigmented nevus, dermatofibroma, syringoadenoma, hydrocystoma*

216.6 Benign neoplasm of skin of upper limb, including shoulder — *including blue nevus, pigmented nevus, dermatofibroma, syringoadenoma, hydrocystoma*

216.7 Benign neoplasm of skin of lower limb, including hip — *including blue nevus, pigmented nevus, dermatofibroma, syringoadenoma, hydrocystoma*

216.8 Benign neoplasm of other specified sites of skin — *not elsewhere classified*

216.9 Benign neoplasm of skin, site unspecified — *unknown*

217 BENIGN NEOPLASM OF BREAST `OK`
Benign neoplasms of the connective, glandular, or soft parts of the male or female breast are classified to this rubric.

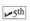

However, adenofibrosis of the breast is reported with 610.2 *Fibroadenosis of breast* and benign cyst of the breast is reported with 610.0 *Solitary cysts of breast*. Fibrocystic disease is reported with 610.1 *Diffuse cystic mastopathy* and benign lesion of the skin of the breast with 216.5 *Benign neoplasm of skin of trunk, except scrotum*. Consult your ICD-9 index for more information.

In ICD-10, there are more than 30 choices for describing benign conditions of the breast, including cystic myopathy, fibroadenosis, other benign dysplasias.

218-222 Benign Neoplasms of Genital Organs

218 UTERINE LEIOMYOMA
Uterine leiomyomas are quite common, found in 20 percent of white women and 50 percent of black women in the United States. Most leiomyomas are detected during the course of routine pelvic exam. there are often no symptoms. If there are symptoms, they might include abdominal discomfort, urinary frequency, and constipation.

Uterine leiomyomas usually occur in multiples. They are classified according to where they establish within the wall of the uterus. They may be called by alternate names such as uterine fibromyoma or, simply, myoma.

218.0 Submucous leiomyoma of uterus — *Submucous fibroid, fibroma, myoma*
218.1 Intramural leiomyoma of uterus — *interstitial fibroid, fibroma, myoma*
218.2 Subserous leiomyoma of uterus — *fibroid, fibroma, myoma on serous membrane*
218.9 Leiomyoma of uterus, unspecified — *unknown*

219 OTHER BENIGN NEOPLASM OF UTERUS
This rubric classifies all benign neoplasms of the uterus, other than leiomyomas, according to site of neoplasm.

219.0 Benign neoplasm of cervix uteri — *including cervical stump, internal and external os*
219.1 Benign neoplasm of corpus uteri — *including endometrium, fundus, myometrium*
219.8 Benign neoplasm of other specified parts of uterus — *not elsewhere classified*
219.9 Benign neoplasm of uterus, part unspecified — *unknown*

220 BENIGN NEOPLASM OF OVARY OK
The ovary is the female gonad and produces the ova. Some ovarian neoplasms are hormone-producing. Use an additional code to report any functional activity associated with the ovarian neoplasm.

221 BENIGN NEOPLASM OF OTHER FEMALE GENITAL ORGANS
Excluded from this rubric is a cyst of the Bartholin's gland or duct, which is classified to 616.2 *Cyst of Bartholin's gland*.

221.0 Benign neoplasm of fallopian tube and uterine ligaments — *including oviduct, parametrium, round and broad ligaments*
221.1 Benign neoplasm of vagina
221.2 Benign neoplasm of vulva — *including clitoris, Bartholin's gland, labia (majora) (minora), pudendum*

M9472/3 Medullomyoblastoma
M9480/3 Cerebellar sarcoma NOS
M9481/3 Monstrocellular sarcoma

M949-M952 Neuroepitheliomatous neoplasms
M9490/0 Ganglioneuroma
M9490/3 Ganglioneuroblastoma
M9491/0 Ganglioneuromatosis
M9500/3 Neuroblastoma NOS
M9501/3 Medulloepithelioma NOS
M9502/3 Teratoid medulloepithelioma
M9503/3 Neuroepithelioma NOS
M9504/3 Spongioneuroblastoma
M9505/1 Ganglioglioma
M9506/0 Neurocytoma
M9507/0 Pacinian tumor
M9510/3 Retinoblastoma NOS
M9511/3 Retinoblastoma, differentiated type
M9512/3 Retinoblastoma, undifferentiated type
M9520/3 Olfactory neurogenic tumor
M9521/3 Esthesioneurocytoma
M9522/3 Esthesioneuroblastoma
M9523/3 Esthesioneuroepithelioma

M953 Meningiomas
M9530/0 Meningioma NOS
M9530/1 Meningiomatosis NOS
M9530/3 Meningioma, malignant
M9531/0 Meningotheliomatous meningioma
M9532/0 Fibrous meningioma
M9533/0 Psammomatous meningioma
M9534/0 Angiomatous meningioma
M9535/0 Hemangioblastic meningioma
M9536/0 Hemangiopericytic meningioma
M9537/0 Transitional meningioma
M9538/1 Papillary meningioma
M9539/3 Meningeal sarcomatosis

M954-M957 Nerve sheath tumor
M9540/0 Neurofibroma NOS
M9540/1 Neurofibromatosis NOS
M9540/3 Neurofibrosarcoma
M9541/0 Melanotic neurofibroma
M9550/0 Plexiform neurofibroma

| 221.8 | Benign neoplasm of other specified sites of female genital organs — *not elsewhere classified, including Mullerian duct (female)* |
| 221.9 | Benign neoplasm of female genital organ, site unspecified — *unknown* |

222 BENIGN NEOPLASM OF MALE GENITAL ORGANS

The testes are a pair of male gonads found in the scrotum and produce spermatozoa for fertilization. Leydig cells in the testes produce testosterone. Few testicular masses are malignant Testicular tumors may cause functional activity problems. If functional activity problems occur, use an additional code to report it.

Benign hyperplasia of the prostate is reported with codes in rubric 600. The codes in rubric 600 describe conditions including adenoma, fibroma, myoma, polyp, cyst or hyperplasia of prostate.

222.0	Benign neoplasm of testis — (Use additional code to identify any functional activity) — *male gonad*
222.1	Benign neoplasm of penis — *including corpus cavernosum, foreskin, prepuce, glans penis*
222.2	Benign neoplasm of prostate — *median or lateral lobes*
222.3	Benign neoplasm of epididymis — *parorchis*
222.4	Benign neoplasm of scrotum — *skin, not contents*
222.8	Benign neoplasm of other specified sites of male genital organs — *not elsewhere classified, including Mullerian duct (male), seminal vesicle, spermatic cord*
222.9	Benign neoplasm of male genital organ, site unspecified — *unknown*

223 BENIGN NEOPLASM OF KIDNEY AND OTHER URINARY ORGANS

Excluded from this rubric are benign neoplasms of the renal calyces (223.1), renal pelvis (223.1), ureteric orifice of the bladder (223.3), and the urethral orifice of the bladder (223.3).

223.0	Benign neoplasm of kidney, except pelvis — *parenchyma*
223.1	Benign neoplasm of renal pelvis — *including calyx, hilus*
223.2	Benign neoplasm of ureter — *except orifice of bladder*
223.3	Benign neoplasm of bladder — *dome, neck, orifice, sphincter, trigone, urachus, wall*
223.81	Benign neoplasm of urethra — *except orifice of bladder*
223.89	Benign neoplasm of other specified sites of urinary organs — *including paraurethral gland*
223.9	Benign neoplasm of urinary organ, site unspecified — *unknown*

224-225 Benign Neoplasms of Nervous System

Benign neoplasms of the brain, eye, spine, meninges, cranial nerves, or sites unknown in the nervous system are classified to rubrics 224 and 225. Peripheral, sympathetic, or parasympathetic nerves are classified to codes in rubric 215.

224 BENIGN NEOPLASM OF EYE

The eye is basically a fluid-filled ball and benign neoplasms can pose two major dangers to sight: neoplasms can disrupt the visual field and cause compression that disrupts the flow of blood or aqueous, leading to permanent tissue damage. In addition, a benign neoplasm can result in significant irritation or pain.

✔5th Needs fifth-digit   **OK** Valid three-digit code

Intraocular pressure in the anterior segment of the eye is maintained through the flow of aqueous humor, or tears. The lacrimal system provides these tears and is also an agent in their disposal. Tears are produced in the lacrimal glands, located bilaterally behind the eyebrow, and the lacrimal ducts carry the tears to the eye, or away from the eye to the nose. Pressure in the posterior segment of the eye is maintained by gel-like vitreous humor.

A thin, vascular, mucous membrane covers the inner eyelids and the white outer shell of the eye (sclera). This membrane is called the conjunctiva. The cornea is the bulging "window" through which we see, and the retina is the light-sensitive "viewing screen" at the back of the eye. The choroid is a vascular layer of the inside of the eyeball.

224.0	Benign neoplasm of eyeball, except conjunctiva, cornea, retina, and choroid — *including ciliary body, iris, sclera, uveal tract, iris,*
224.1	Benign neoplasm of orbit — *soft tissue between eyeball and bony orbit*
224.2	Benign neoplasm of lacrimal gland — *excluding other parts of lacrimal apparatus*
224.3	Benign neoplasm of conjunctiva — *of sclera or inner aspect of eyelid*
224.4	Benign neoplasm of cornea — *including limbus*
224.5	Benign neoplasm of retina — *including pars optica, pars ciliaris, pars iridica*
224.6	Benign neoplasm of choroid — *choroidea, chorioidea*
224.7	Benign neoplasm of lacrimal duct — *including canaliculi, nasal duct, punctum, sac*
224.8	Benign neoplasm of other specified parts of eye — *Other specified parts of eye*
224.9	Benign neoplasm of eye, part unspecified — *unknown*

225 BENIGN NEOPLASM OF BRAIN AND OTHER PARTS OF NERVOUS SYSTEM

All brain tumors are "malignant" in that they may lead to death as they compromise the circulation of fluids in the brain through compression of obstruction. However, neoplasms classified to this rubric are not of a metastasizing nature: they are circumscribed lesions. The incidence of benign and malignant neoplasms of the brain is about the same at 50 percent.

Symptoms of a neoplasm of the brain include headache, seizures, personality changes, impaired mental or physical functions, or in children, an enlarged head. Use an additional code to report any manifestations associated with the neoplasm.

Acoustic neuroma is a common benign tumor of the acoustic nerve, which can cause hearing interruption, dizziness, and tinnitus. It is classified to 225.1 *Benign neoplasm of the cranial nerves.*

225.0	Benign neoplasm of brain — *including cerebrum, cerebellum, hypothalamus, basal ganglia, stem, medulla oblongata*
225.1	Benign neoplasm of cranial nerves — *including acoustic neuroma; cranial, trigeminal, trochlear, vagus nerve*
225.2	Benign neoplasm of cerebral meninges — *including meninges, meningioma*
225.3	Benign neoplasm of spinal cord — *including cauda equina*
225.4	Benign neoplasm of spinal meninges — *including meningioma*
225.8	Benign neoplasm of other specified sites of nervous system — *Other specified sites of nervous system*
225.9	Benign neoplasm of nervous system, part unspecified — *unknown*

M9560/0 Neurilemmoma NOS

M9560/1 Neurinomatosis

M9560/3 Neurilemmoma, malignant

M9570/0 Neuroma NOS

M958 Granular cell tumors and alveolar soft part sarcoma

M9580/0 Granular cell tumor NOS

M9580/3 Granular cell tumor, malignant

M9581/3 Alveolar soft part sarcoma

M959-M963 Lymphomas, NOS or diffuse

M9590/0 Lymphomatous tumor, benign

M9590/3 Malignant lymphoma NOS

M9591/3 Malignant lymphoma, non Hodgkin's type

M9600/3 Malignant lymphoma, undifferentiated cell type NOS

M9601/3 Malignant lymphoma, stem cell type

M9602/3 Malignant lymphoma, convoluted cell type NOS

M9610/3 Lymphosarcoma NOS

M9611/3 Malignant lymphoma, lymphoplasmacytoid type

M9612/3 Malignant lymphoma, immunoblastic type

M9613/3 Malignant lymphoma, mixed lymphocytic-histiocytic NOS

M9614/3 Malignant lymphoma, centroblastic-centrocytic, diffuse

M9615/3 Malignant lymphoma, follicular center cell NOS

M9620/3 Malignant lymphoma, lymphocytic, well differentiated NOS

M9621/3 Malignant lymphoma, lymphocytic, intermediate differentiation NOS

M9622/3 Malignant lymphoma, centrocytic

M9623/3 Malignant lymphoma, follicular center cell, cleaved NOS

M9630/3 Malignant lymphoma, lymphocytic, poorly differentiated NOS

M9631/3 Prolymphocytic lymphosarcoma

M9632/3 Malignant lymphoma,

226-228 Benign Neoplasms of Other and Unspecified Sites

226 BENIGN NEOPLASM OF THYROID GLANDS OK

The thyroid gland is located just below the cricoid cartilage near the larynx. Its purpose is to secrete thyroxine and triiodothyronine, which increase the rate of cell metabolism.

Benign thyroid tumors are adenomas, cysts, or involutionary nodules. A majority is follicular.

In many cases, the patient with a benign thyroid growth undergoes surgery because of suspicion of cancer, to improve cosmetic appearance, or to correct a functional activity. Use an additional code to report any functional activity associated with the neoplasm.

227 BENIGN NEOPLASM OF OTHER ENDOCRINE GLANDS AND RELATED STRUCTURES

The parathyroid glands come in pairs — the superior and inferior pair — and they are embedded in the posterior thyroid. The adrenal glands are situated above each kidney, and the pituitary gland is located in the sella turcica of the sphenoid bone. The pineal gland, located at the base of the corpus callosum, secretes melatonin; and the carotid body, located in the fork of the carotid artery, monitors blood oxygen. The aortic body at the aortic arch and right subclavian artery regulates reflex respiration.

Benign neoplasms of the endocrine glands can create functional activities in those glands. For example, adrenal tumors can cause virilizing or feminizing symptoms. Pituitary cancers can cause gigantism, Cushing's disease, amenorrhea or galactorrhea, or acromegaly. Report these functional activities in addition to the neoplasm.

227.0	Benign neoplasm of adrenal gland — (Use additional code to identify any functional activity) — *including suprarenal gland*
227.1	Benign neoplasm of parathyroid gland — (Use additional code to identify any functional activity) — *inferior or superior*
227.3	Benign neoplasm of pituitary gland and craniopharyngeal duct (pouch) — (Use additional code to identify any functional activity) — *including craniobuccal pouch, Rathke's pouch, hypophysis, sella turcica*
227.4	Benign neoplasm of pineal gland — (Use additional code to identify any functional activity) — *including pineal body*
227.5	Benign neoplasm of carotid body — (Use additional code to identify any functional activity) — *glomus caroticum*
227.6	Benign neoplasm of aortic body and other paraganglia — (Use additional code to identify any functional activity) — *including coccygeal body, para-aortic body, glomus jugulare*
227.8	Benign neoplasm of other endocrine glands and related structures — (Use additional code to identify any functional activity) — *not elsewhere specified*
227.9	Benign neoplasm of endocrine gland, site unspecified — (Use additional code to identify any functional activity) — *unknown*

228 HEMANGIOMA AND LYMPHANGIOMA, ANY SITE

Hemangiomas are neoplasms arising from vascular tissue or malformations of vascular structures. Many are congenital. They can occur topically (on the skin) within any organ system. Common topical hemangiomas include strawberry nevus, nevus vasculosus,

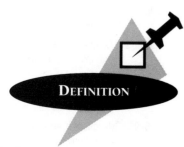

Cystic hygroma of the axilla

Cystic hygromas are large watery growths involving the lymph glands and surrounding tissues

DEFINITION

Angioma: a tumor or mass of the blood vessels.

Hemangioma: most often in the skin and subcutaneous tissue, a vascular mass that resembles a neoplasm.

Lymphangioma: a mass of lymphatic vessels.

↳5th   Needs fifth-digit   **OK**   Valid three-digit code

capillary hemangioma, port wine stain, and nevus flammeus. Classify hemangiomas according to site.

A lymphangioma is a benign, congenital malformation in the lymphatic system. Lymphangiomas may be superficial or deep and all lymphangiomas classify to 228.1 *Hemangioma of the skin and subcutaneous tissue.*

228.00	Hemangioma of unspecified site — *unknown*
228.01	Hemangioma of skin and subcutaneous tissue — *any site*
228.02	Hemangioma of intracranial structures — *brain, brain meninges*
228.03	Hemangioma of retina — *retina*
228.04	Hemangioma of intra-abdominal structures — *including peritoneum, retroperitoneum*
228.09	Hemangioma of other sites — *including choroid, heart, iris, spinal meninges, spinal cord; systemic angiomatosis*
228.1	Lymphangioma, any site — *including congenital lymphangioma, lymphatic nevus*

229 BENIGN NEOPLASM OF OTHER AND UNSPECIFIED SITES

Lymphangiomas are excluded from rubric 229. For intrathoracic or thoracic site not otherwise specified, report 229.8 *Benign neoplasm of other specified sites.*

229.0	Benign neoplasm of lymph nodes — *any site*
229.8	Benign neoplasm of other specified sites — *thoracic or intrathoracic, not otherwise specified*
229.9	Benign neoplasm of unspecified site — *unknown*

230-234 Carcinoma In Situ

Carcinoma in situ is defined as a carcinoma that has not invaded neighboring tissue. Once microscopic extension of malignant cells is found in tissue adjacent to carcinoma in situ, it is no longer "in situ," and malignant neoplasm codes should be used.

230 CARCINOMA IN SITU OF DIGESTIVE ORGANS

Carcinoma in situ in this rubric is classified by site within the digestive system.

230.0	Carcinoma in situ of lip, oral cavity, and pharynx — *including alveolus, gingiva, palate, pharynx, salivary glands, tongue*
230.1	Carcinoma in situ of esophagus — *including distal, proximal, middle*
230.2	Carcinoma in situ of stomach — *including body, cardia, fundus, pylorus, cardiac orifice*
230.3	Carcinoma in situ of colon — *including appendix, cecum, ileocecal valve, large intestine*
230.4	Carcinoma in situ of rectum — *including rectosigmoid junction*
230.5	Carcinoma in situ of anal canal — *including anal sphincter*
230.6	Carcinoma in situ of anus, unspecified — *unknown*
230.7	Carcinoma in situ of other and unspecified parts of intestine — *including duodenum, jejunum, ileum, small intestine*
230.8	Carcinoma in situ of liver and biliary system — *including ampulla of Vater, gallbladder, common bile duct, hepatic duct, cystic duct, sphincter of Oddi*
230.9	Carcinoma in situ of other and unspecified digestive organs — *pancreas, spleen, not elsewhere specified*

centroblastic type NOS

M9633/3 Malignant lymphoma, follicular center cell, noncleaved NOS

M964 Reticulosarcomas

M9640/3 Reticulosarcoma NOS

M9641/3 Reticulosarcoma, pleomorphic cell type

M9642/3 Reticulosarcoma, nodular

M965-M966 Hodgkin's disease

M9650/3 Hodgkin's disease NOS

M9651/3 Hodgkin's disease, lymphocytic predominance

M9652/3 Hodgkin's disease, mixed cellularity

M9653/3 Hodgkin's disease, lymphocytic depletion NOS

M9654/3 Hodgkin's disease, lymphocytic depletion, diffuse fibrosis

M9655/3 Hodgkin's disease, lymphocytic depletion, reticular type

M9656/3 Hodgkin's disease, nodular sclerosis NOS

M9657/3 Hodgkin's disease, nodular sclerosis, cellular phase

M9660/3 Hodgkin's paragranuloma

M9661/3 Hodgkin's granuloma

M9662/3 Hodgkin's sarcoma

M969 Lymphomas, nodular or follicular

M9690/3 Malignant lymphoma, nodular NOS

M9691/3 Malignant lymphoma, mixed lymphocytic-histiocytic, nodular

M9692/3 Malignant lymphoma, centroblastic-centrocytic, follicular

M9693/3 Malignant lymphoma, lymphocytic, well differentiated, nodular

M9694/3 Malignant lymphoma, lymphocytic, intermediate differentiation, nodular

M9695/3 Malignant lymphoma, follicular center cell, cleaved, follicular

M9696/3 Malignant lymphoma, lymphocytic, poorly differentiated, nodular

231 CARCINOMA IN SITU OF RESPIRATORY SYSTEM

Carcinoma in situ in this rubric is classified by site within the respiratory system.

231.0	Carcinoma in situ of larynx — *voice box including cartilage, epiglottis*
231.1	Carcinoma in situ of trachea — *including trachea*
231.2	Carcinoma in situ of bronchus and lung — *including carina, hilus*
231.8	Carcinoma in situ of other specified parts of respiratory system — *including accessory sinus, middle ear, nasal cavities, pleura*
231.9	Carcinoma in situ of respiratory system, part unspecified — *unknown*

232 CARCINOMA IN SITU OF SKIN

Carcinoma in situ in this rubric is classified by site within the skin.

232.0	Carcinoma in situ of skin of lip — *excluding vermilion border, mucosal tissue*
232.1	Carcinoma in situ of eyelid, including canthus — *including cartilage*
232.2	Carcinoma in situ of skin of ear and external auditory canal — *including antitragus, triangular fossa, tragus, lobule, helix, concha*
232.3	Carcinoma in situ of skin of other and unspecified parts of face — *chin and forehead, but not neck or scalp*
232.4	Carcinoma in situ of scalp and skin of neck — *scalp and neck, but not chin and forehead*
232.5	Carcinoma in situ of skin of trunk, except scrotum — *including perianal skin, skin of back, breast, buttock, chest, groin, perineum, umbilicus*
232.6	Carcinoma in situ of skin of upper limb, including shoulder — *including arm, hand, shoulder*
232.7	Carcinoma in situ of skin of lower limb, including hip — *including hip, leg, foot*
232.8	Carcinoma in situ of other specified sites of skin — *not elsewhere classified*
232.9	Carcinoma in situ of skin, site unspecified — *unknown*

233 CARCINOMA IN SITU OF BREAST AND GENITOURINARY SYSTEM

Carcinoma in situ in this rubric is classified by site within the genitourinary system.

In situ carcinoma of the vulva and vagina are linked to human papillomavirus and occur frequently in premenopausal women.

Dysplasias of the cervix are cellular deviations from the normal structure and function of the cells of the cervix of the uterus. Dysplasias are considered a precursor to carcinoma. Cervical dysplasia is classified to one of three levels of cervical intraepithelial neoplasm. CIN 1 and CIN II are reported with 622.1 *Dysplasia of cervix (uteri)*, while CIN III is reported with 233.1 *Carcinoma in situ of cervix uteri*. Vulvar intraepithelial neoplasm VIN III is classified to 233.3 *Carcinoma in situ of other and unspecified female genital organs*.

233.0	Carcinoma in situ of breast — *male or female*
233.1	Carcinoma in situ of cervix uteri — *including cervical stump, internal and external os*
233.2	Carcinoma in situ of other and unspecified parts of uterus — *including endometrium, fundus, myometrium*
233.3	Carcinoma in situ of other and unspecified female genital organs — *other and unspecified female genital organs*
233.4	Carcinoma in situ of prostate — *median or lateral lobes*
233.5	Carcinoma in situ of penis — *including corpus cavernosum, foreskin, prepuce, glans penis*

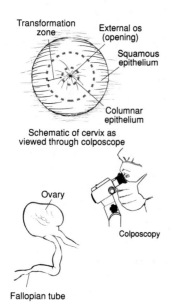

Transformation zone
External os (opening)
Squamous epithelium
Columnar epithelium

Schematic of cervix as viewed through colposcope

Ovary

Colposcopy

Fallopian tube

↵5th   Needs fifth-digit   **OK**   Valid three-digit code

233.6 Carcinoma in situ of other and unspecified male genital organs — *Other and unspecified male genital organs*

233.7 Carcinoma in situ of bladder — *including trigone, ureteral orifice, urethral orifice, urachus, sphincter*

233.9 Carcinoma in situ of other and unspecified urinary organs — *not elsewhere classified or unknown*

234 CARCINOMA IN SITU OF OTHER AND UNSPECIFIED SITES

Carcinoma in this rubric is classified by site as the eye, other, or unspecified. Classify all parts of the eye to 234.0 *Carcinoma in situ of eye*, except eyelid skin (232.1) and eyelid cartilage, optic nerve or orbital bone (234.8). Carcinomas in situ of the adrenal, parathyroid, pituitary, pineal glands and the carotid and pineal bodies are classified to 234.8 Carcinoma in situ of other specified sites.

234.0 Carcinoma in situ of eye — *including retina, conjunctiva, globe, choroid, iris, ciliary body, cornea*

234.8 Carcinoma in situ of other specified sites — *including endocrine glands*

234.9 Carcinoma in situ, site unspecified — *unknown*

235-238 Neoplasms of Uncertain Behavior

Uncertain behavior is a histomorphological determination, as distinguished from unspecified behavior, which indicates a lack of documentation to support a more specific code assignment. Neoplasms of uncertain behavior are classified by site or organ system. Neurofibromatosis, polycythemia vera, and mast cell tumors are classified in this series of rubics.

235 NEOPLASM OF UNCERTAIN BEHAVIOR OF DIGESTIVE AND RESPIRATORY SYSTEMS

Neoplasms in this rubric are classified by site within the digestive or respiratory systems.

235.0 Neoplasm of uncertain behavior of major salivary glands — *parotid, sublingual, submandibular glands*

235.1 Neoplasm of uncertain behavior of lip, oral cavity, and pharynx — *including gingiva, alveolus, pharynx, tongue, minor salivary glands*

235.2 Neoplasm of uncertain behavior of stomach, intestines, and rectum — *including ilium, jejunum, cardia, colon, sigmoid, duodenum*

235.3 Neoplasm of uncertain behavior of liver and biliary passages — *including ampulla of Vater, gallbladder, bile ducts, liver*

235.4 Neoplasm of uncertain behavior of retroperitoneum and peritoneum — *abdominal soft tissue other than organs*

235.5 Neoplasm of uncertain behavior of other and unspecified digestive organs — *including esophagus, pancreas, spleen, anus*

235.6 Neoplasm of uncertain behavior of larynx — *voice box*

235.7 Neoplasm of uncertain behavior of trachea, bronchus, and lung — *all lobes, trachea, bronchi*

235.8 Neoplasm of uncertain behavior of pleura, thymus, and mediastinum — *including thoracic soft tissue other than heart, lungs*

235.9 Neoplasm of uncertain behavior of other and unspecified respiratory organs — *including accessory sinus, middle ear, nasal cavities*

M9697/3 Malignant lymphoma, centroblastic type, follicular

M9698/3 Malignant lymphoma, follicular center cell, noncleaved, follicular

M970 Mycosis fungoides

M9700/3 Mycosis fungoides

M9701/3 Sezary's disease

M971-M972 Miscellaneous reticuloendothelial neoplasms

M9710/3 Microglioma

M9720/3 Malignant histiocytosis

M9721/3 Histiocytic medullary reticulosis

M9722/3 Letterer-Siwe's disease

M973 Plasma cell tumors

M9730/3 Plasma cell myeloma

M9731/0 Plasma cell tumor, benign

M9731/1 Plasmacytoma NOS

M9731/3 Plasma cell tumor, malignant

M974 Mast cell tumors

M9740/1 Mastocytoma NOS

M9740/3 Mast cell sarcoma

M9741/3 Malignant mastocytosis

M975 Burkitt's tumor

M9750/3 Burkitt's tumor

M980-M994 Leukemias
M980 Leukemias NOS

M9800/3 Leukemia NOS

M9801/3 Acute leukemia NOS

M9802/3 Subacute leukemia NOS

M9803/3 Chronic leukemia NOS

M9804/3 Aleukemic leukemia NOS

M981 Compound leukemias

M9810/3 Compound leukemia

M982 Lymphoid leukemias

M9820/3 Lymphoid leukemia NOS

M9821/3 Acute lymphoid leukemia

M9822/3 Subacute lymphoid leukemia

M9823/3 Chronic lymphoid leukemia

M9824/3 Aleukemic lymphoid leukemia

M9825/3 Prolymphocytic leukemia

M983 Plasma cell leukemias

M9830/3 Plasma cell leukemia

M984 Erythroleukemias

M9840/3 Erythroleukemia

M9841/3 Acute erythremia

M9842/3 Chronic erythremia

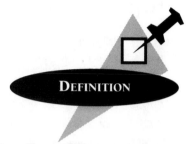

DEFINITION

Neurofibromatosis

Type I: also called von Recklinghausen's disease, a familial condition characterized by formation of disseminated cutaneous lesions and benign tumors of peripheral nerves.

Type II: also called acoustic neurofibromatosis, a familial condition characterized by formation of disseminated cutaneous lesions and benign tumors of peripheral nerves and bilateral 8th nerve masses.

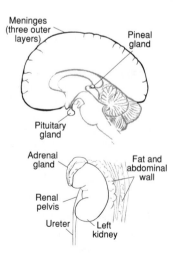

Meninges (three outer layers)
Pineal gland
Pituitary gland
Adrenal gland
Fat and abdominal wall
Renal pelvis
Ureter
Left kidney

236 NEOPLASM OF UNCERTAIN BEHAVIOR OF GENITOURINARY ORGANS

Neoplasms in this rubric are classified by site within the genitourinary system. If a neoplasm of the testis or ovary causes functional changes in hormone levels, report the functional activity in addition to the neoplasm of uncertain behavior.

236.0	Neoplasm of uncertain behavior of uterus — *including endometrium, fundus, myometrium*
236.1	Neoplasm of uncertain behavior of placenta — *including chorioadenoma destruens, malignant hydatidiform mole*
236.2	Neoplasm of uncertain behavior of ovary — (Use additional code to identify any functional activity) — *female gonad*
236.3	Neoplasm of uncertain behavior of other and unspecified female genital organs — *not elsewhere classified or unknown*
236.4	Neoplasm of uncertain behavior of testis — (Use additional code to identify any functional activity) — *male gonad*
236.5	Neoplasm of uncertain behavior of prostate — *median or lateral lobes*
236.6	Neoplasm of uncertain behavior of other and unspecified male genital organs — *not elsewhere classified or unknown*
236.7	Neoplasm of uncertain behavior of bladder — *including trigone, ureteral orifice, urethral orifice, urachus, sphincter*
236.90	Neoplasm of uncertain behavior of urinary organ, unspecified — *unknown*
236.91	Neoplasm of uncertain behavior of kidney and ureter — *including calyx, hilus, pelvis of kidney*
236.99	Neoplasm of uncertain behavior of other and unspecified urinary organs — *including urethra*

237 NEOPLASM OF UNCERTAIN BEHAVIOR OF ENDOCRINE GLANDS AND NERVOUS SYSTEM

If a neoplasm causes functional changes in hormone levels or nervous system functions, report the functional activity or manifestation in addition to the neoplasm of uncertain behavior.

237.0	Neoplasm of uncertain behavior of pituitary gland and craniopharyngeal duct — (Use additional code to identify any functional activity) — *pituitary body, fossa, lobe*
237.1	Neoplasm of uncertain behavior of pineal gland — *pineal body*
237.2	Neoplasm of uncertain behavior of adrenal gland — (Use additional code to identify any functional activity) — *including suprarenal gland*
237.3	Neoplasm of uncertain behavior of paraganglia — *including aortic body, coccygeal body, carotid body, glomus jugulare*
237.4	Neoplasm of uncertain behavior of other and unspecified endocrine glands — *including parathyroid gland, thyroid gland*
237.5	Neoplasm of uncertain behavior of brain and spinal cord — *including frontal lobe, thalamus, cerebrum, cerebellum, temporal lobe and stem*
237.6	Neoplasm of uncertain behavior of meninges — *cerebral or spinal*
237.70	Neurofibromatosis, unspecified — *type unknown*
237.71	Neurofibromatosis, Type 1 (von Recklinghausen's disease) — *"elephant man" syndrome*
237.72	Neurofibromatosis, Type 2 (acoustic neurofibromatosis) — *bilateral 8th nerve masses*
237.9	Neoplasm of uncertain behavior of other and unspecified parts of nervous system — *including cranial, parasympathetic, sympathetic, peripheral nerves or unknown*

✔5th   Needs fifth-digit   **OK**   Valid three-digit code

238 NEOPLASM OF UNCERTAIN BEHAVIOR OF OTHER AND UNSPECIFIED SITES AND TISSUES

Report pancytopenia, panmyelosis, and myelosclerosis with myeloid metaplasia, myelodysplastic syndrome, megakaryocytic myelosclerosis, and idiopathic thrombocythemia with 238.7.

238.0 Neoplasm of uncertain behavior of bone and articular cartilage — *long and short ones and associated cartilage*

238.1 Neoplasm of uncertain behavior of connective and other soft tissue — *including peripheral, sympathetic, and parasympathetic nerves and ganglia*

238.2 Neoplasm of uncertain behavior of skin — *any site*

238.3 Neoplasm of uncertain behavior of breast — *male or female*

238.4 Neoplasm of uncertain behavior of polycythemia vera — *Vaquez-Osler disease*

238.5 Neoplasm of uncertain behavior of histiocytic and mast cells — *mastocytoma NOS*

238.6 Neoplasm of uncertain behavior of plasma cells — *plasmacytoma NOS, solitary myeloma*

238.7 Neoplasm of uncertain behavior of other lymphatic and hematopoietic tissues — *including idiopathic thrombocythemia; megakaryocytic myelosclerosis; myelodysplastic syndrome; panmyelosis; preleukemic syndrome*

238.8 Neoplasm of uncertain behavior of other specified sites — *including eye, heart, nasolacrimal duct, lymph gland, Virchow's gland*

238.9 Neoplasm of uncertain behavior, site unspecified — *unknown*

239 Neoplasms of Unspecified Nature

This rubric classifies neoplasms for unknown or undocumented morphology. Do not use codes from this rubric to classify a "mass." Instead, consult "mass" in the index. Use of any code in this rubric may cause delays in claims processing due to the nonspecific nature of these codes. Classify the neoplasm according to site in this rubric.

239.0 Neoplasm of unspecified nature of digestive system — *including mouth, esophagus, stomach, intestine, pancreas, gallbladder*

239.1 Neoplasm of unspecified nature of respiratory system — *including lungs, pleura, bronchi*

239.2 Neoplasms of unspecified nature of bone, soft tissue, and skin — *including bone, blood vessels, muscles*

239.3 Neoplasm of unspecified nature of breast — *male or female*

239.4 Neoplasm of unspecified nature of bladder — *bladder*

239.5 Neoplasm of unspecified nature of other genitourinary organs — *male or female*

239.6 Neoplasm of unspecified nature of brain — *including cerebellum, cerebrum, stem*

239.7 Neoplasm of unspecified nature of endocrine glands and other parts of nervous system — *including thyroid, pituitary, pineal gland*

239.8 Neoplasm of unspecified nature of other specified sites — *including mediastinum, lymph glands, eye, heart, thymus*

239.9 Neoplasm of unspecified nature, site unspecified — *unknown*

M985 Lymphosarcoma cell leukemias
M9850/3 Lymphosarcoma cell leukemia

M986 Myeloid leukemias
M9860/3 Myeloid leukemia NOS
M9861/3 Acute myeloid leukemia
M9862/3 Subacute myeloid leukemia
M9863/3 Chronic myeloid leukemia
M9864/3 Aleukemic myeloid leukemia
M9865/3 Neutrophilic leukemia
M9866/3 Acute promyelocytic leukemia

M987 Basophilic leukemias
M9870/3 Basophilic leukemia

M988 Eosinophilic leukemias
M9880/3 Eosinophilic leukemia

M989 Monocytic leukemias
M9890/3 Monocytic leukemia NOS
M9891/3 Acute monocytic leukemia
M9892/3 Subacute monocytic leukemia
M9893/3 Chronic monocytic leukemia
M9894/3 Aleukemic monocytic leukemia

M990-M994 Miscellaneous leukemias
M9900/3 Mast cell leukemia
M9910/3 Megakaryocytic leukemia
M9920/3 Megakaryocytic myelosis
M9930/3 Myeloid sarcoma
M9940/3 Hairy cell leukemia

M995-M997 Miscellaneous myeloproliferative and lymphoproliferative disorders
M9950/1 Polycythemia vera
M9951/1 Acute panmyelosis
M9960/1 Chronic myeloproliferative disease
M9961/1 Myelosclerosis with myeloid metaplasia
M9962/1 Idiopathic thrombocythemia
M9970/1 Chronic lymphoproliferative disease

Chapter 3

240-279
Endocrine, Nutritional and Metabolic Diseases, and Immunity Disorders

The endocrine system is a group of specialized organs and body tissues that produces, stores, and secretes chemical substances known as hormones. Hormones provide information and instructions to regulate development, control the function of various tissues, support reproduction, and regulate metabolism.

Hormones from the endocrine system are secreted into the blood, where proteins bind to them to keep them intact as the hormone are disbursed through the body. The proteins also regulate the release of hormones.

Usually, the changes a hormone produces also serve to regulate that hormone's secretion. For example, parathyroid hormone causes the body to increase the level of calcium in the blood. As calcium levels rise, the secretion of parathyroid hormone decreases. Other changes in the body also influence hormone secretions. For example, during illness, the adrenal glands increase the secretions of certain hormones to help the body overcome the stress of illness. The normal regulation of hormone secretion is suspended, allowing for a tolerance of higher levels of hormone in the blood until the illness is resolved.

Nutritional deficiencies in this chapter cover deficiencies in vitamins, minerals, and protein-calorie malnutrition. Deficiencies of anemia are classified to Chapter 4, Disease of the Blood and Blood-Forming Organs.

Metabolic diseases in this chapter cover a wide range of metabolic diseases including problems with amino-acid transport, carbohydrate transport, lipoid metabolism, plasma protein metabolism, gout, mineral metabolism, and fluid, electrolyte and acid-base imbalances. Also covered are cystic fibrosis, porphyrin, purine and pyrimidine metabolism, and obesity.

240-246 Disorders of Thyroid Gland

The thyroid gland is attached to the trachea by loose connective tissue and derives its blood supply from the superior and interior thyroid arteries. The function of the thyroid is to create, store, and secrete thyroxine and triiodothyronine. The thyroid gland secretes hormones in response to stimulation by thyroid stimulating hormone (TSH) from the pituitary gland. The thyroid hormones regulate growth and metabolism and play a role in brain development during childhood.

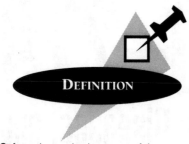

Goiter: abnormal enlargement of the thyroid gland not affecting hormone production.

Nontoxic multinodular goiter: enlargement of thyroid with formation of multiple nodules, due to diminished thyroid hormone production; without clinical hypothyroidism.

Nontoxic uninodular goiter: enlargement of thyroid with formation of single nodule, due to diminished thyroid hormone production; without clinical hypothyroidism.

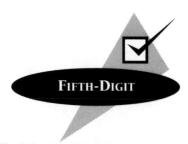

FIFTH-DIGIT

The following fifth-digit subclassification is for use with category 242:

0 without mention of thyrotoxic crisis or storm

1 with metnion of thyrotoxic crisis or storm

240 SIMPLE AND UNSPECIFIED GOITER

In simple goiter, the thyroid gland is enlarged, but the hormone secretions of the thyroid are still within normal limits. Simple goiter can have several causes. Iodine is essential to thyroid hormone secretion. The thyroid of a person whose diet has insufficient iodine will actually become enlarged so that it can produce more thyroid hormone. Iodine deficiency is the most common cause of simple goiter, but as there is no deficiency in the United States, this cause is rarely seen here. Simple goiter can also occur during puberty, pregnancy, or during menses as a result of hormonal imbalances. If a goiter has enough mass, it may cause compression that may lead to airway restriction, swallowing difficulty, or problems with venous flow.

240.0 Goiter, specified as simple — *not affecting hormone production*
240.9 Goiter, unspecified — *extent unknown*

241 NONTOXIC NODULAR GOITER

In nontoxic nodular goiter, the thyroid gland exhibits palpable nodules, though the nodules do not affect thyroid hormone secretion. Goiters in this rubric are classified as having a singular nodule, or multiple nodules. Benign neoplasms of the thyroid are reported with codes in the 226 rubric.

241.0 Nontoxic uninodular goiter — *one node, without clinical hypothyroidism*
241.1 Nontoxic multinodular goiter — *multiple nodes, without clinical hypothyroidism*
241.9 Unspecified nontoxic nodular goiter — *struma nodosa (simplex)*

242 THYROTOXICOSIS WITH OR WITHOUT GOITER

Thyrotoxicosis is an over-secretion of thyroid hormone, and is also called hyperthyroidism. Symptoms include tachycardia, nervousness, termor, weight loss, heat intolerance, goiter, and fatigue. Thyrotoxicosis is eight to 10 times more common in women than in men.

The causes of thyrotoxicosis are varied. Increased hormone secretion can be related to a thyroid nodule or to ectopic thyroid tissue. Thyrotoxicosis can also be the result of a more systemic problem, as in the case of Grave's disease, an autoimmune disorder.

A thyrotoxic storm is a sudden, life-threatening crisis in which symptoms of hyperthyroidism are exacerbated and new symptoms develop. It is most likely to occur at the time of infection, surgical procedure, or trauma in a patient with undertreated hyperthyroidism. The patient may develop a fever, emotional instability or psychosis, heart complications, and an enlarged liver.

Diseases in this rubric are classified first by the cause of hyperthyroidism, and second, by the status of thyrotoxic storm.

If a neoplasm is causing the functional activity, report the appropriate neoplasm code in addition to the hyperthyroidism code. Sequencing varies according to the encounter.

Neonatal thyrotoxicosis is reported with 775.3.

242.0 ⌐5th Toxic diffuse goiter — *Grave's disease, Basedow's disease, Marsh's disease, Parry's syndrome, Parson's disease; exophthalmic goiter*
242.1 ⌐5th Toxic uninodular goiter — *single nodule, toxic, or with hyperthyroidism*
242.2 ⌐5th Toxic multinodular goiter — *multiple nodules, toxic, or with hyperthyroidism*

242.3 ✔5th Toxic nodular goiter, unspecified type — *nodular, unknown type, with hyperthyroidism or toxic; Plummer's disease*

242.4 ✔5th Thyrotoxicosis from ectopic thyroid nodule — *aberrant thyroid tissue as cause*

242.8 ✔5th Thyrotoxicosis of other specified origin — *overproduction of TSH; thyroid toxicosis factitia*

242.9 ✔5th Thyrotoxicosis without mention of goiter or other cause — *not elsewhere specified; Leopold-Levi's syndrome*

243 CONGENITAL HYPOTHYROIDISM OK

The most common cause of congenital hypothyroid is absence of a thyroid gland at birth. This requires lifelong hormone therapy since thyroxine regulates metabolism and growth. Untreated, congenital hypothyroidism causes serious problems in the central nervous system, developmental delay, and problems with somatic growth. Screening programs exist in the United States to test newborns for this disorder. By providing replacement thyroid hormones, almost all of the complications of congenital hypothyroidism are avoidable.

Congenital goiter with an enzyme defect in synthesis of thyroid hormone is reported with 246.1.

244 ACQUIRED HYPOTHYROIDISM

Hypothyroidism is a deficiency of thyroid hormone. Primary hypothyroidism usually develops in older adults, usually after age 40, and causes lethargy, fatigue, and mental sluggishness.

For hypothyroidism complicating pregnancy, see rubric 648.

244.0 Postsurgical hypothyroidism — *athyroidism or part of thyroid removed*

244.1 Other postablative hypothyroidism — *following irradiation*

244.2 Iodine hypothyroidism — (Use additional E code to identify drug) — *resulting from high iodide intake*

244.3 Other iatrogenic hypothyroidism — (Use additional E code to identify drug) — *resulting from: PAS, phenylbutazone, resorcinol*

244.8 Other specified acquired hypothyroidism — *not elsewhere classified, Gull's disease*

244.9 Unspecified hypothyroidism — *unknown; Brissaud-Meige syndrome; Strumipriva cachexia; Hoffmann's syndrome*

245 THYROIDITIS

Diseases in this rubric are classified as acute, subacute, chronic, and iatrogenic. The most common form of thyroiditis in the United States is Hashimoto's thyroiditis (245.2), a chronic condition that usually leads to chronic hypothyroidism and lifetime treatment with synthetic hormone. Hashimoto's thyroiditis is an autoimmune disorder that often presents with other forms of autoimmune disease, including Type 1 diabetes mellitus, hypoparathyroidism, or Addison's disease. Schmidt's syndrome is Addison's disease with hypothyroidism secondary to Hashimoto's thyroiditis, and is reported with 258.1 *Other combinations of endocrine dysfunction*. In diabetes with hypothyroidism, report both conditions rather than this combination code since, as a significant systemic disease, diabetes should always be coded separately.

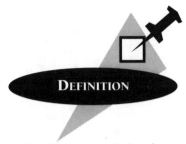

DEFINITION

Hyperthyroidism: overproduction of thyroid hormone.

Hypothyroidism: underproduction of thyroid hormone.

Myxedema: non-pitting edema with dry, waxy appearance and deposits of mucin in the skin, commonly seen in hypothyroidism. Lips and nose typically thicken and facial characteristics change. Some physicians use the term myxedema when they mean adult hypothyroidism.

Thyrotoxic crisis or storm: abrupt onset of florid symptoms including extreme nervousness, insomnia, weight loss, tremors and psychosis, or coma associated with excessive thyroid hormone.

Thyrotoxicosis: the state caused by excessive production of thyroid hormone.

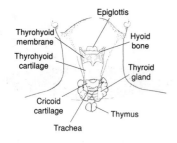

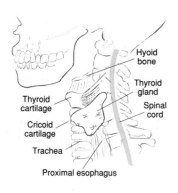

245.0   Acute thyroiditis — (Use additional code to identify organism) — *abscess, pyogenic, suppurative, nonsuppurative*

245.1   Subacute thyroiditis — *de Quervain's, giant cell, granulomatous*

245.2   Chronic lymphocytic thyroiditis — *Hashimoto's disease*

245.3   Chronic fibrous thyroiditis — *Riedel's thyroiditis; struma fibrosa*

245.4   Iatrogenic thyroiditis — (Use additional code to identify cause) — *due to medical treatment other than radiation or excision*

245.8   Other and unspecified chronic thyroiditis — *not elsewhere classified*

245.9   Unspecified thyroiditis — *unknown*

246 OTHER DISORDERS OF THYROID

This rubric captures other disorders of the thyroid, with the exception of neoplasms, which are found in Chapter 2.

246.0   Disorders of thyrocalcitonin secretion — *hypersecretion of calcitonin or thyrocalcitonin*

246.1   Dyshormonogenic goiter — *enzyme defect; congenital dyshormonogenic*

246.2   Cyst of thyroid — *Cyst of thyroid*

246.3   Hemorrhage and infarction of thyroid — *Hemorrhage and infarction of thyroid*

246.8   Other specified disorders of thyroid — *atrophy, TBG defect, degeneration*

246.9   Unspecified disorder of thyroid — *unknown*

250-259 Diseases of Other Endocrine Glands

Included in this section are diseases associated with insulin-producing cells of the pancreas, the islets of Langerhans; parathyroid; pituitary, hypothalamus; adrenals; ovaries; and testes.

250 DIABETES MELLITUS

The pancreas is positioned in the upper abdomen, just under the stomach. The major part of the pancreas, called the exocrine pancreas, secretes digestive enzymes into the gastrointestinal tract. Distributed through the pancreas are clusters of endocrine cells that secrete insulin, glucagon, and somatostatin. These hormones all participate in regulating energy and metabolism in the body.

Diabetes is a systemic disease and, as such, should be codified even in the absence of documented, active intervention during the patient encounter.

Diabetes mellitus has two forms. Diabetes mellitus Type 1 is caused by inadequate secretion of insulin by the pancreas. Diabetes mellitus Type 2 is caused by the body's inability to respond to insulin. Both have similar symptoms, including excessive thirst, hunger, and urination as well as weight loss. Laboratory tests that detect glucose in the urine and elevated levels of glucose in the blood usually confirm the diagnosis.

Treatment of diabetes mellitus Type 1 requires regular injections of insulin. Type 2 can be treated with diet, exercise, oral medication, or injection.

Only about 10 percent of diabetics are Type 1. The primary factor that distinguishes Type 1 from Type 2 is the absence of naturally occurring insulin within the body. Type 1 diabetics require insulin injections to survive. Type 2 diabetics may improve their health with insulin injections, but they would not face immediate crisis without insulin. Therefore, the administration of insulin has no bearing on code selection for diabetes.

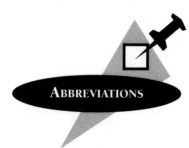

ABBREVIATIONS

DKA: diabetic ketoacidosis, a condition in which accumulation of ketones in diabetes mellitus causes decreased pH and bicarbonate concentration in the body fluids; a complication of high blood glucose levels

IDDM: insulin dependent diabetes mellitus

NIDDM: non-insulin-dependent diabetes mellitus

✓5th   Needs fifth-digit   **OK**   Valid three-digit code

In this rubric, diabetes is classified according to type of complication, as selected by the fourth digit and by Type 1 or Type 2 status and presence of diabetic control, selected by the fifth digit.

Diabetes can cause a variety of complications, including kidney problems, pain due to nerve damage, blindness, and coronary heart disease. Recent studies have shown that controlling blood sugar levels reduces the risk of developing diabetes complications.

Diabetes mellitus should not be classified as out of control unless the physician specifically documents it as such.

For diabetic pregnancy, two codes are required: the pregnancy code from the rubric 648 and also a code from the 250 rubric.

Secondary diabetes should not be reported with this rubric. Instead, the condition causing the diabetes should be reported. For example, in post-pancreatectomy diabetes, assign 251.3 Postsurgical insulinemia.

250.0 ✔5th Diabetes mellitus without mention of complication — *no complications arising from disease*

250.1 ✔5th Diabetes with ketoacidosis — *ketosis, acidosis, without coma*

250.2 ✔5th Diabetes with hyperosmolarity — *Diabetes with hyperosmolarity; increased osmolarity of the body fluids as a complication of diabetes*

250.3 ✔5th Diabetes with other coma — *arising from ketoacidosis or hypoglycemia*

250.4 ✔5th Diabetes with renal manifestations — *kidney disease*

250.5 ✔5th Diabetes with ophthalmic manifestations — *ocular disease*

250.6 ✔5th Diabetes with neurological manifestations — *nerve damage or disease*

250.7 ✔5th Diabetes with peripheral circulatory disorders — *blood vessel damage or disease*

250.8 ✔5th Diabetes with other specified manifestations — (Use additional code to identify manifestation, as: 707.10–707.9, 731.8) — *including hypoglycemic shock*

250.9 ✔5th Diabetes with unspecified complication — *unknown complication*

251 OTHER DISORDERS OF PANCREATIC INTERNAL SECRETION

Diabetes insipidus is caused by a deficiency of vasopressin, one of the antidiuretic hormones (ADH) secreted by the pituitary gland. Symptoms include increased thirst and urination. Treatment is with drugs, such as synthetic vasopressin, that help the body maintain water and electrolyte balance.

251.0 Hypoglycemic coma — (Use additional E code to identify drug, if drug induced) — *Non-diabetic insulin coma*

251.1 Other specified hypoglycemia — (Use additional E code to identify drug, if drug induced) — *including hyperplasia of pancreatic islet beta cells NOS; Harris' syndrome*

251.2 Hypoglycemia, unspecified — *not otherwise specified, including McQuarrie's syndrome*

251.3 Postsurgical hypoinsulinemia — *following complete or partial pancreatectomy*

251.4 Abnormality of secretion of glucagon — *hyperplasia of islet alpha cells with glucagon excess*

251.5 Abnormality of secretion of gastrin — *hyperplasia of alpha cells with gastrin excess; Zollinger-Ellison syndrome*

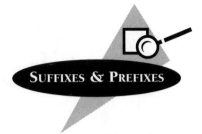

SUFFIXES & PREFIXES

-acidosis: excessive acid in body fluids

-glycemia: presence of sugar in the blood

keto-: compound containing a ketone

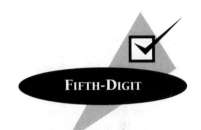

FIFTH-DIGIT

The following fifth-digit subclassification is for use with category 250:

0 type II [non-insulin dependent type] [NIDDM type] [adult-onset type] or unspecified type, not stated as uncontrolled

1 type I [insulin dependent type] [IDDM] [juvenile type], not stated as uncontrolled

2 type II [non-insulin dependent type] [NIDDM type] [adult-onset type] or unspecified type, uncontrolled

3 type I [insulin dependent type] [IDDM] [juvenile type], uncontrolled

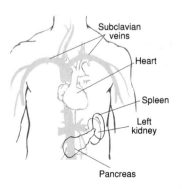

Subclavian veins

Heart

Spleen

Left kidney

Pancreas

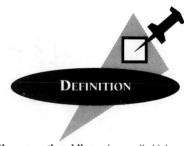

DEFINITION

Hyperparathyroidism: abnormally high secretion of parathyroid hormones causing bone deterioration, reduced frenal function, and kidney stones.

Hyperosmolarity: an increase in the concentration of fluids.

Hypoparathyroidism: abnormally low secretion of parathyroid hormones causing a severe convulsive disorder known as tetany.

Neuropathy: a disorder or disease of the nerve or nervous system, in diabetes, a long-term complication.

251.8	Other specified disorders of pancreatic internal secretion — *including sclerotic islands of Langerhans*
251.9	Unspecified disorder of pancreatic internal secretion — *not elsewhere classified*

252 DISORDERS OF PARATHYROID GLAND

The parathyroid glands are four small glands located at the four corners of the thyroid gland. The hormone secreted, parathyroid hormone, regulates the level of calcium in the blood.

252.0	Hyperparathyroidism — *high secretion of parathyroid hormones causing bone deterioration, reduced renal function, and kidney stones; hyperplasia of parathyroid; osteitis fibrosa cystica generalisata; von Recklinghausen's disease of bone; Jaffe-Lichtenstein (-Uehlinger) syndrome*
252.1	Hypoparathyroidism — *low secretion of parathyroid hormones causing a severe convulsive disorder known as tetany; parathyroiditis; parathyroid tetany*
252.8	Other specified disorders of parathyroid gland — *including cyst, hemorrhage, or infarct*
252.9	Unspecified disorder of parathyroid gland — *unknown*

253 DISORDERS OF THE PITUITARY GLAND AND ITS HYPOTHALAMIC CONTROL

The hypothalamus controls the pituitary gland from deep within the bran. Acting as liaison between the brain and the pituitary gland, the hypothalamus is the primary link between the endocrine and nervous systems.

The pituitary, located in the base of the brain, secretes several hormones that regulate the function of the other endocrine glands. The pituitary gland is divided into two parts, the anterior and posterior lobes, each having separate functions. The anterior lobe regulates the activity of the thyroid, adrenal, and reproductive glands. It also regulates the body's growth and stimulates milk production in women who are breast-feeding. Hormones secreted by the anterior lobe include adrenocorticotropic hormone (ACTH), thyrotropic hormone (TSH), luteinizing hormone (LH), follicle-stimulating hormone (FSH), growth hormone (GH), and prolactin. The anterior lobe also secretes endorphins, chemicals that act on the nervous system to reduce sensitivity to pain.

The posterior lobe of the pituitary gland contains the nerve endings (axons) from the hypothalamus, which stimulate or suppress hormone production. This lobe secretes antidiuretic hormones (ADH), which control water balance in the body, and oxytocin, which controls muscle contractions in the uterus.

253.0	Acromegaly and gigantism — *acromegaly describes unusual growth beginning in middle age; gigantism usually begins in childhood. Both are caused by overproduction of pituitary growth hormone; Erdheim's, Launois', Marie's, syndromes*
253.1	Other and unspecified anterior pituitary hyperfunction — *including Forbes-Albright and Argonz-Del Castillo syndromes*
253.2	Panhypopituitarism — *organic pituitary dysfunction leading to impaired sexual function, fatigue, bradycardia, depression, and impaired growth in children; including cachexia, necrosis, insufficiency; Sheehan's, hypopituitarism, or postpartum-panhypopituitary syndromes*
253.3	Pituitary dwarfism — *with persistence of infantile physical characteristics due to under-secretion of growth hormone and gonadotropin deficiency; HGH deficiency, Lorain-Levi dwarfism, Burnier's syndrome, Nebecourt's syndrome*

✒5th Needs fifth-digit   **OK** Valid three-digit code

253.4 Other anterior pituitary disorders — *including isolated or partial deficiency of an anterior pituitary hormone, other than growth hormone; prolactin deficiency; Kallmann's syndrome*

253.5 Diabetes insipidus — *insufficient diuretic hormone release; symptoms include frequent urination, thirst, and weight loss; vasopressin deficiency*

253.6 Other disorders of neurohypophysis — *including syndrome of inappropriate secretion of antidiuretic hormone [ADH] and Schwartz-Bartter syndrome*

253.7 Iatrogenic pituitary disorders — (Use additional E code to identify cause) — *drug therapy, radiation therapy, or surgery, causing mild to severe symptoms*

253.8 Other disorders of the pituitary and other syndromes of diencephalohypophyseal origin — *including abscess of pituitary; adiposogenital dystrophy; Rathke's pouch, pituitary or intrasellar cyst, empty sella; or hypophyseal, Launois-Cléret syndrome, Fröhlich's syndrome, Rénon-Delille syndrome*

253.9 Unspecified disorder of the pituitary gland and its hypothalamic control — *unknown*

254 DISEASES OF THYMUS GLAND

The thymus gland is comprised of lymphatic and epithelial tissue (Hassall's corpuscles) and is located in the anterior, superior mediastinum. The thymus processes white blood cells (WBC) known as lymphocytes, which kill foreign cells and stimulate other immune cells to produce antibodies. The role of the thymus is not entirely understood, though it seems to be most important during infancy and until puberty, when the lymphatic tissue is chiefly replaced by fat. In adults, the thymus can be removed without significant impact on health.

Thymic disease in this rubric is classified as abscess, hyperplasia, or other specified disease. Excluded from this rubric are aplasia, dysplasia, or hypoplasia of thymus with immunodeficiency (279.2); myasthenia gravis (358.0); and thymoma (212.6); and DiGeorge anomaly (279.11). Congenital absence of thymus is classified to 759.2 *Anomalies of other endocrine glands.*

254.0 Persistent hyperplasia of thymus — *continued, abnormal growth of the twin lymphoid lobes that produce T lymphocytes in the anterior superior mediastinum*

254.1 Abscess of thymus — *pocket of liquid puris caused by infection in the thymus*

254.8 Other specified diseases of thymus gland — *including atrophy, cyst, hemorrhage, necrotic tissue, inflammation, thymicolymphaticus shunt, Kopp's asthma, hyperthymism*

254.9 Unspecified disease of thymus gland — *unknown*

255 DISORDERS OF ADRENAL GLANDS

Located on the kidneys, the adrenal glands have two distinct parts. The outer, called the adrenal cortex, produces a variety of hormones called corticosteroids. Chief among the corticosteroids is cortisol, which regulates salt and water balance in the body, prepares the body for stress, regulates metabolism, interacts with the immune system, and influences sexual function. The inner part, the adrenal medulla, produces catecholamines, such as epinephrine, also called adrenaline, which increases the blood pressure and heart rate during times of stress.

Addison's disease is caused by decreased function of the adrenal cortex. Weakness, fatigue, abdominal pains, nausea, dehydration, fever, and hyperpigmentation (tanning without sun exposure) are among the possible symptoms. Treatment involves providing the body with replacement corticosteroid hormones as well as dietary salt.

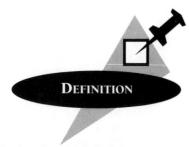

DEFINITION

Corticoadrenal insufficiency: underproduction of adrenal hormones causing low blood pressure.

Cushing's syndrome: oversecretion of adrenal cortisol or the use of glucocorticoid medications causing fat deposits in the head and neck and causing kyphosis.

Dry beriberi: thiamine deficiency with neurologic manifestations including paresthesia of toes, burning of feet, muscle cramps and pains and leading to footdrop and toedrop.

Hyperaldosteronism: oversecretion of aldosterone causing fluid retention and hypertension.

Wernicke-Korsakoff syndrome: thiamine deficiency with cerebral manifestations including mental confusion and loss of hearing, and leading to nystagmus, coma, or death.

Wet beriberi: thiamine deficiency with cardiovascular manifestations including tachycardia and edema and leading to heart failure.

Primary Cushing's syndrome is caused by excessive secretion of glucocorticoids, the subgroup of corticosteroid hormones that includes hydrocortisone, by the adrenal glands. Symptoms may develop over many years prior to diagnosis and may include obesity, physical weakness, easily bruised skin, acne, hypertension, and psychological changes. Treatment may include surgery, radiation therapy, chemotherapy, or blockage of hormone production with drugs. A secondary form of the disease can occur as a side effect of drug therapy, and is reported with the same code, 255.0 Cushing's syndrome. In ICD-10-CM separate codes are available to report Cushing's syndrome due to ectopic ACTH syndrome, drug therapy, pituitary dysfunction, or alcohol use.

Acromegaly and gigantism both are caused by a pituitary tumor that stimulates production of excessive growth hormone, causing abnormal growth in particular parts of the body. Acromegaly is rare and usually develops over many years in adult subjects. Gigantism occurs when the excess of growth hormone begins in childhood.

255.0	Cushing's syndrome — (Use additional E code to identify drug, if drug induced) — *over-secretion of adrenal cortisol or use of glucocorticoid medications causing fat deposits in the head and neck and kyphosis; adrenal hyperplasia, ectopic ACTH syndrome*
255.1	Hyperaldosteronism — *over-secretion of aldosterone causing fluid retention and hypertension; Bartter's or Conn's syndrome*
255.2	Adrenogenital disorders — *congenital or acquired disorders of the genitals due to adrenal dysfunction; Achard-Thiers syndrome, Apert-Gallais syndrome, Cooke-Apert-Gallais syndrome, Corticosexual syndrome, and Hercules syndrome*
255.3	Other corticoadrenal overactivity — *including acquired benign adrenal androgenic overactivity; Schroeder's syndrome or Slocum's syndrome*
255.4	Corticoadrenal insufficiency — *underproduction of adrenal hormones causing low blood pressure; Addisonian crisis, Bernard-Sergent syndrome*
255.5	Other adrenal hypofunction — *including adrenal medullary insufficiency*
255.6	Medulloadrenal hyperfunction — *including catecholamine secretion by pheochromocytoma*
255.8	Other specified disorders of adrenal glands — *including abnormality of cortisol-binding globulin, Adrenal collapse; adrenal/suprarenal cyst; adrenal obesity, inflammation, necrosis, sclerosis, swelling*
255.9	Unspecified disorder of adrenal glands — *unknown*

256 OVARIAN DYSFUNCTION

Female gonads secrete sex hormones in response to stimulation from the pituitary gland. Located in the pelvis, the ovaries produce eggs. They also secrete female sex hormones, estrogen and progesterone, which regulate development of the reproductive organs, female secondary sex characteristics, and menstruation and pregnancy.

256.0	Hyperestrogenism — *over-secretion by the ovary of estrogen*
256.1	Other ovarian hyperfunction — *including hypersecretion of ovarian androgens*
256.2	Postablative ovarian failure — *including iatrogenic, postsurgical, postirradiation*
256.3	Other ovarian failure — *including premature menopause not otherwise specified; primary ovarian failure*
256.4	Polycystic ovaries — *containing multiple follicular cysts filled with serous fluid; isosexual virilization; Stein-Leventhal syndrome*
256.8	Other ovarian dysfunction — *including hyperthecosis, ovary*
256.9	Unspecified ovarian dysfunction — *unknown*

✔5th   Needs fifth-digit   **OK**   Valid three-digit code

257 TESTICULAR DYSFUNCTION

Male gonads produce sperm and secrete androgens. The androgens, the most important of which is testosterone, regulate development of the reproductive organs, male secondary sex characteristics, and muscle.

257.0	Testicular hyperfunction — *over-secretion by the testicles of testosterone*
257.1	Postablative testicular hypofunction — *including iatrogenic, postsurgical, postirradiation*
257.2	Other testicular hypofunction — *including eunuchoidism; defective biosynthesis of testicular androgen; failure of Leydig's cell, adult; fertile eunuch, Reifenstein's syndrome*
257.8	Other testicular dysfunction — *including male pseudohermaphroditism with testicular feminization; Goldberg-Maxwell syndrome, Morris syndrome*
257.9	Unspecified testicular dysfunction — *unknown*

258 POLYGLANDULAR DYSFUNCTION AND RELATED DISORDERS

Autoimmune disorders affecting endocrine glands often occur in multiples. Hashimoto's thyroiditis, for example, often presents with Type 1 diabetes mellitus, hypoparathyroidism, or Addison's disease. Schmidt's syndrome is Addison's disease with hypothyroidism secondary to Hashimoto's thyroiditis, and is reported with 258.1 *Other combinations of endocrine dysfunction.* In diabetes with hypothyroidism, report both conditions rather than this combination code since, as a significant systemic disease, diabetes should always be codified separately.

258.0	Polyglandular activity in multiple endocrine adenomatosis — *abnormal production of hormones by two or more endocrine glands due to hyperplasia; caused by genetic defects; Wermer's syndrome*
258.1	Other combinations of endocrine dysfunction — *including Lloyd's syndrome, Schmidt's syndrome, Pierre Mauriac's syndrome*
258.8	Other specified polyglandular dysfunction — *including atrophy pluriglandular; polyglandular sclerosis*
258.9	Unspecified polyglandular dysfunction — *unknown*

259 OTHER ENDOCRINE DISORDERS

Obesity due to underlying endocrine disease is reported with 259.9 *Unspecified endocrine disorder.*

259.0	Delay in sexual development and puberty, not elsewhere classified — *delayed puberty*
259.1	Precocious sexual development and puberty, not elsewhere classified — *whether cryptogenic, constitutional, idiopathic*
259.2	Carcinoid syndrome — *including Argentaffin syndrome, Björk (-Thorson) syndrome, Cassidy (-Scholte) syndrome, Hedinger's syndrome*
259.3	Ectopic hormone secretion, not elsewhere classified — *arising from an abnormal site or tissue: antidiuretic hormone secretion [ADH], hyperparathyroidism*
259.4	Dwarfism, not elsewhere classified — *constitutional*
259.8	Other specified endocrine disorders — *including pineal dysfunction, pineal calcification; Werner's syndrome, Donohue's syndrome, Gilford (-Hutchinson) syndrome, Pellizzi's, Progeria trigeminal plate syndrome; progeria, leprechaunism*
259.9	Unspecified endocrine disorder — *unknown*

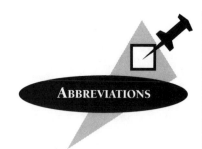

PEM: Protein-energy malnutrition, or protein-calorie malnutrition, characterized by a deficit in energy and nutrients

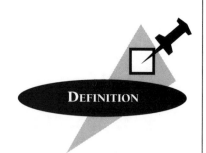

DEFINITION

Malnutrition: undernourishment caused by poor eating habits or malassimilation. Malnutrition is categorized by severity: mild or first degree, moderate or second degree, and severe or third degree.

Marasmus: withering, wasting, weight loss.

260-269 Nutritional Deficiencies

In the United States, nutritional and vitamin deficiencies usually are the result of poverty, prolonged parenteral feeding, chronic substance abuse, or food fads or extreme diets. Malnutrition results from insufficiency in the body's total intake of energizing nutrients and proteins, and vitamin or mineral deficiencies are the result of insufficient intake of very specific nutrients. While patients with malnutrition may also commonly have vitamin or mineral deficiencies, it is also possible to develop a vitamin or mineral deficiency without malnutrition.

This group of rubrics excludes deficiency anemias, which are reported with 280.0-281.9.

260 KWASHIORKOR OK

Kwashiorkor is an African word meaning "first-child, second-child." It refers to the protein-deficit illness that affects the first child when it is weaned to make room for the second child. Instead of protein-rich breast milk, the first child is fed a thin gruel made from sweet potato, banana, or cassava. The gruel is starchy, so there is no energy deficit, but the lack of protein causes edema, lethargy, and impaired growth. Kwashiorkor is considered a third-degree malnutrition disorder.

261 NUTRITIONAL MARASMUS OK

Marasmus results from near starvation with a deficit in protein and nonprotein intake. Typically, marasmus is a childhood disease in underdeveloped countries, and occurs when the mother is unable to breast-feed. The child is very thin, with little muscle or body fat. Marasmus is considered a third-degree malnutrition disorder.

262 OTHER SEVERE, PROTEIN-CALORIE MALNUTRITION OK

Classified malnutrition to this rubric if there is nutritional edema without mention of dyspigmentation of skin and hair.

263 OTHER AND UNSPECIFIED PROTEIN-CALORIE MALNUTRITION

Malnutrition results from inadequate intake or malabsorption of nutrients. Infants and children are at highest risk for malnutrition, since there is a high demand for nutrients during the growth years. Pregnancy and old age also pose other significant risks for malnutrition, as does the presence of chronic disease or adherence to some diets. Substance abuse is also a risk factor for malnutrition.

263.0   Malnutrition of moderate degree — *second degree malnutrition characterized by superimposed biochemical changes in electrolytes, lipids, blood plasma.*

263.1   Malnutrition of mild degree — *first degree malnutrition characterized by tissue wasting in an adult or growth failure in a child, but few or no biochemical changes.*

263.2   Arrested development following protein-calorie malnutrition — *physical retardation due to malnutrition*

263.8   Other protein-calorie malnutrition — *not elsewhere specified*

263.9   Unspecified protein-calorie malnutrition — *unknown*

⌐5th   Needs fifth-digit   **OK**   Valid three-digit code

264 VITAMIN A DEFICIENCY

Vitamin A is found in green, leafy vegetables, fish, and dairy products, and serious deficiency can cause growth retardation in children, blindness, and increased susceptibility to infection. Vitamin A deficiency is common in kwashiorkor and is endemic in areas in which rice is the staple.

264.0	Vitamin A deficiency with conjunctival xerosis — *vitamin A deficiency with conjunctival dryness*
264.1	Vitamin A deficiency with conjunctival xerosis and Bitot's spot — *vitamin A deficiency with conjunctival dryness and superficial spots of keratinized epithelium; Bitot's spot in young child*
264.2	Vitamin A deficiency with corneal xerosis — *vitamin A deficiency with corneal dryness*
264.3	Vitamin A deficiency with corneal ulceration and xerosis — *vitamin A deficiency with corneal dryness and epithelial ulceration*
264.4	Vitamin A deficiency with keratomalacia — *vitamin A deficiency creating corneal dryness progressing to corneal insensitivity, softness, necrosis; usually bilateral*
264.5	Vitamin A deficiency with night blindness — *vitamin A deficiency causing failure of vision in dim light*
264.6	Vitamin A deficiency with xerophthalmic scars of cornea — *vitamin A deficiency with corneal scars caused by dryness*
264.7	Other ocular manifestations of vitamin A deficiency — *xerophthalmia due to vitamin A deficiency*
264.8	Other manifestations of vitamin A deficiency — *including follicular keratosis, xeroderma, phrynoderma*
264.9	Unspecified vitamin A deficiency — *unknown*

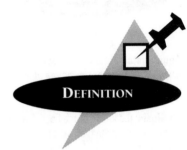

DEFINITION

Bitot's spots: symptom of advanced deficiency of vitamin A, superficial patches of epithelial debris on the exposed bulbar conjunctiva.

265 THIAMINE AND NIACIN DEFICIENCY STATES

Alcoholism is the main cause of thiamine deficiency in the United States. In other countries, it can result from eating a diet of highly polished rice. Infants can develop a thiamine deficiency when breast-fed by thiamine-deficient mothers. Thiamine deficiency causes beriberi, with its manifestations of neuritis, edema, and heart disease.

Niacin deficiency is called pellagra, and is characterized by a light-sensitive rash, diarrhea, glossitis, and psychosis. Pellagra is most common in countries in which corn is the main food source, and is rare in the United States.

265.0	Beriberi — *vitamin B_1 deficiency characterized by neuritis, edema, and heart disease*
265.1	Other and unspecified manifestations of thiamine deficiency — *including Gayet-Wernicke's syndrome*
265.2	Pellagra — *niacin deficiency causing disturbances in skin, digestion, psyche*

266 DEFICIENCY OF B-COMPLEX COMPONENTS

Ariboflavinosis is riboflavin, or vitamin B_2, deficiency that causes inflammation of the lips, tongue fissures, corneal vascularization, and anemia. Ariboflavinosis is associated with deficiency of milk in the diet, though the disease can also occur secondarily in patients with chronic diseases affecting nutritional absorption.

Vitamin B_6 is important in blood, central nervous system, and skin metabolism. It is uncommon to find a primary deficiency in vitamin B_6, but secondary deficiency can result

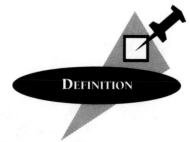

Angular stomatosis: raw tissue at the angles of the mouth, a symptom of vitamin B_2 deficiency.

Cheilosis: reddening of the lipstick area of the lips, a symptom of vitamin B_2 deficiency.

in chronic diseases affecting nutritional absorption, in patients using oral contraceptives, or in alcoholism. Report vitamin B_6 responsive sideroblastic anemia with 285.0.

266.0	Ariboflavinosis — *vitamin B_2 deficiency causing inflammation of the lips, tongue fissures, corneal vascularization, anemia.*
266.1	Vitamin B_6 deficiency — *vitamin B_6 deficiency causing skin, lip, and tongue disturbances, peripheral neuropathy, and in infants, convulsions*
266.2	Other B-complex deficiencies — *including B_{12}, burning feet syndrome, Gopalan's syndrome*
266.9	Unspecified vitamin B deficiency — *unspecified vitamin B deficiency*

267 ASCORBIC ACID DEFICIENCY OK

Vitamin C, or ascorbic acid, is essential for wound healing and connective tissue health and it facilitates absorption of iron. A deficiency in this vitamin is commonly called scurvy or Cheadle-Moller-Barlow syndrome. Vitamin C is common to many fruits and vegetables. Symptoms of scurvy include bleeding gums, weight loss, myalgias, and slowing of the healing process. The symptoms are reversed with ascorbic acid therapy. Anemia related to vitamin C deficiency is reported with 281.8 *Anemia associated with other specified nutritional deficiency.*

268 VITAMIN D DEFICIENCY

Vitamin D is found in yeast, eggs, and dairy products, fish liver oils, and is also created when skin is exposed to sunlight. Deficiency is commonly called "rickets" in children and osteomalacia in adults. The disease is rare in the United States, though seen occasionally in immigrants from India. Demineralization of bone and bone deformity are the most common side effects of vitamin D deficiency.

Diseases in this rubric are classified as active or late effect, and as rickets or adult osteomalacia. Renal rickets are reported with 588.0 *Renal osteodystrophy* and celiac rickets are reported with 579.0 *Celiac disease.*

Rickets or osteomalacia can also be caused by a metabolic resistance to absorb vitamin D, rather than a deficiency in intake. If this is the case, report the resistance with 275.3 *Disorders of phosphorus metabolism.*

268.0	Rickets, active — *vitamin D deficiency causing metabolic bone disease in children; rosary, rachitic*
268.1	Rickets, late effect — (Use additional code to identify the nature of late effect) — *distorted or demineralized bones as a result of vitamin D deficiency and stated to be a late effect or sequela of rickets*
268.2	Osteomalacia, unspecified — *vitamin D deficiency causing metabolic bone disease in adults; Looser-Debray syndrome, Milkman-Looser syndrome, Miller's disease*
268.9	Unspecified vitamin D deficiency — *unknown; viosterol deficiency*

269 OTHER NUTRITIONAL DEFICIENCIES

Vitamin K deficiencies associated with hypoprothrombinemia and depression of coagulation are reported with 286.7. Vitamin K deficiency of newborn is reported with 776.0 *Hemorrhagic disease of newborns.*

Do not use codes from this rubric to report failure to thrive or feeding problems. These conditions are classified to rubric 783. Deficiencies of calcium, potassium, and sodium are classified to rubrics 275 or 276.

269.0	Deficiency of vitamin K — *deficiency of vitamin K*
269.1	Deficiency of other vitamins — *including vitamins E and P*
269.2	Unspecified vitamin deficiency — *multiple vitamin deficiency not specified*
269.3	Mineral deficiency, not elsewhere classified — *including dietary calcium, iodine*
269.8	Other nutritional deficiency — *not elsewhere classified*
269.9	Unspecified nutritional deficiency — *unknown*

270-279 Other Metabolic and Immunity Disorders

Use additional code to identify any associated mental retardation.

270 DISORDERS OF AMINO-ACID TRANSPORT AND METABOLISM

Excluded from this rubric are abnormal findings without manifest disease (790.0-796.9); disorders of purine and pyrimidine metabolism (277.1-277.2); and gout (274.0-274.9).

270.0	Disturbances of amino-acid transport — *including cystinosis, renal glycinuria, cystinuria, Hartnup disease, Fanconi (-de Toni) (-Debré) or Hart's syndrome*
270.1	Phenylketonuria (PKU) — *inherited error of metabolism affecting phenylalanine; early diagnosis through screening blood test prevents mental retardation; hyperphenylalaninemia*
270.2	Other disturbances of aromatic amino-acid metabolism — *including albinism, hypertyrosinemia, alkaptonuria, Oasthouse urine disease, Mende's syndrome, Smith-Strang disease, van der Hoeve-Halbertsma-Waardenburg syndrome*
270.3	Disturbances of branched-chain amino-acid metabolism — *in metabolism of leucine, isoleucine, and valine; hypervalinemia; intermittent branched-chain ketonuria; leucine-induced hypoglycemia; methylmalonic aciduria*
270.4	Disturbances of sulphur-bearing amino-acid metabolism — *including cystathioninuria, cystathioninuria; disturbances of metabolism of methionine, homocystine, and cystathionine, homocystinuria*
270.5	Disturbances of histidine metabolism — *including carnosinemia, histidinemia, hyperhistidinemia, imidazole aminoaciduria*
270.6	Disorders of urea cycle metabolism — *including argininosuccinic aciduria; citrullinemia; disorders of metabolism of ornithine, citrulline, argininosuccinic acid, arginine, and ammonia*
270.7	Other disturbances of straight-chain amino-acid metabolism — *including glucoglycinuria; hyperglycinemia and other disturbances of metabolism of glycine, threonine, serine, glutamine, and lysine; pipecolic acidemia, methylmalonic aciduria with glycinemia*
270.8	Other specified disorders of amino-acid metabolism — *including alaninemia, aminoacidopathy, ethanolaminuria, prolinemia, glycoprolinuria, prolinuria, hydroxyprolinemia, sarcosinemia familial iminoglycinuria, and Lowe-Terrey-MacLachlan syndrome*
270.9	Unspecified disorder of amino-acid metabolism — *unknown*

271 DISORDERS OF CARBOHYDRATE TRANSPORT AND METABOLISM

Excluded from this rubric are abnormality of secretion of glucagon (251.4); diabetes mellitus (rubric 250); hypoglycemia not otherwise specified (251.2); and mucopolysaccharidosis (277.5).

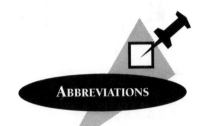

ABBREVIATIONS

PKU: phenylketonuria, an inherited error of metabolism affecting phenylalanine production; early diagnosis through a blood test prevents mental retardation

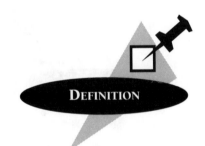

DEFINITION

Amino acid: an acid that is found in proteins and aid in metabolism.

Histidine: a type of amino acid.

Metabolism: chemical changes occurring in various tissues in the body.

Urea: the end product of nitrogen metabolism.

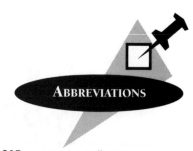

ABBREVIATIONS

CAD: coronary artery disease

HDL: high density lipoproteins, associated with increased CAD

LDL: low density lipoproteins

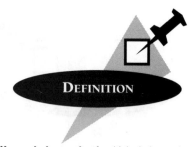

DEFINITION

Hypercholesterolemia: high cholesterol in the blood.

Hyperglyceridemia: elevated level of glyceride, a natural and fatty acid in the blood.

Hyperlipidemia: elevated level of lipoprotein, a complex of fats and proteins, in the blood.

Lipodystrophy: disturbance in fat metabolism causing abnormal distribution of the body's fatty tissue.

271.0	Glycogenosis — *excessive storage of glycogen; amylopectinosis, glucose-6-phosphatase deficiency, McArdle's disease, Pompe's disease, von Gierke's disease*
271.1	Galactosemia — *galactose-1-phosphate uridyl transferase deficiency, galactosuria*
271.2	Hereditary fructose intolerance — *essential benign fructosuria, fructosemia*
271.3	Intestinal disaccharidase deficiencies and disaccharide malabsorption — *intolerance or malabsorption: glucose, lactose, or sucrose*
271.4	Renal glycosuria — *abnormally large amount of sugar in the urine with normal blood sugar, caused by failure of the renal tubules to reabsorb glucose; renal diabetes*
271.8	Other specified disorders of carbohydrate transport and metabolism — *including essential benign pentosuria, mannosidosis, fucosidosis, oxalosis, xylosuria, Bird's disease, glycolic aciduria*
271.9	Unspecified disorder of carbohydrate transport and metabolism — *unknown*

272 DISORDERS OF LIPOID METABOLISM

Excluded from this rubric is localized cerebral lipidoses (330.1).

272.0	Pure hypercholesterolemia — *high cholesterol in the blood; familial, Fredrickson Type II A hyperlipoproteinemia; low-density-lipoid-type [LDL] hyperlipoproteinemia*
272.1	Pure hyperglyceridemia — *elevated level of glyceride, a natural fatty acid, in the blood; endogenous hyperglyceridemia; Fredrickson Type IV hyperlipoproteinemia; very-low-density-lipoid-type [VLDL] hyperlipoproteinemia*
272.2	Mixed hyperlipidemia — *elevated level of lipoprotein, a complex of fats and proteins, in the blood due to an inherited lipoprotein metabolism disorder; Fredrickson Type IIb or III hyperlipoproteinemia, hypercholesterolemia with endogenous hyperglyceridemia; tubo-eruptive xanthoma*
272.3	Hyperchylomicronemia — *including Bürger-Grütz syndrome; Fredrickson type I or V hyperlipoproteinemia; Hyperlipidemia, Group D*
272.4	Other and unspecified hyperlipidemia — *elevated level of chylomicrons in the blood. Chylomicrons are a form of lipoproteins which transport dietary cholesterol and triglycerides from the small intestine to the blood; Seeley-Klionsky disease*
272.5	Lipoprotein deficiencies — *abnormally low level of lipoprotein, a complex of fats and proteins, in the blood; abetalipoproteinemia, hypoalphalipoproteinemia; Bassen-Kornzweig syndrome; high-density lipoid deficiency*
272.6	Lipodystrophy — (Use additional E code to identify cause) — *disturbance in fat metabolism causing abnormal distribution of the body's fatty tissue; Barraquer-Simons disease, Simons' syndrome*
272.7	Lipidoses — *including chemically-induced; Anderson's disease, Fabry's disease, Gaucher's disease, Niemann-Pick disease, pseudo-Hurler's or mucolipidosis III disease, Wolman's disease; Ruiter-Pompen (-Wyers) syndrome, sea-blue histiocyte syndrome*
272.8	Other disorders of lipoid metabolism — *including Hoffa's, Launois-Bensaude's, Anders' syndrome, Dercum's syndrome, Farber (-Uzman) syndrome, Madelung's disease; neurolipomatosis, proteinosis lipoid multicentric reticulohistiocytosis*
272.9	Unspecified disorder of lipoid metabolism — *unknown*

273 DISORDERS OF PLASMA PROTEIN METABOLISM

Excluded from this rubric are agammaglobulinemia and hypogammaglobulinemia (279.0-279.2); coagulation defect (286.0-286.9); and hereditary hemolytic anemias (282.0-282.9).

273.0	Polyclonal hypergammaglobulinemia — *elevated level of gamma globulins in the blood, frequently observed in patients with chronic infectious diseases, including Waldenström's*

✔5th Needs fifth-digit   **OK** Valid three-digit code

273.1   Monoclonal paraproteinemia — *presence of abnormal proteins in the blood plasma; benign monoclonal hypergammaglobulinemia [BMH], monoclonal gammopathy associated with lymphoplasmacytic dyscrasias, paraproteinemia secondary to malignant or inflammatory disease*

273.2   Other paraproteinemias — *including cryoglobulinemic purpura, vasculitis, mixed cryoglobulinemia*

273.3   Macroglobulinemia — *elevated level of macroglobulins in the blood. Macroglobulins are plasma globulins with an unusually high molecular weight; Waldenström's macroglobulinemia*

273.8   Other disorders of plasma protein metabolism — *including bisalbuminemia; hyperglobulinemia; hypoalbuminemia; hypoproteinemia; pyroglobulinemia*

273.9   Unspecified disorder of plasma protein metabolism — *unknown*

274 GOUT

Deposits of monosodium urate or monohydrate crystals cause gout. The most common site for these deposits is around the joints, especially around the big toe. However, these deposits may be found in organ systems, too. Gout is classified according to site. Pseudogout is classified to rubric 275.

Gout is reclassified in ICD-10-CM as a disease of the musculoskeletal system rather than as a metabolic disease. In ICD-10-CM, the cause of the gout is also classified as idiopathic, drug-induced, due to renal impairment, or secondary to other disease.

Excluded from this rubric is lead gout, which is classified to 984.0-984.9.

274.0   Gouty arthropathy — *acute inflammatory arthritis caused by deposits of monosodium urate monohydrate crystals in the joints*

274.10   Gouty nephropathy, unspecified — *any kidney disease characterized by abnormal production and excretion of uric acid*

274.11   Uric acid nephrolithiasis — *with sodium urate stones in the kidney*

274.19   Other gouty nephropathy — *not otherwise specified*

274.81   Gouty tophi of ear — *deposit of sodium urate inflaming external ear*

274.82   Gouty tophi of other sites — *including heart*

274.89   Gout with other specified manifestations — (Use additional code to identify manifestation, as: 357.4, 364.11) — *including dermatitis, eczema, episcleritis, iritis, neuritis, phlebitis*

274.9   Gout, unspecified — *unknown, including podagra, thesaurismosis urate, uric acid diathesis*

275 DISORDERS OF MINERAL METABOLISM

Hypercalcemia includes symptoms of nausea, vomiting, anorexia, fever, and constipation. Pseudogout is chondrocalcinosis, a disorder of calcium metabolism. Joint disease is due to deposits of dicalcium phosphate or pyrophosphate crystals.

275.0   Disorders of iron metabolism — *including bronzed diabetes, pigmentary cirrhosis, hemochromatosis, Troisier-Hanot-Chauffard syndrome, von Recklinghausen-Applebaum disease*

275.1   Disorders of copper metabolism — *including hepatolenticular degeneration; Wilson's disease; amyostatic syndrome, chorea-athetosis-agitans syndrome, Westphal-Strümpel syndrome*

275.2   Disorders of magnesium metabolism — *including hypermagnesemia, hypomagnesemia*

275.3   Disorders of phosphorus metabolism — *including familial hypophosphatemia, vitamin D-resistant osteomalacia or rickets*

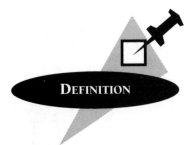

DEFINITION

Podagra: acute, inflammatory gouty arthralgia of the metatarsophalangeal joint of the great toe.

Tophi: monosodium urate crystal aggregates, sometimes large enough to be palpated as subcutaneous nodules.

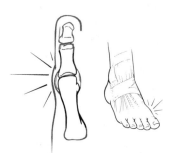

A classic gout symptom is extremely painful inflammation of the first metatarsophalangeal joint, although other joints may also be affected

275.40	Unspecified disorder of calcium metabolism — *unknown*	
275.41	Hypocalcemia — *ow level of calcium in the blood with possible symptoms including muscle or abdominal cramps, tendon reflex anomalies, or carpopedal spasms*	
275.42	Hypercalcemia — *elevated level of calcium in the blood with possible symptoms including fatigue, nausea, constipation, depression*	
275.49	Other disorders of calcium metabolism — *including nephrocalcinosis; pseudohypoparathyroidism; pseudopseudohypoparathyroidism; and Martin-Albright syndrome, Seabright-Bantam syndromes*	
275.8	Other specified disorders of mineral metabolism — *not elsewhere classified*	
275.9	Unspecified disorder of mineral metabolism — *unknown*	

276 DISORDERS OF FLUID, ELECTROLYTE, AND ACID-BASE BALANCE

Dehydration is the depletion of total body water and sodium. Dehydration may follow bouts of diarrhea, vomiting, or profuse sweating. It is often a manifestation of the patient's illness (for example gastroenteritis), and in such cases, the code for dehydration would not be sequenced first. However, if the patient's dehydration becomes significant enough to warrant separate treatment for rehydration, the dehydration code would be sequenced first.

When reporting volume depletion due to chemotherapy, also report E879.9 *Unspecified procedure* to indicate that drug therapy is the cause of dehydration.

In ICD-9-CM, the same code, 276.5 *Volume depletion*, reports dehydration and hypovolemia. Dehydration is the depletion of total body water and sodium; hypovolemia speaks specifically to a reduction of volume and concentration of contents of the blood seen as a result of dehydration. In ICD-10-CM, separate codes will be available for hypovolemia and dehydration under a rubric titled "volume depletion."

276.0	Hyperosmolality and/or hypernatremia — *sodium [Na] excess or overload*
276.1	Hyposmolality and/or hyponatremia — *sodium [Na] deficiency*
276.2	Acidosis — *accumulation of acid or depletion of alkali in blood and body tissues; metabolic or respiratory*
276.3	Alkalosis — *accumulation of base or loss of acid without relative loss of base in body fluids, caused by increased arterial plasma bicarbonate concentration or by abnormal loss of carbon dioxide due to hyperventilation; metabolic or respiratory*
276.4	Mixed acid-base balance disorder — *hypercapnia with mixed acid-base disorder*
276.5	Volume depletion — *dehydration, hypovolemia, Luetscher's syndrome*
276.6	Fluid overload — *fluid retention*
276.7	Hyperpotassemia — *elevated level of potassium in the blood with symptoms including abnormal EKG readings and weakness; often associated with defective renal excretion; hyperkalemia, potassium [K] intoxication*
276.8	Hypopotassemia — *decreased level of potassium in the blood with symptoms including neuromuscular disorders; often associated with potassium loss through vomiting and diarrhea; hypokalemia*
276.9	Electrolyte and fluid disorders not elsewhere classified — *including electrolyte imbalance, hypochloremia, hyperchloremia, disequilibrium syndrome*

277 OTHER AND UNSPECIFIED DISORDERS OF METABOLISM

Cystic fibrosis is a hereditary disorder in which the body secretes thick, sticky mucus that clogs organs and leads to problems with breathing and digestion. About 30,000 children and young adults in the United States have cystic fibrosis. The disease affects one in 2,500 Caucasians and one in 17,000 African-Americans.

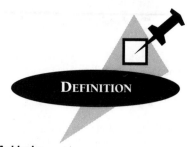

DEFINITION

Acidosis:

Metabolic: a lowered pH and bicarbonate level in the body fluids caused by acids accumulating or by losses of fixed base.

Respiratory: inadequate ventilation causing a retention of carbon dioxide in the body fluids.

Lactic: a lowered pH and bicarbonate level in the body fluids caused by lactic acid accumulating. Is often due to a drug reaction or hypoxia.

Alkalosis:

Respiratory: a lowered bicarbonate level in the body fluids caused by hyperventilation.

Metabolic: an elevation of the bicarbonate level in the body fluids caused by an excessive loss of acid in the urine or by vomiting or caused by an excessive intake of alkaline substances.

Volume depletion: principal causes of volume depletion are vomiting, diarrhea, sweating, dialysis, burns, trauma, diuretic use, diabetes, kidney disease, adrenal disease, or Bartter's syndrome.

Cystic fibrosis is caused by a defect in the manufacture of cystic fibrosis transmembrane conductance regulator (CFTR). Normally, CFTR forms a channel through which chloride ions traverse the cells lining the lungs, pancreas, sweat glands, and small intestine. With cystic fibrosis, malfunctioning CFTR precludes chloride from entering or leaving cells, resulting in production of thick, sticky mucus. In the lungs, this mucus blocks airways. In the digestive system, the mucus prevents enzymes produced in the pancreas from reaching the intestines, impairing digestion. In addition, the malfunctioning CFTR causes excessive amounts of salt to escape in the sweat.

Cystic fibrosis is an autosomal recessive genetic disorder. To have cystic fibrosis, both parents must carry the disease. One in 31 people in the United States carries the gene. With two carriers, there is a 25 percent change of producing a child with cystic fibrosis.

Cystic fibrosis symptoms may be apparent soon after birth, or the symptoms may go undiagnosed for years. In 20 percent of cases, the first symptom is meconium ileus, intestinal blockage in newborns, which may require surgery.

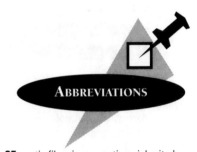

ABBREVIATIONS

CF: cystic fibrosis, a genetic or inherited disorder causing pancreatic and respiratory deficiencies.

277.00   Cystic fibrosis without mention of meconium ileus — *genetic disorder causing pancreatic and respiratory deficiencies.*

277.01   Cystic fibrosis with meconium ileus — *inherited disorder causing pancreatic and respiratory deficiencies; with meconium ileus present at birth*

277.1   Disorders of porphyrin metabolism — *including hematoporphyria, hematoporphyrinuria, hereditary coproporphyria, porphyrinuria, protocoproporphyria, Günther's syndrome*

277.2   Other disorders of purine and pyrimidine metabolism — *including hypoxanthine-guanine-phosphoribosyltransferase deficiency [HG-PRT deficiency], Lesch-Nyhan syndrome, xanthinuria*

277.3   Amyloidosis — *accumulation of insoluble fibrillar proteins compromising organ function; familial Mediterranean fever, hereditary cardiac amyloidosis, Reimann's periodic disease, Siegal-Cattan-Mamou disease*

277.4   Disorders of bilirubin excretion — *including hyperbilirubinemia; Dubin-Johnson syndrome, Gilbert's syndrome, Rotor's syndrome, Crigler-Najjar syndrome*

277.5   Mucopolysaccharidosis — *including gargoylism; osteochondrodystrophy; lipochondrodystrophy; Morquio-Brailsford disease, Hunter's syndrome, Hurler's syndrome, Sanfilippo's syndrome, Scheie's syndrome, Maroteaux-Lamy syndrome*

277.6   Other deficiencies of circulating enzymes — *including alpha 1-antitrypsin deficiency, hereditary angioedema*

277.8   Other specified disorders of metabolism — *including Hand-Schüller-Christian disease, histiocytosis, acatalasemia, reticulohistiocytoma, and craniohypophyseal xanthomatosis*

277.9   Unspecified disorder of metabolism

278 OBESITY AND OTHER HYPERALIMENTATION

Obesity is defined as a condition in which the body weight of the patient is at least 30 percent above the ideal weight as seen on standardized weight charts. Codes from this rubric are reported to classify obesity when no underlying condition exists, for instance, underlying endocrine disease (259.9).

Obesity is epidemic in the United States. It is more common among women than among men and more common among African-Americans than Caucasians. Obesity occurs when caloric intake chronically outpaces the energy required. Obesity puts patients at risk for diabetes, hypertension, and coronary artery disease.

Obesity is classified in this rubric as morbid obesity or unspecified obesity. Morbid obesity is defined as obesity in which the patient weighs at least double the ideal weight as seen on standardized weight charts.

Excluded from this rubric are hyperalimentation not otherwise specified (783.6), poisoning by vitamins (rubric 963) and polyphagia (783.6).

278.00	Obesity, unspecified — *not elsewhere classified*
278.01	Morbid obesity — *double or more the normal body weight*
278.1	Localized adiposity — *fat pad*
278.2	Hypervitaminosis A
278.3	Hypercarotinemia — *elevated blood carotene levels due to ingestion of excessive amounts of carotenoids or from an inability to convert carotenoids to vitamin A*
278.4	Hypervitaminosis D — *ingestion of an excessive amount of vitamin D resulting in weakness, fatigue, loss of weight, and other symptoms.*
278.8	Other hyperalimentation — *including cardiopulmonary obesity syndrome, Pickwickian syndrome*

279 DISORDERS INVOLVING THE IMMUNE MECHANISM

Transplant failure or rejection is classified to the rubric 996 rather than to this rubric.

279.00	Unspecified hypogammaglobulinemia — *abnormally low levels of immunoglobulins in the blood; agammaglobulinemia or antibody deficiency syndrome*
279.01	Selective IgA immunodeficiency — *selective IgA immunodeficiency*
279.02	Selective IgM immunodeficiency — *selective IgM immunodeficiency*
279.03	Other selective immunoglobulin deficiencies — *including selective deficiency of IgG*
279.04	Congenital hypogammaglobulinemia — *including Bruton's type, x-linked agammaglobulinemia, congenital antibody deficiency syndrome*
279.05	Immunodeficiency with increased IgM — *including autosomal recessive and x-linked immunodeficiency with hyper-IgM*
279.06	Common variable immunodeficiency — *including dysgammaglobulinemia and hypogammaglobulinemia*
279.09	Other deficiency of humoral immunity — *including transient hypogammaglobulinemia of infancy*
279.10	Unspecified immunodeficiency with predominant T-cell defect — *unknown*
279.11	DiGeorge's syndrome — *including pharyngeal pouch syndrome and thymic hypoplasia*
279.12	Wiskott-Aldrich syndrome — *eczema-thrombocytopenia syndrome*
279.13	Nezelof's syndrome — *cellular immunodeficiency with abnormal immunoglobulin deficiency*
279.19	Other deficiency of cell-mediated immunity — *not elsewhere classified*
279.2	Combined immunity deficiency — *including agammaglobulinemia; severe combined immunodeficiency [SCID]; thymic alymphoplasia, aplasia or dysplasia with immunodeficiency*
279.3	Unspecified immunity deficiency — *unknown*
279.4	Autoimmune disease, not elsewhere classified — *not elsewhere classified*
279.8	Other specified disorders involving the immune mechanism — *including single complement [C1-C9] deficiency or dysfunction, hypocomplementemia*
279.9	Unspecified disorder of immune mechanism — *unknown*

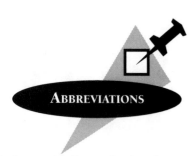

DEFINITION

Hypogammaglobulinemia: a state of having a decreased quantity of immunoglobulins.

Immunodeficiency: a condition caused by a problem within the immune mechanism, could also have been caused by another disease.

ABBREVIATIONS

Ig: immunoglobulin, one of a class of proteins that is classified according to the amounts present in normal human serum.

IgA-(10-15%)

IgG-(80%)

IgM-(5-10%)

⤷5th Needs fifth-digit   **OK** Valid three-digit code

Chapter 4

280–289
Diseases of the Blood and Blood-Forming Organs

This chapter classifies diseases and disorders of blood and blood-forming (hemopoietic) organs, including anemias, coagulation defects, purpura and other hemorrhagic conditions, diseases of white blood cells, other diseases of blood, and blood-forming organs.

Bone marrow is the principal site for hemopoietic cell proliferation and differentiation. One of the largest organs in the human body, hemopoietic tissue is responsible for producing erythrocytes (red blood cells), neutrophils, eosinophils, basophils, monocytes, platelets, and lymphocytes.

The term "anemia" refers to a lower than normal erythrocyte count or level of hemoglobin in the circulating blood. A clinical sign rather than a diagnostic entity, anemia can be classified by three morphological variations of the erythrocyte: size (volume), hemoglobin content, and shape. These variations give clinicians clues to the specific type of anemia.

In laboratory blood tests, erythrocyte size is gauged by estimating the volume of red cells in the circulating blood. Red cell volume, or mean corpuscular volume, is estimated by dividing the patient's hematocrit (percentage of red blood cells in whole blood) by the red blood cell (count) (RBC). Normal values are normocytic; abnormally low values are microcytic; and abnormally high values are macrocytic.

Hemoglobin content refers to the average amount of hemoglobin in each red blood cell. This value, called the mean cell hemoglobin, is calculated by dividing the patient's hemoglobin by the number of red blood cells. Normal values are normochromic; less than normal values are hypochromic; and greater than normal values are hyperchromic.

Shape is determined by microscopy. Normally, red blood cells have a smooth concave shape. Erythrocytes with irregular shapes are called poikilocytes, a general term meaning abnormally shaped. Terms referring to specific abnormal cell shapes include acanthocytes, leptocytes, nucleated erythrocytes, macro-ovalocytes, schistocytes, helmet cells, teardrop cells, sickle cells, and target cells.

Once the cell morphology is determined, the anemia can be further classified based on certain physiological and pathological criteria. For example, constitutional aplastic anemia (284.0) is classified physiologically as an anemia of hypoproliferation and pathologically as inborn error of heredity.

The term "coagulation defect" refers to deficiencies or disorders of hemostasis. A complicated process involving substances in the injured tissues, formed elements of blood (platelets, monocytes) and the coagulation proteins, coagulation requires the production of

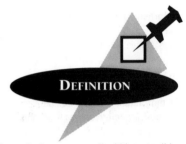

DEFINITION

Coagulation: to turn a liquid into a solid; clot formation of the blood, normally associated with hemostasis.

Erythrocyte: red blood cell (corpuscles).

Haema (or heme): blood.

Hemoglobin: the oxygen-laden portion of the erythrocyte.

Hemostasis: a halt to bleeding, by coagulation, vasoconstriction, or surgical intervention.

Leukocyte: white blood cell (corpuscles).

Sanguis: blood.

Thrombocytes: blood platelets, which serve a role in coagulation.

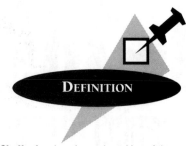

DEFINITION

Cheilosis: chapping and cracking of the lips.

Chlorosis: green/yellow discoloration of the skin usually associated with hypochromic erythrocytes.

Dyspnea: labored respiration.

Fe deficiency anemia: iron deficiency anemia, also referred to as hypochromic-microcytic anemia, low iron levels in the red blood cells.

Glossitis: inflammation of the tongue.

Koilonychia: fingernails that are thin, concave, or otherwise dystrophic, associated with iron deficiency.

Pagophagia: a craving and ingestion of ice, associated with iron deficiency.

Pica: craving and ingestion of nonnutritive substance sometimes associated with iron or zinc deficiency.

Somnolence: abnormal sleepiness.

Tinnitus: ringing in the ears.

Vertigo: dizziness.

thrombin, a substance that stabilizes the platelet plug and forms the fibrin clot. Together, they mechanically block the extravasation of blood from ruptured vessels.

The coagulation process can be interrupted by a genetic or disease-caused protein deficiency, interrupted by an increase in the catabolism of coagulation proteins or inhibited by antibodies directed against the coagulation proteins. There are many proteins involved in coagulation, many of which are identified by the term "factor" followed by a Roman numeral. The appropriate Roman numeral followed by the suffix "a" indicates the activated form of a coagulation factor. For example, when the protein Factor II (prothrombin) is activated by the enzyme thrombin, it is designated Factor IIa.

The term "purpura" refers to a condition characterized by hemorrhage, or extravasation of blood, into the tissues, producing bruises and small red patches on the skin. Purpura may be associated with thrombocytopenia or can occur in a nonthrombocytopenic form. Thrombocytopenia is a decrease of the number of platelets in the circulating blood and may be primary (hereditary or idiopathic) or secondary to a known cause.

Diseases of white blood cells refers to increases, decreases, or genetic or idiopathic anomalies of white blood cells not associated with malignant disease classified to categories 200-208.

Excluded from this rubric is anemia complicating pregnancy and the puerperium, classified to category 648.2.

280 IRON DEFICIENCY ANEMIAS

Classified to this rubric are chronic hypochromic, and microcytic anemias characterized by small, pale erythrocytes and a depletion of iron stores. In adults, iron deficiency anemia is almost always due to blood loss; with loss of as little as 2 ml to 4 ml of blood per day enough to deplete iron stores. This condition also is known as hypoferric anemia, hypochromic, or microcytic anemia and chlorosis.

Signs and symptoms of iron deficiency anemias include pallor, lassitude, somnolence, pica, pagophagia, vertigo, headache, tinnitus, behavioral changes, dyspnea, palpitations, anginal chest pains, and brittle hair and nails. Blood work shows hypochromia, microcytosis, and erythrocyte count less reduced than hemoglobin, serum ferritin below 12 ng/ml, low serum iron, and increased total iron-binding capacity. Bone marrow biopsy shows absence of hemosiderin. Associated conditions include Plummer-Vinson syndrome, glossitis, cheilosis, and koilonychia. Therapies include iron supplementation, either dietary (ferrous sulfate, ferrous gluconate) or parenteral (iron dextran, such as Imferon or similar agent), and blood or blood product transfusion in severe cases.

Excluded from this rubric is familial microcytic anemia (282.4).

280.0   Iron deficiency anemia secondary to blood loss (chronic) — *normocytic anemia due to blood loss*

This subclassification classifies iron deficiency anemia due to prolonged blood loss, usually from a chronically bleeding lesion in the gastrointestinal tract, such as a gastric ulcer or diverticulitis, or a urologic or gynecologic site.

⤶5th   Needs fifth-digit   **OK**   Valid three-digit code

Signs and symptoms of iron deficiency anemias secondary to blood loss (chronic) include history of a chronically bleeding lesion, pallor, lassitude, somnolence, pica, pagophagia, vertigo, headache, tinnitus, behavioral changes, dyspnea, palpitations, anginal chest pains, and brittle hair and nails. Guaiac test reveals occult bleeding. Blood work shows hypochromia, microcytosis, erythrocyte count less reduced than hemoglobin, serum ferritin below 12 ng/ml, low serum iron, and increased total iron-binding capacity. Bone marrow biopsy shows absence of hemosiderin. Therapies include endoscopy to determine bleeding site; iron supplementation, either dietary (ferrous sulfate, ferrous gluconate) or parenteral (iron dextran, such as Imferon or similar agent); and blood or blood product transfusion in severe cases.

Excluded from this subclassification is acute posthemorrhagic anemia (285.1).

280.1   Iron deficiency anemia secondary to inadequate dietary iron intake — *dietary anemia*

This subclassification classifies iron deficiency anemia due to excretion of iron that exceeds normal dietary intake. Iron is recycled metabolically so that less than one milligram is lost through excretion per day. A normal diet consists of 12 mg to 15 mg of iron, of which 0.6 mg to 1.5 mg are absorbed. Neonates and young children may develop iron deficiency anemia due to new blood formation and increased iron utilization that exceeds dietary intake.

280.8   Other specified iron deficiency anemias — *including Paterson-Kelly syndrome, Plummer-Vinson syndrome, Waldenström-Kjellberg syndrome; sideropenic dysphagia*

This subclassification classifies iron deficiency anemias of other specified types and causes, such as gastrectomy, excessive blood donation, and upper small-bowel malabsorption syndromes.

280.9   Unspecified iron deficiency anemia — *including achlorhydric, chlorotic, idiopathic hypochromic Witt's anemias; sideropenia, Hayem-Faber syndrome*

Use this subclassification only when other, more specific codes are not appropriate. Typically classified to 280.9 are microcytic or hypochromic anemias not otherwise specified and iron deficiency anemia due to impaired iron absorption not otherwise specified.

281 OTHER DEFICIENCY ANEMIAS

281.0   Pernicious anemia — *chronic progressive anemia caused by failure to absorb vitamin B_{12}; Addison's anemia, Biermer's anemia; Dana-Putnam syndrome, Lichtheim's syndrome, Runeberg's disease*

Use this subclassification to report chronic, progressive anemia of vitamin B_{12} deficiency due to an absorption defect. Also known as Addison or Biermer anemia, it rarely occurs before the fourth decade of life. The condition may be due to an inherited genetic defect characterized by a deficiency of intrinsic factor, a substance essential for B_{12} absorption.

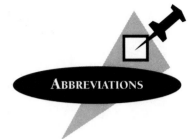

ABBREVIATIONS

CBC: complete blood count

LDH: lactic dehydrogenase

MCH: mean corpuscular Hb

MCHC: mean corpuscular Hb concentration

MCV: mean corpuscular volume

RBC: red blood cell (count)

RIA: radioimmunoassay

WBC: white blood cell (count)

Signs and symptoms of pernicious anemia include anorexia, dyspepsia, pallor with trace of jaundice, weakness, numbness and tingling of extremities, gingival bleeding, smooth, and sore tongue. Blood work reveals oval macrocytes, pancytopenia, hypersegmented neutrophils, elevated serum gastrin, elevated LDH, high serum iron, and absent haptoglobin. Gastric analysis shows no free gastric acid, reveals pH above 7; Schilling test measures absorption of vitamin B_{12}; bone marrow aspiration and analysis shows bone marrow to be megaloblastic. Therapies include parenteral vitamin B_{12}.

Excluded from this subclassification are combined system disease without mention of anemia (266.2) and subacute degeneration of spinal cord without mention of anemia (266.2).

281.1   Other vitamin B_{12} deficiency anemia — *including vegan's anemia; selective vitamin B_{12} malabsorption with proteinuria; Imerslund's syndrome, Imerslund-Gräsbeck syndrome*

Use this subclassification only when other, more specific codes are not appropriate. Clinical vitamin B_{12} deficiency may be caused by dietary deficiency, gastrectomy, regional ileitis, diseases of malformation involving the ileum, ileum resection, and fish tapeworm disease.

Excluded from this subclassification are combined system disease without mention of anemia (266.2) and subacute degeneration of spinal cord without mention of anemia (266.2).

281.2   Folate-deficiency anemia — (Use additional E code to identify drug) — *including congenital, dietary, drug-induced, Zuelzer-Ogden syndrome*

Use this subclassification to report anemia due to deficient stores of folic acid (pteroylmonoglutamic acid), a water-soluble B complex vitamin essential for cell growth and reproduction. Folate is a salt of folic acid.

Signs and symptoms of folate-deficiency anemia include history of poor nourishment or alcoholism, weight loss, glossitis, and blunt masklike facies. Blood work reveals low serum folate levels, decreased red cell folate levels, and peripheral blood smear shows megaloblastic anemia. Therapies include oral or parenteral folic acid.

Associated conditions include nontropical sprue, malabsorption syndrome, alcoholism, and complicated pregnancy.

Folate deficiency can be the result of drug therapy. If a drug causes the folate deficiency anemia, use an additional E code to identify that drug.

281.3   Other specified megaloblastic anemias not elsewhere classified — *predominance of megaloblasts in bone marrow with few normoblasts; combined B12 and folate-deficiency anemia, refractory megaloblastic anemia*

281.4   Protein-deficiency anemia — *amino-acid-deficiency anemia*

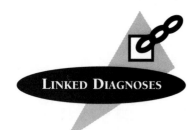

LINKED DIAGNOSES

E codes for drugs commonly associated with folate-deficiency anemia:

E931.0 Sulfonamides causing adverse effects in therapeutic use (Sulfamethoxazole)

E932.2 Ovarian hormones and synthetic substitutes causing adverse effects in therapeutic use (oral contraceptives)

E933.1 Antineoplastic and immunosuppressive drugs causing adverse effects in therapeutic use (Methotrexate)

E936.1 Hydantoin derivatives causing adverse effects in therapeutic use (Dilantin)

✔5th   Needs fifth-digit   **OK**   Valid three-digit code

281.8　Anemia associated with other specified nutritional deficiency — *including scorbutic anemia and achrestic anemia*

281.9　Unspecified deficiency anemia — *unknown*

282 HEREDITARY HEMOLYTIC ANEMIAS

282.0　Hereditary spherocytosis — *genetic hemolytic anemia characterized by jaundice, splenomegaly, and abnormally fragile sphere-shaped erythrocytes; acholuric (familial) jaundice; congenital hemolytic anemia (spherocytic); congenital spherocytosis; Minkowski-Chauffard syndrome; spherocytosis (familial)*

Excluded from this subclassification is hemolytic anemia of newborn (773.0-773.5).

282.1　Hereditary elliptocytosis — *genetic hemolytic anemia characterized by an excessive proportion of abnormally fragile rod-shaped erythrocytes; elliptocytosis, ovalocytosis, Dresbach's syndrome*

282.2　Anemias due to disorders of glutathione metabolism — *including 6-phosphogluconic dehydrogenase deficiency; drug-induced enzyme deficiency; erythrocytic glutathione deficiency; glucose-6-phosphate dehydrogenase [G-6-PD] deficiency; disorder of pentose phosphate pathway; favism*

282.3　Other hemolytic anemias due to enzyme deficiency — *including hemolytic nonspherocytic (hereditary), type II; hexokinase deficiency; pyruvate kinase [PK] deficiency; triosephosphate isomerase deficiency*

282.4　Thalassemias — *hereditary anemias characterized by impaired or decreased synthesis of the polypeptide chains of hemoglobin, occurring primarily in Mediterranean or Southeast Asian populations; Cooley's anemia; sickle-cell thalassemia; Dameshek's syndrome, Rietti-Greppi-Micheli syndrome, Silvestroni-Bianco syndrome*

This subclassification reports microcytic, hypochromic hemolytic anemias that result from a hereditary defect causing deficient hemoglobin synthesis. The severity, treatment, and prognosis of thalassemia depend on the globin gene arrangement and deletion type. Thalassemia major, the most severe form, is evident soon after birth and requires lifelong blood transfusions. Life expectancy rarely exceeds the second decade.

Excluded from this subclassification is sickle-cell anemia (282.60-282.69) and sickle-cell trait (282.5).

282.5　Sickle-cell trait — *Hb-AS genotype*

This subclassification reports a heterozygous carrier of both the hemoglobin S and hemoglobin A genes. The condition rarely is associated with a clinical disorder. Couples in which both individuals carry the sickle-cell trait should be counseled about the possibility of having a child with sickle-cell disease.

Excluded from this subclassification is sickle-cell trait with other hemoglobinopathy (282.60-282.69) or that with thalassemia (282.4).

282.6　Sickle-cell anemia

This subclassification reports severe, chronic, and incurable form of anemia occurring in-patients who inherit hemoglobin S genes from both their parents. Less severe variations of

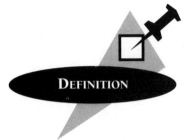

DEFINITION

Hereditary hemolytic anemia: any hereditary anemia characterized by an escalated rate of erythrocyte destruction.

Sickle-cell anemia: Hereditary, genetically determined anemia which symptoms include painful joints, abdominal pain, and skin ulcers.

Thalassemias: a group of hereditary anemias occurring primarily in Mediterranean or Southeast Asian populations.

Normal red
blood cells

Misshapen sickle
red blood cells

the disease occur when the patient inherits hemoglobin S gene from one parent and hemoglobin C, D, or E gene from the other.

Signs and symptoms of sickle-cell anemia include joint pain, fever, lethargy, weakness, and splenomegaly. Blood work reveals hematocrit of 20 percent to 30 percent, hemoglobin of 6.5-10 g/dl, reticulocyte count markedly elevated at 10 percent to 25 percent. Microscopic exam of erythrocytes reveals characteristic "sickling" deformity. Screening tests, such as sodium metabisulfite test and dithionite solubility test, detect sickle-cell anemia or trait. Hemoglobin electrophoresis or chromatography reveal specific hemoglobin abnormalities such as hemoglobin S. Therapies include IV hydration, analgesics for pain, oxygen for hypoxemia, antibiotics for concomitant infection, blood transfusions, and experimental drugs, such as hydroxyurea, to induce fetal hemoglobin synthesis.

Associated conditions include frequent concomitant infections; dehydration; peripheral vaso-occlusion; multisystem involvement, e.g., bone (aseptic necrosis), spleen (splenic infarction), pulmonary (pneumonia), neurological (cerebral ischemia), and ophthalmic (retinopathy).

Sickle-cell crisis refers to recurring acute episodes of pain involving any body system, but usually the chest, bones, or abdomen. In children, vaso-occlusive crisis is the most common form, although the term "sickle-cell crisis" may refer to any one of a variety of sudden and potentially serious conditions.

Excluded from this subclassification are sickle-cell thalassemia (282.4) and sickle-cell trait (282.5).

282.60	Unspecified sickle-cell anemia — *splenic sequestration syndrome*
282.61	Hb-S disease without mention of crisis — *Herrick's syndrome*
282.62	Hb-S disease with mention of crisis — *acute abdominal pain, arthralgia, and leg ulcers in sickle cell anemia; atrophy of the spleen may occur with increased susceptibility to bacterial infection; sickle-cell crisis*
282.63	Sickle-cell/Hb-C disease — *Hb-S/Hb-C disease*
282.69	Other sickle-cell anemia — *including Hb-S/Hb-D; Hb-S/Hb-E*
282.7	Other hemoglobinopathies — *including congenital Heinz-body anemia; hereditary persistence of Hb-Bart's [HPFH], hemoglobin C [Hb-C], hemoglobin D [Hb-D], hemoglobin E [Hb-E], hemoglobin Zurich [Hb-Zurich]*

Excluded from this subclassification are familial polycythemia (289.6), hemoglobin M (Hb-M) disease (289.7), and high-oxygen-affinity hemoglobin (289.0).

282.8	Other specified hereditary hemolytic anemias — *including stomatocytosis*
282.9	Unspecified hereditary hemolytic anemia — *unknown*

283 ACQUIRED HEMOLYTIC ANEMIAS

This rubric reports anemia characterized by the premature destruction of erythrocytes, exclusive of an inherited erythrocyte disorder. Hemolytic anemias may be acquired through infection, injury, drugs, blood transfusions (autoimmune), or other intrinsic or extrinsic causes. Hemolytic uremic syndrome (hemolytic anemia and thrombocytopenia occurring with acute renal failure) is a common manifestation of nonautoimmune hemolytic anemia.

Use an additional E code to identify cause, as appropriate. Excluded from this rubric are Evan's syndrome (287.3) and hemolytic disease of newborn (773.0-773.5).

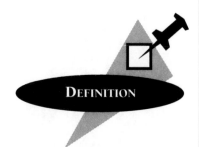

DEFINITION

Hemolysis: disruption in the outer membrane of a red blood cell, causing release of hemoglobin.

✔5th   Needs fifth-digit   **OK**   Valid three-digit code

283.0 Autoimmune hemolytic anemias — (Use additional E code to identify drug, if drug induced) — *including hemolytic anemia: cold, warm, or drug-induced*

283.10 Unspecified non-autoimmune hemolytic anemia — (Use additional E code to identify cause) — *unknown*

283.11 Hemolytic-uremic syndrome

283.19 Other non-autoimmune hemolytic anemias — (Use additional E code to identify cause) — *including mechanical, microangiopathic, toxic; erythrocyte fragmentation syndrome, Lederer-Brill syndromes*

283.2 Hemoglobinuria due to hemolysis from external causes — (Use additional E code to identify cause) — *including acute intravascular hemolysis; hemoglobinuria from exertion or due to hemolysis; Marchiafava-Micheli syndrome, Murri's disease*

283.9 Acquired hemolytic anemia, unspecified — *unknown*

284 APLASTIC ANEMIA

This rubric reports failure of bone marrow to generate blood cells, resulting in a deficiency of all of the formed elements of the blood (erythrocytes, platelets, and leukocytes).

Signs and symptoms of aplastic anemia include bleeding gums (early), oropharyngeal ulcerations (late), fever, waxy pallor, easily fatigued, weakness, frequent infections, bruising easily, increased menstrual flow, and frequent nosebleeds. Blood work reveals pancytopenia (e.g., thrombocytopenia, neutropenia). Bone marrow biopsy shows aplasia or hypocellularity. Therapies include packed red blood cells and platelet transfusions, bone marrow transplants, splenectomy, and drugs such as androgens and adrenal corticosteroids, to stimulate hematopoiesis and marrow regeneration.

Associated conditions include concomitant infections.

284.0 Constitutional aplastic anemia — *including Blackfan-Diamond syndrome, Kaznelson's syndrome*

This subclassification reports an inherited form of aplastic anemia, both planocellular and unicellular. The etiology is believed to be a fundamental intrinsic abnormality of the stem cells.

284.8 Other specified aplastic anemias — (Use additional E code to identify cause) — *including aplastic anemias due to drugs, infection, radiation, toxins, infections, chronic system disease*

This subclassification reports acquired or secondary forms of aplastic anemia. Etiologies include radiation, chronic systemic disease, infections, drugs, toxic chemicals, and red cell aplasia secondary to thymoma.

284.9 Unspecified aplastic anemia — *unknown*

285 OTHER AND UNSPECIFIED ANEMIAS

285.0 Sideroblastic anemia — (Use additional E code to identify drug, if drug induced) — *including pyridoxine-responsive anemia, sideroblastic anemia, sideroblastic hypochromic with iron loading anemia*

285.1 Acute posthemorrhagic anemia — *secondary to acute blood loss*

This subclassification reports anemia due to frank, rapid blood loss. The etiology may be trauma, spontaneous rupture of a blood vessel, surgical procedures involving major blood vessels, pathology such as bleeding peptic ulcers or neoplasms, or extravasation secondary to a bleeding

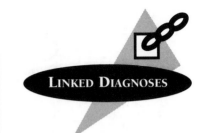

LINKED DIAGNOSES

E codes for drugs commonly associated with hemolytic anemia:

E934.7 Natural blood and blood products causing adverse effects in therapeutic use

E934.8 Other agents affecting blood constituents

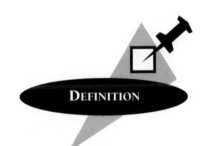

DEFINITION

Aplastic anemia: defective regeneration of red blood cells.

Sideroblastic anemia: an anemia where the iron within the red blood cells is underutilized.

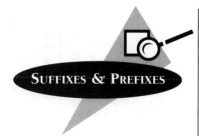

SUFFIXES & PREFIXES

Erythro - red

Hemo - blood

Hypo - lower than normal

Leuko - white

Pan - involving all

Poly - many

Post - after

Thrombo - clot, blood clot

Uni - one

Vaso - vessel, blood vessel

diathesis such as hemophilia. The anemia is usually normochromic and normocytic in an otherwise healthy patient; blood cells can show morphological changes indicative of other concomitant forms of anemia since the condition can occur with any other form of anemia.

Signs and symptoms of acute posthemorrhagic anemia include faintness, dizziness, thirst, weak, rapid pulse, rapid respirations, orthostatic changes in blood pressure, hypovolemic shock. Blood work during and immediately after the hemorrhage may reveal high erythrocyte, hemoglobin, and hematocrit levels due to vasoconstriction. Within a few hours, blood work shows evidence of hemodilution with abnormally low blood indices, polymorphonuclear leukocytosis, and increased thrombocyte production. Therapies include rapid identification of bleeding site and establishment of hemostasis, blood transfusions and IV hydration to restore blood volume, iron supplementation, and monitoring for hypovolemic shock.

Associated conditions include angina and hypovolemic shock. Excluded from this rubric is anemia due to chronic blood loss or not specified as acute blood loss (280.0).

285.2 Anemia in chronic illness

Report codes in this subclassification in conjunction with codes describing the underlying disease as a specific end stage renal disease (ESRD), neoplastic disease, or other chronic illness. Sequencing of the codes depends on the presenting patient complaint and clinical circumstances.

285.21	Anemia in end-stage renal disease — *secondary to early stage renal disease [ESRD]*
285.22	Anemia in neoplastic disease — *secondary to neoplastic disease*
285.29	Anemia of other chronic illness — *secondary to other chronic illness*
285.8	Other specified anemias — *not elsewhere classified, including von Jaksch's anemia, and Brühl's disease; dyserythropoietic anemia, infantile pseudoleukemia*
285.9	Unspecified anemia — *unknown*

Use this subclassification to report normochromic, normocytic anemia of unspecified type, including anemia of chronic disease characterized by shortened red cell survival, suboptimal marrow compensation (sometimes referred to as "relative marrow failure"), defective reutilization of iron, and, occasionally, reduced production of erythropoietin. Such anemias normally do not require treatment unless other characteristics develop, such as iron deficiency anemia (code 280.9) or folic acid deficiency anemia (code 281.2).

Excluded from this subclassification are anemias due to chronic blood loss (280.0), acute blood loss (285.1), or iron deficiency (280.0-280.9).

✔5th   Needs fifth-digit   **OK**   Valid three-digit code

286 COAGULATION DEFECTS

Use an additional E code if the coagulation defect is drug induced.

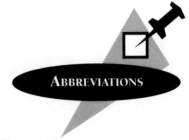

ABBREVIATIONS

286.0   Congenital factor VIII disorder — *abnormal coagulation characterized by subcutaneous and intramuscular hemorrhage and caused by a mutant gene on the X chromosome; classical, familial, hereditary hemophilia A*

286.1   Congenital factor IX disorder — *abnormality of coagulation characterized by subcutaneous and intramuscular hemorrhage and caused by a mutant gene on the X chromosome; Christmas disease, hemophilia B*

286.2   Congenital factor XI deficiency — *Rosenthal's disease; hemophilia C*

286.3   Congenital deficiency of other clotting factors — *congenital afibrinogenemia; Owren's disease, Stuart-Prower disease; dysfibrinogenemia, parahemophilia*

286.4   Von Willebrand's disease — *angiohemophilia (A) (B); factor VIII deficiency with vascular defect*

286.5   Hemorrhagic disorder due to circulating anticoagulants — (Use additional E code to identify drug, if drug induced) — *acquired abnormality of coagulation caused by presence of tissue factor activity (TFA) which initiates coagulation. Manifestation may be blood clot formation (subacute) or serious bleeding (acute)*

286.6   Defibrination syndrome — *consumption coagulopathy; disseminated intravascular coagulation [DIC syndrome], ICF syndrome, IVC syndrome; pathologic fibrinolysis*

286.7   Acquired coagulation factor deficiency — (Use additional E code to identify drug, if drug induced) — *deficiency of coagulation factor due to liver disease or vitamin K deficiency*

286.9   Other and unspecified coagulation defects — *including delay in coagulation or hemostasis disorder*

Abs: antibodies

AF: antifibrinolytic

Ag: antigen

PT: prothrombin time

PTT: partial thromboplastin time

SLE: systemic lupus erythematosus

TFA: tissue factor activity

VWF: von Willebrand factor

287 PURPURA AND OTHER HEMORRHAGIC CONDITIONS

Excluded from this rubric are hemorrhagic thrombocythemia (238.7) and purpura fulminans (286.6).

287.0   Allergic purpura — *small hemorrhage into the skin, mucous membrane, or serosal surface caused by sensitization to foods, drugs, insect bites; peliosis rheumatica rheumataica; Schönlein-Henoch purpura*

The definition of allergic purpura is acute and chronic vasculitis. Also known as anaphylactoid purpura and Schönlein-Henoch purpura, allergic purpura affects small vessels of skin, joints, gastrointestinal tract, and kidney.

Signs and symptoms of allergic purpura include rash on extensor surfaces of arms, legs and feet and across buttocks, fever, polyarthralgia, periauricular tenderness and swelling of joints, edema of hands and feet, colicky abdominal pain, tenderness, melena, hematuria, and proteinuria. Therapies include corticosteroids to control edema, joint and abdominal pain, and eliminating the offending drug.

Excluded from this subclassification are hemorrhagic purpura (287.3) and purpura annularis telangiectodes (709.1).

287.1   Qualitative platelet defects — *including thrombasthenia; thrombocytasthenia, and Bernard-Soulier thrombopathy*

Excluded from this subclassification is von Willebrand's disease (286.4).

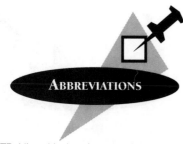

ABBREVIATIONS

ITP: idiopathic thrombocytopenia purpura, a decreased number of platelets circulating in the blood, which in children is usually following an infection and in adults is chronic and has no apparent cause.

287.2 Other nonthrombocytopenic purpuras — *including Diamond-Gardener syndrome*

287.3 Primary thrombocytopenia — *reduced number of platelets in the circulating blood as the principle disease or condition; Evans' syndrome, Kasabach-Merritt syndrome, thrombopenia-hemangioma syndrome, Werlhof-Wichmann syndrome*

This subclassification reports abnormally small number of platelets in the circulating blood as a result of increased platelet destruction without an identifiable exogenous cause or underlying disease. The condition, also known as Werlhof Wichmann Syndrome and idiopathic thrombocytopenia purpura (ITP), is characterized by the sudden onset of signs and symptoms.

Signs and symptoms of primary thrombocytopenia include petechiae; epistaxis; hematuria or abnormal bleeding of gums, vagina, gastrointestinal tract, and bruising easily. Blood work shows decreased platelet count, abnormal bleeding time, and normal prothrombin time (PT) and partial thromboplastin time (PTT). Bone marrow biopsy and analysis reveal increased megakaryocytes without surrounding platelets. Therapies include drugs such as corticosteroids, immunosuppressive therapy (e.g., vincristine or vinblastine) or IV immunoglobulin; splenectomy; and avoidance of any activity that would expose patient to bleeding.

Associated conditions include fatal cerebral hemorrhage, hemorrhage of other sites, acute leukemia, macroglobulinemia, and hematoma formation occasionally causing nerve damage. Excluded from this subclassification are thrombotic thrombocytopenic purpura (446.6) and transient thrombocytopenia of newborn (776.1).

287.4 Secondary thrombocytopenia — (Use additional E code to identify cause) — *reduced number of platelets in the circulating blood as a consequence of an underlying disease or condition; posttransfusion purpura, thrombocytopenia due to drugs, extracorporeal circulation of blood, or platelet alloimmunization*

This subclassification reports thrombocytopenia due to an identifiable exogenous cause or underlying condition, such as congestive splenomegaly, Felty's syndrome, Gaucher's disease, tuberculosis, sarcoidosis, myelofibrosis, lupus erythematosus, Wiskott-Aldrich syndrome, chronic alcoholism, and scurvy. It also may occur as a result of overhydration, blood transfusions, or drug therapy. Use an additional E code to identify cause.

Excluded from this subclassification is transient thromboecytopenia of newborn (776.1).

287.5 Unspecified thrombocytopenia — *unknown*

287.8 Other specified hemorrhagic conditions — *including capillary fragility (hereditary) and vascular pseudohemophilia*

287.9 Unspecified hemorrhagic conditions — *unknown*

✔5th Needs fifth-digit   **OK** Valid three-digit code

288 DISEASES OF WHITE BLOOD CELLS

Excluded from this rubric is leukemia, reported with codes from the series 204.0-208.9.

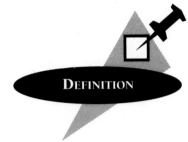

288.0   Agranulocytosis — (Use additional E code to identify drug) — *sudden, severe condition characterized by significant reduction in white blood cells with ulceration of the throat, intestinal tract, and skin; Kostmann's syndrome, Doan-Wiseman syndrome, Werner-Schultz syndrome, Shwachman's syndrome*

This subclassification reports absolute neutrophil count of less than 1,500/cu ml. Also known as neutropenia, agranulocytosis frequently leads to increased susceptibility to bacterial and fungal infections.

Signs and symptoms of agranulocytosis include fever, chills, sore throat, prostration, regional adenopathy, jaundice with liver damage, mucosal ulceration of throat, vagina, or respiratory tract. Peripheral blood smear reveals absence of granulocytes, reduced monocytes, and lymphocytes. Repeated total and differential white blood cell (counts) determine if the neutropenia is acute or chronic. Bone marrow aspiration and biopsy typically appear hypoplastic and may reveal bone marrow involvement by leukemia or infiltrative disorders. Serial blood counts and repeat bone marrow exam five days to seven days typically define the mechanism. Blood and tissue cultures identify infection resulting from agranulocytosis. Therapies include broad-spectrum antibiotics (e.g., penicillin or cephalosporin, as well as aminoglycosides such as gentamicin or tobramycin). If determined to be drug induced, the recommended therapy includes cessation of causative drug and antipyretics for fever. Associated conditions include sepsis and septicemia, pneumonia, hemorrhagic necrosis of mucous membranes, perirectal abscess, and parenchymal liver damage. Use an additional E code to identify the drug or other cause of agranulocytosis. Excluded from this subclassification is transitory neonatal neutropenia (776.7).

288.1   Functional disorders of polymorphonuclear neutrophils — *including chronic childhood granulomatous disease, congenital dysphagocytosis, Job's syndrome, lipochrome histiocytosis, and progressive septic granulomatosis*

288.2   Genetic anomalies of leukocytes — *including Alder's (-Reilly) syndrome, Chédiak-Steinbrinck (-Higashi) syndrome, Jordan's syndrome, May-Hegglin syndrome, Pelger-Huet syndrome; Döhle body-panmyelopathic syndrome*

288.3   Eosinophilia — *elevated proportion of a type of white blood cell readily stained with eosin; allergic, hereditary, idiopathic, secondary*

This subclassification reports absolute eosinophil count of more than 500/cu ml. Counts of 500/ cu ml to 1,000/cu ml are nonspecific and normally are not viewed as a clinical problem. Associated conditions include allergic disorders, parasitic infestation with tissue invasion, skin diseases, tumors, Hodgkin's disease, granulomatous disease, eosinophilic leukemia, fibroplastic endocarditis, systemic vasculitis, and tropical eosinophilia.

Excluded from this rubric are Loffler's syndrome and pulmonary eosinophilia (518.3).

Agranulocytosis: usually referred to as neutropenia, a sudden, severe condition characterized by a significant reduction in white blood cells.

Eosinophilia: elevated proportion of a type of white blood cell readily stained with eosin, a fluorescent acid dye.

Leukocytosis: an increased amount of white blood cells, often seen in acute infections.

288.8 Other specified disease of white blood cells — *including lymphocytopenia, lymphocytosis, monocytosis, leukocytosis, plasmacytosis, hyperleukocytosis, hypoeosinophilia*

288.9 Unspecified disease of white blood cells — *unknown*

289 OTHER DISEASES OF BLOOD AND BLOOD-FORMING ORGANS

289.0 Polycythemia, secondary — *elevated number of red blood cells in the circulating blood occurring as a result to reduced oxygen supply to the tissues; Gaisböck's syndrome*

This subclassification reports an increase in the normal number of red blood cells. Secondary polycythemia also is known as secondary erythrocytosis, spurious polycythemia, and reactive polycythemia. Spurious polycythemia, which is characterized by increased hematocrit and normal or increased erythrocyte total mass, results from a decrease in plasma volume and hemoconcentration. Reactive polycythemia is a condition characterized by excessive production of circulating erythrocytes due to an identifiable secondary condition, such as hypoxia, or an underlying disease, such as a neoplasm.

Excluded from this subclassification are neonatal polycythemia (776.4) and primary polycythemia and polycythemia vera (238.4).

289.1 Chronic lymphadenitis — *persistent inflammation of one or more lymph nodes except mesenteric*

This subclassification reports inflammation of lymph nodes. Any pathogen can cause lymphadenitis. Lymphadenitis may be generalized or restricted to regional lymph nodes and may occur with systemic infections. Excluded from this subclassification are acute lymphadenitis (683), mesenteric lymphadenitis (289.2), and enlarged glands not otherwise specified (785.6).

289.2 Nonspecific mesenteric lymphadenitis — *inflammation of one or more lymph nodes in the peritoneal fold that encases the abdominal organs; Brennemann's syndrome*

This subclassification reports lymphadenitis occurring in a double layer of peritoneum attached to the abdominal wall that encloses a portion or all of one of the mesentery (abdominal viscera).

289.3 Lymphadenitis, unspecified, except mesenteric — *unknown and other than mesenteric*

289.4 Hypersplenism — *cellular components of blood or platelets are removed at an accelerated rate causing deficiency of peripheral blood elements; "big spleen" syndrome; hypoleukemia splenica*

This subclassification reports a clinical syndrome characterized by splenic hyperactivity and splenomegaly. The condition results in a peripheral blood cell deficiency because the spleen traps and destroys the circulating peripheral blood cells.

Signs and symptoms of hypersplenism include history of frequent infection and bruising easily, and abnormal bleeding from mucous

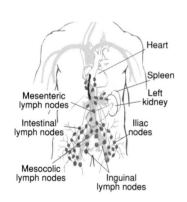

Heart
Spleen
Left kidney
Mesenteric lymph nodes
Intestinal lymph nodes
Iliac nodes
Mesocolic lymph nodes
Inguinal lymph nodes

✔5th   Needs fifth-digit   **OK**   Valid three-digit code

membranes, genitourinary tract, or gastrointestinal tract. There may be ulcers of the mouth, legs, or feet, fever, weakness, and palpitations. Blood work reveals mild, normochromic, and normocytic anemia with elevated reticulocyte count and markedly decreased platelets and granulocytes. Radionuclide scan of chromium-labeled erythrocytes or platelets demonstrates increased splenic activity, while splenic angiography demonstrates portal obstruction or hypertension. Biopsy of spleen reveals pathology such as infiltrative disease (e.g., lymphoma, Gaucher's amyloidosis).

Therapies include medical treatment of underlying etiology or splenectomy, if medical treatment ineffective.

Associated conditions include recurrent infections such as persistent leg ulcers, Gaucher disease, Niemann-Pick disease, congestive cirrhosis (portal hypertension) or thrombosis, hemolytic anemia, polycythemia vera, Felty's syndrome, subacute bacterial endocarditis, Letterer-Siwe disease, tuberculosis, cystic or neoplastic disease, such as leukemia, lymphoma, myelofibrosis, or Boeck's sarcoidosis.

Excluded from this subclassification is primary splenic neutropenia (288.0).

289.50	Unspecified disease of spleen — *unknown*
289.51	Chronic congestive splenomegaly — *chronic congestive splenomegaly*
289.59	Other diseases of spleen — *including fibrosis, infarct, rupture, infection, abscess, cyst, atrophy, prolapse, ptosis, torsion, splenocele, wandering spleen*
289.6	Familial polycythemia — *elevation of the number of red blood cells in the blood; benign polycythemia; erythrocytosis*
289.7	Methemoglobinemia — (Use additional E code to identify cause) — *presence in the blood of methemoglobin, a chemically altered form of hemoglobin useless for respiration, causing cyanosis, headache, dizziness, ataxia dyspnea, tachycardia, nausea, stupor, coma, and rarely, death; NADH, DPNH-methemoglobin-reductase deficiency; Stokvis' disease, van den Bergh's disease*
289.8	Other specified diseases of blood and blood-forming organs — *including hypergammaglobulinemia, myelofibrosis, pseudocholinesterase deficiency, hypercoagulation syndrome, hyperprothrombinemia, lipophagocytosis, macrocytosis, myeloid metaplasia, necrotic bone marrow, nitrosohemoglobinemia, normoblastosis, osteosclerosis myelofibrosis, osteosclerotic anemia*
289.9	Unspecified diseases of blood and blood-forming organs — *unknown*

Chapter 5

290–319
Mental Disorders

The World Health Organization (WHO) offers the following guidelines that apply to this chapter: when classifying behavioral disorders, organically based illnesses should get precedence over functional ones, and within the functional group, the order then may be psychoses, neuroses, personality disorders and others. When coding mental illnesses associated with physical conditions, assign as many codes as necessary to fully describe the clinical picture.

290-299 Psychoses

The term "psychoses" has been applied to many non-psychotic mental disorders historically. For this classification, the definition of psychoses includes only conditions that interfere with activities of daily living and include a gross impairment of reality. Codes in this section represent disorders that exhibit delusions, hallucinations, markedly incoherent speech, disorganized behaviors, and the inability on the part of the patient to comprehend the inappropriateness of this behavior.

290-294 Organic Psychotic Conditions

Included in this section are senile and presenile dementia, arteriosclerotic dementia, dementia, and hallucinosis associated with substance abuse and organic brain syndromes. Assign a code from these rubrics only when the specific organic clinical feature of a confused state, dementia, or delirium is present. Do not use a code from these categories to report the organic etiology of a psychotic mental state that is coded elsewhere in this chapter.

290 SENILE AND PRESENILE ORGANIC PSYCHOTIC CONDITIONS

Arteriosclerotic dementia is attributable to degenerative arterial disease of the brain. Symptoms suggesting a focal lesion in the brain are common. There may be a fluctuating or patchy intellectual defect with insight, and an intermittent course is common. Clinical differentiation from senile or presenile dementia, which may coexist with it, may be very difficult or impossible. Cerebral atherosclerosis should also be reported in addition to the code for the psychosis.

Senile dementia usually occurs after the age of 65 in which any cerebral pathology other than that of senile atrophic change can be reasonably excluded. Presenile dementia occurs before age 65, and is usually associated with diffuse or lobar cerebral atrophy.

In delirium, a superimposed reversible episode of acute confusional state exists; in the delusional type, delusions, varying from simple poorly formed paranoid delusions to highly formed paranoid delusional states, and hallucinations are also present in a progressive

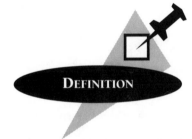

DEFINITION

Arteriosclerotic dementia: also referred to as multi-infarct dementia, is brought on by the hardening of the blood vessels.

Delirium: confused state of having false beliefs and judgments.

Delusional: the state of having false beliefs and judgments.

Presenile: dementia: mental deterioration before age 65.

Senile dementia: mental deterioration brought on by aging.

disease of persons in advanced age. Senile dementia, depressed type, is characterized by development in advanced old age, progressive in nature, in which depressive features, ranging from mild to severe forms of manic-depressive affective psychosis, are also present. Disturbance of the sleep-waking cycle and preoccupation with the deceased often particularly prominent.

In addition to the appropriate code from this rubric, also code any associated neurological condition such as Pick's disease, Alzheimer's disease, or Jakob-Creutzfeldt disease. Pick's disease, while present in the senile period, may primarily affect the frontal and temporal lobes. Alzheimer's disease is due to a large loss of cells from brain areas such as the cerebral cortex. Jakob-Creutzfeldt disease is a rare, progressive, fatal virus of the central nervous system.

Excluded from this rubric are dementias associated with other cerebral conditions (294.10-294.11), psychoses occurring in old age without dementia or delirium (295.0-298.8), senility with mental changes of nonpsychotic severity (310.1), and transient organic psychotic conditions (293.0-293.9).

If mental or behavioral problems are unspecified, report V40.9 *Unspecified mental or behavioral problem*. However, this code is not an acceptable principal diagnosis.

290.0	Senile dementia, uncomplicated — (Use additional code to identify associated (condition)) — *senile dementia, not otherwise specified*
290.10	Presenile dementia, uncomplicated — *simple type*
290.11	Presenile dementia with delirium — *with acute confusional state*
290.12	Presenile dementia with delusional features — *paranoid type, including Binswanger's dementia*
290.13	Presenile dementia with depressive features — *depressed type*
290.20	Senile dementia with delusional features — *paranoid type or senile psychosis not otherwise specified*
290.21	Senile dementia with depressive features
290.3	Senile dementia with delirium — (Use additional code to identify associated (condition)) — *with acute confusional state*
290.40	Arteriosclerotic dementia, uncomplicated — (Use additional code to identify associated (condition) 437.0) — *simple type*
290.41	Arteriosclerotic dementia with delirium — (Use additional code to identify associated (condition) 437.0) — *with acute confusional state*
290.42	Arteriosclerotic dementia with delusional features — (Use additional code to identify associated (condition) 437.0) — *paranoid type*
290.43	Arteriosclerotic dementia with depressive features — (Use additional code to identify associated (condition) 437.0) — *depressed type*
290.8	Other specified senile psychotic conditions
290.9	Unspecified senile psychotic condition

291 ALCOHOLIC PSYCHOSES

Alcoholic psychoses are organic psychotic states due mainly to excessive consumption of alcohol. Defects of nutrition are thought to play an important role in alcoholic psychoses. Alcoholic psychoses are classified according to the complex of presenting symptoms.

Alcohol withdrawal delirium is an acute or subacute organic psychotic state in alcoholics characterized by clouded consciousness, disorientation, fear, illusions, delusions, hallucinations of any kind, notably visual and tactile, and restlessness, tremor, and

✎5th   Needs fifth-digit   **OK**   Valid three-digit category sometimes fever. Alcohol amnestic syndrome is a syndrome of prominent and lasting reduction of memory span, including striking loss of recent memory, disordered time appreciation, and confabulation, occurring in alcoholics as the sequel to an acute alcoholic psychosis (especially delirium tremens) or, more rarely, in the course of chronic alcoholism. It is usually accompanied by peripheral neuritis and may be associated with Wernicke's encephalopathy.

291.0	Alcohol withdrawal delirium — *delirium tremens*
291.1	Alcohol amnestic syndrome — *Korsakoff's psychosis, alcoholic polyneuritic psychosis*
291.2	Other alcoholic dementia — *chronic alcoholic brain syndrome*
291.3	Alcohol withdrawal hallucinosis — *psychosis with hallucinosis*
291.4	Idiosyncratic alcohol intoxication — *pathologic drunkenness*
291.5	Alcoholic jealousy — *psychosis, paranoid type*
291.81	Alcohol withdrawal — *withdrawal symptoms*
291.89	Other specified alcoholic psychosis — *not elsewhere specified*
291.9	Unspecified alcoholic psychosis — *chronic alcoholism with psychosis, not otherwise specified*

292 DRUG PSYCHOSES

Drug psychoses are organic mental syndromes which are due to consumption of drugs (notably amphetamines, barbiturates, and opiate and LSD groups) and solvents. Some of the syndromes in this group are not as severe as most conditions labeled "psychotic," but they are included here for practical reasons. Drug psychoses are classified according to the complex of presenting symptoms. In drug withdrawal syndrome, convulsions, tremor, disorientation, and memory disturbances may occur. In hallucinatory/paranoid states, the patient may experience auditory hallucinations and anxiety.

Use an additional code from rubric 304 to report any associated drug dependence, and an E code to identify the drug.

292.0	Drug withdrawal syndrome — (Use additional code to identify any associated (condition) 304.00–304.93) — *abstinence syndrome or symptoms*
292.11	Drug-induced organic delusional syndrome — *paranoid state induced by drugs*
292.12	Drug-induced hallucinosis — *hallucinatory state induced by drugs*
292.2	Pathological drug intoxication — (Use additional code to identify any associated (condition) 304.00–304.93) — *reaction resulting in brief psychotic state*
292.81	Drug-induced delirium
292.82	Drug-induced dementia
292.83	Drug-induced amnestic syndrome — *memory loss*
292.84	Drug-induced organic affective syndrome — *depressive state induced by drugs*
292.89	Other specified drug-induced mental disorder — *including drug-induced organic personality syndrome, amotivational syndrome, and drug flashback syndrome*
292.9	Unspecified drug-induced mental disorder — (Use additional code to identify any associated (condition) 304.00–304.93) — *not otherwise specified*

293 TRANSIENT ORGANIC PSYCHOTIC CONDITIONS

Transient organic psychotic conditions are conditions characterized by clouded consciousness, confusion, disorientation, illusions, and frequently vivid hallucinations. Typically, they are due to some intra- or extracerebral toxic, infectious, metabolic, or other systemic disturbance and generally are reversible.

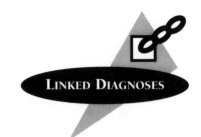

LINKED DIAGNOSES

The following E Codes can be used with 292 Drug Psychoses:

Accidental poisoning by drugs
E850.0 Heroin

E850.1 Methadone

E850.2 Other opiates and related narcotics

E851 Accidental poisoning by barbiturates

E852.3 Methaqualone compounds

E852.5 Mixed sedatives not elsewhere classified

E854.0 Antidepressants

E854.1 Psychodysleptic

E854.2 Psychostimulants

Drugs causing adverse effects in therapeutic use
E935.0 Heroin

E935.1 Methadone

E935.2 Other opiates and related narcotics

E937.0 Barbiturates

E937.4 Methaqualone compounds

E937.6 Mixed sedatives not elsewhere classified

E939.0 Antidepressants

E939.1 Phenothiazine-based tranquilizers

E939.6 Psychodysleptic

E939.7 Psychostimulants

When using a code from this category, assign an additional code to identify the associated physical or neurological condition.

Acute delirium has an acute or rapid onset and is characterized by extreme disturbances of arousal, attention, orientation, perception, intellectual functions, and affect. These conditions are accompanied commonly by fear and agitation.

Organic affective syndrome is similar to depressive or manic-depressive disorder, but occurs in the presence of specific organic factors such as head trauma, endocranial tumors, exocranial tumors (such as pancreatic carcinoma), steroid overuse, Cushing's syndrome, and other endocrine disorders.

293.0	Acute delirium — (Code first the associated condition) — *including postoperative confusion state, psycho-organic syndrome*
293.1	Subacute delirium — (Code first the associated condition) — *organic in origin*
293.81	Organic delusional syndrome — *transient psychotic condition, paranoid type*
293.82	Organic hallucinosis syndrome — *transient psychotic condition, hallucinatory type*
293.83	Organic affective syndrome — *transient psychotic condition, depressive type*
293.84	Organic anxiety syndrome
293.89	Other specified transient organic mental disorder — *including Alice in Wonderland syndrome*
293.9	Unspecified transient organic mental disorder

294 OTHER ORGANIC PSYCHOTIC CONDITIONS (CHRONIC)

Amnestic syndrome presents with a prominent and lasting reduction of memory span, including striking loss of recent memory, disordered time appreciation, and confabulation. The commonest causes are chronic alcoholism [alcohol amnestic syndrome, Korsakoff's alcoholic psychosis], chronic barbiturate dependence, and malnutrition. An amnestic syndrome may be the predominating disturbance in the early states of presenile and senile dementia, arteriosclerotic dementia, and in encephalitis and other inflammatory and degenerative diseases in which there is particular bilateral involvement of the temporal lobes, and certain temporal lobe tumors.

Other specified chronic organic brain syndromes include conditions that present a clinical picture of organic psychosis but do not take the shape of a confusional state (293), a nonalcoholic Korsakoff's psychosis (294.0), or demential due to an underlying physical condition (294.1).

294.0	Amnestic syndrome — *Korsakoff's psychosis or syndrome (nonalcoholic)*
294.10	Dementia in conditions classified elsewhere without behavioral disturbance — *secondary to organic disease*
294.11	Dementia in conditions classified elsewhere with behavioral disturbance — *secondary to organic disease*
294.8	Other specified organic brain syndromes (chronic) — (Use additional code for associated (condition) 345.00–345.91) — *including mixed paranoid and affective organic psychotic state*
294.9	Unspecified organic brain syndrome (chronic) — *chronic organic psychosis*

✔5th Needs fifth-digit   **OK** Valid three-digit category

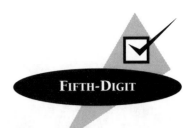

295-299 Other Psychoses

Use an additional code to identify any associated physical disease, injury, or condition affecting the brain with psychoses classifiable to these rubrics.

295 SCHIZOPHRENIC DISORDERS

Schizophrenia is not diagnosed unless there is characteristic disturbance of at least two of these areas: thought, perception, mood, conduct, and personality. Paranoid type schizophrenia includes delusions of persecution or grandeur, thought disorder and hallucinations with less personality disintegration than in other subtypes of schizophrenia. Latent schizophrenia is sometimes called borderline schizophrenia, and is a condition in which there is potential for developing schizophrenia under emotional distress. This term is not recommended for patient diagnosis because a general consensus of its description has not been reached.

Residual schizophrenia presents with symptoms from the acute phrase, but the symptoms have lost their prominence or sharpness. Schizoaffective type schizophrenia is a mixture of symptoms form schizophrenia and affective psychoses.

- **295.0** ✔5th Simple type schizophrenia — *schizophrenia simplex*
- **295.1** ✔5th Disorganized type schizophrenia — *hebephrenic type schizophrenia*
- **295.2** ✔5th Catatonic type schizophrenia — *catatonic schizophrenia*
- **295.3** ✔5th Paranoid type schizophrenia — *paraphrenic schizophrenia*
- **295.4** ✔5th Acute schizophrenic episode — *oneirophrenia, schizophreniform psychosis, confusional*
- **295.5** ✔5th Latent schizophrenia — *prodromal, pseudoneurotic, borderline, incipient, prepsychotic*
- **295.6** ✔5th Residual schizophrenia — *chronic undifferentiated, Restzustand schizophrenia*
- **295.7** ✔5th Schizo-affective type schizophrenia — *cyclic, mixed*
- **295.8** ✔5th Other specified types of schizophrenia — *acute, atypical, cenesthopathic*
- **295.9** ✔5th Unspecified schizophrenia — *not otherwise specified, including Morel-Kraepelin disease*

296 AFFECTIVE PSYCHOSES

Affective psychoses are recurrent, severe disturbances of mood accompanied by one or more of the following: delusions, perplexity, disturbed attitude to self, disorder of perception and behavior. Patients with affective psychoses have a strong characteristic inclination toward suicide. This category includes mild disorders of mood if the symptoms closely match the descriptions.

Manic disorder, as a single episode, is characterized by elation, excitement, rapid thought process, increased psychomotor activity, and emotional instability. Diminished interest in activities, fatigue, insomnia or hypersomnia, and change in weight characterize a major depressive disorder as a single episode. In bipolar disorder, the patient cycles between the two states: manic and depressive.

- **296.0** ✔5th Manic disorder, single episode — *hypomania, single episode or unspecified*
- **296.1** ✔5th Manic disorder, recurrent episode — *hypomania, recurrent*
- **296.2** ✔5th Major depressive disorder, single episode — *endogenous depression, single episode or unspecified*
- **296.3** ✔5th Major depressive disorder, recurrent episode — *endogenous depression, recurrent*

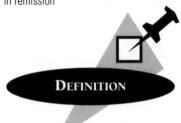

The following fifth-digit subclassification is for use with category 295:
0 unspecified
1 subchronic
2 chronic
3 subchronic with acute exacerbation
4 chronic with acute exacerbation
5 in remission

Types of Schizophrenia:
Catatonic: schizophrenia with a change in activity by either an increase or inhibition.
Disorganized: severe schizophrenia with incoherent and inappropriate behavior.
Paranoid: schizophrenia in which the affected has delusions of being persecuted.
Simple: schizophrenia with indifference and withdrawal.

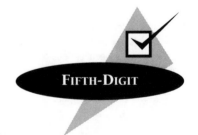

The following fifth-digit subclassification is for use with categories 296.0-296.6:
0 unspecified
1 mild
2 moderate
3 severe, without mention of psychotic behavior
4 severe, specified as with psychotic behavior
5 in partial or unspecified remission
6 in full remission

FIFTH-DIGIT

The following fifth-digit subclassification is for use with categories 296.0-296.6:

0 unspecified
1 mild
2 moderate
3 severe, without mention of psychotic behavior
4 severe, specified as with psychotic behavior
5 in partial or unspecified remission
6 in full remission

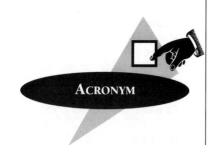

ACRONYM

BAD: bipolar affective disorder, a disorder in which the mood fluctuates between depression and mania. When feeling an emotion, it is usually very intense.

MDD: manic-depressive disorder, the same disorder as BAD except that either state occurs in a single episode or reaction.

296.4 ✔5th Bipolar affective disorder, manic — *circular manic depressive psychosis, in manic state*
296.5 ✔5th Bipolar affective disorder, depressed — *circular manic depressive psychosis, in depressed state*
296.6 ✔5th Bipolar affective disorder, mixed — *circular manic depressive psychosis, mixed state*
296.7 Bipolar affective disorder, unspecified — *circular manic depressive psychosis, current state unspecified*
296.80 Manic-depressive psychosis, unspecified — *atypical manic depressive psychosis, current state unspecified*
296.81 Atypical manic disorder — *atypical manic only*
296.82 Atypical depressive disorder — *atypical depressive only*
296.89 Other manic-depressive psychosis — *atypical manic depressive psychosis, mixed status*
296.90 Unspecified affective psychosis — *not otherwise specified*
296.99 Other specified affective psychoses — *mood swings: brief compensatory, rebuond*

297 PARANOID STATES (DELUSIONAL DISORDERS)

Excluded from this rubric are acute paranoid reaction (298.3), alcoholic jealousy or paranoid state (291.5), and paranoid schizophrenia (295.3).

Cotard's syndrome, characterized by suicidal tendencies and sensory disturbances, is classified to 297.1.

297.0 Paranoid state, simple — *simple*
297.1 Paranoia — *chronic, Sander's disease, Cotard's syndrome, systematized delusions*
297.2 Paraphrenia — *involutional paranoid state, late paraphrenia, paraphrenia (involutional)*
297.3 Shared paranoid disorder — *folie à deux, induced psychosis or paranoid disorder*
297.8 Other specified paranoid states — *including paranoia querulans, sensitiver Beziehungswahn, psyche passionelle; tarantism*
297.9 Unspecified paranoid state — *unknown, including Lasegue's disease*

298 OTHER NONORGANIC PSYCHOSES

Classified to this rubric are a small group of psychotic conditions that are attributable largely to a recent life experience. They should not be used for the wider range of psychoses in which environmental factors play some, but not a major, part in the etiology.

Lycanthropy, the delusion that the patient believes himself to be a wolf, is classified in the ICD-9-CM index to 298.9, as is nosomania, a delusion of being infected by disease.

298.0 Depressive type psychosis — *psychogenic depressive psychosis*
298.1 Excitative type psychosis — *acute hysterical psychosis; reactive excitation*
298.2 Reactive confusion — *psychogenic confusion/twilight state*
298.3 Acute paranoid reaction — *acute psychogenic paranoid psychosis; Bouffée délirante*
298.4 Psychogenic paranoid psychosis — *protracted reactive paranoid psychosis*
298.8 Other and unspecified reactive psychosis — *hysterical psychosis, psychogenic stupor*
298.9 Unspecified psychosis — *including lycanthropy, nosomania, parergasia, vesania*

✔5th   Needs fifth-digit   **OK**   Valid three-digit category

299 PSYCHOSES WITH ORIGIN SPECIFIC TO CHILDHOOD

Excluded from this rubric are adult type psychoses occurring in childhood, as in affective disorders (296.0-296.9); manic-depressive disorders (296.0-296.9), and schizophrenia (295.0-295.9).

Infantile autism is a syndrome present from birth or beginning almost invariably in the first 30 months. Responses to auditory and sometimes to visual stimuli are abnormal, and there are usually severe problems in the understanding of spoken language. Speech is delayed and, if it develops, is characterized by echolalia, the reversal of pronouns, immature grammatical structure, and inability to use abstract terms. There is generally an impaired social use of both verbal and gestural language. Problems in social relationships are most severe before the age of five years and include an impaired development of eye-to-eye gaze, social attachments, and cooperative play. Ritualistic behavior is usual and may include abnormal routines, resistance to change, attachment to odd objects, and stereotyped patterns of play. The capacity for abstract or symbolic thought and for imaginative play is diminished. Intelligence ranges from severely subnormal to normal or above. Performance is usually better on tasks involving rote memory or visuospatial skills than on those requiring symbolic or linguistic skills.

299.0 ✔5th Infantile autism — *childhood autism; Kanner's syndrome*
299.1 ✔5th Disintegrative psychosis — (Use additional code to identify any associated (condition)) — *Heller's syndrome*
299.8 ✔5th Other specified early childhood psychoses — *atypical childhood psychosis; borderline psychosis of childhood*
299.9 ✔5th Unspecified childhood psychosis — *unknown*

300-316 Neurotic Disorders, Personality Disorders, and Other Nonpsychotic Mental Disorders

300 NEUROTIC DISORDERS

Neurotic disorders have no obvious evidence of an organic etiology, and there is no lost sense of reality or disorganized personality. Symptoms may include anxiety, hysteria, obsession, compulsion, depression, or phobia. Behavior may be greatly affected although usually remaining within socially acceptable limits.

In psychogenic amnesia, there is a temporary disturbance in the ability to recall important personal information that has already been registered and stored in memory. The sudden onset of this disturbance in the absence of an underlying organic mental disorder, and the extent of the disturbance being too great to be explained by ordinary forgetfulness are the essential features.

In factitious illness, there are physical or psychological symptoms that are not real, genuine, or natural, which are produced by the individual and are under voluntary control. The presentation of physical symptoms may be fabricated, self-inflicted, an exaggeration or exacerbation of a pre-existing physical condition, or any combination or variation of these.

In phobia, the patient experiences abnormal intense dread of certain objects or specific situations. If the anxiety tends to spread from a specified situation or object to a wider range of circumstances, it becomes akin to or identical with an anxiety state, and should be classified as such. Excluded from phobic disorders are anxiety states not associated with a specific situation or object (300.00-300.09) and obsessional phobia (300.3).

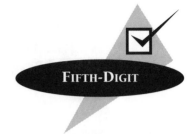

FIFTH-DIGIT

The following fifth-digit subclassification is for use with category 299:

0 current or active state

1 residual state

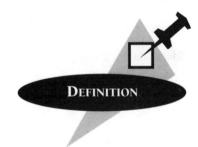

DEFINITION

Anxiety: a feeling of distress or apprehension. Can cause difficulty breathing, restlessness, and tension.

Conversion: where emotions are transformed into a physical condition.

Hysteria: psychogenic symptoms affecting the ability to function.

Neurotic: suffering from a neurosis, in which the affected is tense, irritable, and anxious.

Panic: extreme fearfulness.

Phobia: an unfounded fear.

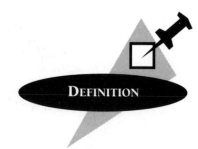

DEFINITION

Acrophobia: fear of heights.

Agoraphobia: fear of leaving the familiar setting of the home.

Ailurophobia/galeophobia: fear of cats.

Algophobia: fear of pain.

Bromidrosiphobia: fear of body odor.

Brontophobia: fear of thunderstorms.

Claustrophobia: fear of closed spaces.

Cynophobia: fear of dogs.

Mysophobia: fear of germs.

Ophidiophobia: fear of snakes.

Panphobia: fear of everything.

Sitophobia: fear of eating.

In obsessive-compulsive behavior, the outstanding symptom is a feeling of subjective compulsion, which must be resisted. The obsessional urge or idea is recognized as alien to the personality but as coming from within the self. Obsessional actions may be quasi-ritual performances designed to relieve anxiety. Attempts to dispel the unwelcome thoughts or urges may lead to a severe inner struggle, with intense anxiety.

300.00	Anxiety state, unspecified — *anxiety neurosis; asphyctic syndrome*
300.01	Panic disorder — *panic attack*
300.02	Generalized anxiety disorder
300.09	Other anxiety states — *not elsewhere classified*
300.10	Hysteria, unspecified
300.11	Conversion disorder — *astasia-abasia; hysterical blindness/deafness; Bergeron's disease*
300.12	Psychogenic amnesia — *hysterical amnesia*
300.13	Psychogenic fugue — *hysterical fugue*
300.14	Multiple personality — *dissociative identity disorder*
300.15	Dissociative disorder or reaction, unspecified — *unknown*
300.16	Factitious illness with psychological symptoms — *compensation neurosis; Ganser's hysterical syndrome*
300.19	Other and unspecified factitious illness — *including factitious illness with physical symptoms, NOS*
300.20	Phobia, unspecified — *unknown*
300.21	Agoraphobia with panic attacks — *fear of open spaces, streets, travel; with panic attacks*
300.22	Agoraphobia without mention of panic attacks — *fear of open spaces, streets, travel; without mention of panic attacks*
300.23	Social phobia — *fear of eating, washing, speaking in public*
300.29	Other isolated or simple phobias — *including acrophobia, claustrophobia, animal phobias*
300.3	Obsessive-compulsive disorders — *including anancastic neurosis, any obsessional phobia, compulsive neurosis*
300.4	Neurotic depression — *anxiety depression, reactive depression*
300.5	Neurasthenia — (Use additional code to identify any associated (condition)) — *fatigue neurosis, general fatigue, psychogenic asthenia*
300.6	Depersonalization syndrome — *neurotic derealization*
300.7	Hypochondriasis — *body dysmorphic disorder*
300.81	Somatization disorder — *Briquet's disorder, severe somatoform disorder*
300.82	Undifferentiated somatoform disorder — *atypical somatoform disorder*
300.89	Other neurotic disorders — *including occupational neurosis, including writers' cramp, psychasthenia, Janet's disease*
300.9	Unspecified neurotic disorder — *including neurosis NOS, merergasia, self-mutilation, suicide risk*

301 PERSONALITY DISORDERS

Personality disorders include character neuroses, but excludes nonpsychotic personality disorders associated with organic brain syndromes (310.0-310.9). Use an additional code to identify an associated neurosis or psychosis, or physical condition.

A dependent personality disorder allows a patient to permit another individual to take control of his or her life. This patient also allows the needs of the person to supersede personal needs. A borderline personality is characterized by instability in interpersonal relationships, behavior, mood, and perception of self-image.

✔5th   Needs fifth-digit   **OK**   Valid three-digit category

301.0	Paranoid personality disorder — (Use additional code to identify any associated (condition)) — *fanatic personality; paranoid traits*
301.10	Hysteria, unspecified
301.11	Chronic hypomanic personality disorder — *chronic hypomanic disorder*
301.12	Chronic depressive personality disorder — *chronic depressive disorder*
301.13	Cyclothymic disorder — *cycloid personality; cyclothymia*
301.20	Schizoid personality disorder, unspecified — *schizoid personality disorder, unspecified*
301.21	Introverted personality
301.22	Schizotypal personality
301.3	Explosive personality disorder — (Use additional code to identify any associated (condition)) — *excessive emotional instability; pathological emotionality*
301.4	Compulsive personality disorder — (Use additional code to identify any associated (condition)) — *compulsive personality disorder; obsessional personality*
301.50	Histrionic personality disorder, unspecified — *not elsewhere classified*
301.51	Chronic factitious illness with physical symptoms — *including hospital addiction syndrome; Munchausen syndrome*
301.59	Other histrionic personality disorder — *emotionally unstable; psychoinfantile; labile*
301.6	Dependent personality disorder — (Use additional code to identify any associated (condition)) — *asthenic or passive personality*
301.7	Antisocial personality disorder — (Use additional code to identify any associated (condition)) — *amoral or sociopathic personality*
301.81	Narcissistic personality
301.82	Avoidant personality
301.83	Borderline personality
301.84	Passive-aggressive personality
301.89	Other personality disorder — *including eccentric, masochistic or psychoneurotic*
301.9	Unspecified personality disorder — (Use additional code to identify any associated (condition)) — *including Witzelsucht; psychopathic constitutional*

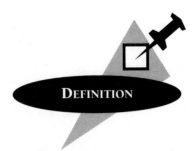

DEFINITION

Personality Disorders:

Affective: a personality disorder in which the emotions (either depression or mania) affect relationships.

Paranoid: suspicious, jealous, and sensitive behavior in relationships.

Schizoid: coldness, withdrawal, and indifference in relationships.

Witzelsucht: mental disorder in which the patient is highly amused at own pointless jokes, puns, or stories; the condition is usually associated with frontal lobe lesions. Witzelsucht is reported with 301.9.

302 SEXUAL DEVIATIONS AND DISORDERS

The limits and features of normal sexual behavior have not been stated absolutely in different societies and cultures, but applied broadly serve as approved social and biological purposes. The sexual activities of patients with deviant disorders are directed primarily toward sexual acts not associated with coitus normally, or toward coitus performed under abnormal circumstances. If the anomalous behavior becomes manifest only during psychosis or other mental illness, the condition should be classified under the major illness. Gender identity disorder and trans-sexualism are considered to be psychosexual gender identity disorders and are not included in this rubric. Also excluded from psychosexual dysfunction are organic causes for impotence (607.84); occasional or transient failures of erection or sexual excitement; or other dysfunction with organic cause.

302.0	Ego-dystonic homosexuality — *ego-dystonic lesbianism; homosexual conflict disorder*
302.1	Zoophilia
302.2	Pedophilia
302.3	Transvestism
302.4	Exhibitionism
302.50	Trans-sexualism with unspecified sexual history
302.51	Trans-sexualism with asexual history

302.52	Trans-sexualism with homosexual history
302.53	Trans-sexualism with heterosexual history
302.6	Disorders of psychosexual identity — *feminism in boys*
302.70	Psychosexual dysfunction, unspecified — *unknown*
302.71	Psychosexual dysfunction with inhibited sexual desire
302.72	Psychosexual dysfunction with inhibited sexual excitement — *frigidity or impotence*
302.73	Psychosexual dysfunction with inhibited female orgasm
302.74	Psychosexual dysfunction with inhibited male orgasm
302.75	Psychosexual dysfunction with premature ejaculation
302.76	Psychosexual dysfunction with functional dyspareunia
302.79	Psychosexual dysfunction with other specified psychosexual dysfunctions — *not elsewhere classified*
302.81	Fetishism
302.82	Voyeurism
302.83	Sexual masochism
302.84	Sexual sadism
302.85	Gender identity disorder of adolescent or adult life — *gender identity disorder of adult life*
302.89	Other specified psychosexual disorder — *including nymphomania, satyriasis, frotteurism, coprophilia and necrophilia*
302.9	Unspecified psychosexual disorder

303 ALCOHOL DEPENDENCE SYNDROME

Alcohol dependence syndrome is both a psychic and physical state, resulting from excessive alcohol consumption. The syndrome is characterized by behavioral and other responses that always include a compulsion to take alcohol on a continuous or periodic basis in order to experience its psychic effects, and sometimes to avoid the discomfort of its absence; tolerance may or may not be present. A person may be dependent on alcohol and other drugs; if so, also record the diagnosis of drug dependence to identify the agent. If alcohol dependence is associated with alcoholic psychosis or with physical complications, both diagnoses should be recorded. Use an additional code to identify any associated conditions, as in alcoholic psychosis (291.0-291.9), drug dependence (304.0-304.9), or physical complications of alcohol, including gastritis (535.3), cirrhosis (571.2), hepatitis (571.1), or cerebral degeneration (331.7).

Axes in this rubric classify the alcohol dependence as acute or chronic, and according to the nature of the dependence during the episode of care. When drunkenness is not otherwise specified, report with 305.0, which reports nondependent abuse of alcohol.

303.0 ✔5th Acute alcoholic intoxication — *acute drunkenness in alcoholism*
303.9 ✔5th Other and unspecified alcohol dependence — *chronic alcoholism; dipsomania*

304 DRUG DEPENDENCE

Drug dependence is both a psychic and physical state, resulting from taking a drug. It is characterized by behavioral and other responses that always include a compulsion to take a drug on a continuous or periodic basis in order to experience its psychic effects, and sometimes to avoid the discomfort of its absence. Tolerance may be present. A person may be dependent on more than one drug. This rubric excludes nondependent abuse of drugs, which is reported with codes in the 305 rubric.

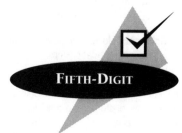

FIFTH-DIGIT

The following fifth-digit subclassification is for use with categories 303, 304, and 305.0, 305.2-305.9:

0 unspecified

1 continuous

2 episodic

3 in remission

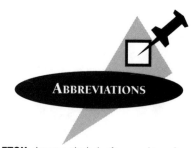

ABBREVIATIONS

ETOH: denotes alcohol, often used to refer to alcoholism or alcohol abuse.

✔5th Needs fifth-digit   **OK** Valid three-digit category

304.0 ✔5th Opioid type dependence — *including heroin, opium alkaloids and their derivatives, meperidine, methadone*

304.1 ✔5th Barbiturate and similarly acting sedative or hypnotic dependence — *including nonbarbiturate sedatives and tranquilizers with similar effect: chlordiazepoxide, meprobamate, diazepam, methaqualone, glutethimide*

304.2 ✔5th Cocaine dependence — *including coca leaves, crack cocaine, coke*

304.3 ✔5th Cannabis dependence — *including hashish, marijuana, pot*

304.4 ✔5th Amphetamine and other psychostimulant dependence — *including methylphenidate, phenmetrazine*

304.5 ✔5th Hallucinogen dependence — *including dimethyltryptamine [DMT], lysergic acid diethylamide [LSD], mescaline, psilocybin*

304.6 ✔5th Other specified drug dependence — *including absinthe; glue sniffing*

304.7 ✔5th Combinations of opioid type drug with any other drug dependence

304.8 ✔5th Combinations of drug dependence excluding opioid type drug

304.9 ✔5th Unspecified drug dependence — *drug addiction NOS*

305 NONDEPENDENT ABUSE OF DRUGS

Drug abuse includes cases where the individual, for whom no other diagnosis is possible, has come under medical care because of the maladaptive effect of a drug on which the patient is not dependent. In nondependent abuse of drugs the individual generally has taken the drug on personal initiative to the detriment of health or social functioning. When drug abuse is secondary to a psychiatric disorder, record the disorder as a primary diagnosis.

Codes in this rubric are classified according to the drug being abused, and whether the abuse is continuous, episodic, or in remission.

Cases in which tobacco is used to the detriment of a person's health or social functioning or in which there is tobacco dependence are classified to codes in 305.1, which requires a fifth digit. Dependence is included here rather than under drug dependence because tobacco differs from other drugs of dependence in its psychotoxic effects. Excluded from the code for tobacco dependence is history of tobacco use, V15.82.

305.0 ✔5th Nondependent alcohol abuse — *drunkenness NOS*

305.1 Nondependent tobacco use disorder — *tobacco dependence*

305.2 ✔5th Nondependent cannabis abuse — *abuse of hashish, marijuana, pot*

305.3 ✔5th Nondependent hallucinogen abuse — *abuse of dimethyltryptamine [DMT], lysergic acid diethylamide [LSD], mescaline, psilocybin*

305.4 ✔5th Nondependent barbiturate and similarly acting sedative or hypnotic abuse — *abuse of including nonbarbiturate sedatives and tranquilizers with similar effect: chlordiazepoxide, meprobamate, diazepam, methaqualone, glutethimide*

305.5 ✔5th Nondependent opioid abuse — *abuse of heroin, opium alkaloids, meperidine, methadone*

305.6 ✔5th Nondependent cocaine abuse — *abuse of coca leaves, crack cocaine, coke*

305.7 ✔5th Nondependent amphetamine or related acting sympathomimetic abuse — *abuse of methylphenidate, phenmetrazine*

305.8 ✔5th Nondependent antidepressant type abuse

305.9 ✔5th Other, mixed, or unspecified nondependent drug abuse — *including laxative habit, nonprescribed drugs or patent medicinals*

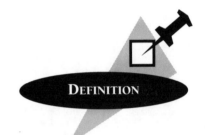

DEFINITION

Caffeine intoxication: consumption of at least 150 mg caffeine with five or more of the following symptoms: restlessness, nervousness, twitching, rambling speech, cardiac arrhythmia, diuresis, excitement, insomnia, agitation, or gastrointestinal disturbance, coupled with clinically significant impairment social or professional function.

306 PHYSIOLOGICAL MALFUNCTION ARISING FROM MENTAL FACTORS

This rubric includes psychogenic physical and physiological malfunctions that do not include tissue damage. If there is tissue damage, see rubric 316. Also excluded are hysteria (300.11-300.19) and specific nonpsychotic mental disorders following organic brain damage (310.0-310.9).

306.0	Musculoskeletal malfunction arising from mental factors — *psychogenic paralysis or torticollis*
306.1	Respiratory malfunction arising from mental factors — *including psychogenic hyperventilation; cough, yawn, or hiccough*
306.2	Cardiovascular malfunction arising from mental factors — *cardiac neurosis*
306.3	Skin malfunction arising from mental factors — *psychogenic pruritus or hyperhidrosis*
306.4	Gastrointestinal malfunction arising from mental factors — *including aerophagy, psychogenic vomiting or diarrhea*
306.50	Psychogenic genitourinary malfunction, unspecified — *unknown*
306.51	Psychogenic vaginismus — *vaginal spasm*
306.52	Psychogenic dysmenorrhea — *painful menstruation*
306.53	Psychogenic dysuria — *painful urination*
306.59	Other genitourinary malfunction arising from mental factors — *specified psychogenic pain*
306.6	Endocrine malfunction arising from mental factors — *pancreas, thyroid,*
306.7	Malfunction of organs of special sense arising from mental factors — *eyes, ears*
306.8	Other specified psychophysiological malfunction — *including bruxism, teeth grinding*
306.9	Unspecified psychophysiological malfunction — *not otherwise specified*

307 SPECIAL SYMPTOMS OR SYNDROMES, NOT ELSEWHERE CLASSIFIED

This category is intended for psychopathology manifested by a single specific symptom or group of symptoms not part of an organic illness or other mental disorder classified elsewhere.

In anorexia nervosa, the symptoms include persistent active refusal to eat and marked loss of weight. The level of activity and alertness is characteristically high in relation to the degree of emaciation. Typically the disorder begins in teenage girls but it may begin before puberty. It rarely occurs in males. Amenorrhea is usual and, in advanced cases, slowed pulse and respiration, low body temperature, dependent edema, and heart rhythm abnormalities. Manifestations of anorexia nervosa should be reported additionally.

307.0	Stammering and stuttering
307.1	Anorexia nervosa — *fear of obesity, usually in females, resulting in emaciation*
307.20	Tic disorder, unspecified — *unknown*
307.21	Transient tic disorder of childhood
307.22	Chronic motor tic disorder — *blink, shrug, grimace, cough, jerk*
307.23	Gilles de la Tourette's disorder — *motor-verbal tic disorder; Brissaud's motor-verbal tic*
307.3	Stereotyped repetitive movements — *body-rocking; spasmus nutans; head banging*
307.40	Nonorganic sleep disorder, unspecified — *unknown*
307.41	Transient disorder of initiating or maintaining sleep — *associated with intermittent emotional reactions or conflicts*

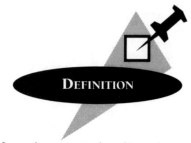

DEFINITION

Anorexia nervosa: a fear of becoming obese that often results in life threatening loss of weight.

Bulimia: a disorder of repetitive bingeing and purging to control weight gain.

✔5th   Needs fifth-digit   **OK**   Valid three-digit category

307.42	Persistent disorder of initiating or maintaining sleep — *associated with anxiety, depression, psychosis*
307.43	Transient disorder of initiating or maintaining wakefulness — *associated with acute or intermittent emotional reactions or conflicts*
307.44	Persistent disorder of initiating or maintaining wakefulness — *associated with depression*
307.45	Phase-shift disruption of 24-hour sleep-wake cycle — *jet lag syndrome; shifting sleep-work schedule*
307.46	Somnambulism or night terrors — *sleepwalking*
307.47	Other dysfunctions of sleep stages or arousal from sleep — *nightmares*
307.48	Repetitive intrusions of sleep — *environmental disturbances or repeated REM-interruptions*
307.49	Other specific disorder of sleep of nonorganic origin — *subjective "short-sleeper;" pseudoinsomnia*
307.50	Eating disorder, unspecified — *unknown*
307.51	Bulimia — *including binge/purge*
307.52	Pica — *perverted appetite of nonorganic origin*
307.53	Psychogenic rumination — *regurgitation, of nonorganic origin, of food with reswallowing*
307.54	Psychogenic vomiting — *no physical cause*
307.59	Other disorder of eating — *no physical cause*
307.6	Enuresis — *of nonorganic origin*
307.7	Encopresis — *of nonorganic origin*
307.80	Psychogenic pain, site unspecified — *unknown*
307.81	Tension headache — *stress headache*
307.89	Other psychalgia — *not elsewhere classified*
307.9	Other and unspecified special symptom or syndrome, not elsewhere classified — *including hair plucking, masturbation, lalling, nail-biting, lisping, thumb-sucking*

308 ACUTE REACTION TO STRESS

This rubric is reserved for acute reactions as a response to exceptional physical or mental distress, which usually subside within hours or days. Some examples include catastrophic stress, combat fatigue, or gross stress reaction. Excluded from this rubric are adjustment reaction disorders (309.0-309.9) and chronic stress reaction (309.1-309.9).

308.0	Predominant disturbance of emotions — *anxiety, emotional crisis, panic*
308.1	Predominant disturbance of consciousness as reaction to stress — *fugues*
308.2	Predominant psychomotor disturbance as reaction to stress — *agitation or stupor*
308.3	Other acute reactions to stress — *brief or acute posttraumatic stress disorder*
308.4	Mixed disorders as reaction to stress — *combination of reactions classified to 308*
308.9	Unspecified acute reaction to stress — *unknown, and including combat fatigue*

309 ADJUSTMENT REACTION

An adjustment or adaptation reaction is a mild or transient disorders lasting longer than acute stress reactions and occurring in individuals of any age without any apparent pre-existing mental disorder. Such disorders are often relatively circumscribed or situation-specific, are generally reversible, and usually last only a few months. They are usually closely related in time and content to stresses such as bereavement, migration, or other experiences. Reactions to major stress that last longer than a few days are also included. In children such disorders are associated with no significant distortion of development.

Excluded from this rubric are acute reactions to major stress (308.0-308.9) and neurotic disorders (300.1-300.9).

309.0	Brief depressive reaction as adjustment reaction — *including grief reaction*
309.1	Prolonged depressive reaction as adjustment reaction — *as an adjustment reaction*
309.21	Separation anxiety disorder — *abnormal stress upon leaving another person*
309.22	Emancipation disorder of adolescence and early adult life
309.23	Specific academic or work inhibition as adjustment reaction
309.24	Anxious mood as adjustment reaction
309.28	Mixed emotional features as adjustment reaction — *adjustment reaction with anxiety and depression*
309.29	Other adjustment reaction with predominant disturbance of other emotions — *including culture shock*
309.3	Predominant disturbance of conduct as adjustment reaction — *conduct disturbance or destructiveness as an adjustment reaction*
309.4	Mixed disturbance of emotions and conduct as adjustment reaction
309.81	Prolonged posttraumatic stress disorder — *chronic posttraumatic stress disorder; concentration camp syndrome*
309.82	Adjustment reaction with physical symptoms
309.83	Adjustment reaction with withdrawal — *elective mutism, hospitalism*
309.89	Other specified adjustment reaction — *homesickness*
309.9	Unspecified adjustment reaction — *adaptation reaction NOS*

310 SPECIFIC NONPSYCHOTIC MENTAL DISORDERS DUE TO ORGANIC BRAIN DAMAGE

Postconcussion syndrome occurs after generalized contusion of the brain, resembling the overall symptoms found in frontal lobe syndrome or any of the neurotic disorders, but in which headache, giddiness, fatigue, insomnia, and a subjective feeling of impaired intellectual ability are also prominent. Mood may fluctuate, and quite ordinary stress may produce exaggerated fear and apprehension. There may be marked intolerance of mental and physical exertion, undue sensitivity to noise, and hypochondriacal preoccupation. The symptoms are more common in persons who have previously suffered from neurotic or personality disorders. This syndrome is particularly associated with the closed type of head injury when signs of localized brain damage are slight or absent, but it may also occur in other conditions.

Frontal lobe syndrome presents with changes in behavior following damage to the frontal areas of the brain or following interference with the connections of those areas. There is a general diminution of self-control, foresight, creativity, and spontaneity, which may be manifest as increased irritability, selfishness, restlessness, and lack of concern for others. Conscientiousness and powers of concentration are often diminished, but measurable deterioration of intellect or memory is not necessarily present. The overall picture is often one of emotional dullness, lack of drive, and slowness; but, particularly in persons previously with energetic, restless, or aggressive characteristics, there may be a change towards impulsiveness, boastfulness, temper outbursts, silly fatuous humor, and the development of unrealistic ambitions. The direction of change usually depends upon the previous personality. A considerable degree of recovery is possible and may continue over the course of several years.

↙5th Needs fifth-digit   **OK** Valid three-digit category

310.0 Frontal lobe syndrome — *postleucotomy syndrome, Klüver-Bucy (-Terzian) syndrome*

310.1 Organic personality syndrome — *cognitive or personality change of other type, of nonpsychotic severity; mild memory disturbance; presbyophrenia NOS*

310.2 Postconcussion syndrome — *postconcussion syndrome or encephalopathy*

310.8 Other specified nonpsychotic mental disorder following organic brain damage — *postencephalitic syndrome*

310.9 Unspecified nonpsychotic mental disorder following organic brain damage — *unknown*

311 DEPRESSIVE DISORDER, NOT ELSEWHERE CLASSIFIED

This rubric is reserved for depressive disorders not classified in other sections of this chapter, or depressive orders not assigned a more specific diagnosis.

312 DISTURBANCE OF CONDUCT, NOT ELSEWHERE CLASSIFIED

This rubric is reserved for psychosocial and other conduct disorders not classified in other sections of this chapter, or that cannot be assigned a more specific diagnosis. Conduct disorders mainly involve aggressive and destructive behavior and disorders involving delinquency. Codes in this rubric should be used for abnormal behavior, in individuals of any age, which gives rise to social disapproval although not part of any other psychiatric condition. Minor emotional disturbances may also be present. To be included, the behavior, as judged by its frequency, severity, and type of associations with other symptoms, must be abnormal in its context. Disturbances of conduct are distinguished from an adjustment reaction by a longer duration and by a lack of close relationship in time and content to some stress. They differ from a personality disorder by the absence of deeply ingrained maladaptive patterns of behavior present from adolescence or earlier.

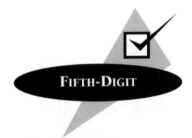

The following fifth-digit subclassification is for use with categories 312.0-312.2:

0 unspecified

1 mild

2 moderate

3 severe

312.0 ✔5th Undersocialized conduct disorder, aggressive type — *aggressive outburst, anger reaction; unsocialized, aggressive disorder*

312.1 ✔5th Undersocialized conduct disorder, unaggressive type — *childhood truancy; tantrums, solitary, stealing; unsocialized*

312.2 ✔5th Socialized conduct disorder — *childhood truancy socialized, group delinquency*

312.30 Impulse control disorder, unspecified — *impulse control disorder, unspecified*

312.31 Pathological gambling

312.32 Kleptomania — *compulsive theft*

312.33 Pyromania — *compulsive fire starting*

312.34 Intermittent explosive disorder

312.35 Isolated explosive disorder

312.39 Other disorder of impulse control — *not elsewhere specified, trichotillomania*

312.4 Mixed disturbance of conduct and emotions — *neurotic delinquency*

312.81 Conduct disorder, childhood onset type

312.82 Conduct disorder, adolescent onset type

312.89 Other specified disturbance of conduct, not elsewhere classified

312.9 Unspecified disturbance of conduct

313 DISTURBANCE OF EMOTIONS SPECIFIC TO CHILDHOOD AND ADOLESCENCE

This rubric excludes adjustment reactions (309.0-309.9), neurotic emotional disorders (300.0-300.9), and isolated symptoms including masturbation, nail biting, thumb-sucking (307.0-307.9).

Academic underachievement disorder (313.83) presents as a failure to achieve in most school tasks despite adequate intellectual capacity, a supportive and encouraging social environment, and apparent effort. The failure occurs in the absence of a demonstrable specific learning disability and is caused by emotional conflict not clearly associated with any other mental disorder.

313.0	Overanxious disorder specific to childhood and adolescence — *anxiety and fearfulness in childhood*
313.1	Misery and unhappiness disorder specific to childhood and adolescence
313.21	Shyness disorder of childhood
313.22	Introverted disorder of childhood
313.23	Elective mutism specific to childhood and adolescence
313.3	Relationship problems specific to childhood and adolescence
313.81	Oppositional disorder of childhood or adolescence
313.82	Identity disorder of childhood or adolescence
313.83	Academic underachievement disorder of childhood or adolescence
313.89	Other emotional disturbance of childhood or adolescence
313.9	Unspecified emotional disturbance of childhood or adolescence

314 HYPERKINETIC SYNDROME OF CHILDHOOD

Hyperkinetic syndromes of childhood are disorders in which the essential features are short attention span and distractibility. In early childhood the most striking symptom is disinhibited, poorly organized and poorly regulated extreme overactivity but in adolescence this may be replaced by underactivity. Impulsiveness, marked fluctuations in mood, and aggression are also common symptoms. Delays in the development of specific skills are often present and disturbed, poor relationships are common. If the hyperkinesis is symptomatic of an underlying disorder, the diagnosis of the underlying disorder is recorded instead. This rubric excludes hyperkinesis as a symptom of an underlying disorder.

314.00	Attention deficit disorder of childhood without mention of hyperactivity
314.01	Attention deficit disorder of childhood with hyperactivity
314.1	Hyperkinesis of childhood with developmental delay
314.2	Hyperkinetic conduct disorder of childhood — *without developmental delay*
314.8	Other specified manifestations of hyperkinetic syndrome of childhood
314.9	Unspecified hyperkinetic syndrome of childhood

315 SPECIFIC DELAYS IN DEVELOPMENT

This rubric classifies a group of disorders in which a specific delay in development is the main feature. For many, the delay is not explicable in terms of general intellectual delay or of inadequate schooling. In each case, development is related to biological maturation, but it is also influenced by nonbiological factors. A diagnosis of a specific developmental delay carries no etiological implications. A diagnosis of specific delay in development should not be made if it is due to a known neurological disorder. Excluded from this rubric are delays in development that are due to neurological disorders (320.0-389.9).

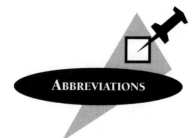

ABBREVIATIONS

ADD: attention deficit disorder, characterized by lack of attention and impulse behavior.

ADHD: attention deficit hyperactivity disorder, the above plus an inability to stay put.

✔5th Needs fifth-digit   **OK** Valid three-digit category

315.00	Developmental reading disorder, unspecified — *unknown*
315.01	Alexia — *inability to comprehend words*
315.02	Developmental dyslexia — *impaired reading ability*
315.09	Other specific developmental reading disorder — *specific spelling difficulty*
315.1	Developmental arithmetical disorder — *dyscalculia*
315.2	Other specific developmental learning difficulties — *specific spelling difficulty*
315.31	Developmental language disorder — *expressive language disorder*
315.32	Receptive language disorder (mixed) — *receptive, expressive language disorder*
315.39	Other developmental speech or language disorder — *dyslalia*
315.4	Developmental coordination disorder — *clumsiness/dyspraxia syndrome*
315.5	Mixed development disorder
315.8	Other specified delay in development
315.9	Unspecified delay in development — *unknown*

316 PSYCHIC FACTORS ASSOCIATED WITH DISEASES CLASSIFIED ELSEWHERE OK

This rubric is used to report psychological factors in physical conditions classified elsewhere. Use an additional code to report the associated physical condition, as in psychogenic ulcerative colitis (556); eczema (691.8, 692.9); paroxysmal tachycardia (427.2) or psychosocial dwarfism (259.4). Do not use this rubric to report physical symptoms and physiological malfunctions not involving tissue damage or mental origin. For those cases, see 306.0-306.9.

317-319 Mental Retardation

Mental retardation is defined as general intellectual functioning at least two standard deviations below the norm as measured in a standardized intelligence test, when it is accompanied by significant limitation in communication, self-care, home living, interpersonal skills, self-direction, work, leisure, health, or safety. The onset must occur before adulthood.

Use additional codes to identify any associated psychiatric or physical conditions.

317 MILD MENTAL RETARDATION OK

In mild mental retardation, the patient has an IQ of 50-70. Individuals with this level of retardation are usually educable. During the preschool period they can develop social and communication skills, have minimal delay in sensorimotor areas, and often are not distinguished from normal children until a later age. During the school age period they can learn academic skills up to approximately the sixth-grade level. During the adult years, they can usually achieve social and vocational skills adequate for minimum self-support, but may need guidance and assistance when under social or economic stress.

318 OTHER SPECIFIED MENTAL RETARDATION

In moderate mental retardation, the patient has an IQ of 35-49. Individuals with this level of retardation are usually trainable. During the preschool period they can talk or learn to communicate. They have poor social awareness and fair motor development. During the school age period they can profit from training in social and occupational skills, but are unlikely to progress beyond the second-grade level in academic subjects. During their adult years they may achieve self-maintenance in unskilled or semi-skilled work under sheltered conditions. They need supervision and guidance when under mild social or economic stress.

In severe mental retardation, the patient has an IQ of 20-34. Individuals with this level of retardation evidence poor motor development, minimal speech, and are generally unable to profit from training and self-help during the preschool period. During the school age period they can talk or learn to communicate, can be trained in elementary health habits, and may profit from systematic habit training. During the adult years they may contribute partially to self-maintenance under complete supervision.

In profound mental retardation, the patient has an IQ under 20. Individuals with this level of retardation evidence minimal capacity for sensorimotor functioning and need nursing care during the preschool period. During the school age period some further motor development may occur, and they may respond to minimal or limited training in self-help. During the adult years some motor and speech development may occur, and they may achieve very limited self-care and need nursing care.

318.0	Moderate mental retardation — *IQ 35-49*	
318.1	Severe mental retardation — *IQ 20-34*	
318.2	Profound mental retardation — *IQ under 20*	

319 UNSPECIFIED MENTAL RETARDATION OK

This rubric is reserved for patients who evidence obvious mental retardation, but the severity of the condition has not been measured with standardized testing.

✔5th Needs fifth-digit   **OK** Valid three-digit category

Chapter 6

320-389
Diseases of the Nervous System and Sense Organs

This chapter classifies diseases and disorders of the nervous system including meninges (the coverings of the brain and spinal cord, central nervous system, and peripheral nervous system (the nerves that relay signals between the central nervous system and the organs of the body). This chapter also classifies conditions affecting the eye and ear.

320-326 Inflammatory Diseases of the Central Nervous System

These categories include meningitis, encephalitis, cerebral abscesses, late effects of infections of the central nervous system, and other types of inflammations such as meningitis due to sarcoidosis and lead poisoning (toxic) encephalitis. However, many infections of the central nervous system are excluded.

320 BACTERIAL MENINGITIS

Bacterial meningitis is inflammation of the covering of the meninges due to a bacterial organism. Bacterial meningitis can be caused by a variety of pyogenic bacterial organisms, most commonly *Haemophilus influenzae* (type B), Streptococcus pneumoniae, *Pneumococcus*, *Neisseria meningitidis*, *Staphylococcus aureus*, *Klebsiella*, *Pseudomonas* and *Escherichia coli*. Code selection is based upon the infective agent.

Signs and symptoms of bacterial meningitis include fever and chills, headache, stiff neck, nausea and vomiting, alterations in sensorium, seizure, positive Kernig's and Brudzinski's signs, and rash. These signs and symptoms in addition to chronically draining ear are associated with pneumococcal meningitis.

Diagnostic tests include lumbar puncture to obtain cerebrospinal fluid for verifying elevated fluid pressure. Culture of cerebrospinal fluid is performed to identify organism and gram stain of cerebrospinal fluid reveals polymorphonuclear leukocytes, elevated white blood cell count, decreased glucose level, and elevated protein content. In addition, a limulus lysate assay test may be performed to detect endotoxins due to gram-negative bacteria and a cranial CT scan may indicate cerebral edema early and subdural effusion or empyema later. Therapies include isolation, avoidance of temperature extremes, antimicrobials administered intravenously in large doses, IV hydration, medication such as Dilantin to control seizures, diuretics or withdrawal of cerebrospinal fluid through an intraventricular catheter to reduce intracranial pressure, oxygen therapy for hypoxia, and intubation and ventilation for hypoventilation with hypercapnia.

Associated conditions include seizures due to increased intracranial pressure, respiratory distress or failure, altered state of consciousness, vasomotor collapse or shock, intravascular coagulation, syndrome of inappropriate antidiuretic hormone secretion (SIADH), dehydration, or various electrolyte imbalances.

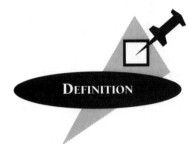

DEFINITION

Alert: consciousness that is wakeful and responsive.

Brudzinski's sign: flexion of the neck results in flexion of the knee and hip. This is a sign of meningitis.

Coma: consciousness fails to respond to stimulation.

Kernig's sign: patient can completely extend the leg in dorsal decubitus but cannot extend the leg from a sitting or lying position. This is a sign of meningitis.

Stuporous: consciousness is only aroused by vigorous stimulation.

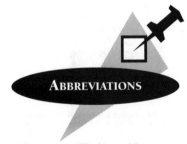

ABBREVIATIONS

H. influenzae or Hib: *Hemophilus influenza* infection

Staph: *Staphylococcal* infection

Strep: *Streptococcal* infection

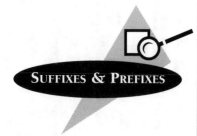
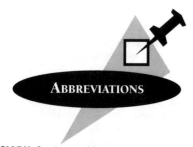
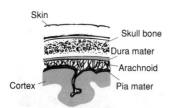

Skin
Skull bone
Dura mater
Arachnoid
Cortex
Pia mater

The meninges constitute the three layers that cover the brain and spinal cord: the dura mater, pia mater, and arachnoid

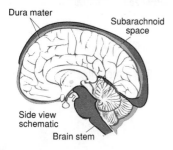

Dura mater
Subarachnoid space
Side view schematic
Brain stem

If the medical documentation indicates aseptic, viral, or nonbacterial meningitis without further specification, see category 047 *Meningitis due to enterovirus*. When meningitis is a manifestation of another disease process (320.7), code the underlying disease first.

320.0	Hemophilus meningitis — *meningitis due to Hemophilus influenzae [H. influenzae]*
320.1	Pneumococcal meningitis — *pneumococcal infection causing inflammation of the membranes enveloping the brain and/or spinal cord*
320.2	Streptococcal meningitis — *streptococcal infection causing inflammation of the membranes enveloping the brain and/or spinal cord*
320.3	Staphylococcal meningitis — *staphylococcal infection causing inflammation of the membranes enveloping the brain and/or spinal cord*
320.7	Meningitis in other bacterial diseases classified elsewhere — (Code first underlying disease, as: 002.0, 027.0, 033.0–033.9, 039.8) — *including actinomycosis, listeriosis, typhoid fever, and whooping cough*

320.8   Meningitis due to other specified bacteria

Anaerobic bacteria are organisms that thrive only in the absence of free oxygen and can be either gram negative or gram positive. *Clostridium tetani* is an example of a gram-positive anaerobe, and *Proteus vulgaris* is an example of a gram-negative anaerobe.

The terms "gram negative" and "gram positive" refer to a method of differential staining of bacteria for bacterial taxonomy and identification. Gram-positive bacteria retain the basic dye crystal violet, and gram-negative bacteria lose the crystal violet dye to become colorless. Counterstains colors gram-negative bacteria pink to red and leaves gram-positive bacteria dark purple.

320.81	Anaerobic meningitis — *bacteroides (fragilis); gram-negative anaerobes*
320.82	Meningitis due to gram-negative bacteria, not elsewhere classified — *including Aerobacter aerogenes; Klebsiella pneumoniae; Proteus morganii; Pseudomonas*
320.89	Meningitis due to other specified bacteria — *including Bacillus pyocyaneus*
320.9	Meningitis due to unspecified bacterium — *including arachnoiditis, leptomeningitis, pachymeningitis due to organisms other than bacteria*

321 MENINGITIS DUE TO OTHER ORGANISMS

The definition of meningitis due to other organisms is inflammation of the covering of the meninges due to organisms other than bacteria. These can be fungal organisms, viruses not classified elsewhere, or other nonbacterial organisms.

Signs and symptoms of meningitis due to other organisms vary according to infectious agent. Therapies include specific treatment depending on infectious agent (e.g., antifungal agents such as amphotericin B for fungal meningitis and corticosteroids for sarcoid meningitis).

Since meningitis classified to this category is a manifestation of another disease process, code the underlying disease first. If the medical documentation indicates aseptic, viral, or nonbacterial meningitis without further specification, see category 047.

321.0	Cryptococcal meningitis — (Code first underlying disease 117.5) — *including cryptococcus infection causing inflammation of the membranes enveloping the brain and/or spinal cord*
321.1	Meningitis in other fungal diseases

✔5th   Needs fifth-digit   **OK**   Valid three-digit category

321.2   Meningitis due to viruses not elsewhere classified — (Code first underlying disease, as: 060.0–066.9)

321.3   Meningitis due to trypanosomiasis — (Code first underlying disease 086.0–086.9) — *trypanosomiasis infection causing inflammation of the membranes enveloping the brain and/or spinal cord*

321.4   Meningitis in sarcoidosis — (Code first underlying disease 135) — *sarcoidosis causing inflammation of the membranes enveloping the brain and/or spinal cord; code first underlying disease (135)*

321.8   Meningitis due to other nonbacterial organisms classified elsewhere — (Code first underlying disease)

322 MENINGITIS OF UNSPECIFIED CAUSE

322.0   Nonpyogenic meningitis — *inflammation of the membranes enveloping the brain and/or spinal cord*

322.1   Eosinophilic meningitis — *presence of cells readily stained with eosin causing inflammation of the membranes enveloping the brain and/or spinal cord*

322.2   Chronic meningitis — *persistent inflammation of the membranes enveloping the brain and/or spinal cord*

322.9   Unspecified meningitis — *unspecified; leptomeningopathy; ventriculitis, cerebral*

323 ENCEPHALITIS, MYELITIS, AND ENCEPHALOMYELITIS

Encephalitis, myelitis, and encephalomyelitis are inflammations of the central nervous system that alter the function of various portions of the brain (encephalitis), spinal cord (myelitis), or both (encephalomyelitis). The inflammation usually results from either a direct invasion of the central nervous system by a virus or postinfection involvement of the central nervous system after a viral disease. Bacteria, medications, toxic substances, and parasites also may cause it. Arthropod-borne viruses as seen in mosquitoes most often cause encephalitis. Myelitis infection results from direct invasion or tick bites classified to categories 062 and 063.

Signs and symptoms of encephalitis, myelitis and encephalomyelitis, with mild benign forms, is malaise, fever, headache, dizziness, apathy, neck stiffness, nausea and vomiting, ataxia, tremors, hyperactivity, speech difficulties. With severe central nervous system involvement it is high fever, stupor, seizures, disorientation, ocular palsies, paralysis, spasticity, coma that may proceed to death.

Diagnostic tests include lumbar puncture with analysis of cerebrospinal fluid to show lymphocytes, moderate rises in protein, and markedly elevated specific viral antibody titers with acute encephalitis. Cultures (i.e., cerebrospinal fluid, blood, and saliva) may identify the specific virus (except arboviruses that rarely are detected in the blood or spinal fluid). A brain biopsy may rule out herpes simplex.

Therapies include IV hydration, control of temperature, specific treatment depends on etiology (e.g., chelation therapy for lead poisoning encephalitis and chloroquine for malarial encephalitis).

Diseases in this rubric are classified according to causative organism. Sequence the underlying disease first. If the organism is unspecified or the encephalitis has a noninfectious or toxic etiology, see codes 323.5, 323.8 and 323.9.

323.0 Encephalitis in viral diseases classified elsewhere — (Code first underlying disease, as: 073.7, 075, 078.3) — *including cat-scratch disease, infectious mononucleosis, and ornithosis*

323.1 Encephalitis in rickettsial diseases classified elsewhere — (Code first underlying disease 080–083.9) — *inflammation of the brain caused by rickettsial disease carried by louse, tick or mite; code first underlying disease*

323.2 Encephalitis in protozoal diseases classified elsewhere — (Code first underlying disease, as: 084.0–084.9, 086.0–086.9) — *including malaria and trypanosomiasis*

323.4 Other encephalitis due to infection classified elsewhere — (Code first underlying disease)

323.5 Encephalitis following immunization procedures

323.6 Postinfectious encephalitis — (Code first underlying disease) — *infection and inflammation of the brain several weeks following outbreak of a systemic infection; code first underlying disease*

323.7 Toxic encephalitis — (Code first underlying disease, as: 961.3, 982.1, 984.0–84.9, 985.0, 985.8) — *inflammation of the brain due to toxic effect of exposure to a chemical; code first underlying disease*

323.8 Other causes of encephalitis

323.9 Unspecified cause of encephalitis — *including syringomyelitis*

324 INTRACRANIAL AND INTRASPINAL ABSCESS

The definition of intracranial and intraspinal abscess is the localized collection of pus in a cavity involving the brain or spinal column, respectively.

324.0 Intracranial abscess — *cerebellar (embolic) abscess; abscess (embolic) of brain [any part]*

Intracranial abscess is the localized collection of purulent material and liquified brain tissue involving the many layers of the brain, including the epidural or subdural spaces, or within the substance of the brain itself. The etiology is usually bacterial and occurs through direct extension from a contiguous focus, blood-borne metastases, or by penetrating injury. The most common cause of direct extension in a brain abscess is a contiguous infection such as in the middle ear, mastoid, or sinuses. The most common site of origin for blood-borne metastasis is the lung (empyema, bronchiectasis). When the abscess is due to trauma, a skull fracture or penetrating injury is usually involved. The most common organisms are streptococci, pneumococci, and staphylococci.

Signs and symptoms of intracranial abscess, with brain abscess, include headache, altered sensorium (lethargy, irritability, confusion or coma), nausea and vomiting, fever, seizures, multiple alternation nerve palsies, and other neurologic deficits. Signs and symptoms of intracranial abscess, with subdural abscess, include headache, sinusitis, altered sensorium (lethargy, obtundation or coma), seizures, fever and chills, hemiparesis, and aphasia. Signs and symptoms of intracranial abscess, with cerebral epidural abscess, involve limited localized symptoms.

Diagnostic tests include MRI and radionuclide or CT scans to identify the location and size of abscess. With subdural abscess, plain skull x-rays reveal underlying sinus or mastoid disease, while cerebral arteriography shows space between cerebral vessels and the inner surface of cranium.

ᴸ5th Needs fifth-digit   **OK** Valid three-digit category

Therapies include antimicrobials for early abscess, and incision and drainage or excision of abscess.

324.1 Intraspinal abscess — *abscess (embolic) of spinal cord [any part]; epidural, extradural or subdural*

The definition of intraspinal abscess is the localized collection of pus in a cavity involving the layers of the spinal cord, including the epidura, extradura, and subdura. It is usually bacterial, and the most common organisms are *streptococci, pneumococci,* and *staphylococci.* The etiology is usually due to blood-borne spread, direct extension from contiguous sites, or as a consequence of an invasive procedure. Most spinal abscesses are epidural.

Signs and symptoms of intraspinal abscess include spinal ache, root pain, weakness, paresthesias, and eventually paralysis. Diagnostic tests include lumbar puncture with analysis of cerebrospinal fluid to show elevated protein, xanthochromia, and normal glucose. Culture identifies bacterial agent. Myelography, CT scan, and MRI visualize abscess. Therapies include antimicrobials for early abscess, and incision and drainage or excision for fully established intraspinal abscess.

324.9 Intracranial and intraspinal abscess of unspecified site — *extradural or subdural abscess NOS*

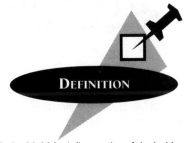

325 PHLEBITIS AND THROMBOPHLEBITIS OF INTRACRANIAL VENOUS SINUSES OK

Excluded from this rubric is phlebitis and thrombophlebitis of intracranial venous sinuses associated with pregnancy (671.5) or of nonpyogenic origin (437.6).

326 LATE EFFECTS OF INTRACRANIAL ABSCESS OR PYOGENIC INFECTION OK

Late effects of intracranial abscess or pyogenic infection are the late effects of meningitis, encephalitis, myelitis, encephalomyelitis, intracranial and intraspinal abscess, and phlebitis or thrombophlebitis of the intracranial sinuses except when these conditions are manifestations of another disease process identified by italics in the ICD-9-CM tabular list. Use an additional code to describe the condition, as in hydrocephalus (331.4) or paralysis (rubrics 342 and 344).

Endophlebitis: inflammation of the inside of the vein.

Phlebitis: inflammation of a vein.

Thrombophlebitis: inflammation and formation of a blood clot in a vein.

Thrombosis: presence of blood clot in a blood vessel.

330-337 Hereditary and Degenerative Diseases of the Central Nervous System

Excluded from this section are hepatolenticular degeneration (275.1); multiple sclerosis (340); and other demyelinating diseases of the central nervous system (rubric 341).

330 CEREBRAL DEGENERATIONS USUALLY MANIFEST IN CHILDHOOD

Report Rett's syndrome with 330.8. For 330.2 and 330.3, sequence first the underlying disease, as in Fabry's, Gaucher's, Niemann-Pick, or sphingolipidosis (272.7); or Hunter's disease or mucopolysaccharidosis (277.5).

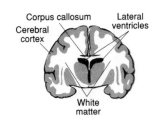

Frontal cross section

330.0 Leukodystrophy — (Use additional code to identify associated (condition)) — *including Krabbe's disease; globoid cell or metachromatic leukodystrophy; sulfatide lipidosis*

330.1 Cerebral lipidoses — (Use additional code to identify associated (condition)) — *including amaurotic (familial) idiocy; Batten disease; gangliosidosis; Tay-Sachs disease*

330.2 Cerebral degeneration in generalized lipidoses — (Code first underlying disease, as: 272.7) — *including Fabry's disease*

330.3 Cerebral degeneration of childhood in other diseases classified elsewhere — (Code first underlying disease, as: 277.5) — *including Hunter's disease, mucopolysaccharidosis*

330.8 Other specified cerebral degenerations in childhood

330.9 Unspecified cerebral degeneration in childhood — *including childhood cerebral degeneration NOS*

331 OTHER CEREBRAL DEGENERATIONS

331.0 Alzheimer's disease — *including a chronic, progressive form of dementia, characterized by plaque formations in the brain, eventually leading to total dependence on others*

Alzheimer's disease is a form of presenile dementia caused by the destruction of the subcortical white matter of the brain and characterized by increasing loss of intellectual functioning beginning with minor memory loss and eventually resulting in total loss of ability to function.

Signs and symptoms of Alzheimer's disease include loss of interest in usual pursuits and marked changes of habits. CT scan of the brain shows shrinkage of white matter and an increase in size of ventricles. Microscopic exam of brain tissue shows neuronal loss with neurofibrillar and granulovacuolar degeneration and may also show amyloid plaques in cerebral cortex tissue. Neurochemical studies show changes in cholinergic system (reduced acetylcholine and choline acetyltransferase) and noradrenergic system (decreased norepinephrine) and may reveal low serotonin levels in caudate and hippocampus nuclei.

Therapies include sedatives, such as chloral hydrate or phenhydramine, for sleep disorders; benzodiazapines, such as lorazepam or oxazepam, for aggressive or assaultive behavior; neuroleptics, such as chlorpromazine or haloperidol, for extreme aggressiveness.

Associated conditions include trisomy 21, aspiration pneumonia, and urinary and fecal incontinence.

Assign an additional code to identify any mental condition, such as presenile dementia in rubric 290, associated with the current condition.

331.1 Pick's disease — *including presenile dementia due to atrophy of frontal and temporal lobes of the brain*

331.2 Senile degeneration of brain — *decline in intellectual function due to brain deterioration*

331.3 Communicating hydrocephalus — *including acquired hydrocephalus NOS*

331.4 Obstructive hydrocephalus

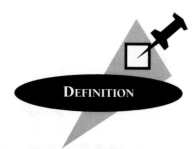

DEFINITION

Communication hydrocephalus: excess cerebrospinal fluid in dilated brain cavities, caused by acquired, abnormal non-absorption of fluid back into fluid pathways.

Obstructive hydrocephalus: excess cerebrospinal fluid filling dilated cavities of the brain, caused by an acquired obstruction of the cerebrospinal fluid pathways.

 5th   Needs fifth-digit   **OK**   Valid three-digit category

331.7 Cerebral degeneration in diseases classified elsewhere

331.81 Reye's syndrome — *occurs in children under age 15, and is marked by acute encephalopathy and fatty infiltrates of multiple organs*

331.89 Other cerebral degeneration — *including cerebral ataxia*

331.9 Unspecified cerebral degeneration

332 PARKINSON'S DISEASE

332.0 Paralysis agitans — *including Parkinson's disease*

Paralysis agitans is an idiopathic neurological disease causing degeneration and dysfunction of the basal ganglia. This disease, also known as Parkinsonism or Parkinson's disease, is due to a toxic degeneration of the nigral neurons, a group of specialized cells in the midbrain that contain neuromelanin and manufacture the neurotransmitter substance dopamine. When 75 percent to 80 percent of the dopamine innervation is destroyed, signs and symptoms of Parkinsonism appear.

Signs and symptoms of paralysis agitans include tremor, rigidity, difficulty starting movement or slowness in movement, "pill-rolling" movement of fingers, shuffling gait with short steps and dragging feet, drooling, and problems of articulation.

Therapies include Levodopa or anticholinergic agents, transplantation of catecholamine tissue (autologous adrenal medulla) into brain adjacent to striatum, and surgery to destroy areas controlling specific functions to control severe tremor.

This disease is associated with mental disorders such as dementia, depression, and delirium. True dementia affects 20 percent to 30 percent of patients.

332.1 Secondary Parkinsonism — (Use additional E code to identify drug, if drug induced) — *including Parkinsonism due to drugs*

Secondary Parkinsonism is a neurologic disease that similar to paralysis agitans affects the central nervous system. It is caused by a number of other diseases or by the adverse affect of certain drugs and chemicals.

Associated conditions include Wilson's disease, postencephalic Parkinsonism, midbrain injury or trauma (dementia pugalistica), neoplasms, vascular malformations, Binswanger's disease, etat lacunaire, and hypertensive cerebrovascular disease with normal pressure hydrocephalus. Use the appropriate E code to identify the causative drug or chemical such as carbon monoxide, manganese, methylphenyltetrahydropyridine (MPTP), or reserpine.

If the medical record documentation indicates Huntington's disease, see 333.4. For progressive supranuclear palsy, striatonigral degeneration, corticodentationigral degeneration with neuronal achromasia, olivopontocerebellar atrophy, Shy-Drager syndrome, or multiple system atrophy, see 333.0. If the Parkinsonism is secondary to syphilis, see 094.82.

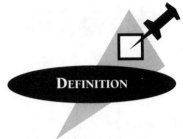

DEFINITION

Akinesia: inability to initiate movement.

Bradykinesia: slowness of movement.

Festination: involuntary tendency to take short, quick steps when walking.

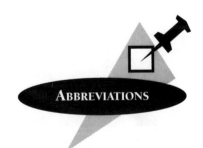

ABBREVIATIONS

PD: Parkinson's disease, also called Parkinsonism, a progressive disease causing neurological and muscular abnormalities including tremors, weakness, and other physical anomalies.

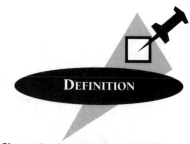

DEFINITION

Chorea: involuntary spasms of the limbs or facial muscles.

Dystonia: a state of abnormal spasms in which the muscles are hypertonic when in spasm and hypotonic when at rest.

Myoclonus: twitching muscle or group of muscles.

Tic: a habitual or involuntary spasm of a group of muscles.

Tremor: an involuntary shaking or trembling.

333 OTHER EXTRAPYRAMIDAL DISEASE AND ABNORMAL MOVEMENT DISORDERS

333.0   Other degenerative diseases of the basal ganglia — *including progressive supranuclear ophthalmoplegia; Parkinsonian syndrome associated with idiopathic orthostatic hypotension or symptomatic orthostatic hypotension*

333.1   Essential and other specified forms of tremor — (Use additional E code to identify drug, if drug induced) — *including benign essential tremor; familial tremor*

333.2   Myoclonus — (Use additional E code to identify drug, if drug induced) — *including familial essential myoclonus; progressive myoclonic epilepsy*

333.3   Tics of organic origin — (Use additional E code to identify drug, if drug induced) — *use E code to identify drug if drug-induced*

333.4   Huntington's chorea — *including inherited, progressive disease involving CNS, leading to involuntary movements and deterioration of mental faculties ending in dementia*

Huntington's chorea is a fatal hereditary disease affecting the basal ganglia and cerebral cortex. The onset varies but usually begins in the fourth decade of life. Death usually follows within 15 years. Signs and symptoms of Huntington's chorea include family history of Huntington's chorea; weight loss; facial grimacing; ceaseless rapid, complex, jerky movements; personality changes, including irritability and indifference; mental deterioration until dementia is reached; and, in children, rigid rather than choreic movements and seizures.

Diagnostic tests include MRI or CT scan of head to reveal gross atrophy and neuronal loss in caudate with lesser changes elsewhere in the brain. Microscopic exam of tissue identifies gliosis and loss of intrinsic neurons. Neurochemical studies reveal loss of gamma-aminobutyric acid (GABA), acetylcholine, substance P (a tachykinin of 11 amino acids), and enkephalin.

333.5   Other choreas — (Use additional E code to identify drug, if drug induced) — *including hemiballism; paroxysmal choreo-athetosis; use additional E code to identify drug if drug-induced*

333.6   Idiopathic torsion dystonia — *including deformans progressiva or musculorum deformans dystonia*

333.7   Symptomatic torsion dystonia — (Use additional E code to identify drug, if drug induced) — *including athetoid cerebral palsy (Vogt's disease); double athetosis syndrome; use additional E code to identify drug if drug-induced*

333.81   Blepharospasm — (Use additional E code to identify drug, if drug induced) — *including spasmodic contraction of orbicularis oculi muscle caused by a number of conditions*

333.82   Orofacial dyskinesia — (Use additional E code to identify drug, if drug induced) — *including defect in voluntary movement of orofacial muscles*

333.83   Spasmodic torticollis — (Use additional E code to identify drug, if drug induced) — *including impermanent condition in which head tilts to one side*

333.84   Organic writers' cramp — (Use additional E code to identify drug, if drug induced) — *including cramp affecting thumb, index finger and third finger due to prolonged writing*

333.89   Other fragments of torsion dystonia — (Use additional E code to identify drug, if drug induced)

⌐5th   Needs fifth-digit   **OK**   Valid three-digit category

333.90 Unspecified extrapyramidal disease and abnormal movement disorder — *including extrapyramidal disorder NOS*

333.91 Stiff-man syndrome — *including disease of the CNS marked by progressive muscle rigidity and spasms*

333.92 Neuroleptic malignant syndrome — (Use additional E code to identify drug) — *use additional E code to identify drug if drug-induced*

333.93 Benign shuddering attacks — *including protracted period of convulsive tremors*

333.99 Other extrapyramidal disease and abnormal movement disorder — *including restless legs*

334 SPINOCEREBELLAR DISEASE

334.0 Friedreich's ataxia — *including inherited disease marked by dorsal and lateral columnar sclerosis of the spinal cord*

334.1 Hereditary spastic paraplegia — *including paralysis of lower half of body marked by increased muscle tone and heightened tendon reflexes*

334.2 Primary cerebellar degeneration — *including Sanger-Brown cerebellar ataxia; dyssynergia cerebellaris myoclonica; primary cerebellar degeneration NOS*

334.3 Other cerebellar ataxia — (Use additional E code to identify drug, if drug induced) — *including cerebellar ataxia NOS; use additional E code to identify drug if drug-induced*

334.4 Cerebellar ataxia in diseases classified elsewhere — (Code first underlying disease, as: 140.0–239.9, 244.0–244.9, 303.00–303.93) — *code first underlying disease as: alcoholism, myxedema or neoplastic disease*

334.8 Other spinocerebellar diseases — *including ataxia-teleangiectasis [Louis-Bar syndrome]; corticostriatal-spinal degeneration*

334.9 Unspecified spinocerebellar disease — *unknown*

335 ANTERIOR HORN CELL DISEASE

335.0 Werdnig-Hoffmann disease — *including infantile spinal muscular atrophy; progressive muscular atrophy of infancy*

335.10 Unspecified spinal muscular atrophy — *including muscular atrophy of the spine NOS*

335.11 Kugelberg-Welander disease — *including familial spinal muscular atrophy*

335.19 Other spinal muscular atrophy — *including adult spinal muscular atrophy*

335.20 Amyotrophic lateral sclerosis — *including motor neuron disease (bulbar)(mixed type); Lou Gehrig's disease*

335.21 Progressive muscular atrophy — *including Duchenne-Aran muscular atrophy; progressive muscular atrophy (pure)*

335.22 Progressive bulbar palsy — *degeneration of the nuclear cells of lower cranial nerves leading to paralysis*

335.23 Pseudobulbar palsy — *condition in which balance and walking are affected by arteriosclerosis-mediated mini-strokes that damage the pertinent areas of the brain*

335.24 Primary lateral sclerosis — *sclerosis of lateral column of spinal cord*

335.29 Other motor neuron diseases

335.8 Other anterior horn cell diseases

335.9 Unspecified anterior horn cell disease — *unknown*

336 OTHER DISEASES OF SPINAL CORD

336.0 Syringomyelia and syringobulbia — *progressive spinal cord disease marked by cavitation and gliosis of surrounding tissues*

336.1 Vascular myelopathies — *including acute infarction of spinal cord (embolic) (nonembolic); arterial thrombosis of spinal cord; hematomyelia*

336.2 Subacute combined degeneration of spinal cord in diseases classified elsewhere — (Code first underlying disease, as: 266.2, 281.0, 281.1) — *code first underlying disease as: pernicious anemia (281.0), other vitamin B12 deficiency anemia (281.1) or vitamin B12 deficiency (266.2)*

336.3 Myelopathy in other diseases classified elsewhere — (Code first underlying disease, as: 140.0–239.9) — *code first underlying disease as: myelopathy in neoplastic disease*

336.8 Other myelopathy — (Use additional E code to identify cause) — *including drug-induced myelopathy; radiation-induced myelopathy; use additional E code to identify cause*

336.9 Unspecified disease of spinal cord — *including cord compression NOS; myelopathy NOS*

337 DISORDERS OF THE AUTONOMIC NERVOUS SYSTEM

337.0 Idiopathic peripheral autonomic neuropathy — *including carotid sinus syncope or syndrome; cervical sympathetic dystrophy or paralysis*

337.1 Peripheral autonomic neuropathy in disorders classified elsewhere — (Code first underlying disease, as: 250.6, 277.3) — *code first underlying disease as: amyloidosis, diabetes*

Peripheral autonomic neuropathy in disorders classified elsewhere are the chronic and progressive disorders of the peripheral autonomic nerves most often associated with diabetes mellitus, usually insulin dependent or of long-standing duration. Other common etiologies include amyloidosis, botulism, porphyria, and multiple endocrine adenomas.

Signs and symptoms of peripheral autonomic neuropathy in disorders classified elsewhere include impotence, bladder atony, nocturnal diarrhea, orthostatic hypotension, hypersensitivity to cold, and gustatory sweating.

Diagnostic tests include voiding cystometrogram to study urinary neuropathy and motility studies for esophagus, stomach, and duodenum. Therapies include rigorous control of blood glucose for diabetic autonomic polyneuropathy and symptomatic therapies such as stool bulking agents for diabetic diarrhea, bladder neck resection for urinary bladder dysfunction, and penile implants for impotence.

Associated conditions include foot ulcers, gangrene, other diabetic complications such as diabetic nephropathy, Charcot's joint, or diabetic gastroparesis.

Code first the etiology of the peripheral autonomic neuropathy (e.g., diabetes mellitus (250.6) or amyloidosis (277.3)).

337.20 Unspecified reflex sympathetic dystrophy — *unspecified*

337.21 Reflex sympathetic dystrophy of the upper limb — *reflex sympathetic dystropy (RSD) of upper limb*

337.22 Reflex sympathetic dystrophy of the lower limb — *reflex sympathetic dystropy (RSD) of lower limb*

337.29 Reflex sympathetic dystrophy of other specified site — *reflex sympathetic dystropy (RSD), unspecified*

5th Needs fifth-digit   **OK** Valid three-digit category

337.3 Autonomic dysreflexia — (Use additional code to identify the underlying cause, such as: 560.39, 599.0, 707.0) — *use additional code to identify the underlying cause, such as decubitus ulcer, fecal impaction or urinary tract infection*

337.9 Unspecified disorder of autonomic nervous system — *unspecified*

340-349 Other Disorders of the Central Nervous System

340 MULTIPLE SCLEROSIS OK

Multiple sclerosis is chronic demyelinating disease affecting the white matter of the spinal cord and brain. Multiple sclerosis is characterized by the breaking down of the myelin fibers of the nervous system; patches of scarred nervous fibers develop at these sites. The etiology is unknown, but recent studies suggest the condition may be a cell-mediated autoimmune disease due to an inherited disorder of immune regulation. The disease affects adults between the ages of 20 years and 40 years and occurs more often in women.

Signs and symptoms of multiple sclerosis include acute optic neuritis, diplopia, internuclear ophthalmoplegia, frequent dropping of articles, stumbling or falling for no reason, Lhermitte's phenomenon (flexion of the neck producing tingling and paresthesias of legs), and mental changes.

Lab work shows cerebrospinal fluid with five to 100 lymphocytes per cubic millimeter, elevated gamma globulin level (IgG), abnormal gold curve, evoked-potential testing of the visual evoked response, brainstem auditory evoked response, and somatosensory evoked response is abnormally delayed. Therapies include corticosteroids to lessen intensity and duration of acute exacerbations; physical and occupational therapy to preserve muscle strength and maintain motor function; and muscle relaxant and transcutaneous electrical nerve stimulation (TENS) units to treat spasm and pain. Immunosuppressive therapy with agents such as oral azathioprine and high dose IV cyclophosphamide is in the experimental phase.

Associated conditions include poor bladder tone (atonic and neurogenic) and urinary incontinence.

341 OTHER DEMYELINATING DISEASES OF CENTRAL NERVOUS SYSTEM

341.0 Neuromyelitis optica — *syndrome involving demyelination of spinal cord, optic nerves and optic chiasma*

341.1 Schilder's disease — *including Balo's concentric sclerosis; encephalitis periaxialis diffusa*

341.8 Other demyelinating diseases of central nervous system — *including central demyelination of corpus callosum; central pontine myelinosis*

341.9 Unspecified demyelinating disease of central nervous system — *unspecified*

342 HEMIPLEGIA AND HEMIPARESIS

342.0 ✔5th Flaccid hemiplegia — *hemiplegia (paralysis of half the body) with absent or defective muscle tone*

Flaccid hemiplegia is the loss of muscle tone in the paralyzed body parts with absence of tendon reflex. It may be caused by disease or trauma affecting the nerves associated with the involved muscles.

342.1 ✔5th Spastic hemiplegia — *hemiplegia (paralysis of half the body) with increased muscular tone*

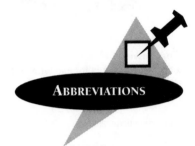

ABBREVIATIONS

MS: Multiple Sclerosis, patches of plaque in the brain or spinal cord causing paralysis, speech disturbances, and tremors.

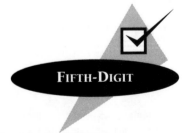

FIFTH-DIGIT

The following fifth-digit subclassification is for use with codes 342.0-342.9:

0 affecting unspecified side

1 affecting dominant side

2 affecting nondominant side

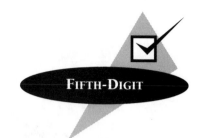

FIFTH-DIGIT

The following fifth-digit subclassification is for use with codes 342.0-342.9:

0 affecting unspecified side

1 affecting dominant side

2 affecting nondominant side

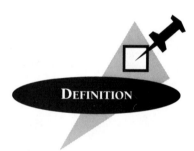

DEFINITION

Diplegia: paralysis affecting corresponding extremities on both sides of the body.

Flaccid: a state of hemiplegia in which the affected muscles are without tone or are flabby.

Hemiparesis: the state of paralysis affecting part or all of just one side of the body.

Hemiplegia: the state of paralysis of just one side of the body.

Monoplegia: paralysis affecting one extremity.

Paraplegia: paralysis affecting the lower extremities and the lower trunk.

Quadriplegia: also referred to as tetraplegia, paralysis affecting all four extremities.

Spastic: a state of hemiplegia in which the affected muscles have increased tonicity.

Spastic hemiplegia is muscle spasm within paralyzed parts of the body with increased tendon reflexes. It may be caused by disease or trauma affecting the nerves associated with the involved muscles.

342.8 ↳5th Other specified hemiplegia — *hemiplegia (paralysis of half the body) NEC*

342.9 ↳5th Unspecified hemiplegia — *hemiplegia (paralysis of half the body NOS*

343 INFANTILE CEREBRAL PALSY

The definition of infantile cerebral palsy is chronic nonprogressive disorders, present from birth, due to damage to the motor function of the brain. The functional impairment may range from disorders of movement or coordination to paresis.

343.0 Diplegic infantile cerebral palsy — *including congenital paraplegia; stiffness is greater in legs than in arms*

Diplegic infantile cerebral palsy — *including congenital paraplegia; stiffness is greater in legs than in arms*

The term "congenital diplegia" is used to include a group of cases characterized by bilateral and symmetrical disturbances or motility present from birth and that remain stationary or tend to improve. Traditionally, the term "diplegia" is used when all four limbs are affected, but weakness and spasticity are more severe in the lower limbs. Quadriplegia or tetraplegia is the term used when all four limbs are affected to an equal extent.

343.1 Hemiplegic infantile cerebral palsy — *including congenital hemiplegia*

Congenital hemiplegia refers to conditions demonstrated at birth while infantile hemiplegia is the term applied to hemiplegia that develops during the first few years of life. Clinically, the distinction between congenital and infantile hemiplegia is academic.

343.2 Quadriplegic infantile cerebral palsy

343.3 Monoplegic infantile cerebral palsy — *infantile cerebral palsy which affects a single limb or a single group of muscles*

343.4 Infantile hemiplegia — *including infantile hemiplegia (postnatal) NOS*

343.8 Other specified infantile cerebral palsy — *including congenital or infantile triplegia*

343.9 Unspecified infantile cerebral palsy — *including cerebral palsy NOS*

344 OTHER PARALYTIC SYNDROMES

344.00 Unspecified quadriplegia — *including quadriplegia NOS*

344.01 C1-C4, complete — *paralysis at least below the level of C4 and lesion that lesion transects cord*

344.02 C1-C4, incomplete — *paralysis at least below the level of C4 and lesion that does not completely transect the cord*

344.03 C5-C7, complete — *paralysis at least below the level of C7 and lesion that lesion transects cord*

344.04 C5-C7, incomplete — *incomplete; paralysis at least below the level of C7 and lesion that does not completely transect the cord*

344.09 Other quadriplegia and quadriparesis — *Other quadriplegia and quadriparesis*

344.1 Paraplegia — *including paralysis of both lower limbs; paraplegia (lower)*

344.2 Diplegia of upper limbs — *including diplegia (upper); paralysis of both upper limbs*

344.30 Monoplegia of lower limb affecting unspecified side — *including paralysis of lower limb NOS*

344.31 Monoplegia of lower limb affecting dominant side — *affecting dominant side*

↳5th   Needs fifth-digit   **OK**   Valid three-digit category

344.32	Monoplegia of lower limb affecting nondominant side — *affecting nondominant side*
344.40	Monoplegia of upper limb affecting unspecified side — *monoplegia of upper limb NOS*
344.41	Monoplegia of upper limb affecting dominant side — *upper limb affecting dominant side*
344.42	Monoplegia of upper limb affecting nondominant side — *upper limb affecting nondominant side*
344.5	Unspecified monoplegia — *unknown*
344.60	Cauda equina syndrome without mention of neurogenic bladder — *without mention of neurogenic bladder*
344.61	Cauda equina syndrome with neurogenic bladder — *including acontractile bladder; autonomic hyperreflexia of bladder; cord bladder*
344.81	Locked-in state — *victim cannot communicate except sometimes through eye-blinking, that he is fully conscious*
344.89	Other specified paralytic syndrome — *including alternating oculomotor paralysis, Avellis' syndrome, Babinski-Nageotte syndrome, Benedikt's paralysis, Brown-Sequard syndrome, Cestan-Chenais syndrome, tegmental syndrome, triplegia, Weber-Leyden syndrome*
344.9	Unspecified paralysis

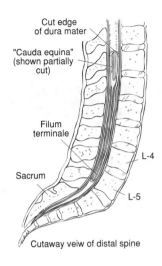

Cut edge of dura mater

"Cauda equina" (shown partially cut)

Filum terminale

L-4

Sacrum

L-5

Cutaway veiw of distal spine

345 EPILEPSY

Epilepsy is a disorder characterized by recurrent transient disturbances of the cerebral function. An abnormal paroxysmal neuronal discharge in the brain usually results in convulsive seizures, but may result in loss of consciousness, abnormal behavior, and sensory disturbances in any combination. Epilepsy may be secondary to prior trauma, hemorrhage, intoxication (toxins), chemical imbalances, anoxia, infections, neoplasms, or congenital defects.

Signs and symptoms of epilepsy include momentary interruption of activity, staring, and mental blankness. More severe symptoms include complete loss of consciousness, sudden momentary loss or contracture of muscle tone, rolling of the eyes, stiffness, violent jerking movements, and incontinence of urine and feces.

Diagnostic tests include lab work such as CBC for signs of infection and serum lead levels for signs of lead poisoning. Lumbar puncture may rule out suspected cerebrospinal infection or trauma, while CT scan of brain may rule out intracranial lesions, and an EEG may detect abnormal electrical activity in the brain.

Therapies include anticonvulsives such as phenobarbital, Tegretol, phenytoin (Dilantin), and surgery (temporal lobectomy, extratemporal cortical resections, hemispherectomy, and CT- or MRI-based stereotactic resections of epileptogenic lesions) for severe, intractable, or life-threatening disease.

This category includes seizure disorders described as repetitive or recurrent. Patients with history of seizure disorders maintained on anticonvulsive medications are most likely epileptics and should be classified to category 345 with physician verification.

Assign a fourth digit to indicate the type of epilepsy. If the physician does not indicate the type of epilepsy in the medical record, report 345.9 with the appropriate fifth digit.

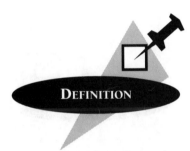

DEFINITION

Generalized convulsive epilepsy: also called tonic-clonic epilepsy, abnormalities in the brain's electrical activity cause convulsive seizures with tension of limbs (tonic) or rhythmic contractions (clonic).

Grand mal status: extended convulsive seizures with tension of limbs and/or rhythmic contractions.

Partial epilepsy: also referred to as focal epilepsy, a partial seizure.

Petit mal status: refers to the current absence of seizures.

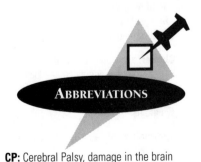

ABBREVIATIONS

CP: Cerebral Palsy, damage in the brain interrupting coordination and motor skills.

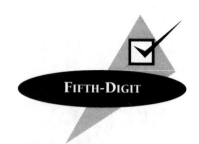

FIFTH-DIGIT

The following fifth-digit subclassification is for use with categories 345.0, 345.1, and 345.4-345.9:

0 without mention of intractable epilepsy

1 with intractable epilepsy

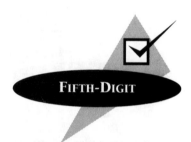

FIFTH-DIGIT

The following fifth-digit subclassification is for use with category 346:

0 without mention of intractable migraine

1 with intractable migraine, so stated

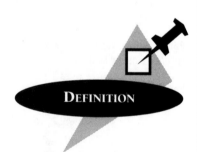

DEFINITION

Forms of Migraine:

Classical: a headache with an early visual symptom

Cluster: also called histamine or Horton's, severe one-sided headache

Common: a headache without early symptoms

Intractable: a headache resistant to treatment

A series of seizures at intervals too brief to allow consciousness between attacks is known as status epilepticus and can result in death. Status epilepticus not otherwise specified is classified to code 345.3, grand mal status, but status epilepticus can occur in other specified forms of epilepsy.

345.0 ✔5th Generalized nonconvulsive epilepsy — *including atonic absences; minor epilepsy; petit mal; atonic seizures*

345.1 ✔5th Generalized convulsive epilepsy — *including clonic, tonic, myoclonic epileptic seizures; grand mal; major epilepsy*

345.2 Epileptic petit mal status — *including epileptic absence status*

345.3 Epileptic grand mal status — *including status epilepticus NOS*

345.4 ✔5th Partial epilepsy with impairment of consciousness — *including limbic system epilepsy; partial secondarily graded epilepsy; psychomotor epilepsy; epileptic automatism*

345.5 ✔5th Partial epilepsy without mention of impairment of consciousness — *including Bravais-Jacksonian epilepsy NOS; motor partial epilepsy; sensory-induced epilepsy; visceral epilepsy; temporal lobe epilepsy*

345.6 ✔5th Infantile spasms — *including hypsarrhythmia; lightning spasms*

345.7 ✔5th Epilepsia partialis continua — *including Kojevnikov's epilepsy*

345.8 ✔5th Other forms of epilepsy — *including cursive or gelastic epilepsy*

345.9 ✔5th Unspecified epilepsy — *including epileptic convulsions, fits or seizures NOS*

346 MIGRAINE

346.0 ✔5th Classical migraine — *migraine preceded or accompanied by transient focal neurological symptoms; migraine with aura*

346.1 ✔5th Common migraine — *including atypical migraine; sick headache*

346.2 ✔5th Variants of migraine — *including cluster headache; histamine cephalgia; abdominal migraine; migrainous or ciliary neuralgia*

346.8 ✔5th Other forms of migraine — *including hemiplegic or ophthalmoplegic migraine*

346.9 ✔5th Unspecified migraine — *unspecified*

347 CATAPLEXY AND NARCOLEPSY OK

Cataplexy is defined as abrupt attacks of muscular weakness, while narcolepsy is defined as uncontrollable sleep.

348 OTHER CONDITIONS OF THE BRAIN

348.0 Cerebral cysts — *including arachnoid cyst; pseudoporencephaly*

348.1 Anoxic brain damage — (Use additional E code to identify cause) — *use additional E code to identify cause*

348.2 Benign intracranial hypertension — *including pseudotumor cerebri*

348.3 Unspecified encephalopathy — *unspecified*

348.4 Compression of brain — *including brain (stem) compression or herniation*

348.5 Cerebral edema — *swelling of the brain*

348.8 Other conditions of brain — *including cerebral fungus or calcification*

348.9 Unspecified condition of brain — *unspecified*

349 OTHER AND UNSPECIFIED DISORDERS OF THE NERVOUS SYSTEM

349.0 Reaction to spinal or lumbar puncture — *including headache following lumbar puncture*

349.1 Nervous system complications from surgically implanted device — *Nervous system complications from surgically implanted device*

349.2 Disorders of meninges, not elsewhere classified — *including meningeal adhesions, (cerebral), (spinal); acquired meningocele; acquired pseudomeningocele*

✔5th Needs fifth-digit   OK Valid three-digit category

349.81 Cerebrospinal fluid rhinorrhea — *escape of CSF through nose*

349.82 Toxic encephalopathy — *(Use additional E code to identify cause)* — *use additional E code to identify cause*

349.89 Other specified disorder of nervous system — *including nervous system disorders NEC*

349.9 Unspecified disorders of nervous system — *including disorder of nervous system (central) NOS*

350-359 Disorders of the Peripheral Nervous System

350 TRIGEMINAL NERVE DISORDERS

350.1 Trigeminal neuralgia — *including tic douloureux; trifacial neuralgia*

350.2 Atypical face pain

350.8 Other specified trigeminal nerve disorders — *including auriculotemporal syndrome; compression fifth cranial nerve; Frey's syndrome; gustatory sweating syndrome; lesion of gasserian ganglion*

350.9 Unspecified trigeminal nerve disorder — *unknown*

351 FACIAL NERVE DISORDERS

351.0 Bell's palsy — *including facial palsy*

351.1 Geniculate ganglionitis — *including geniculate ganglionitis NOS*

351.8 Other facial nerve disorders — *including facial myokymia; Melkersson's syndrome*

351.9 Unspecified facial nerve disorder — *including facial nerve disorder NOS*

352 DISORDERS OF OTHER CRANIAL NERVES

352.0 Disorders of olfactory (1st) nerve — *disorders of olfactory [1st] nerve*

352.1 Glossopharyngeal neuralgia — *pain between the throat and the ear along the petrosal and jugular ganglia*

352.2 Other disorders of glossopharyngeal (9th) nerve — *disorders of glossopharyngeal [9th] nerve*

352.3 Disorders of pneumogastric (10th) nerve — *disorders of pneumogastric [10th] nerve; disorders of vagal nerve*

352.4 Disorders of accessory (11th) nerve — *disorder in the nerves affecting the palate, pharynx, larynx, thoracic viscera, and sternocleidomastoid and trapezius muscles*

352.5 Disorders of hypoglossal (12th) nerve — *disorder in the nerves affecting the muscles of the tongue*

352.6 Multiple cranial nerve palsies — *including Collet-Sicard syndrome; polyneuritis cranialis*

352.9 Unspecified disorder of cranial nerves — *Unspecified*

353 NERVE ROOT AND PLEXUS DISORDERS

353.0 Brachial plexus lesions — *including cervical rib syndrome; thoracic outlet syndrome; scalenus anticus syndrome*

353.1 Lumbosacral plexus lesions — *acquired defect in tissue along the network of nerves in the lower back, causing corresponding motor and sensory dysfunction*

353.2 Cervical root lesions, not elsewhere classified — *including cervicodorsal outlet syndrome*

353.3 Thoracic root lesions, not elsewhere classified — *not elsewhere classified*

353.4 Lumbosacral root lesions, not elsewhere classified — *not elsewhere classified*

353.5 Neuralgic amyotrophy — *including Parsonage-Aldren-Turner syndrome*

353.6 Phantom limb (syndrome) — *including postamputation neural disorder causing itch, ache, or pain as if in the nerves of the amputated limb*

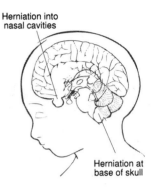

Herniation into nasal cavities

Herniation at base of skull

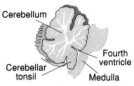

Cerebellum

Cerebellar tonsil

Fourth ventricle

Medulla

Detail of section through brain stem showing part of cerebellum herniating into the brain stem

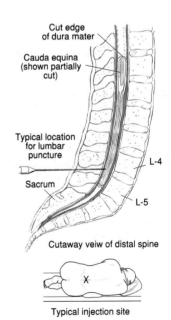

Cut edge of dura mater

Cauda equina (shown partially cut)

Typical location for lumbar puncture

Sacrum

L-4

L-5

Cutaway veiw of distal spine

Typical injection site

353.8	Other nerve root and plexus disorders — *other*
353.9	Unspecified nerve root and plexus disorder — *unspecified*

354 MONONEURITIS OF UPPER LIMB AND MONONEURITIS MULTIPLEX

354.0	Carpal tunnel syndrome — *including median nerve entrapment; partial thenar atrophy*
354.1	Other lesion of median nerve — *acquired defect in tissue in the ulnar nerve, causing corresponding motor and sensory dysfunction in the forearm and hand; cubital tunnel syndrome; tardy ulnar nerve palsy*
354.2	Lesion of ulnar nerve
354.3	Lesion of radial nerve — *acquired defect in tissue in the radial nerve, causing corresponding motor and sensory dysfunction in the forearm and hand; acute radial nerve palsy*
354.4	Causalgia of upper limb — *dysfunction of peripheral nerve of upper limb, usually due to injury, causing burning pain and trophic skin changes*
354.5	Mononeuritis multiplex — *combinations of single conditions classifiable to 354 or 355*
354.8	Other mononeuritis of upper limb — *including paralysis nerve phrenic (acquired); paralysis subscapularis; subcostal nerve compression syndrome*
354.9	Unspecified mononeuritis of upper limb — *unspecified*

355 MONONEURITIS OF LOWER LIMB AND UNSPECIFIED SITE

355.0	Lesion of sciatic nerve — *acquired defect in tissue in the sciatic nerve, causing corresponding motor and sensory dysfunction in the back, buttock, and leg; pyriformis syndrome*
355.1	Meralgia paresthetica — *including lateral cutaneous femoral nerve of thigh compression or syndrome*
355.2	Other lesion of femoral nerve
355.3	Lesion of lateral popliteal nerve — *lesion of common peroneal nerve*
355.4	Lesion of medial popliteal nerve — *lesion of medial popliteal nerve*
355.5	Tarsal tunnel syndrome — *neuropathy of distal tibial nerve*
355.6	Lesion of plantar nerve — *including Morton's metatarsalgia, neuralgia or neuroma*
355.71	Causalgia of lower limb — *causalgia of lower limb*
355.79	Other mononeuritis of lower limb
355.8	Unspecified mononeuritis of lower limb — *unspecified*
355.9	Mononeuritis of unspecified site — *unspecified; causalgia NOS*

356 HEREDITARY AND IDIOPATHIC PERIPHERAL NEUROPATHY

356.0	Hereditary peripheral neuropathy — *including Dejerine-Sottas disease*
356.1	Peroneal muscular atrophy — *including Charcot-Marie-Tooth disease; neuropathic muscular atrophy*
356.2	Hereditary sensory neuropathy — *inherited defect in dorsal root ganglia, optic nerve, and cerebellum causing sensory losses, shooting pains, foot ulcers*
356.3	Refsum's disease — *including heredopathia atactica polyneuritiformis*
356.4	Idiopathic progressive polyneuropathy — *advancing disease or dysfunction of multiple nerves; cause unknown*
356.8	Other specified idiopathic peripheral neuropathy — *including supranuclear paralysis*
356.9	Unspecified hereditary and idiopathic peripheral neuropathy — *unspecified*

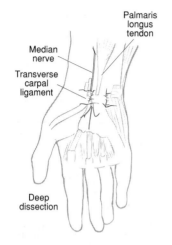

Palmaris longus tendon

Median nerve

Transverse carpal ligament

Deep dissection

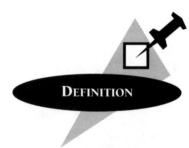

DEFINITION

Carpal tunnel syndrome: compression of the median nerve causing pain, tingling, or burning in the affected hand.

Cubital tunnel syndrome: acquired defect in tissue in the ulnar nerve, causing corresponding motor and sensory dysfunction in the forearm and hand.

Mononeuritis: inflammation of one nerve

Radial nerve palsy: acquired defect in the radial nerve causing motor and sensory dysfunction in the forearm and hand.

↙5th   Needs fifth-digit   **OK**   Valid three-digit category

357 INFLAMMATORY AND TOXIC NEUROPATHY

Inflammatory and toxic neuropathy is pain, swelling, and loss of function of the peripheral nerves in response to another disease process, injury or unknown etiology (inflammatory neuropathy), or in response to a toxic substance (toxic neuropathy).

357.0 Acute infective polyneuritis — *including Guillain-Barre syndrome; postinfectious polyneuritis*

Acute infective polyneuritis is polyneuropathy due to an infective organism, usually viral or bacterial. The most common infective organism causing polyneuritis is herpes zoster, which is classified to code 053.13. Guillain-Barre syndrome, the most common diagnosis classified here, is characterized by rapid development of symmetrical weakness or flaccid paralysis affecting the lower extremities. The upper extremities and face are less often affected.

Signs and symptoms of acute infective polyneuritis include history of recent herpesvirus (cytomegalovirus, Epstein-Barr virus) infection or immunization, paresthesia and tingling, depressed respirations in severe disease, weakness of hands and feet, and inability to perform fine movements.

Diagnostic tests include lumbar puncture with analysis of cerebrospinal fluid to show elevated protein level, often in normal cell counts. Therapies include plasmapheresis (plasma exchange), immunoglobulins in high doses, IV corticosteroids, and respiratory assistance.

Use an additional code to identify the organism causing the infection. Human immunodeficiency virus (HIV) is becoming a common cause of acute or infective polyneuropathy and is coded 357.0 with an appropriate code from categories 042-044.

357.1 Polyneuropathy in collagen vascular disease — (Code first underlying disease, as: 446.0, 710.0, 714.0) — *code first underlying disease as: disseminated lupus erythematosus, polyarteritis nodosa, rheumatoid arthritis*

357.2 Polyneuropathy in diabetes — (Code first underlying disease 250.6) — *code first underlying disease*

Polyneuropathy in diabetes is neuropathy involving the long sensory nerves supplying the hands and feet. The axons of the sensory nerves degenerate from the most distal sites and gradually spread more proximally.

Signs and symptoms of polyneuropathy in diabetes include loss of sensation to body part involved, thin and shiny skin, hair loss, "stocking and glove" effect, decreased sensation, and paresthesias.

Therapies include strict control of blood glucose levels, vitamin B and thiamine, drugs such as phenytoin, carbamazepine, amitriptyline, and fluphenazine.

Associated conditions include complications of diabetes mellitus such as diabetic nephropathy, ulcers, gangrene, and frequent infections of hands and feet.

Code the underlying diabetes, rubric 250, first. Sensory polyneuropathy rarely occurs in diabetic patients without involving the autonomic nervous system as well (337.1).

357.3 Polyneuropathy in malignant disease — (Code first underlying disease) — *code first underlying disease (140.0-208.9)*

357.4 Polyneuropathy in other diseases classified elsewhere — (Code first underlying disease, as: 032.0–032.9, 135, 251.2, 265.0, 265.2, 266.0–266.9, 277.1, 277.3, 585) — *code first underlying disease as: amyloidosis, sarcoidosis, hypoglycemia*

357.5 Alcoholic polyneuropathy — *Alcoholic polyneuropathy*

Alcoholic polyneuropathy, also called polyneuritis potatorum, is due to thiamine and other vitamin deficiency caused by chronic alcohol abuse. In addition, alcohol is believed to be neurotoxic.

Signs and symptoms of alcoholic polyneuropathy is pain, particularly in midcalf and soles of foot, tingling, loss of sensation, weakness of hands and feet, inability to perform fine movements, diminished tendon reflexes, excessive perspiration, and atrophy of lower limbs.

Diagnostic tests include EMG to show axonal sensorimotor neuropathy. Lab work reveals low vitamin B levels, anemia (chronic alcoholism interferes with eating balanced meals), and elevated liver enzymes (SGOT, SGPT, and bilirubin). Therapies include control of alcohol intake, correction of nutritional deficiencies, and physiotherapy in severe cases.

Associated conditions include cirrhosis of the liver, foot drop and wrist drop, and Korsakoff's psychosis.

357.6 Polyneuropathy due to drugs — (Use additional E code to identify drug) — *use additional E code to identify drug*

357.7 Polyneuropathy due to other toxic agents — (Use additional E code to identify toxic agent) — *use additional E code to identify toxic agent*

357.8 Other inflammatory and toxic neuropathy — *including chronic inflammatory demyelinating polyneuritis; actinoneuritis*

357.9 Unspecified inflammatory and toxic neuropathy — *unspecified*

358 MYONEURAL DISORDERS

358.0 Myasthenia gravis — *including Erb (-Oppenheim)-Goldflam syndrome*

Myasthenia gravis is a disorder of neuromuscular transmission due to the presence of autoimmune antibodies at the neuromuscular junction.

Signs and symptoms of myasthenia gravis include skeletal muscle weakness and fatigability, dysarthria, chewing fatigue, dysphagia, fever, respiratory distress, ptosis, and ocular muscle weakness.

✔5th Needs fifth-digit   **OK** Valid three-digit category

Diagnostic tests include blood serum with AChR-ab (gamma globulin antibody found in 90 percent of patients). CT scan of mediastinum or chest x-ray may show thymoma or prominent thymus gland, while an EMG shows abnormalities in muscle fiber performance. Therapies include drugs such as anticholinesterase, and adrenal corticosteroids, and immunosuppressants such as azathioprine, thymectomy, plasmapheresis, and leukoplasmapheresis.

Associated conditions include thymus gland abnormalities, osteoporosis, cataracts, frequent infections, and cholinergic crisis (primarily respiratory depression and paroxysmal atrial tachycardia) due to anticholinesterase medications.

If the documentation states that the patient's myasthenic symptoms are due to another underlying condition, see subcategory 358.1.

358.1 Myasthenic syndromes in diseases classified elsewhere — (Code first underlying disease, as: 005.1, 140.0–208.9, 242.00–242.91, 244.0–244.9, 250.6, 281.0) — *including amyotrophy or Eaton-Lambert syndrome from stated cause classified elsewhere; code first underlying disease, as: botulism, diabetes mellitus*

358.2 Toxic myoneural disorders — (Use additional E code to identify toxic agent) — *use additional E code to identify toxic agent*

358.8 Other specified myoneural disorders — *including amyotonia congenita; Oppenheim's disease*

358.9 Unspecified myoneural disorders — *unspecified*

359 MUSCULAR DYSTROPHIES AND OTHER MYOPATHIES

Muscular dystrophies and other myopathies are disease processes that are genetic in origin and cause the degeneration of muscle and nerve fibers.

359.0 Congenital hereditary muscular dystrophy — *including benign congenital myopathy; central core disease; centronuclear myopathy*

359.1 Hereditary progressive muscular dystrophy — *including Gower's or Duchenne's muscular dystrophy*

Hereditary progressive muscular dystrophy is a disease process that is genetic in origin and causes the degeneration of muscle and nerve fibers. This condition usually has an early onset, primarily affects males, and has a relentless progression until death. In the final stages, wasting of the muscles of the diaphragm and respiratory system causes respiratory failure. Classified here are any of the X-linked recessive types of dystrophy such as Duchenne's, Erb's dystrophy, Landouzy-Dejerine disease, or Gower's dystrophy.

Signs and symptoms of hereditary progressive muscular dystrophy include wasting of muscles, and deformities of small and large joints.

Diagnostic tests include serum enzyme measurements that may reveal extremely high levels of serum creatine phosphokinase, aldolase, and glutamic-oxaloacetic transaminase in the first two years, diminishing (but not returning to normal) as disease progresses. A muscle biopsy shows

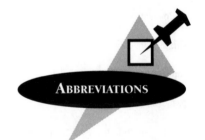

ABBREVIATIONS

MD: Muscular dystrophy, progressive weakness and wasting of muscle without nerve involvement; caused by genetic, degenerative muscle disease.

degeneration of muscle fibers and an EMG reveals decrease in amplitude and duration of motor unit potentials. Therapies include physical and occupational therapy to maintain muscle function, and treatment of complications such as heart failure or concomitant infection.

Associated conditions include atrophy of the liver, frequent infections, contracture deformities, heart failure, and respiratory failure.

359.2	Myotonic disorders — *including dystrophia myotonica; Thomsen's disease*
359.3	Familial periodic paralysis — *including hypokalemic familial periodic paralysis*
359.4	Toxic myopathy — (Use additional E code to identify toxic agent) — *muscle disorder caused by toxic agent; use additional E code to identify toxic agent*
359.5	Myopathy in endocrine diseases classified elsewhere — (Code first underlying disease, as: 242.00–242.91, 244.0–244.9, 253.2, 255.0, 255.4) — *first underlying disease as: Addison's disease or Cushing's syndrome*
359.6	Symptomatic inflammatory myopathy in diseases classified elsewhere — (Code first underlying disease, as: 135, 277.3, 446.0, 710.0, 710.1, 710.2, 714.0) — *code first underlying disease as: amyloidosis, rheumatoid arthritis*
359.8	Other myopathies — *unknown*
359.9	Unspecified myopathy — *unspecified*

360-379 Disorders of the Eye and Adnexa

360 DISORDERS OF THE GLOBE

360.00	Unspecified purulent endophthalmitis — *unspecified*
360.01	Acute endophthalmitis — *sudden, severe infection of the eyeball, with pus*
360.02	Panophthalmitis — *sudden, severe infection throughout the eyeball*
360.03	Chronic endophthalmitis — *persistent infection and inflammation of the eyeball*
360.04	Vitreous abscess — *a pocket of pus in the gel-like fluid that fills the eyeball*
360.11	Sympathetic uveitis — *inflammation of the vascular layer of the uninjured eye following an injury to the patient's other eye*
360.12	Panuveitis — *inflammation of the entire vascular layer of the eye, including the choroid, iris and ciliary body*
360.13	Parasitic endophthalmitis NOS — *inflammation of the entire eye in a parasitic infection*
360.14	Ophthalmia nodosa — *inflammation of the conjunctiva of the eye caused by embedded caterpillar hairs*
360.19	Other endophthalmitis — *not elsewhere classified*
360.20	Unspecified degenerative disorder of globe — *unspecified*
360.21	Progressive high (degenerative) myopia — *including malignant myopia*
360.23	Siderosis of globe — *deposits of iron pigment within the tissues of the eyeball, caused by high iron content of blood*
360.24	Other metallosis of globe — *including chalcosis*
360.29	Other degenerative disorders of globe — *not elsewhere classified*
360.30	Unspecified hypotony of eye — *unspecified*
360.31	Primary hypotony of eye — *low intraocular pressure without apparent cause*
360.32	Ocular fistula causing hypotony — *low intraocular pressure due to leak through abnormal passage*
360.33	Hypotony associated with other ocular disorders — *associated with other ocular disorders*
360.34	Flat anterior chamber of eye — *including obliteration of the eye, anterior chamber*
360.40	Unspecified degenerated globe or eye — *unspecified*

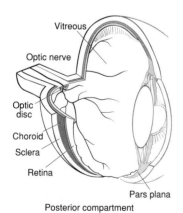

SUFFIXES & PREFIXES

endo-: within, inside

-itis: inflammation

-ophthal-: pertaining to the eye

pan-: all, encompassing

uve-: referring to the uveal tract which includes the iris, ciliary body, and choroid of the eye

Vitreous
Optic nerve
Optic disc
Choroid
Sclera
Retina
Pars plana
Posterior compartment

✍5th Needs fifth-digit   **OK** Valid three-digit category

360.41	Blind hypotensive eye — *including atrophy of globe; phthisis bulbi*
360.42	Blind hypertensive eye — *including absolute glaucoma*
360.43	Hemophthalmos, except current injury — *pool of blood within the eyeball, not from current injury*
360.44	Leucocoria — *reflection from mass behind lens, so that the pupil may look white, often indicative of retinoblastoma*
360.50	Foreign body, magnetic, intraocular, unspecified — *unspecified*
360.51	Foreign body, magnetic, in anterior chamber of eye — *in anterior chamber*
360.52	Foreign body, magnetic, in iris or ciliary body — *in iris or ciliary body*
360.53	Foreign body, magnetic, in lens — *in lens*
360.54	Foreign body, magnetic, in vitreous — *in vitreous*
360.55	Foreign body, magnetic, in posterior wall — *in posterior wall*
360.59	Intraocular foreign body, magnetic, in other or multiple sites — *in other or multiple sites*
360.60	Foreign body, intraocular, unspecified — *unspecified*
360.61	Foreign body in anterior chamber — *in anterior chamber*
360.62	Foreign body in iris or ciliary body — *in iris or ciliary body*
360.63	Foreign body in lens — *in lens*
360.64	Foreign body in vitreous — *in vitreous*
360.65	Foreign body in posterior wall of eye — *in posterior wall*
360.69	Foreign body in other or multiple sites of eye — *in other or multiple sites*
360.81	Luxation of globe — *including double whammy syndrome*
360.89	Other disorders of globe — *including acquired deformity of globe; adhesion of globe*
360.9	Unspecified disorder of globe — *unspecified*

361 RETINAL DETACHMENTS AND DEFECTS

361.00	Retinal detachment with retinal defect, unspecified — *unspecified*
361.01	Recent retinal detachment, partial, with single defect — *partial, with single defect*
361.02	Recent retinal detachment, partial, with multiple defects — *partial, with multiple defects*
361.03	Recent retinal detachment, partial, with giant tear — *partial, with giant tear*
361.04	Recent retinal detachment, partial, with retinal dialysis — *partial, with retinal dialysis; dialysis (juvenile) of retina (with detachment)*
361.05	Recent retinal detachment, total or subtotal — *total or subtotal*
361.06	Old retinal detachment, partial — *partial; delimited old retinal detachment*
361.07	Old retinal detachment, total or subtotal — *total or subtotal*

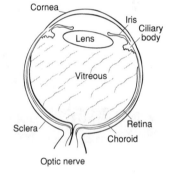

361.1   Retinoschisis and retinal cysts

Retinoschisis and retinal cysts involve the splitting of the retina due to microcystoid degeneration (retinoschisis) and development of fluid-filled sacs on the retina (retinal cysts). Retinoschisis often is bilateral and is seen in older persons. Retinal detachment is an occasional complication.

This subcategory excludes juvenile retinoschisis (362.73) and cystic or cytoid degeneration of the retina (362.62).

361.10	Unspecified retinoschisis — *unspecified*
361.11	Flat retinoschisis — *slowly progressive split of retinal sensory layers*
361.12	Bullous retinoschisis — *fluid retention between split retinal sensory layers*
361.13	Primary retinal cysts — *abnormal fluid-filled cavities or sacs within the retina*
361.14	Secondary retinal cysts — *abnormal fluid-filled cavities or sacs within the retina, caused by another condition or disease*
361.19	Other retinoschisis and retinal cysts — *including cyst of ora serrata*

361.2   Serous retinal detachment

Serous retinal detachment is separation of the retina from the choroid. Usually spontaneous, although it may be due to a trauma, this condition usually occurs in patients 50 years of age or older. Aging may cause the vitreous to shrink, which causes the retina to tear.

Signs and symptoms of serous retinal detachment include reduced vision, flashing lights (photopsia), vitreous floaters, with total detachment, and no light perception.

Diagnostic tests include exam with an ophthalmoscope and a scleral depressor, which allows visualization of tear. Therapies include scleral buckling.

Retinal defects that predispose a patient to retinal detachment classified elsewhere include peripheral cystoid degeneration, senile retinoschisis, peripheral chorioretinal degeneration, lattice degeneration, and dialysis of retina.

361.30	Unspecified retinal defect — *unspecified*
361.31	Round hole of retina without detachment — *hole of retina*
361.32	Horseshoe tear of retina without detachment — *including operculum of retina*
361.33	Multiple defects of retina without detachment — *multiple defects*
361.81	Traction detachment of retina — *traction detachment with vitreoretinal organization*
361.89	Other forms of retinal detachment — *not elsewhere classified*
361.9	Unspecified retinal detachment — *unspecified*

362 OTHER RETINAL DISORDERS

362.01	Background diabetic retinopathy — (Code first the associated condition 250.5) — *diabetic macular edema; diabetic retina microaneurysm*
362.02	Proliferative diabetic retinopathy — (Code first the associated condition 250.5) — *neovascularization, vitreous hemorrhage and detachment in a diabetic retina*
362.10	Unspecified background retinopathy — *unspecified*
362.11	Hypertensive retinopathy — *retinal irregularities caused by systemic hypertension*
362.12	Exudative retinopathy — *including Coat's syndrome*
362.13	Changes in vascular appearance of retina — (Use additional code to identify any associated (condition) 440.8) — *including vascular sheathing of retina; use additional code for any associated atherosclerosis*
362.14	Retinal microaneurysms NOS — *microscopic dilation of retinal vessels in nondiabetic*
362.15	Retinal telangiectasia — *permanent dilation of blood vessels of the retina*
362.16	Retinal neovascularization NOS — *including choroidal or subretinal revascularization*
362.17	Other intraretinal microvascular abnormalities — *including retinal varices*
362.18	Retinal vasculitis — *including Eales' disease; retinal arteritis or endarteritis*
362.21	Retrolental fibroplasia — *including Terry's syndrome*
362.29	Other nondiabetic proliferative retinopathy — *other*
362.30	Unspecified retinal vascular occlusion — *unspecified*
362.31	Central artery occlusion of retina — *central retinal arterial occlusion*
362.32	Arterial branch occlusion of retina
362.33	Partial arterial occlusion of retina — *including Hollenhorst plaque; retinal microembolism*
362.34	Transient arterial occlusion of retina — *including amaurosis fugax*
362.35	Central vein occlusion of retina — *central retinal vein occlusion*

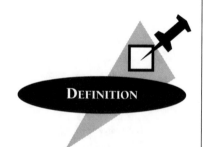

DEFINITION

Background diabetic retinopathy: microaneurysms and macular edema in a diabetic retina.

Exudative retinopathy: disease of the retina caused by destructive deposits on the posterior eye.

Hypertensive retinopathy: disease of the retina caused by systemic hypertension.

Proliferative diabetic retinopathy: neovascularization, vitreous hemorrhage, and detachment in a diabetic retina.

✔5th Needs fifth-digit   **OK** Valid three-digit category

362.36 Venous tributary (branch) occlusion of retina — *venous tributary (branch) occlusion*

362.37 Venous engorgement of retina — *including incipient or partial occlusion of retinal vein*

362.40 Unspecified retinal layer separation — *unspecified*

362.41 Central serous retinopathy — *serous-filled blister causing localized detachment of retina from pigment epithelium*

362.42 Serous detachment of retinal pigment epithelium — *exudative detachment of retinal pigment epithelium*

362.43 Hemorrhagic detachment of retinal pigment epithelium — *blood-filled blister causing localized detachment of retina from pigment epithelium*

362.50 Macular degeneration (senile) of retina, unspecified — *including Behr's disease*

362.51 Nonexudative senile macular degeneration of retina — *including atrophic or dry senile macular degeneration*

362.52 Exudative senile macular degeneration of retina — *including Kuhnt-Junius degeneration; disciform or wet senile macular degeneration*

362.53 Cystoid macular degeneration of retina — *including cystoid macular edema*

362.54 Macular cyst, hole, or pseudohole of retina — *break or tear in macula*

362.55 Toxic maculopathy of retina — (Use additional E code to identify drug, if drug induced) — *macular disease caused by toxic substance; use additional E code to identify drug, if drug induced*

362.56 Macular puckering of retina — *including preretinal fibrosis*

362.57 Drusen (degenerative) of retina — *white hyaline deposits on the retinal pigment epithelium*

362.60 Unspecified peripheral retinal degeneration — *unspecified*

362.61 Paving stone degeneration of peripheral retina — *spots of retinal thinning through which the choroid can be seen*

362.62 Microcystoid degeneration of peripheral retina — *including Blessig's or Iwanoff's cysts*

362.63 Lattice degeneration of peripheral retina — *including palisade degeneration of retina*

362.64 Senile reticular degeneration of peripheral retina — *net-like appearance of retina; a sign of degeneration*

362.65 Secondary pigmentary degeneration of peripheral retina — *including pseudoretinitis pigmentosa*

362.66 Secondary vitreoretinal degenerations peripheral retina — *including non-ocular disease causing vitreoretinal change*

362.70 Unspecified hereditary retinal dystrophy — *unspecified*

362.71 Retinal dystrophy in systemic or cerebroretinal lipidoses — (Code first underlying disease, as: 272.7, 330.1) — *code first underlying disease as: cerebroretinal lipidoses, systemic lipidoses*

362.72 Retinal dystrophy in other systemic disorders and syndromes — (Code first underlying disease, as: 272.5, 356.3) — *code first underlying disease as: Bassen-Kornzweig syndrome, Refsum's disease*

362.73 Vitreoretinal dystrophies — *including juvenile retinoschisis*

362.74 Pigmentary retinal dystrophy — *including retinal dystrophy, albipunctate; retinitis pigmentosa*

362.75 Other dystrophies primarily involving the sensory retina — *including progressive cone (-rod) dystrophy; Stargardt's disease*

362.76 Dystrophies primarily involving the retinal pigment epithelium — *including fundus flavimaculatus; vitelliform dystrophy*

362.77 Retinal dystrophies primarily involving Bruch's membrane — *including hyaline or pseudoinflammatory foveal dystrophy; hereditary drusen*

362.81	Retinal hemorrhage — *including preretinal, retinal (deep) (superficial) or subretinal hemorrhage*
362.82	Retinal exudates and deposits — *fatty fluids or denser deposits leaking into the retina*
362.83	Retinal edema — *including cotton wool retinal spots; retinal edema (localized)(macular) (peripheral)*
362.84	Retinal ischemia — *abnormal reduction of retinal blood supply*
362.85	Retinal nerve fiber bundle defects — *anomalies within the retinal nerves*
362.89	Other retinal disorders — *hyperemian of retina; phakoma; tessellated fundus, retina (tigroid)*
362.9	Unspecified retinal disorder — *unspecified*

363 CHORIORETINAL INFLAMMATIONS, SCARS, AND OTHER DISORDERS OF CHOROID

363.00	Unspecified focal chorioretinitis — *unspecified*
363.01	Focal choroiditis and chorioretinitis, juxtapapillary — *juxtapapillary*
363.03	Focal choroiditis and chorioretinitis of other posterior pole — *of other posterior pole*
363.04	Focal choroiditis and chorioretinitis, peripheral — *peripheral*
363.05	Focal retinitis and retinochoroiditis, juxtapapillary — *juxtapapillary; neuroretinitis*
363.06	Focal retinitis and retinochoroiditis, macular or paramacular — *macular or paramacular*
363.07	Focal retinitis and retinochoroiditis of other posterior pole — *of other posterior pole*
363.08	Focal retinitis and retinochoroiditis, peripheral — *peripheral*
363.10	Unspecified disseminated chorioretinitis — *unspecified*
363.11	Disseminated choroiditis and chorioretinitis, posterior pole — *posterior pole*
363.12	Disseminated choroiditis and chorioretinitis, peripheral — *peripheral*
363.13	Disseminated choroiditis and chorioretinitis, generalized — (Code first underlying disease, as: 017.3) — *generalized; code first any underlying disease as: tuberculosis*
363.14	Disseminated retinitis and retinochoroiditis, metastatic — *metastatic*
363.15	Disseminated retinitis and retinochoroiditis, pigment epitheliopathy — *unspecified acute posterior multifocal placoid pigment epitheliopathy*
363.20	Unspecified chorioretinitis — *unspecified*
363.21	Pars planitis — *posterior cyclitis*
363.22	Harada's disease — *unspecified uveomeningeal syndrome*
363.30	Unspecified chorioretinal scar — *unspecified*
363.31	Solar retinopathy — *macular damage from staring at the sun*
363.32	Other macular scars of chorioretina — *not elsewhere classified*
363.33	Other scars of posterior pole of chorioretina — *of posterior pole*
363.34	Peripheral scars of the chorioretina — *peripheral scars*
363.35	Disseminated scars of the chorioretina — *disseminated scars*
363.40	Unspecified choroidal degeneration — *unspecified*
363.41	Senile atrophy of choroid — *wasting away of choroid due to advanced age*
363.42	Diffuse secondary atrophy of choroid — *wasting away of choroid in systemic disease*
363.43	Angioid streaks of choroid — *cracks radiating from the optic disk in the layer separating the choriocapillaris from retinal epithelium*
363.50	Unspecified hereditary choroidal dystrophy or atrophy — *unspecified*
363.51	Circumpapillary dystrophy of choroid, partial — *partial*
363.52	Circumpapillary dystrophy of choroid, total — *total; including helicoid dystrophy of choroid*

↙**5th**   Needs fifth-digit   **OK**   Valid three-digit category

363.53 Central dystrophy of choroid, partial — *partial; including central areolar choroidal dystrophy; circinate choroidal dystrophy*

363.54 Central choroidal atrophy, total — *total; including central gyrate choroidal dystrophy; serpiginous choroidal dystrophy*

363.55 Choroideremia — *degeneration of choroid, affecting both sexes, leading to blindness in males*

363.56 Other diffuse or generalized dystrophy of choroid, partial — *partial; including diffuse choroidal sclerosis*

363.57 Other diffuse or generalized dystrophy of choroid, total — *total; including generalized gyrate atrophy, choroid*

363.61 Unspecified choroidal hemorrhage — *unspecified*

363.62 Expulsive choroidal hemorrhage — *expulsive hemorrhage*

363.63 Choroidal rupture — *rupture*

363.70 Unspecified choroidal detachment — *unspecified*

363.71 Serous choroidal detachment — *blister of serous fluid causing localized detachment of choroid from the sclera*

363.72 Hemorrhagic choroidal detachment — *blood-filled blister causing localized detachment of choroid from the sclera*

363.8 Other disorders of choroid — *not elsewhere classified*

363.9 Unspecified disorder of choroid — *unspecified*

364 DISORDERS OF IRIS AND CILIARY BODY

364.00 Unspecified acute and subacute iridocyclitis — *unspecified*

364.01 Primary iridocyclitis — *inflammation of the iris and ciliary body*

364.02 Recurrent iridocyclitis — *repeated bouts of inflammation of the iris and ciliary body*

364.03 Secondary iridocyclitis, infectious — *inflammation of the iris and ciliary body as a result of a primary infection elsewhere*

364.04 Secondary iridocyclitis, noninfectious — *inflammation of the iris and ciliary body as a result of a other systemic disease or disorder; aqueous fibrin or flare*

364.05 Hypopyon — *accumulation of pus between the cornea and the lens*

364.10 Unspecified chronic iridocyclitis — *persistent inflammation of the iris and ciliary body as a result of an underlying disease or condition*

364.11 Chronic iridocyclitis in diseases classified elsewhere — (Code first underlying disease, as: 017.3, 135) — *code first underlying disease as: sarcoidosis, tuberculosis*

364.21 Fuchs' heterochromic cyclitis — *unilateral inflammation of the ciliary body and iris, making the eyes appear to be different colors*

364.22 Glaucomatocyclitic crises — *uveal inflammation causing acute rise in intraocular pressure*

364.23 Lens-induced iridocyclitis — *immune reaction to proteins in the lens; follows lens trauma or extraction and causes inflammation of the iris*

364.24 Vogt-Koyanagi syndrome — *including oculocutaneous syndrome; uveocutaneous syndrome*

364.3 Unspecified iridocyclitis — *unspecified*

364.41 Hyphema — *hemorrhage of iris or ciliary body*

364.42 Rubeosis iridis — *neovascularization of iris or ciliary body*

364.51 Essential or progressive iris atrophy — *weakened and defective iris of unknown cause*

364.52 Iridoschisis — *splitting of the iris into two layers*

364.53 Pigmentary iris degeneration — *including acquired heterochromia of iris; translucency of iris*

364.54 Degeneration of pupillary margin — *including atrophy of sphincter of iris; ectropion of pigment epithelium of iris*

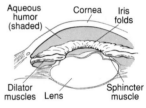

Sideview of iris and lens

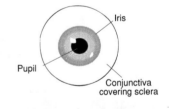

364.55	Miotic cysts of pupillary margin — *cysts of pupillary margin*
364.56	Degenerative changes of chamber angle — *changes of chamber angle*
364.57	Degenerative changes of ciliary body — *changes of ciliary body*
364.59	Other iris atrophy — *including iris atrophy (generalized) (sector shaped)*
364.60	Idiopathic cysts of iris, ciliary body, and anterior chamber — *fluid-filled sacs of the iris or ciliary body of unknown etiology*
364.61	Implantation cysts of iris, ciliary body, and anterior chamber — *including epithelial down-growth, anterior chamber; implantation cysts (surgical) (traumatic)*
364.62	Exudative cysts of iris or anterior chamber — *protein or fatty fluid-filled sacs of the iris or ciliary body caused by leak of fluid from blood vessels*
364.63	Primary cyst of pars plana — *fluid-filled sacs of the outermost ciliary ring*
364.64	Exudative cyst of pars plana — *protein or fatty fluid-filled sacs of the outermost ciliary ring, caused by leak of fluid from blood vessels*
364.70	Unspecified adhesions of iris — *unspecified*
364.71	Posterior synechiae — *adhesions binding iris to the lens*
364.72	Anterior synechiae — *adhesions binding iris to cornea*
364.73	Goniosynechiae — *peripheral anterior synechiae*
364.74	Adhesions and disruptions of pupillary membranes — *iris bombe; pupillary occlusion or seclusion*
364.75	Pupillary abnormalities — *deformed pupil; rupture of pupillary sphincter; ectopic pupil*
364.76	Iridodialysis — *tear at the base of the iris, separating it from the ciliary body*
364.77	Recession of chamber angle of eye — *recession*
364.8	Other disorders of iris and ciliary body — *including hernia of ciliary body; hernia of iris; iridodonesis*
364.9	Unspecified disorder of iris and ciliary body — *unspecified*

365 GLAUCOMA

Glaucoma is an increase in intraocular pressure due to an abnormal aqueous humor outflow from the anterior chamber or, rarely, from an above normal rate of aqueous humor production by the ciliary body. If untreated, glaucoma ultimately leads to optic nerve damage and loss of vision.

365.00	Unspecified preglaucoma — *unspecified*
365.01	Borderline glaucoma, open angle with borderline findings — *open angle with cupping of optic discs*
365.02	Borderline glaucoma with anatomical narrow angle — *defect restricting aqueous flow in the anterior segment, possibly resulting in high intraocular pressure*
365.03	Borderline glaucoma with steroid responders — *responders*
365.04	Borderline glaucoma with ocular hypertension — *high fluid pressure within the eye due to no apparent cause*

365.1 Open-angle glaucoma

Open-angle glaucoma is an increase in intraocular pressure due to the free access of aqueous humor to the trabecular network in the angle of the anterior chamber. Heredity may play a factor in patients developing primary open-angle glaucoma as well as trauma.

Signs and symptoms of open-angle glaucoma include progressive loss of peripheral vision over a span of years, blurred or foggy vision, seeing halos around lights, reduced night vision, and aching in the eyes.

Diagnostic tests include tonometry using an applanation such as a Schiotz or pneumatic tonometer to measures intraocular pressure. An exam (ophthalmoscope, slit lamp) shows fundus, optic disk, anterior structure of eyes, while a gonioscopy differentiates between

DEFINITION

Air puff device: measures intraocular pressure by evaluation of the force of a reflected amount of air blown against the cornea. A valuable screening tool, but less precise than other methods.

Applanation tonometer: measures intraocular pressure by recording the force required to flatten an area of cornea. It is attached to a slit lamp and is considered the most accurate method.

Schiotz tonometer: measures intraocular pressure by recording the depth of an indentation on the cornea by a plunger of known weight. The degree of indentation is calibrated on the tonometer to correspond to intraocular pressure.

✔5th Needs fifth-digit   **OK** Valid three-digit category

chronic open-angle glaucoma and acute closed-angle glaucoma. Perimetry and visual field tests determine the extent of peripheral vision loss and fundus photography records and monitors changes in optic disk.

Therapies include topical miotic drugs (Pilocarpine, Carcholin), carbonic anhydrase inhibitors (acetazolamide), surgery (iridectomy, trephine procedures, trabeculectomy, posterior lip sclerectomy, thermal sclerotomy) to reduce intraocular pressure, Argon laser trabeculoplasty or iridectomy, and cyclodialysis or cyclocryotherapy.

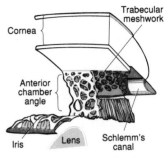

Schematic of anterior chamber

365.10	Unspecified open-angle glaucoma — *unspecified*	
365.11	Primary open-angle glaucoma — *including chronic simple glaucoma*	
365.12	Low tension open-angle glaucoma — *comparatively low rise in intraocular pressure*	
365.13	Pigmentary open-angle glaucoma — *high intraocular pressure due to iris pigment granules breaking free and blocking aqueous flow*	
365.14	Open-angle glaucoma of childhood — *infantile or juvenile glaucoma*	
365.15	Residual stage of open angle glaucoma — *residual stage*	

365.2 Primary angle-closure glaucoma

Primary angle-closure glaucoma is an increase in intraocular pressure due to the iris occluding the anterior chamber structures and preventing the aqueous humor from reaching its usual outflow channel. Acute angle-closure glaucoma is a medical emergency and requires immediate, definitive treatment.

Signs and symptoms of primary angle-closure glaucoma include progressive loss of peripheral vision over a span of years, blurred or foggy vision, seeing colored halos around lights, severe eye pain and headache, corneal epithelial edema, and nausea and vomiting.

Diagnostic tests include exam (flashlight, slit lamp, or ophthalmoscope) to reveal corneal epithelial edema as a fine rough haziness in light and to allow visualization of fundus and optic disk. Gonioscopy confirms angle closure and tonometry using an applanation such as a Schiotz or pneumatic tonometer measures intraocular pressure. Perimetry and visual field tests determine extent of peripheral vision loss and fundus photography records and monitors changes in optic disk.

Therapies include systemic osmotics (glycerol, mannitol, and acetazolamide) to lower intraocular pressure, topical miotic drugs (Pilocarpine, Carcholin), carbonic anhydrase inhibitors (acetazolamide), argon laser iridotomy, and surgical peripheral iridectomy.

365.20	Unspecified primary angle-closure glaucoma — *interval or subacute angle-closure glaucoma*	
365.21	Intermittent angle-closure glaucoma	
365.22	Acute angle-closure glaucoma — *sudden, severe rise in intraocular pressure due to blockage in aqueous drainage*	
365.23	Chronic angle-closure glaucoma — *persistent elevation of intraocular pressure due to continued blockage in aqueous drainage*	
365.24	Residual stage of angle-closure glaucoma — *residual stage*	
365.31	Corticosteroid-induced glaucoma, glaucomatous stage — *glaucomatous stage*	
365.32	Corticosteroid-induced glaucoma, residual stage — *residual stage*	
365.41	Glaucoma associated with chamber angle anomalies — (Code first associated disorder, as: 743.44) — *code first associated disorder as: Axenfeld's anomaly, Rieger's anomaly or syndrome*	

365.42 Glaucoma associated with anomalies of iris — (Code first associated disorder, as: 364.51, 743.45) — *code first associated disorder as: aniridia, essential iris atrophy*

365.43 Glaucoma associated with other anterior segment anomalies — (Code first associated disorder, as: 743.41) — *code first associated disorders as: microcornea*

365.44 Glaucoma associated with systemic syndromes — (Code first associated disease, as: 237.7, 759.6) — *code first associated disease as: neurofibromatosis, Sturge-Weber (-Dimitri) syndrome*

365.51 Phacolytic glaucoma — (Use additional code for associated (condition) 366.18) — *use additional code for associated hypermature cataract*

365.52 Pseudoexfoliation glaucoma — (Use additional code for associated (condition) 366.11) — *use additional code for associated pseudoexfoliation of capsule*

365.59 Glaucoma associated with other lens disorders — (Use additional code for associated disorder, as: 379.33, 379.34, 743.36) — *use additional code for associated disorder as: dislocation of lens, spherophakia*

365.60 Glaucoma associated with unspecified ocular disorder — *unspecified ocular disorder*

365.61 Glaucoma associated with pupillary block — (Use additional code for associated disorder, as: 364.74) — *functional defect of the pupil impeding aqueous flow*

365.62 Glaucoma associated with ocular inflammations — (Use additional code for associated disorder, as: 364.00, 364.01, 364.02, 364.03, 364.04, 364.05, 364.10, 364.11, 364.21, 364.22, 364.22, 364.23, 364.24, 364.3) — *inflammatory disease impeding aqueous flow*

365.63 Glaucoma associated with vascular disorders of eye — (Use additional code for associated disorder, as: 362.35, 364.41) — *blood vessel block or defect impeding aqueous flow*

365.64 Glaucoma associated with tumors or cysts — (Use additional code for associated disorder, as: 190.0–190.9, 224.0–224.9, 364.61) — *aberrant ocular tissue impeding aqueous flow*

365.65 Glaucoma associated with ocular trauma — (Use additional code for associated condition, as: 364.77, 921.3) — *eye injury creating defect and impeding aqueous flow*

365.81 Hypersecretion glaucoma — *hypersecretion*

365.82 Glaucoma with increased episcleral venous pressure — *increased episcleral venous pressure*

365.89 Other specified glaucoma — *unknown*

365.9 Unspecified glaucoma — *Unspecified*

366 CATARACT

Cataract is the partial or total opacity of the crystalline lens or lens capsule. Cataracts form gradually and occur bilaterally in patients over 70 years of age, with the exception of traumatic and congenital cataracts. Cataracts are classified by the zones of the lens involved in the opacity: anterior and posterior cortical, equatorial cortical, and supranuclear and nuclear. They are further subdivided into congenital, degenerative, traumatic, secondary or complicated (due to ocular or systemic disease, radiation, or other external influences), toxic, and after-cataracts (meaning one remaining in the lens or capsule following cataract extraction).

366.0   Infantile, juvenile, and presenile cataract

The definition of infantile, juvenile, and presenile cataract is the partial or total opacity of the lens occurring in an infant, a young child, or a young adult. This type of cataract usually is the result of an injury or associated with conditions such as nutritional deficiencies (e.g., galactosemia), previous inflammation, or convulsions.

Signs and symptoms of infantile, juvenile and presenile cataract include slowly progressing and painless loss of vision, leukocoria, behavioral problems indicative of vision problems, and strabismus.

Diagnostic tests include tests of visual acuity to detect any loss of vision sharpness or clarity. An exam (flashlight, slit lamp, or ophthalmoscope) reveals opacity of lens and pupil, shows anterior portion of the eye, and detects nuclear cataracts. Refraction and retinoscopy detect nuclear myopia and lenticonus. A-scan and B-scan ultrasound measure thickness and location of cataract.

Therapies include cataract extraction, intra- or extracapsular; phacoemulsification and aspiration; lensectomy and phacofragmentation; intraocular lens implantation; and cataract glasses postoperatively.

Associated conditions include galactosemia and galactokinase deficiency, hypoglycemia (neonatal), Lowe's syndrome (oculocerebrorenal syndrome), myotonic dystrophy, congenital ichthyosis, Rothmund-Thomson syndrome, rubella, Werner's syndrome, and Hallermann-Streiff-Francois syndrome.

366.00	Unspecified nonsenile cataract
366.01	Anterior subcapsular polar cataract, nonsenile
366.02	Posterior subcapsular polar cataract, nonsenile
366.03	Cortical, lamellar, or zonular cataract, nonsenile
366.04	Nuclear cataract, nonsenile
366.09	Other and combined forms of nonsenile cataract

366.1   Senile cataract

Senile cataract is partial or total opacity of the lens due to degenerative changes in the lens in patients over 55 years old.

Signs and symptoms of senile cataract include slowly progressing and painless loss of vision, leukocoria, difficulty in night driving, altered color perception, and strabismus.

Diagnostic tests include tests of visual acuity to detect any loss of vision sharpness or clarity. Exams (flashlight, slit lamp, or ophthalmoscope) reveal opacity of lens and pupils, show anterior portion of eyes, and detect nuclear cataracts. Refraction and retinoscopy detect nuclear myopia and lenticonus. A-scan and B-scan ultrasound measure thickness and location of cataract.

Therapies include cataract extraction, intra- or extracapsular; phacoemulsification and aspiration; lensectomy and phacofragmentation; intraocular lens implantation; and cataract glasses postoperatively.

366.10	Unspecified senile cataract
366.11	Pseudoexfoliation of lens capsule
366.12	Incipient cataract
366.13	Anterior subcapsular polar senile cataract

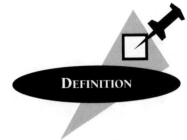

DEFINITION

Haptics: fixation portion of intraocular lenses, typically loops or tension supports. Haptics are usually made of plastic and may be secured by loops, tension, or sutures.

Intraocular lenses: anterior chamber lenses are inserted in conjunction with intracapsular cataract extraction and posterior chamber lenses are inserted in conjunction with extracapsular cataract extraction. Anterior chamber lenses are commonly used for secondary insertion.

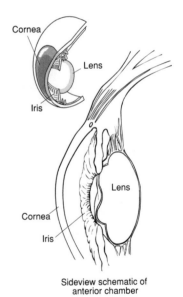

Sideview schematic of anterior chamber

366.14   Posterior subcapsular polar senile cataract
366.15   Cortical senile cataract
366.16   Nuclear sclerosis
366.17   Total or mature senile cataract
366.18   Hypermature senile cataract
366.19   Other and combined forms of senile cataract
366.20   Unspecified traumatic cataract
366.21   Localized traumatic opacities of cataract
366.22   Total traumatic cataract
366.23   Partially resolved traumatic cataract
366.30   Unspecified cataracta complicata
366.31   Cataract secondary to glaucomatous flecks (subcapsular)
366.32   Cataract in inflammatory ocular disorders
366.33   Cataract with ocular neovascularization
366.34   Cataract in degenerative ocular disorders
366.41   Diabetic cataract
366.42   Tetanic cataract
366.43   Myotonic cataract
366.44   Cataract associated with other syndromes
366.45   Toxic cataract
366.46   Cataract associated with radiation and other physical influences
366.50   Unspecified after-cataract
366.51   Soemmering's ring
366.52   Other after-cataract, not obscuring vision
366.53   After-cataract, obscuring vision
366.8   Other cataract
366.9   Unspecified cataract

367 DISORDERS OF REFRACTION AND ACCOMMODATION

367.0   Hypermetropia — *far-sightedness; hyperopia*
367.1   Myopia — *near-sightedness*
367.20   Unspecified astigmatism — *light rays are refracted over a diffuse area, rather than over a focus on the retina*
367.21   Regular astigmatism — *refers to a state of mutual perpendicularity of the sharp (maximum curvatures) and flat (minimum curvatures) of the meridians of the lens and cornea*
367.22   Irregular astigmatism — *axes are irregular, not usually correctable with spherocylinder lens*
367.31   Anisometropia — *refractive errors differing by at least one diopter when eyes are compared*
367.32   Aniseikonia — *unequal retinal image sizes in eyes, usually caused by differing refractive errors*
367.4   Presbyopia — *loss of elasticity of the elderly lens causing errors of accommodation*
367.51   Paresis of accommodation — *including cycloplegia*
367.52   Total or complete internal ophthalmoplegia — *large pupil incapable of focus due to total paralysis of ciliary muscle*
367.53   Spasm of accommodation — *focus dysfunction due to abnormal contraction of ciliary muscle*
367.81   Transient refractive change — *temporary change in refractive error*
367.89   Other disorders of refraction and accommodation — *including drug-induced disorders of refraction and accommodation*
367.9   Unspecified disorder of refraction and accommodation — *unspecified*

✔5th   Needs fifth-digit   **OK**   Valid three-digit category

368 VISUAL DISTURBANCES

368.00	Unspecified amblyopia — *unspecified amblyopia*
368.01	Strabismic amblyopia — *including suppression amblyopia*
368.02	Deprivation amblyopia — *decreased vision associated with suppression of retinal image of one eye*
368.03	Refractive amblyopia — *decreased vision in one eye associated with uncorrected refractive error*
368.10	Unspecified subjective visual disturbance — *unspecified subjective visual disturbance*
368.11	Sudden visual loss — *sudden*
368.12	Transient visual loss — *transient, including concentric fading; scintillating scotoma*
368.13	Visual discomfort — *discomfort, including asthenopia; eye strain*
368.14	Visual distortions of shape and size — *distortions of shape and size, including macropsia; micropsia*
368.15	Other visual distortions and entoptic phenomena — *other distortions and entoptic phenomena, including photopsia; refractive diplopia; visual halos*
368.16	Psychophysical visual disturbances — *including visual agnosia; visual hallucinations; disorientation syndrome; Riddoch's syndrome*
368.2	Diplopia — *Diplopia; double vision*
368.30	Unspecified binocular vision disorder — *unspecified; binocular vision disorder NOS*
368.31	Suppression of binocular vision — *suppression of binocular vision*
368.32	Simultaneous visual perception without fusion — *Simultaneous visual perception without fusion*
368.33	Fusion with defective stereopsis — *fusion with defective stereopsis*
368.34	Abnormal retinal correspondence — *abnormal retinal correspondence*
368.40	Unspecified visual field defect — *unspecified visual field defect*
368.41	Scotoma involving central area in visual field — *including centrocecal scotoma; chiasmatic syndrome*
368.42	Scotoma of blind spot area in visual field — *including enlarged angioscotoma; paracecal scotoma*
368.43	Sector or arcuate defects in visual field — *including Bjerrum scotoma*
368.44	Other localized visual field defect — *including scotoma NOS; nasal step visual field defect*
368.45	Generalized contraction or constriction in visual field — *contraction or constriction*
368.46	Homonymous bilateral field defects in visual field — *including hemianopsia (altitudinal) (homonymous); quadrant anopia*
368.47	Heteronymous bilateral field defects in visual field — *including binasal hemianopsia; bitemporal hemianopsia*
368.51	Protan defect in color vision — *including protanomaly; protanopia*
368.52	Deutan defect in color vision — *including deuteranomaly; deuteranopia*
368.53	Tritan defect in color vision — *including tritanomaly; tritanopia*
368.54	Achromatopsia — *including monochromatism (cone) (rod)*
368.55	Acquired color vision deficiencies — *acquired*
368.59	Other color vision deficiencies — *including anomalous trichromatopsia (congenital)*
368.60	Unspecified night blindness — *unspecified night blindness*
368.61	Congenital night blindness — *including hereditary night blindness; Oguchi's disease*
368.62	Acquired night blindness — *acquired*
368.63	Abnormal dark adaptation curve — *including abnormal threshold of cones or rods; delayed adaptation of cones or rods*

368.69	Other night blindness — *other night blindness*
368.8	Other specified visual disturbances — *unspecified*
368.9	Unspecified visual disturbance — *unspecified*

369 BLINDNESS AND LOW VISION

Classification		Levels of Visual Impairment					Additional descriptors which may be encountered
"Legal"	WHO	Visual acuity and/or visual field limitation (whichever is worse)					
Legal Blindness (U.S.A.) Both Eyes	(Near-) Normal Vision	Range of Normal Vision 20/10　20/13　20/16　20/20　20/25 2.0　　1.6　　1.25　　1.0　　0.8					
		Near-Normal Vision 　　20/30　20/40　20/50　20/60 0.7　0.6　　0.5　　0.4　　0.3					
	Low Vision	Moderate Visual Impairment 20/70　20/80　20/100　20/125　20/160 　　　0.25　　0.20　　0.16　　0.12					Moderate low vision
		Severe Visual Impairment 　　20/200　20/250　20/320　20/400 　　　0.10　　0.08　　0.06　　0.05 Visual field: 20 degrees or less					Severe low vision, "Legal" blindness
	Blindness (WHO) One or Both Eyes	Profound Visual Impairment 　　20/500　20/630　20/800　20/1000 　　　0.04　　0.03　　0.025　　0.02 Count fingers at: less than 3m (10 ft.) Visual field: 10 degrees or less					Profound low vision, Moderate blindness
		Near-Total Visual Impairment Visual acuity: less than 0.02 (20/1000) Count fingers at: 1m (3 ft.) or less Hand movements: 5m (15 ft.) or less Light projection, light perception Visual field: 5 degrees or less					Severe blindness, Near-total blindness
		Total Visual Impairment No light perception (NLP)					Total blindness

Visual acuity refers to best achievable acuity with correction.
Non-listed Snellen fractions may be classified by converting to the nearest decimal equivalent, e.g., 10/200 = 0.05, 6/30 = 0.20.
CF (count fingers) without designation of distance, may be classified to profound impairment.
HM (hand motion) without designation of distance, may be classified to near-total impairment.
Visual field measurements refer to the largest field diameter for a 1/100 white test object.

369.00	Blindness of both eyes, impairment level not further specified — *blindness, both eyes*
369.01	Better eye: total vision impairment; lesser eye: total vision impairment — *total impairment; lesser eye: total impairment*
369.02	Better eye: near-total vision impairment; lesser eye: not further specified — *near-total impairment; lesser eye: not further specified*
369.03	Better eye: near-total vision impairment; lesser eye: total vision impairment — *near-total impairment; lesser eye total impairment*
369.04	Better eye: near-total vision impairment; lesser eye: near-total vision impairment — *near-total impairment; lesser eye near-total impairment*
369.05	Better eye: profound vision impairment; lesser eye: not further specified — *profound impairment; lesser eye not further specified*
369.06	Better eye: profound vision impairment; lesser eye: total vision impairment — *profound impairment; lesser eye: total impairment*
369.07	Better eye: profound vision impairment; lesser eye: near-total vision impairment — *profound impairment; lesser eye: near-total impairment*
369.08	Better eye: profound vision impairment; lesser eye: profound vision impairment — *profound impairment; lesser eye: profound impairment*
369.10	Profound, moderate or severe vision impairment, not further specified — *blindness, one eye, low vision other eye*
369.11	Better eye: severe vision impairment; lesser eye: blind, not further specified — *severe impairment; lesser eye: blind, not further specified*
369.12	Better eye: severe vision impairment; lesser eye: total vision impairment — *severe impairment; lesser eye: total impairment*
369.13	Better eye: severe vision impairment; lesser eye: near-total vision impairment — *severe impairment; lesser eye: near-total impairment*
369.14	Better eye: severe vision impairment; lesser eye: profound vision impairment — *severe impairment; lesser eye: profound impairment*

✔5th　Needs fifth-digit　　　　**OK**　Valid three-digit category

369.15 Better eye: moderate vision impairment; lesser eye: blind, not further specified — *moderate impairment; lesser eye: blind, not further specified*

369.16 Better eye: moderate vision impairment; lesser eye: total vision impairment — *moderate impairment; lesser eye: total impairment*

369.17 Better eye: moderate vision impairment; lesser eye: near-total vision impairment — *moderate impairment; lesser eye: near-total impairment*

369.18 Better eye: moderate vision impairment; lesser eye: profound vision impairment — *moderate impairment; lesser eye: profound impairment*

369.20 Vision impairment, both eyes, impairment level not further specified — *not further specified*

369.21 Better eye: severe vision impairment; lesser eye; impairment not further specified — *severe impairment; lesser eye: not further specified*

369.22 Better eye: severe vision impairment; lesser eye: severe vision impairment — *severe impairment; lesser eye: severe impairment*

369.23 Better eye: moderate vision impairment; lesser eye: impairment not further specified — *moderate impairment; lesser eye; not further specified*

369.24 Better eye: moderate vision impairment; lesser eye: severe vision impairment — *moderate impairment; lesser eye; severe impairment*

369.25 Better eye: moderate vision impairment; lesser eye: moderate vision impairment — *moderate impairment; lesser eye: moderate impairment*

369.3 Unqualified visual loss, both eyes — *unqualified*

369.4 Legal blindness, as defined in USA — *blindness according to U.S.A. definition*

369.60 Impairment level not further specified — *including blindness one eye*

369.61 One eye: total vision impairment; other eye: not specified — *other eye not specified*

369.62 One eye: total vision impairment; other eye: near-normal vision — *other eye: near normal vision*

369.63 One eye: total vision impairment; other eye: normal vision — *total impairment; other eye: normal vision*

369.64 One eye: near-total vision impairment; other eye: vision not specified — *near total impairment; other eye: not specified*

369.65 One eye: near-total vision impairment; other eye: near-normal vision — *near-total impairment; other eye: near-normal vision*

369.66 One eye: near-total vision impairment; other eye: normal vision — *near-total impairment; other eye: normal vision*

369.67 One eye: profound vision impairment; other eye: vision not specified — *profound impairment; other eye: not specified*

369.68 One eye: profound vision impairment; other eye: near-normal vision — *profound impairment; other eye: near normal vision*

369.69 One eye: profound vision impairment; other eye: normal vision — *profound impairment; other eye: normal vision*

369.70 Low vision, one eye, not otherwise specified — *not further specified*

369.71 One eye: severe vision impairment; other eye: vision not specified — *severe impairment; other eye: not specified*

369.72 One eye: severe vision impairment; other eye: near-normal vision — *severe impairment; other eye: near-normal vision*

369.73 One eye: severe vision impairment; other eye: normal vision — *severe impairment; other eye: normal vision*

369.74 One eye: moderate vision impairment; other eye: vision not specified — *moderate impairment; other eye, not specified*

369.75 One eye: moderate vision impairment; other eye: near-normal vision — *moderate impairment; other eye: normal vision*

369.76 One eye: moderate vision impairment; other eye: normal vision

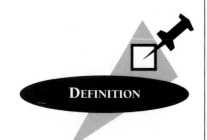

DEFINITION

Fluorescein staining: staining may enhance visualization of a corneal defect. A fluorescein strip is moistened with sterile saline and the strip is then touched to the inside of the patient's lower eyelid. After several seconds, the strip is removed and the patient's eye is closed. Cobalt blue illumination will cause the defects to stain green.

Ethylenediaminetetraacetic acid (EDTA): inhibits damage to the cornea by collagenase. EDTA is especially effective in alkali burns since it neutralizes soluble alkali, including lye.

369.8	Unqualified visual loss, one eye — *unqualified, one eye*	
369.9	Unspecified visual loss — *unspecified*	

370 KERATITIS

Keratitis is inflammation of the cornea, the transparent membrane at the front of the eye, with or without associated conjunctivitis (keratoconjunctivitis). Keratitis usually is due to type 1 herpes simplex virus (dendritic keratitis, code 054.42), but may be due to bacteria, fungus, amoeba, radiation, trauma, or other source of inflammatory reaction.

Signs and symptoms of keratitis include impaired vision (early) or blindness (late), opacity of the cornea, irritation and tearing, and photophobia.

Diagnostic tests include exam (flashlight, slit lamp) to reveal exudate and hypopyon, which are typical of corneal ulcer, and to confirm keratitis. Instillation of fluorescein dye outlines corneal ulcers. Culture and sensitivity of corneal exudate or hypopyon identify causative organism. For corneal ulcer, superficial keratectomy may provide culture material.

Therapies include antimicrobials for infection, eye lubricants, plastic bubble eye shield or eye patch, and replacement of cornea from a cadaver (keratoplasty) for corneal scarring.

370.00	Unspecified corneal ulcer — *unspecified corneal ulcer*
370.01	Marginal corneal ulcer — *tissue loss and inflammation in the margins of the cornea*
370.02	Ring corneal ulcer — *continuous, peripheral tissue loss ringing the cornea*
370.03	Central corneal ulcer — *corneal tissue loss in the center of the cornea*
370.04	Hypopyon ulcer — *including serpiginous ulcer*
370.05	Mycotic corneal ulcer — *including fungal infection causing corneal tissue loss*
370.06	Perforated corneal ulcer — *tissue loss through all layers of the cornea*
370.07	Mooren's ulcer — *painful chronic inflammation and tissue loss at the junction of the cornea and sclera; seen in elderly*
370.20	Unspecified superficial keratitis — *unspecified superficial keratitis*
370.21	Punctate keratitis — *including Thygeson's superficial punctate keratitis*
370.22	Macular keratitis — *including nummular or areolar keratitis*
370.23	Filamentary keratitis — *painful and inflamed cornea due to flaking of corneal cells*
370.24	Photokeratitis — *including snow blindness; welders' keratitis*
370.31	Phlyctenular keratoconjunctivitis — (Use additional code for any associated (condition) 017.3) — *including phlyctenulosis; use additional code for any associated tuberculosis*
370.32	Limbar and corneal involvement in vernal conjunctivitis — (Use additional code for associated (condition) 372.13) — *corneal itching and inflammation in conjunctivitis usually limited to the lining of the eyelids; use additional code for vernal conjunctivitis*
370.33	Keratoconjunctivitis sicca, not specified as Sjögren's — *inadequate tear production causing dry, burning eye*
370.34	Exposure keratoconjunctivitis — *incomplete closure of eyelid causing dry, inflamed eye*
370.35	Neurotrophic keratoconjunctivitis — *corneal and conjunctival inflammation, insensitivity, and nerve damage following injury*
370.40	Unspecified keratoconjunctivitis — *unspecified; superficial keratitis with conjunctivitis*

370.44   Keratitis or keratoconjunctivitis in exanthema — (Code first underlying condition 050.0–052.9) — *corneal inflammation accompanying infection and rash; code first underlying condition*

370.49   Other unspecified keratoconjunctivitis — *other keratoconjunctivitis*

370.50   Unspecified interstitial keratitis — *unspecified*

370.52   Diffuse interstitial keratitis — *including Cogan's syndrome*

370.54   Sclerosing keratitis — *chronic corneal inflammation leading to opaque scarring*

370.55   Corneal abscess — *pocket of pus and inflammation on the cornea*

370.59   Other interstitial and deep keratitis — *other interstitial and deep keratitis*

370.60   Unspecified corneal neovascularization — *unspecified corneal neovascularization*

370.61   Localized vascularization of cornea — *limited infiltration of the cornea by new blood vessels*

370.62   Pannus (corneal) — *shallow infiltration of the cornea by new blood vessels*

370.63   Deep vascularization of cornea — *deep infiltration of the cornea by new blood vessels*

370.64   Ghost vessels (corneal) in corneal neovascularization — *transparent, empty blood vessels remaining in cornea after the inflammation that created them has resolved*

370.8   Other forms of keratitis — *other forms*

370.9   Unspecified keratitis — *unspecified*

371 CORNEAL OPACITY AND OTHER DISORDERS OF CORNEA

371.00   Unspecified corneal opacity — *unspecified corneal scar*

371.01   Minor opacity of cornea — *corneal nebula*

371.02   Peripheral opacity of cornea — *corneal macula not interfering with central vision*

371.03   Central opacity of cornea — *corneal leucoma or macula interfering with central vision*

371.04   Adherent leucoma — *dense, opaque corneal growth adhering to the iris*

371.05   Phthisical cornea — *code first underlying tuberculosis*

371.10   Unspecified corneal deposit — *unspecified corneal deposit*

371.11   Anterior pigmentations of cornea — *including Stähli's lines*

371.12   Stromal pigmentations of cornea — *including hematocornea*

371.13   Posterior pigmentations of cornea — *including Krukenberg spindle*

371.14   Kayser-Fleischer ring — *copper deposits forming ring at outer edge of cornea*

371.15   Other deposits of cornea associated with metabolic disorders — *other deposits*

371.16   Argentous deposits of cornea — *silver deposits in cornea*

371.20   Unspecified corneal edema — *unspecified corneal edema*

371.21   Idiopathic corneal edema — *corneal swelling and fluid retention of unknown cause*

371.22   Secondary corneal edema — *corneal swelling and fluid retention caused by underlying disease, injury or condition*

371.23   Bullous keratopathy — *small blisters formed on swollen corneal epithelium*

371.24   Corneal edema due to wearing of contact lenses — *wearing of contact lenses*

371.30   Unspecified corneal membrane change — *unspecified corneal membrane change*

371.31   Folds and rupture of Bowman's membrane — *folds and rupture in the second outermost layer of the cornea*

371.32   Folds in Descemet's membrane — *folds in the second innermost layer of the cornea*

371.33   Rupture in Descemet's membrane — *rupture in the second innermost layer of the cornea*

371.40	Unspecified corneal degeneration — *unspecified corneal degeneration*	
371.41	Senile corneal changes — *including arcus senilis; Hassall-Henle bodies*	
371.42	Recurrent erosion of cornea — *recurrent erosion*	
371.43	Band-shaped keratopathy — *horizontal bands of superficial corneal calcium deposits*	
371.44	Other calcerous degenerations of cornea — *other calcerous degenerations*	
371.45	Keratomalacia NOS — *corneal softening with the development of opacities*	
371.46	Nodular degeneration of cornea — *including Salzmann's nodular dystrophy*	
371.48	Peripheral degenerations of cornea — *marginal degeneration of cornea [Terrien's]*	
371.49	Other corneal degenerations — *including discrete colliquative keratopathy*	
371.50	Unspecified hereditary corneal dystrophy — *unspecified corneal dystrophy*	
371.51	Juvenile epithelial corneal dystrophy — *juvenile*	
371.52	Other anterior corneal dystrophies — *including microscopic, cystic corneal dystrophy*	
371.53	Granular corneal dystrophy — *granular*	
371.54	Lattice corneal dystrophy — *lattice*	
371.55	Macular corneal dystrophy — *macular*	
371.56	Other stromal corneal dystrophies — *including crystalline corneal dystrophy*	
371.57	Endothelial corneal dystrophy — *including combined corneal dystrophy; cornea guttata; Fuchs' endothelial dystrophy*	
371.58	Other posterior corneal dystrophies — *including polymorphous corneal dystrophy*	
371.60	Unspecified keratoconus — *unspecified keratoconus*	
371.61	Keratoconus, stable condition — *stable condition*	
371.62	Keratoconus, acute hydrops — *acute hydrops*	
371.70	Unspecified corneal deformity — *unspecified*	
371.71	Corneal ectasia — *bulging protrusion of a thinned, scarred cornea*	
371.72	Descemetocele — *protrusion of Descemet's membrane into the cornea*	
371.73	Corneal staphyloma — *protrusion of the cornea into surrounding tissue*	
371.81	Corneal anesthesia and hypoesthesia — *decreased or absent sensitivity of the cornea*	
371.82	Corneal disorder due to contact lens — *due to contact lens*	

Corneal disorders due to contact lens are corneal disorders not elsewhere classifiable due to contact lens use. Complications associated with contact lens use include, but are not limited to, foreign body sensation and irritation, infectious and noninfectious infiltrates, anterior chamber reaction, peripheral vascularization, corneal distortion, corneal perforations, and giant papillary conjunctivitis.

371.89	Other corneal disorder — *including hypertrophic cornea*	
371.9	Unspecified corneal disorder — *unspecified corneal disorder*	

372 DISORDERS OF CONJUNCTIVA

372.0 Acute conjunctivitis

Acute conjunctivitis is an acute inflammation of the conjunctiva, the mucous membrane covering the anterior surface of the eyeball and the lining of the eyelids. Acute conjunctivitis usually is due to bacteria such as *Staphylococcus aureus*, *Staphylococcus epidermidis*, *Streptococcus pneumoniae*, *Streptococcus pyogenes*, *Moraxella lacunata*, and *Neisseria gonorrhoeae* (098.40). Acute conjunctivitis also may be due to viruses and chlamydiae (rubric 077), and to allergies (atopic).

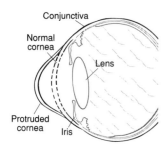

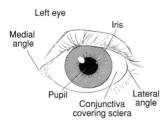

Depiction of keratoconus, a noninflammatory protruding deformity of the cornea

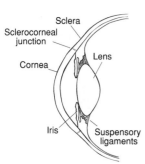

✔5th Needs fifth-digit   **OK** Valid three-digit category

Signs and symptoms of acute conjunctivitis include hyperemia of conjunctiva, pain and itching, tearing, sticky mucopurulent discharge, injection of bulbar conjunctival vessels, and history of contact lens wear.

Diagnostic tests include culture and sensitivity of discharge to identify infective organism. Stain may show predominant eosinophils if allergy related, neutrophils if bacterial, and monocytes if caused by a virus (category 077).

Therapies include topical antibiotics for bacterial conjunctivitis, corticosteroid drops, antihistamines and cold compresses for allergic conjunctivitis, and eye lubricants.

372.00	Unspecified acute conjunctivitis — *unspecified acute conjunctivitis*
372.01	Serous conjunctivitis, except viral — *severe conjunctival inflammation with watery discharge*
372.02	Acute follicular conjunctivitis — *including conjunctival folliculitis NOS; Parinaud's oculoglandular syndrome*
372.03	Other mucopurulent conjunctivitis — *including catarrhal conjunctivitis*
372.04	Pseudomembranous conjunctivitis — *including membranous conjunctivitis*
372.05	Acute atopic conjunctivitis — *sudden severe conjunctivitis due to allergies*

372.1   Chronic conjunctivitis

Chronic conjunctivitis is chronic inflammation of the conjunctiva characterized by acute exacerbations and remissions occurring over months or years. Degenerative changes or damage may occur from repeated acute attacks. The clinical presentation is similar in most respects to acute conjunctivitis except that it is more innocuous at the onset and runs a more protracted course.

372.10	Unspecified chronic conjunctivitis — *unspecified chronic conjunctivitis*
372.11	Simple chronic conjunctivitis — *persistent conjunctival inflammation*
372.12	Chronic follicular conjunctivitis — *persistent conjunctival inflammation with dense, localized infiltrations of lymphoid tissues of inner eyelids*
372.13	Vernal conjunctivitis — *persistent seasonal conjunctival inflammation in childhood*
372.14	Other chronic allergic conjunctivitis — *chronic*
372.15	Parasitic conjunctivitis — (Code first underlying disease, as: 085.5, 125.0–125.9) — *parasitic, code first underlying disease as: filariasis, mucocutaneous leishmaniasis*
372.20	Unspecified blepharoconjunctivitis — *unspecified blepharoconjunctivitis*
372.21	Angular blepharoconjunctivitis — *inflammation at the junction where the upper and lower eyelids meet; usually blocks lacrimal secretions*
372.22	Contact blepharoconjunctivitis — *inflammation of the eyelid margin and conjunctiva due to an allergic reaction*
372.30	Unspecified conjunctivitis — *unspecified*
372.31	Rosacea conjunctivitis — (Code first underlying condition 695.3) — *conjunctival inflammation associated with rosacea; code first underlying rosacea dermatitis*
372.33	Conjunctivitis in mucocutaneous disease — (Code first underlying disease, as: 099.3, 695.1) — *conjunctival inflammation associated with other mucous membrane or skin disease; code first underlying disease as: erythema multiforme or Reiter's disease*
372.39	Other and unspecified conjunctivitis — *other conjunctivitis*
372.40	Unspecified pterygium — *unspecified pterygium*
372.41	Peripheral ptergium, stationary — *stationary*
372.42	Peripheral pterygium, progressive — *progressive*

372.43	Central pterygium — *central*
372.44	Double pterygium
372.45	Recurrent pterygium — *recurrent*
372.50	Unspecified conjunctival degeneration — *degeneration, unspecified*
372.51	Pinguecula — *benign subconjunctival elevation on either side of the cornea*
372.52	Pseudopterygium
372.53	Conjunctival xerosis — *conjunctival dryness due to insufficient secretions*
372.54	Conjunctival concretions — *hard masses in the conjunctiva*
372.55	Conjunctival pigmentations — *conjunctival argyrosis*
372.56	Conjunctival deposits — *deposits*
372.61	Granuloma of conjunctiva — *abnormal dense collection of cells in the conjunctiva*
372.62	Localized adhesions and strands of conjunctiva — *abnormal fibrous connections in conjunctiva*
372.63	Symblepharon — *extensive adhesions of conjunctiva*
372.64	Scarring of conjunctiva — *contraction of eye socket (after enucleation)*
372.71	Hyperemia of conjunctiva — *conjunctival blood vessel congestion causing eye redness*
372.72	Conjunctival hemorrhage — *including hyposphagma; subconjunctival hemorrhage*
372.73	Conjunctival edema — *subconjunctival edema*
372.74	Vascular abnormalities of conjunctiva — *including aneurysm (ata) of conjunctiva*
372.75	Conjunctival cysts — *abnormal thin-walled sacs of fluid in the conjunctiva*
372.81	Conjunctivochalasis
372.89	Other disorders of conjunctiva — *other disorders*
372.9	Unspecified disorder of conjunctiva — *unspecified disorder*

373 INFLAMMATION OF EYELIDS

The patient presenting with a chalazion differs from the patient presenting with a hordeolum (stye) in that the chalazion is usually painless after a few days, while discomfort from a hordeolum usually escalates. A chalazion will usually resolve within a few months and can be treated with hot compresses to hasten resolution. Intrachalazion administration of corticosteroid is another method of treatment.

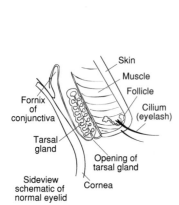

Skin
Muscle
Follicle
Cilium (eyelash)
Fornix of conjunctiva
Tarsal gland
Opening of tarsal gland
Sideview schematic of normal eyelid
Cornea

373.00	Blepharitis, unspecified — *unspecified blepharitis*
373.01	Ulcerative blepharitis — *inflammation of the eyelid with erosion of tissue*
373.02	Squamous blepharitis — *inflammation of eyelid margin with scaling of tissue*
373.11	Hordeolum externum — *including hordeolum NOS; stye*
373.12	Hordeolum internum — *including infection of meibomian gland; stye*
373.13	Abscess of eyelid — *including furuncle of eyelid*
373.2	Chalazion — *including meibomian (gland) cyst*
373.31	Eczematous dermatitis of eyelid — *including itchy inflammation of eyelid*
373.32	Contact and allergic dermatitis of eyelid — *inflammation of the eyelid due to allergic reaction*
373.33	Xeroderma of eyelid — *rough, dry, and scaly skin of the eyelid*
373.34	Discoid lupus erythematosus of eyelid — *swollen eyelids from discoid lupus erythematosus*
373.4	Infective dermatitis of eyelid of types resulting in deformity — (Code first underlying disease, as: 017.0, 030.0–030.9, 102.0–102.9) — *code first underlying disease as: leprosy, lupus vulgaris (tuberculous), yaws*
373.5	Other infective dermatitis of eyelid — (Code first underlying disease, as: 039.3, 051.0, 110.0–111.9, 684, 999.0) — *code first underlying disease as: actinomycosis, impetigo, mycotic dermatitis*

✒5th Needs fifth-digit   **OK** Valid three-digit category

373.6	Parasitic infestation of eyelid — (Code first underlying disease, as: 085.0–085.9, 125.2, 125.3, 132.0) — *code first underlying disease as: leishmaniasis, loiasis, onchocerciasis, pediculosis*
373.8	Other inflammations of eyelids — *including inflammations of eyelids NEC*
373.9	Unspecified inflammation of eyelid — *unspecified*

374 OTHER DISORDERS OF EYELIDS

374.00	Unspecified entropion — *including entropion NOS*
374.01	Senile entropion — *eyelid margin curves inward in an elderly eye*
374.02	Mechanical entropion — *eyelid margin curves inward due to external forces*
374.03	Spastic entropion — *eyelid margin curves inward intermittently and involuntarily*
374.04	Cicatricial entropion — *eyelid margin curves inward due to scarring*
374.05	Trichiasis of eyelid without entropion — *eyelashes curve inward, without eyelid margin defect*
374.10	Unspecified ectropion — *including ectropion NOS*
374.11	Senile ectropion — *lower eyelid droops away from the elderly eye*
374.12	Mechanical ectropion — *lower eyelid droops away from eye due to external forces*
374.13	Spastic ectropion — *lower eyelid droops away from eye intermittently and involuntarily*
374.14	Cicatricial ectropion — *cicatricial*
374.20	Unspecified lagophthalmos — *including lagophthalmos NOS*
374.21	Paralytic lagophthalmos — *full closure of eyelid prevented by nerve defect*
374.22	Mechanical lagophthalmos — *outside force prevents full closure of eyelids*
374.23	Cicatricial lagophthalmos — *scar tissue prevents full closure of eyelids*
374.30	Unspecified ptosis of eyelid — *unspecified*
374.31	Paralytic ptosis — *drooping of upper eyelid due to nerve defect*
374.32	Myogenic ptosis — *drooping of upper eyelid due to muscular defect*
374.33	Mechanical ptosis — *outside force causes drooping of upper eyelid*
374.34	Blepharochalasis — *drooping or relaxation of upper eyelid due to atrophy of intercellular tissue*
374.41	Eyelid retraction or lag — *retraction or lag*
374.43	Abnormal innervation syndrome of eyelid — *including jaw-blinking; paradoxical facial movements*
374.44	Sensory disorders of eyelid — *sensory*
374.45	Other sensorimotor disorders of eyelid — *including deficient blink reflex*
374.46	Blepharophimosis — *including ankyloblepharon*
374.50	Unspecified degenerative disorder of eyelid — *unspecified*
374.51	Xanthelasma of eyelid — (Code first underlying condition 272.0–272.9) — *xanthoma (planum) (tuberosum) of eyelid*
374.52	Hyperpigmentation of eyelid — *including chloasma; dyspigmentation*
374.53	Hypopigmentation of eyelid — *including vitiligo of eyelid*
374.54	Hypertrichosis of eyelid — *excessive eyelash growth*
374.55	Hypotrichosis of eyelid — *including less than normal amount, or absence of, eyelashes; madarosis of eyelid*
374.56	Other degenerative disorders of skin affecting eyelid — *other degenerative skin disorders affecting eyelid NEC*
374.81	Hemorrhage of eyelid — *bleeding eyelid*
374.82	Edema of eyelid — *including hyperemia of eyelid*
374.83	Elephantiasis of eyelid — *filarial disease causing dermatitis and enlargement of eyelid*
374.84	Cysts of eyelids — *sebaceous cyst of eyelid*
374.85	Vascular anomalies of eyelid — *vascular anomalies*
374.86	Retained foreign body of eyelid — *retained foreign body*

374.87	Dermatochalasis — *loss of elasticity causing skin under eye to sag*
374.89	Other disorders of eyelid — *including blepharoplegia; granuloma of eyelid*
374.9	Unspecified disorder of eyelid — *unspecified disorder*

375 DISORDERS OF LACRIMAL SYSTEM

The lacrimal system produces and distributes the tears that lubricate and clean the eye and keep nasal tissues moist. Excluded from this rubric are congenital disorders of the lacrimal system.

375.00	Unspecified dacryoadenitis — *unspecified dacryoadenitis*
375.01	Acute dacryoadenitis — *severe, sudden inflammation of the lacrimal gland*
375.02	Chronic dacryoadenitis — *persistent inflammation of the lacrimal gland*
375.03	Chronic enlargement of lacrimal gland — *chronic enlargement*
375.11	Dacryops — *overproduction and constant flow of tears*
375.12	Other lacrimal cysts and cystic degeneration — *other cysts and cystic degeneration*
375.13	Primary lacrimal atrophy — *wasting away of the lacrimal gland*
375.14	Secondary lacrimal atrophy — *wasting away of the lacrimal gland due to other disease process*
375.15	Unspecified tear film insufficiency — *including dry eye syndrome*
375.16	Dislocation of lacrimal gland — *dislocation*
375.20	Epiphora, unspecified as to cause — *unspecified epiphora*
375.21	Epiphora due to excess lacrimation — *overflow of tears due to overproduction*
375.22	Epiphora due to insufficient drainage — *overflow of tears due to blocked drainage*
375.30	Unspecified dacryocystitis — *unspecified dacryocystitis*
375.31	Acute canaliculitis, lacrimal — *including sudden, severe inflammation of the tear drainage system*
375.32	Acute dacryocystitis — *including acute peridacryocystitis*
375.33	Phlegmonous dacryocystitis — *infection of the tear sac with pockets of pus*
375.41	Chronic canaliculitis — *persistent inflammation of the tear drainage system*
375.42	Chronic dacryocystitis — *persistent inflammation of the tear sac*
375.43	Lacrimal mucocele — *enlarged pocket of mucus in lacrimal system*
375.51	Eversion of lacrimal punctum — *abnormal turning outward of the tear duct*
375.52	Stenosis of lacrimal punctum — *abnormal narrowing of tear duct*
375.53	Stenosis of lacrimal canaliculi — *abnormal narrowing of the tear drainage system*
375.54	Stenosis of lacrimal sac — *abnormal narrowing of tear sac*
375.55	Obstruction of nasolacrimal duct, neonatal — *acquired narrowing of the tear drainage system from the eye to the nose*
375.56	Stenosis of nasolacrimal duct, acquired
375.57	Dacryolith — *concretion of stone anywhere in lacrimal system*
375.61	Lacrimal fistula — *abnormal communication from the lacrimal system*
375.69	Other change of lacrimal passages — *changes of lacrimal passage NOS*
375.81	Granuloma of lacrimal passages — *abnormal nodules within the tear drainage system*
375.89	Other disorder of lacrimal system — *including disorders of lacrimal system NOS*

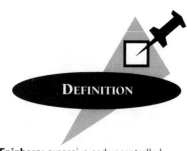

DEFINITION

Epiphora: excessive and uncontrolled tears in the eye due to blocked drainage passages or due to overproduction of tears

Dacryops: overproduction and constant flow of tears

Dacryoadenitis: inflammation of the lacrimal gland

Dacryocystitis: inflammation of the lacrimal sac

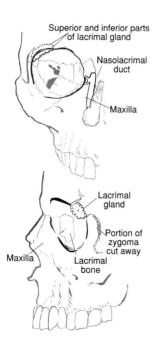

Superior and inferior parts of lacrimal gland

Nasolacrimal duct

Maxilla

Lacrimal gland

Portion of zygoma cut away

Maxilla

Lacrimal bone

↙5th   Needs fifth-digit   **OK**   Valid three-digit category

376 DISORDERS OF THE ORBIT

When an underlying disease causes the orbital disorder, sequence the underlying disease code first and a code from this rubric secondarily.

376.0   Acute inflammation of orbit

Codes in this subclassification are selected by site. In orbital cellulitis, the infection is between the orbital bone and the eyeball. In orbital periostitis, the infection is in the connective tissue covering the orbital bone. In orbital osteomyelitis, the bone is infected; and in tenonitis, the infection is in the Tenon's capsule, the thin membrane that envelops the eyeball. In all cases, a second code from Infectious and Parasitic Diseases (001-139) can be reported to identify the infective agent.

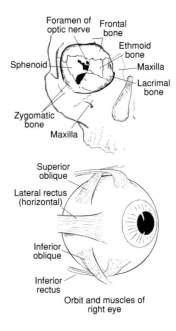

Orbit and muscles of right eye

376.00	Unspecified acute inflammation of orbit — *acute orbital inflammation NOS*
376.01	Orbital cellulitis — *abscess of orbit*
376.02	Orbital periostitis — *inflammation of connective tissue covering the orbital bone*
376.03	Orbital osteomyelitis — *inflammation of the orbital bone*
376.04	Orbital tenonitis — *inflammation of Tenon's capsule, the thin membrane that envelops the eyeball*
376.10	Unspecified chronic inflammation of orbit — *chronic orbital inflammation NOS*
376.11	Orbital granuloma — *including pseudotumor (inflammatory) of orbit*
376.12	Orbital myositis — *painful inflammation of the muscles of the eye*
376.13	Parasitic infestation of orbit — *code first underlying disease, as: hydatid infestation of orbit, myiasis of orbit*
376.21	Thyrotoxic exophthalmos — *bulging eyes as a result of hyperthyroidism*
376.22	Exophthalmic ophthalmoplegia — *inability to rotate eyes as a result of bulging eyes*
376.30	Unspecified exophthalmos — *unspecified exophthalmos*
376.31	Constant exophthalmos — *continuous, abnormal protrusion or bulging of eyeball*
376.32	Orbital hemorrhage — *bleeding behind the eyeball, causing it to bulge forward*
376.33	Orbital edema or congestion — *fluid retention behind eyeball, causing it to bulge forward*
376.34	Intermittent exophthalmos — *separate incidences of abnormal bulging of the eyeball*
376.35	Pulsating exophthalmos — *throbbing bulge or protrusion of the eyeball, usually associated with a carotid-cavernous fistula*
376.36	Lateral displacement of globe of eye — *abnormal displacement of the eyeball away from the nose, toward the temple*
376.40	Unspecified deformity of orbit — *unspecified orbital deformity*
376.41	Hypertelorism of orbit — *congenital anomaly in which the eyes are widely placed*
376.42	Exostosis of orbit — *abnormal bony growth of orbit*
376.43	Local deformities of orbit due to bone disease — *acquired abnormalities of the orbit due to bone disease*
376.44	Orbital deformities associated with craniofacial deformities — *including congenital malformation of the orbital bone*
376.45	Atrophy of orbit — *wasting away of bone tissue of orbit*
376.46	Enlargement of orbit — *enlargement*
376.47	Deformity of orbit due to trauma or surgery — *trauma or surgery*
376.50	Enophthalmos, unspecified as to cause — *recession of eyeball deep into eye socket*
376.51	Enophthalmos due to atrophy of orbital tissue — *recession of eyeball deep into eye socket due to atrophy of orbital tissue*
376.52	Enophthalmos due to trauma or surgery — *due to trauma or surgery*
376.6	Retained (old) foreign body following penetrating wound of orbit — *retrobulbar foreign body*

376.81	Orbital cysts — *encephalocele of orbit; mucocele of orbit*
376.82	Myopathy of extraocular muscles — *disease in one or more of the six muscles that control eyeball movement*
376.89	Other orbital disorder — *emphysema of eye; retrobulbar hemorrhage*
376.9	Unspecified disorder of orbit — *unspecified*

377 DISORDERS OF OPTIC NERVE AND VISUAL PATHWAYS

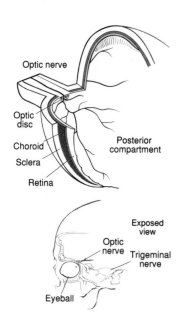

Optic nerve

Optic disc

Choroid

Sclera

Retina

Posterior compartment

Exposed view

Optic nerve

Trigeminal nerve

Eyeball

377.00	Unspecified papilledema — *unspecified*
377.01	Papilledema associated with increased intracranial pressure — *pressure within the brain causes swelling and engorgement of the optic disc and its blood vessels*
377.02	Papilledema associated with decreased ocular pressure — *reduced pressure within the eyeball causes swelling and engorgement of the optic disc and its blood vessels*
377.03	Papilledema associated with retinal disorder — *retinal disease or dysfunction causes swelling and engorgement of optic disc and its blood vessels*
377.04	Foster-Kennedy syndrome — *including basofrontal syndrome*
377.10	Unspecified optic atrophy — *unspecified*
377.11	Primary optic atrophy — *disc is grayish white with sharp edges*
377.12	Postinflammatory optic atrophy — *eye wastes away due to inflammation*
377.13	Optic atrophy associated with retinal dystrophies — *wasting away of eye due to progressive changes in retinal tissue due to metabolic defects*
377.14	Glaucomatous atrophy (cupping) of optic disc — *wasting away of eye as a result of high intraocular pressure*
377.15	Partial optic atrophy — *including temporal pallor of optical disc*
377.16	Hereditary optic atrophy — *including Leber's optic atrophy*
377.21	Drusen of optic disc — *glistening white nodules within optic nerve head*
377.22	Crater-like holes of optic disc — *crater-like holes*
377.23	Coloboma of optic disc — *congenital cleft, or defect in continuity of the optic disc*
377.24	Pseudopapilledema — *optic nerve head deformity resembling a choked optic disc*
377.30	Unspecified optic neuritis — *unspecified*
377.31	Optic papillitis — *swelling and inflammation of the optic disc*
377.32	Retrobulbar neuritis (acute) — *inflammation of optic nerve in the orbit behind the eye*
377.33	Nutritional optic neuropathy — *optic nerve disorder caused by malnutrition*
377.34	Toxic optic neuropathy — *including toxic amblyopia*
377.39	Other optic neuritis — *including optic neuritis NEC*
377.41	Ischemic optic neuropathy — *optic nerve disorder due to decreased blood flow*
377.42	Hemorrhage in optic nerve sheaths — *bleeding in optic nerve sheaths*
377.49	Other disorder of optic nerve — *compression of optic nerve*
377.51	Disorders of optic chiasm associated with pituitary neoplasms and disorders — *disruption in nerve chain from retina to brain, caused by abnormal pituitary growth*
377.52	Disorders of optic chiasm associated with other neoplasms — *disruption in nerve chain from retina to brain, caused by abnormal growth, other than pituitary*
377.53	Disorders of optic chiasm associated with vascular disorders — *disruption in nerve chain from retina to brain, caused by a vascular disorder*
377.54	Disorders of optic chiasm associated with inflammatory disorders — *disruption in nerve chain from retina to brain, caused by inflammatory disease*
377.61	Disorders of other visual pathways associated with neoplasms — *associated with neoplasms*
377.62	Disorders of other visual pathways associated with vascular disorders — *associated with vascular disorders*

⤲5th   Needs fifth-digit   **OK**   Valid three-digit category

377.63 Disorders of other visual pathways associated with inflammatory disorders — *associated with inflammatory disorders*

377.71 Disorders of visual cortex associated with neoplasms — *associated with neoplasms*

377.72 Disorders of visual cortex associated with vascular disorders — *associated with vascular disorders*

377.73 Disorders of visual cortex associated with inflammatory disorders — *associated with inflammatory disorders*

377.75 Disorders of visual cortex associated with cortical blindness — *associated with cortical blindness; blindness due to brain disorder, not eye disorder*

377.9 Unspecified disorder of optic nerve and visual pathways — *unspecified*

378 STRABISMUS AND OTHER DISORDERS OF BINOCULAR EYE MOVEMENTS

378.00 Unspecified esotropia — *unspecified*

378.01 Monocular esotropia — *one eye turns inward*

378.02 Monocular esotropia with A pattern — *one eye turns inward with A pattern*

378.03 Monocular esotropia with V pattern — *one eye turns inward with V pattern*

378.04 Monocular esotropia with other noncomitancies — *monocular esotropia with X or Y pattern*

378.05 Alternating esotropia — *each eye takes turns deviating toward inner eye*

378.06 Alternating esotropia with A pattern — *each eye takes turns deviating toward inner eye with A pattern*

378.07 Alternating esotropia with V pattern — *each eye takes turns deviating toward inner eye with V pattern*

378.08 Alternating esotropia with other noncomitancies — *each eye takes turns deviating toward inner eye with X or Y pattern*

378.10 Unspecified exotropia — *unspecified*

378.11 Monocular exotropia — *one eye turns outward*

378.12 Monocular exotropia with A pattern — *one eye turns outward with A pattern*

378.13 Monocular exotropia with V pattern — *one eye turns outward with V pattern*

378.14 Monocular exotropia with other noncomitancies — *monocular exotropia with X or Y pattern*

378.15 Alternating exotropia — *each eye takes turns deviating outward*

378.16 Alternating exotropia with A pattern — *each eye takes turns deviating outward with A pattern*

378.17 Alternating exotropia with V pattern — *each eye takes turns deviating outward with V pattern*

378.18 Alternating exotropia with other noncomitancies — *each eye takes turns deviating outward with X or Y pattern*

378.20 Unspecified intermittent heterotropia — *intermittent esotropia NOS or intermittent exotropia NOS*

378.21 Intermittent esotropia, monocular — *monocular*

378.22 Intermittent esotropia, alternating — *alternating*

378.23 Intermittent exotropia, monocular — *monocular*

378.24 Intermittent exotropia, alternating — *alternating*

378.30 Unspecified heterotropia — *unspecified*

378.31 Hypertropia — *vertical heterotropia (constant) (intermittent)*

378.32 Hypotropia

378.33 Cyclotropia

378.34 Monofixation syndrome — *including microtropia*

378.35 Accommodative component in esotropia — *accommodative*

378.40 Unspecified heterophoria — *unspecified*

378.41 Esophoria

378.42 Exophoria

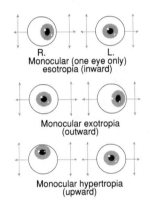

R.   L.
Monocular (one eye only)
esotropia (inward)

Monocular exotropia
(outward)

Monocular hypertropia
(upward)

The various heterophorias present when the visual axis fails upon removal of the fusioning stimuli. The eye then wanders in the indicated direction

378.43	Vertical heterophoria — *vertical*
378.44	Cyclophoria
378.45	Alternating hyperphoria — *alternating*
378.50	Unspecified paralytic strabismus — *unspecified*
378.51	Paralytic strabismus, third or oculomotor nerve palsy, partial — *partial*
378.52	Paralytic strabismus, third or oculomotor nerve palsy, total — *total including Nothnagel's syndrome; ophthalmoplegia-cerebellar ataxia syndrome*
378.53	Paralytic strabismus, fourth or trochlear nerve palsy — *fourth or trochlear*
378.54	Paralytic strabismus, sixth or abducens nerve palsy — *sixth or abducens*
378.55	Paralytic strabismus, external ophthalmoplegia — *including Tolosa-Hunt syndrome*
378.56	Paralytic strabismus, total ophthalmoplegia — *total*
378.60	Unspecified mechanical strabismus — *unspecified*
378.61	Mechanical strabismus from Brown's (tendon) sheath syndrome — *unilateral defect in sheath of superior oblique muscle, mimicking palsy*
378.62	Mechanical strabismus from other musculofascial disorders — *other musculofascial disorders*
378.63	Mechanical strabismus from limited duction associated with other conditions — *associated with other conditions*
378.71	Duane's syndrome — *eye retraction syndrome*
378.72	Progressive external ophthalmoplegia — *including von Graefe's syndrome*
378.73	Strabismus in other neuromuscular disorders — *other neuromuscular disorders*
378.81	Palsy of conjugate gaze — *including oculomotor syndrome' Parinaud's syndrome*
378.82	Spasm of conjugate gaze — *muscle contractions impairing parallel movement of eyes*
378.83	Convergence insufficiency or palsy in binocular eye movement — *insufficiency or palsy*
378.84	Convergence excess or spasm in binocular eye movement — *overcompensation in parallel movement of eye*
378.85	Anomalies of divergence in binocular eye movement — *divergence*
378.86	Internuclear ophthalmoplegia — *eye movement anomaly attributed to brainstem lesion*
378.87	Other dissociated deviation of eye movements — *skew deviation*
378.9	Unspecified disorder of eye movements — *unspecified*

379 OTHER DISORDERS OF EYE

Aphakia is classified to this rubric. Report aphakia as a condition warranting treatment with 379.31, while aphakia (pseudophakia) as a post-cataract extraction status is reported with V45.61. Congenital aphakia is reported with 743.35.

379.00	Unspecified scleritis — *including episcleritis NOS*
379.01	Episcleritis periodica fugax — *inflammation of outermost layer of the sclera, with blood engorgement*
379.02	Nodular episcleritis — *inflammation of outermost layer of the sclera, with nodular formations*
379.03	Anterior scleritis — *scleritis adjacent to corneal limbus*
379.04	Scleromalacia perforans — *softening and thinning of sclera*
379.05	Scleritis with corneal involvement — *including scleroperikeratitis*
379.06	Brawny scleritis — *severe scleral inflammation with thickening corneal margins*
379.07	Posterior scleritis — *including sclerotenonitis*
379.09	Other scleritis and episcleritis — *including scleral abscess; scleral ulcer*
379.11	Scleral ectasia — *including scleral staphyloma NOS*
379.12	Staphyloma posticum — *stretched, bulging sclera and uveal tissue at the posterior pole of eye*

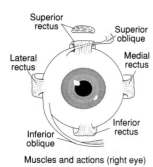

Muscles and actions (right eye)

✔5th Needs fifth-digit   **OK** Valid three-digit category

379.13   Equatorial staphyloma — *stretched, bulging sclera and uveal tissue midway between anterior and posterior portions of eye*

379.14   Anterior staphyloma, localized — *stretched, bulging sclera and uveal tissue at the anterior pole of eye*

379.15   Ring staphyloma — *stretched, bulging sclera and uveal tissue in ring shape*

379.16   Other degenerative disorders of sclera — *other degenerative disorders*

379.19   Other scleral disorder — *other disorders of sclera*

379.21   Vitreous degeneration — *including vitreous cavitation, detachment or liquefaction*

379.22   Crystalline deposits in vitreous — *including asteroid hyalitis; synchysis scintillans*

379.23   Vitreous hemorrhage — *bleeding into the vitreous*

379.24   Other vitreous opacities — *including vitreous floaters*

379.25   Vitreous membranes and strands — *membranes and strands*

379.26   Vitreous prolapse — *vitreous slippage from normal position*

379.29   Other disorders of vitreous — *other disorders*

379.31   Aphakia — *condition of being without natural optical lens*

379.32   Subluxation of lens — *partial dislocation of natural lens*

379.33   Anterior dislocation of lens — *anterior displacement of natural lens toward iris*

379.34   Posterior dislocation of lens — *backward displacement of natural lens toward vitreous*

379.39   Other disorders of lens — *other disorders*

379.40   Unspecified abnormal pupillary function — *unspecified*

379.41   Anisocoria — *unequal pupils, differing by 1mm or more*

379.42   Miosis (persistent), not due to miotics — *sustained, abnormal contraction of pupil*

379.43   Mydriasis (persistent), not due to mydriatics — *sustained, abnormal dilation of pupil*

379.45   Argyll Robertson pupil, atypical — *including Argyll Robertson phenomenon or pupil, nonsyphilitic*

379.46   Tonic pupillary reaction — *including Adie's pupil or syndrome; Saenger's syndrome*

379.49   Other anomaly of pupillary function — *including pupillary paralysis*

379.50   Unspecified nystagmus — *unspecified nystagmus*

379.52   Latent nystagmus

379.51   Congenital nystagmus — *oscillating eye movements, congenital*

379.53   Visual deprivation nystagmus — *oscillating eye movements caused by darkness*

379.54   Nystagmus associated with disorders of the vestibular system — *oscillating eye movements due to inner ear disease*

379.55   Dissociated nystagmus — *oscillating eye movements independent of each other*

379.56   Other forms of nystagmus — *other forms*

379.57   Nystagmus with deficiencies of saccadic eye movements — *abnormal optokinetic response*

379.58   Nystagmus with deficiencies of smooth pursuit movements — *dysfunction in normal tracking focus and movement of eyes*

379.59   Other irregularities of eye movements — *including opsoclonus*

379.8   Other specified disorders of eye and adnexa

379.90   Unspecified disorder of eye — *unspecified eye disorder*

379.91   Pain in or around eye — *pain*

379.92   Swelling or mass of eye — *swelling or mass*

379.93   Redness or discharge of eye — *redness or discharge*

379.99   Other ill-defined disorder of eye — *other ill-defined disorders*

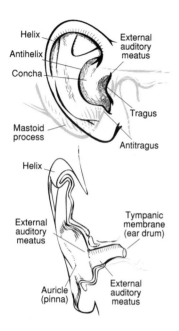

Helix

Antihelix

Concha

External auditory meatus

Mastoid process

Tragus

Antitragus

Helix

External auditory meatus

Tympanic membrane (ear drum)

Auricle (pinna)

External auditory meatus

380-389 Diseases of the Ear and Mastoid Process

380 DISORDERS OF EXTERNAL EAR

Disorders of external ear occur in the external ear including the auricle (pinna) and external auditory meatus. The auricle consists of the helix, anthelix, scapha, concha, tragus, antitragus, intertragic notch, and lobule. The auricle is a single, elastic cartilage covered in skin and normal adnexal features (hair follicles, sweat glands, and sebaceous glands). The ridged nature of the auricle is to channel sounds into the acoustic meatus. The semicircular depression leading to the ear is named the concha, Latin for shell. The external auditory meatus consists of cartilaginous and osseous portions with the canal lined with epidermis, hair, and ceruminous glands that extend to the tympanic membrane.

380.00	Unspecified perichondritis of pinna — *unspecified pinnal perichondritis*
380.01	Acute perichondritis of pinna — *sudden, severe inflammation of the connective tissue of the cartilage of the outer ear*
380.02	Chronic perichondritis of pinna — *persistent inflammation of the connective tissue of outer ear*

380.1   Infective otitis externa

Infective otitis externa is inflammation and infection of the auricle and external meatus. Bacteria, such as *Pseudomonas*, *Proteus vulgaris*, *Streptococci*, and *Staphylococcus aureus*, or fungal infections such as *Candida albicans* can cause this condition.

Signs and symptoms of infective otitis externa include redness and swelling that can obstruct the meatus, serous or purulent drainage, external ear tenderness, and enlarged regional lymph nodes.

Diagnostic tests include culture and sensitivity to identify infective organism. An otoscopy reveals inflammation and ceruminous impaction.

Therapies include antimicrobials (topically, systemically, or both), heat therapy to relieve pain, and gentle ear cleansing.

Assign a fifth digit to indicate the exact nature and/or location of the inflammation.

380.10	Unspecified infective otitis externa — *including unspecified otitis externa (acute), otitis externa (acute), circumscribed; otitis externa (acute), hemorrhagica*
380.11	Acute infection of pinna — *sudden, severe infection of outer ear canal*
380.12	Acute swimmers' ear — *including beach ear; tank ear*
380.13	Other acute infections of external ear — (Code first underlying disease, as: 035, 684, 690.10–690.18) — *code first underlying disease, as: erysipelas, impetigo, seborrheic dermatitis*
380.14	Malignant otitis externa — *severe infection of outer ear canal with some tissue destruction*
380.15	Chronic mycotic otitis externa — (Code first underlying disease, as: 111.9, 117.3) — *code first underlying disease as: aspergillosis, otomycosis NOS*
380.16	Other chronic infective otitis externa — *including chronic infective otitis externa NOS*
380.21	Cholesteatoma of external ear — *including keratosis obturans of external ear (canal)*
380.22	Other acute otitis externa — *including acute otitis external, actinic, chemical, contact, eczematoid, reactive*
380.23	Other chronic otitis externa — *including chronic otitis externa NOS*

✔5th   Needs fifth-digit   **OK**   Valid three-digit category

380.30	Unspecified disorder of pinna — *unspecified pinnal disorder NOS*
380.31	Hematoma of auricle or pinna — *collection of blood in the tissue of the fleshy external ear*
380.32	Acquired deformities of auricle or pinna — *acquired*
380.39	Other noninfectious disorder of pinna — *including ossification ear*
380.4	Impacted cerumen — *wax in ear*
380.50	Acquired stenosis of external ear canal unspecified as to cause — *unspecified as to cause*
380.51	Acquired stenosis of external ear canal secondary to trauma — *narrowing of the external ear canal due to trauma*
380.52	Acquired stenosis of external ear canal secondary to surgery — *postsurgical narrowing of external ear canal*
380.53	Acquired stenosis of external ear canal secondary to inflammation — *narrowing of the external ear canal due to inflammation*
380.81	Exostosis of external ear canal
380.89	Other disorder of external ear — *including auricular calcification; cicatrix of auricle; fistula of ear canal*
380.9	Unspecified disorder of external ear — *unspecified*

381 NONSUPPURATIVE OTITIS MEDIA AND EUSTACHIAN TUBE DISORDERS

Suppurative and unspecified otitis media are infections of the middle ear due to pyogenic organisms such as *staphylococci, pneumococci, Haemophilus influenzae, beta-hemolytic streptococci*, and gram-negative bacteria.

Signs and symptoms of suppurative and unspecified otitis media include chills and fever, malaise, deep throbbing ear pain, nausea and vomiting, dulled or impaired hearing, ear drainage, bulging of tympanic membrane, signs of upper respiratory infection, and a tender and swollen mastoid process.

Diagnostic tests include otoscopy to reveal obscured or distorted bony landmarks of tympanic membrane, with scarring and thickening in chronic otitis media. A pneumatoscope shows decreased tympanic membrane motility. Culture and sensitivity of purulent material identify infective organism.

Therapies include systemic antibiotics, nasal decongestants, and analgesics such as aspirin to control pain and fever, and myringotomy with aspiration of the middle ear fluid if tympanic membrane is in danger of rupture. Surgery may be performed (tympanoplasty, myringoplasty, mastoidectomy, excision of cholesteatomas) for chronic otitis media.

Associated conditions include adenoiditis or tonsillitis, colds or sinusitis, cholesteatoma, adhesions or scarring of middle ear structures, conductive hearing loss, abscesses, meningitis, mastoiditis, suppurative labyrinthitis, facial paralysis, otitis externa, sigmoid sinus, and jugular vein thrombosis.

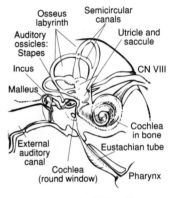

Exposed view of middle and inner ear

381.00	Unspecified acute nonsuppurative otitis media — *unspecified acute nonsuppurative otitis media*
381.01	Acute serous otitis media — *acute or subacute secretory otitis media*
381.02	Acute mucoid otitis media — *including acute or subacute seromucinous otitis media; blue drum syndrome*
381.03	Acute sanguinous otitis media — *sudden, severe infection of the middle ear, with blood*
381.04	Acute allergic serous otitis media — *allergic serous*
381.05	Acute allergic mucoid otitis media — *allergic mucoid*

381.06	Acute allergic sanguinous otitis media — *allergic sanguinous*
381.10	Simple or unspecified chronic serous otitis media — *persistent infection of the middle ear, without pus*
381.19	Other chronic serous otitis media — *including serosanguinous chronic otitis media*
381.20	Simple or unspecified chronic mucoid otitis media — *simple or unspecified*
381.29	Other chronic mucoid otitis media — *mucosanguineous chronic otitis media*
381.3	Other and unspecified chronic nonsuppurative otitis media — *including otitis media, chronic - allergic, exudative, secretory, transudative, with effusion*
381.4	Nonsuppurative otitis media, not specified as acute or chronic — *including allergic, catarrhal, exudative, secretory, serous, transudative, with effusion, otitis media*
381.50	Unspecified Eustachian salpingitis — *unspecified*
381.51	Acute Eustachian salpingitis — *sudden, severe inflammation of the Eustachian tube*
381.52	Chronic Eustachian salpingitis — *persistent inflammation of the Eustachian tube*
381.60	Unspecified obstruction of Eustachian tube — *unspecified; obstruction of Eustachian tube NOS*
381.61	Osseous obstruction of Eustachian tube — *obstruction of Eustachian tube from cholesteatoma, polyp, or other osseous lesion*
381.62	Intrinsic cartilagenous obstruction of Eustachian tube — *Eustachian tube blockage caused by Eustachian cartilage overgrowth*
381.63	Extrinsic cartilagenous obstruction of Eustachian tube — *including compression of Eustachian tube; Eustachian tube blockage caused by other cartilage overgrowth*
381.7	Patulous Eustachian tube — *distended, oversized*
381.81	Dysfunction of Eustachian tube — *dysfunction*
381.89	Other disorders of Eustachian tube — *including adhesion of Eustachian tube; diverticula of Eustachian tube*
381.9	Unspecified Eustachian tube disorder — *unspecified*

382 SUPPURATIVE AND UNSPECIFIED OTITIS MEDIA

382.00	Acute suppurative otitis media without spontaneous rupture of eardrum — *severe inflammation of middle ear, with pus*
382.01	Acute suppurative otitis media with spontaneous rupture of eardrum — *sudden, severe inflammation of middle ear, with pressure tearing ear drum tissue, with pus*
382.02	Acute suppurative otitis media in diseases classified elsewhere — (Code first underlying disease, as: 034.1, 487.8) — *code first underlying disease, as: influenza, scarlet fever*
382.1	Chronic tubotympanic suppurative otitis media — *benign chronic suppurative otitis media or chronic tubotympanic disease with anterior perforation of ear drum*
382.2	Chronic atticoantral suppurative otitis media — *chronic atticoantral disease or persistent mucosal disease with posterior or superior marginal perforation of ear drum*
382.3	Unspecified chronic suppurative otitis media — *including chronic purulent otitis media*
382.4	Unspecified suppurative otitis media — *including purulent otitis media NOS*
382.9	Unspecified otitis media — *including otitis media NOS, acute otitis media NOS; chronic otitis media NOS*

✓5th Needs fifth-digit   **OK** Valid three-digit category

383 MASTOIDITIS AND RELATED CONDITIONS

Mastoiditis and related conditions describe inflammation and/or infection of the mastoid bone or an abscess in the mastoid antrum. The infections usually are due to *Pneumococcus, Haemophilus influenzae,* beta-hemolytic *Streptococci,* and gram-negative organisms.

Signs and symptoms of mastoiditis and related conditions include dull ache and tenderness over mastoid process, low-grade fever, thick and purulent discharge, postauricular edema, erythema, and conductive hearing loss.

Diagnostic tests include x-rays of mastoid area to reveal hazy signs of infection and an otoscopy to reveal dull and thick edematous tympanic membrane.

Therapies include antibiotics, myringotomy and drainage of purulent fluid, mastoidectomy (simple or radical), sequestrectomy, or debridement of necrotic bone.

Associated conditions include meningitis, facial paralysis, brain abscess, suppurative labyrinthitis, chronic otitis media, and conductive hearing loss.

383.00	Acute mastoiditis without complications — *sudden, severe inflammation of the mastoid air cells*
383.01	Subperiosteal abscess of mastoid — *including von Bezold's abscess*
383.02	Acute mastoiditis with other complications — *including Gradenigo's syndrome*
383.1	Chronic mastoiditis — *caries of mastoid; fistula of mastoid*
383.20	Unspecified petrositis — *unspecified*
383.21	Acute petrositis — *sudden, severe inflammation of the dense bone behind the ear*
383.22	Chronic petrositis — *persistent inflammation of the dense bone behind the ear*
383.30	Unspecified postmastoidectomy complication — *including postmastoidectomy complication NOS*
383.31	Mucosal cyst of postmastoidectomy cavity — *mucous-lined cyst cavity following removal of mastoid bone*
383.32	Recurrent cholesteatoma of postmastoidectomy cavity — *cystlike mass of cell debris in cavity following removal of mastoid bone*
383.33	Granulations of postmastoidectomy cavity — *chronic inflammation of postmastoidectomy cavity*
383.81	Postauricular fistula — *abnormal passage behind mastoid cavity*
383.89	Other disorder of mastoid — *including perforation of mastoid (antrum) (cell)*
383.9	Unspecified mastoiditis

384 OTHER DISORDERS OF TYMPANIC MEMBRANE

384.00	Unspecified acute myringitis — *unspecified*
384.01	Bullous myringitis — *including myringitis bullosa hemorrhagica*
384.09	Other acute myringitis without mention of otitis media — *other acute*
384.1	Chronic myringitis without mention of otitis media — *including chronic tympanitis*
384.20	Unspecified perforation of tympanic membrane — *unspecified*
384.21	Central perforation of tympanic membrane — *central perforation*
384.22	Attic perforation of tympanic membrane — *attic perforation including pars flaccida*
384.23	Other marginal perforation of tympanic membrane — *other marginal perforation*
384.24	Multiple perforations of tympanic membrane — *multiple perforations*
384.25	Total perforation of tympanic membrane — *total perforation*
384.81	Atrophic flaccid tympanic membrane — *healed perforation of ear drum*

384.82	Atrophic nonflaccid tympanic membrane — *atrophic nonflaccid*
384.9	Unspecified disorder of tympanic membrane — *unspecified disorder*

385 OTHER DISORDERS OF MIDDLE EAR AND MASTOID

385.00	Tympanosclerosis, unspecified as to involvement — *unspecified as to involvement*
385.01	Tympanosclerosis involving tympanic membrane only — *tough fibrous tissue impeding functions of the ear drum*
385.02	Tympanosclerosis involving tympanic membrane and ear ossicles — *tough fibrous tissue impeding functions of the eardrum and middle ear bones (stapes, malleus, and incus)*
385.03	Tympanosclerosis involving tympanic membrane, ear ossicles, and middle ear — *tough fibrous tissue impeding functions of the ear drum, middle ear bones, and middle ear canal*
385.09	Tympanosclerosis involving other combination of structures — *other combination of structures*
385.10	Adhesive middle ear disease, unspecified as to involvement — *unspecified as to involvement*
385.11	Adhesions of drum head to incus — *drum head to incus*
385.12	Adhesions of drum head to stapes — *drum head to stapes*
385.13	Adhesions of drum head to promontorium — *drum head to promontorium*
385.19	Other middle ear adhesions and combinations — *other*
385.21	Impaired mobility of malleus — *including ankylosis of malleus*
385.22	Impaired mobility of other ear ossicles — *including ankylosis of ear ossicles, except malleus*
385.23	Discontinuity or dislocation of ear ossicles — *including disruption in the auditory chain created by the malleus, incus, and stapes*
385.24	Partial loss or necrosis of ear ossicles — *loss of tissue in the malleus, incus, or stapes*

385.3   Cholesteatoma of middle ear and mastoid

Cholesteatoma of middle ear and mastoid is an abnormal growth of squamous epithelial cells within the middle ear extending from the external meatus. The dead epithelial tissue, which usually is forced to the exterior of the ear with the movement of the earwax, forms a sac and produces keratin.

Signs and symptoms of cholesteatoma of middle ear and mastoid include hearing loss and history of acute or chronic otitis media.

Otoscopy reveals white debris in middle ear and destruction of external auditory canal bone; x-rays of middle ear and mastoid show tumor formation.

Therapies include control of concomitant infection, excision of cholesteatoma in extreme cases, tympanoplasty (reconstruction of ossicles), and myringoplasty.

Associated conditions include acute or chronic otitis media, hearing loss due to bony destruction of ossicles, middle ear hemorrhage, attic and marginal perforations of tympanic membrane, aural polyps, purulent labyrinthitis, facial paralysis, and intracranial abscess.

385.30	Unspecified cholesteatoma — *unspecified*
385.31	Cholesteatoma of attic — *cystlike mass of cell debris in upper portion of middle ear*
385.32	Cholesteatoma of middle ear — *cystlike mass of cell debris in middle ear*

✔5th   Needs fifth-digit   **OK**   Valid three-digit category

385.33 Cholesteatoma of middle ear and mastoid — *cystlike mass of cell debris in middle ear and mastoid air cells behind ear*

385.35 Diffuse cholesteatosis of middle ear and mastoid — *cystlike masses of cell debris throughout middle ear*

385.82 Cholesterin granuloma of middle ear — *fatty granulations in the middle ear*

385.83 Retained foreign body of middle ear — *retained foreign body of middle ear*

385.89 Other disorders of middle ear and mastoid — *including caries of middle ear; cicatrix of middle ear; hemotympanum; neuralgic mastoid; fistula of middle ear*

385.9 Unspecified disorder of middle ear and mastoid — *including disorder of middle ear or mastoid NOS*

386 VERTIGINOUS SYNDROMES AND OTHER DISORDERS OF VESTIBULAR SYSTEM

386.00 Unspecified Meniere's disease — *including Menière's disease (active); Lermoyez' syndrome*

386.01 Active Meniere's disease, cochleovestibular — *cochleovestibular*

386.02 Active Meniere's disease, cochlear — *cochlear*

386.03 Active Meniere's disease, vestibular — *vestibular*

386.04 Inactive Meniere's disease — *Menière's disease in remission*

386.10 Unspecified peripheral vertigo — *unspecified*

386.11 Benign paroxysmal positional vertigo — *benign paroxysmal positional nystagmus*

386.12 Vestibular neuronitis — *including Pedersen's (epidemic) vertigo*

386.19 Other and unspecified peripheral vertigo — *including aural vertigo; otogenic vertigo; otolith syndrome*

386.2 Vertigo of central origin — *including central positional nystagmus; malignant positional vertigo*

386.30 Unspecified labyrinthitis — *unspecified*

386.31 Serous labyrinthitis — *Serous labyrinthitis; diffuse labyrinthitis; inflammation with fluid buildup*

386.32 Circumscribed labyrinthitis — *including focal labyrinthitis; localized inflammation*

386.33 Suppurative labyrinthitis — *including purulent labyrinthitis; inflammation with pus*

386.34 Toxic labyrinthitis — *inflammation caused by toxic reaction*

386.35 Viral labyrinthitis — *inflammation caused by virus*

386.40 Unspecified labyrinthine fistula — *unspecified*

386.41 Round window fistula — *round*

386.42 Oval window fistula — *oval window*

386.43 Semicircular canal fistula — *semicircular canal*

386.48 Labyrinthine fistula of combined sites — *combined sites*

386.50 Unspecified labyrinthine dysfunction — *unspecified*

386.51 Hyperactive labyrinth, unilateral — *oversensitivity of labyrinth, one ear*

386.52 Hyperactive labyrinth, bilateral — *bilateral; oversensitivity of labyrinth, both ears*

386.53 Hypoactive labyrinth, unilateral — *reduced sensitivity of labyrinth, one ear*

386.54 Hypoactive labyrinth, bilateral — *reduced sensitivity of labyrinth, both ears*

386.55 Loss of labyrinthine reactivity, unilateral — *reduced reaction of labyrinth, one ear*

386.56 Loss of labyrinthine reactivity, bilateral — *bilateral; reduced reaction of labyrinth, both ears*

386.58 Other forms and combinations of labyrinthine dysfunction — *other*

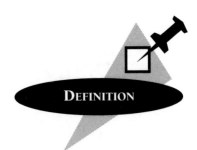

DEFINITION

Dysdiadochokinesia: inability or impairment in performing rapidly alternating movements.

Dysmetria: condition in which distance is distorted in the performance of muscular movement.

COWS: cold to the opposite, and warm to the same, in reference to caloric testing of the labyrinth with warm and cold water to test for nystagmus.

Air conduction: transportation of sound from the air, through the external auditory canal, to the tympanic membrane, and ossicular chain, ending at, but not including, the cochlea. Testing air conduction establishes the patency or nonpatency of these mechanisms.

Bone conduction: transportation of sound through bone. The source of sound is placed on the skull or teeth, and the vibration stimulates the cochlea, bypassing normal air conduction routes. Bone conduction requires operational sensorineural hearing mechanisms.

Sensorineural conduction: transportation of sound from the cochlea to the acoustic nerve and central auditor pathway to the brain.

Rinne test: compares air conduction with bone conduction using tuning fork held near patient's ear.

Weber test: tests bone conduction with tuning fork held on the teeth or midline to stimulate both cochleas simultaneously.

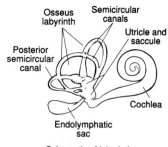

Osseus labyrinth
Semicircular canals
Utricle and saccule
Posterior semicircular canal
Cochlea
Endolymphatic sac

Schematic of labyrinth
and semicircular ducts

386.8 Other disorders of labyrinth — *including caries of labyrinth; hemorrhage of cochlea; otoconia*

386.9 Unspecified vertiginous syndromes and labyrinthine disorders — *including vertiginous syndrome or labyrinthine disorder NOS*

387 OTOSCLEROSIS

387.0 Otosclerosis involving oval window, nonobliterative — *tough, fibrous tissue impeding functions of the oval window*

387.1 Otosclerosis involving oval window, obliterative — *tough, fibrous tissue blocking the oval window*

387.2 Cochlear otosclerosis — *otosclerosis involving otic capsule or round window*

387.8 Other otosclerosis — *other*

387.9 Unspecified otosclerosis — *including ossification of middle ear; otoporosis; otospongiosis*

388 OTHER DISORDERS OF EAR

388.00 Unspecified degenerative and vascular disorders — *including degenerative and vascular disorders NOS*

388.01 Presbyacusis — *loss of hearing associated with aging process*

388.02 Transient ischemic deafness — *temporary loss of hearing due to restricted blood flow to auditory organs*

388.10 Unspecified noise effects on inner ear — *including effects on inner ear NOS*

388.11 Acoustic trauma (explosive) to ear — *otitic blast injury*

388.12 Noise-induced hearing loss — *noise-induced loss*

388.2 Unspecified sudden hearing loss — *sudden hearing loss NOS*

388.30 Unspecified tinnitus — *unspecified*

388.31 Subjective tinnitus — *noises heard only by patient - usually biochemical in nature*

388.32 Objective tinnitus — *noises originating within patient and audible to others*

388.40 Unspecified abnormal auditory perception — *abnormal auditory perception NOS*

388.41 Diplacusis — *Cochlear dysfunction causing patient to hear a single auditory stimulus as two sounds*

388.42 Hyperacusis — *acute hearing sensitivity - not necessarily painful*

388.43 Impairment of auditory discrimination — *impairment in ability to distinguish sound*

388.44 Other abnormal auditory perception, recruitment — *impairment in ability to distinguish volume of sound*

388.5 Disorders of acoustic nerve — *including acoustic neuritis; degeneration or disorder of acoustic or eighth nerve*

388.60 Unspecified otorrhea — *including discharging ear NOS*

388.61 Cerebrospinal fluid otorrhea — *spinal fluid leakage from ear*

388.69 Other otorrhea — *including otorrhagia*

388.70 Unspecified otalgia — *including earache NOS*

388.71 Otogenic pain — *ear pain caused by a condition within the ear*

388.72 Referred otogenic pain — *ear pain caused by a condition outside the ear*

388.8 Other disorders of ear — *including swelling ear*

388.9 Unspecified disorder of ear — *including atrophic ear*

389 HEARING LOSS

389.00 Unspecified conductive hearing loss — *unspecified*

389.01 Conductive hearing loss, external ear — *external ear*

389.02 Conductive hearing loss, tympanic membrane — *tympanic membrane*

389.03 Conductive hearing loss, middle ear — *middle ear*

389.04 Conductive hearing loss, inner ear — *inner ear*

✔5th Needs fifth-digit   **OK** Valid three-digit category

389.08   Conductive hearing loss of combined types — *combined types*
389.10   Unspecified sensorineural hearing loss — *unspecified*
389.11   Sensory hearing loss — *sensory*
389.12   Neural hearing loss — *neural*
389.14   Central hearing loss — *central*
389.18   Sensorineural hearing loss of combined types — *sensorineural of combined type*
389.2   Mixed conductive and sensorineural hearing loss — *deafness or hearing loss of type classifiable to 389.1*
389.7   Deaf mutism, not elsewhere classifiable — *including deaf, nonspeaking*
389.8   Other specified forms of hearing loss — *other specified*
389.9   Unspecified hearing loss — *including deafness NOS*

Chapter 7

390-459
Diseases of the Circulatory System

Coding diseases of the circulatory system can be complex for several reasons, some of which are among the following:

- Interrelationship of conditions
- Specificity of coding guidelines
- Varied medical lexicon used to describe circulatory conditions

390-392 Acute Rheumatic Fever

Acute rheumatic fever is defined as a systemic disease/nonsuppurative acute complication, generally affecting joints (arthritis), subcutaneous tissue (nodules), skin (erythema marginatum), heart (carditis) and brain (chorea). The fever usually follows a throat infection by Group A Streptococci. Therapies include medications such as antibiotics (including subsequent antistreptococcal prophylaxis), analgesics, and anti-inflammatory agents.

Rheumatic fever is classified according to the site of inflammation. In acute rheumatic fever, the infection is active. Excluded from these rubrics are chronic heart conditions caused by rheumatic fever (393.0-398.9).

390 RHEUMATIC FEVER WITHOUT MENTION OF HEART INVOLVEMENT OK

This rubric is limited to rheumatic fever that may have acute or subacute arthritis, but no heart involvement.

391 RHEUMATIC FEVER WITH HEART INVOLVEMENT

Acute rheumatic pericarditis is an acute rheumatic fever with fibrinous involvement of the pericardium without mention of other cardiac involvement. It is uncommon in adults.

Acute rheumatic endocarditis is an acute rheumatic fever with involvement of the endocardium. This form of acute rheumatic fever principally involves one or more of the heart valves. Echocardiography of a patient with acute rheumatic endocarditis reveals large, friable "vegetations" on the heart valves or chordae tendineae.

Acute rheumatic myocarditis is an acute rheumatic fever with involvement of the heart muscle. Signs and symptoms may include tachycardia out of proportion to fever, cardiac manifestations such as heart blocks and arrhythmias, or a history of recent upper respiratory infection, pharyngitis, or tonsillitis. Diagnostic tests such as stool and throat cultures may identify the bacteria present, while endomyocardial biopsy provides a definite diagnosis. Disorders associated with acute rheumatic myocarditis may include cardiac arrhythmias, congestive heart failure, thromboembolism, or pericarditis. Therapies include antibiotics for bacterial infection, anti-arrhythmics for cardiac arrhythmias, and/or anticoagulants for possible thromboembolism.

391.0 Acute rheumatic pericarditis — *sudden, severe inflammation of the lining of the heart*

391.1 Acute rheumatic endocarditis — *sudden, severe inflammation of the heart cavities*

391.2 Acute rheumatic myocarditis — *sudden, severe inflammation of the heart muscle*

391.8 Other acute rheumatic heart disease — *sudden, severe inflammation of multiple sites in heart*

391.9 Unspecified acute rheumatic heart disease — *sudden, severe inflammation of unknown site of heart*

392 RHEUMATIC CHOREA

Rheumatic chorea is an inflammatory complication of Group A streptococcal infection involving the central nervous system. It is also known as chorea minor, chorea dance, Sydenham's chorea, and Saint Vitus dance. It generally affects children and young adults. Signs and symptoms may include involuntary, irregular, jerky movements of the face (excluding eyes), neck, or limbs.

392.0 Rheumatic chorea with heart involvement — *involuntary muscle movement and weakness*

392.9 Rheumatic chorea without mention of heart involvement — *involuntary muscle movement and weakness*

393-398 Chronic Rheumatic Heart Disease

Chronic rheumatic heart disease is a chronic disease resulting from single or repeated attacks of acute rheumatic fever that produce late effects in the structure of the heart, usually the endocardium. Sequelae include rigidity and deformity of the valvular cusps, fusion of the commissures, or shortening and fusion of the chordae tendinea. Damage also may occur in the myocardium following severe bouts of acute rheumatic myocarditis affecting cardiac performance. Associated conditions may include valvular stenosis and/or insufficiency and, usually, mitral and myocardial damage.

393 CHRONIC RHEUMATIC PERICARDITIS **OK**

Chronic rheumatic pericarditis is a set of conditions such as adhesive pericarditis and constrictive pericarditis when specified as a manifestation following an acute rheumatic infection. Adhesive pericarditis (chronic) occurs when adhesions develop between the two-pericardial layers, or between the pericardium and the heart or other neighboring structures. Constrictive pericarditis (chronic) is a thickening of the pericardial membrane with constriction of the cardiac chambers.

394 DISEASES OF MITRAL VALVE

Mitral stenosis, mitral valve disease (unspecified) and mitral valve failure are presumed to be rheumatic origin for classification purposes and need not be stated as rheumatic. Other manifestations, such as insufficiency, incompetence, or regurgitation (without stenosis) must be specified as due to rheumatic heart disease for classification under rubric 394.

Mitral stenosis is a narrowing of the orifice of the mitral valve due to (presumed) rheumatic heart disease that impedes left ventricular filling. Signs and symptoms include left or

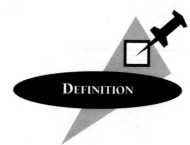

DEFINITION

Sydenham's chorea is a childhood disease featuring irregular, spasmodic, involuntary movements of the limbs and fascial muscles, psychic symptoms, and irritability. It is also called juvenile chorea, St. Vitus' dance, and rheumatic chorea.

Failure: inability to function.

Incompetence: inability of the valve to perform normal function.

Insufficiency: inadequate closure of the valve, allowing abnormal backflow of blood.

Regurgitation: abnormal backflow of blood.

Obstruction: blockage preventing normal function of valve.

Stenosis: narrowing or stricture of a valve that interferes with blood flow.

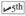 5th   Needs fifth-digit   **OK**   Valid three-digit code

combined left and right heart failure, hemoptysis, systematic embolism, hoarseness, atrial fibrillation, or pulmonary rales and increased S1/S2 heart sounds.

Rheumatic mitral insufficiency is a reflux of a portion of blood back into the left atrium instead of forward into the aorta, resulting in increased atrial pressure and decreased forward cardiac output. Signs and symptoms may include dyspnea due to left ventricular failure (which may be combined with right heart failure in severe cases), pulmonary hypertension, holosystolic apical murmur, S3 heart sound, or brisk carotid upstroke. An EKG may show left ventricular hypertrophy and left atrial enlargement in cases of rheumatic mitral insufficiency, and a chest x-ray usually shows heart enlargement and vascular congestion when the insufficiency has resulted in heart failure. Echocardiography may visualize scarring and retraction of the mitral leaflets. Cardiac catheterization with a pulmonary capillary wedge monitor (Swan-Ganz) may reveal systolic volume overload, which is characterized by a large V wave on right heart catheterization, and left ventriculography demonstrates systolic regurgitation of contrast material into the left atrium. Therapies for rheumatic mitral insufficiency may include medications (digitalis, diuretics, or vasodilators) to increase forward cardiac output and reduce pulmonary venous hypertension. Anticoagulants may be prescribed for patients with atrial fibrillation or surgery such as annuloplasty or replacement of the mitral valve for chronic mitral valve insufficiency and sometimes in cases demonstrating relatively mild symptoms to forestall significant ventricular muscle dysfunction. Conditions associated with rheumatic mitral insufficiency include atrial fibrillation, pulmonary hypertension, left or congestive heart failure, and systemic embolism.

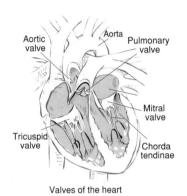

Valves of the heart

394.0	Mitral stenosis — *obstruction*
394.1	Rheumatic mitral insufficiency — *incompetence, regurgitation*
394.2	Mitral stenosis with insufficiency — *obstruction with incompetence or regurgitation*
394.9	Other and unspecified mitral valve diseases — *unknown or not otherwise specified*

395 DISEASES OF AORTIC VALVE

Rheumatic aortic stenosis is a pathological narrowing of the aortic valve orifice due to fibrosis of the commissures and/or degenerative distortion of the aortic valve cusps. Commissural fusion and scarring may be present early in the progression of the disease, and calcification of the valve is often a late complication. The resulting stenosis produces a pressure overload on the left ventricle due to the increased pressure needed to force the blood through the narrowed aortic valve orifice. Signs and symptoms of rheumatic aortic stenosis include angina, syncope, heart failure, delayed carotid upstroke, and/or a sustained forceful apex beat, systolic ejection murmur, or softened singular S2 heart sound with S4 heart sound. An EKG normally shows left ventricular hypertrophy in cases of rheumatic aortic stenosis, and cardiac catheterization provides definitive diagnosis and evaluation of the condition. Echocardiography and fluoroscopy may be of limited value in assessing the severity of the stenosis. Therapies include medications (digitalis, diuretics, and antiarrhythmics) as temporary symptomatic measures, or aortic valve replacement. Associated conditions include left heart failure, mitral valve disease, angina (exertional), heart blocks due to calcification of the conduction system, and atrial and ventricular arrhythmias.

Rheumatic aortic insufficiency is the reflux of blood into the left ventricle during diastole due to an incompetent aortic valve. Chronic aortic insufficiency eventually leads to left

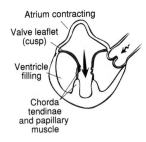

Atrium contracting
Valve leaflet (cusp)
Ventricle filling
Chorda tendinae and papillary muscle

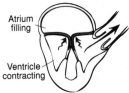

Atrium filling
Ventricle contracting

Normal heart valve function

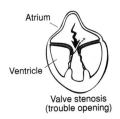

Atrium
Ventricle

Valve stenosis (trouble opening)

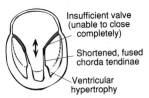

Insufficient valve (unable to close completely)
Shortened, fused chorda tendinae
Ventricular hypertrophy

Ventricular hypertrophy. Insufficient or incompetent valve allows backflow of blood from the aorta to the left ventricle causing ventricular hypertrophy

ventricular dysfunction and failure. The condition is also known as rheumatic aortic regurgitation and rheumatic aortic incompetence. Signs and symptoms include left ventricular failure, syncope, angina, diastolic murmur along the left sternal border or an Austin Fling murmur, and/or stroke volume increase. An EKG normally shows left ventricular hypertrophy in cases of rheumatic aortic insufficiency. Chest x-rays show cardiac enlargement in severe chronic cases. Echocardiography demonstrates an enlarged left ventricular cavity and frequently reveals diastolic vibration of the mitral valve. Cardiac catheterization and arteriography demonstrate regurgitation of contrast material back into the left ventricle. Therapies include medications (digitalis, diuretics, and vasodilators) for symptomatic relief, and aortic valve replacement in severe cases. Associated conditions include angina and left heart failure, and congestive heart failure.

395.0	Rheumatic aortic stenosis — *obstruction*	
395.1	Rheumatic aortic insufficiency — *incompetence or regurgitation*	
395.2	Rheumatic aortic stenosis with insufficiency — *obstruction with incompetence or regurgitation*	
395.9	Other and unspecified rheumatic aortic diseases — *unknown or not otherwise specified*	

396 DISEASES OF MITRAL AND AORTIC VALVES

When both the mitral and aortic valves are involved, ICD-9-CM presumes an etiology of rheumatic heart disease for classification purposes. In all cases, when both the aortic and mitral valves are diseased, the ICD-9-CM index will lead you to rubric 396. For more information about the subcategories of this rubric, refer to the detailed descriptions of the individual components of combined aortic and mitral valve disease.

396.0	Mitral valve stenosis and aortic valve stenosis — *narrowing of both valves*
396.1	Mitral valve stenosis and aortic valve insufficiency — *narrowing of mitral valve with incompetence or regurgitation of aortic valve*
396.2	Mitral valve insufficiency and aortic valve stenosis — *incompetence or regurgitation of mitral valve with narrowing of aortic valve*
396.3	Mitral valve insufficiency and aortic valve insufficiency — *incompetence or regurgitation of both valves*
396.8	Multiple involvement of mitral and aortic valves — *stenosis and insufficiency of mitral or aortic valve with stenosis or insufficiency, or both, of the other valve*
396.9	Unspecified mitral and aortic valve diseases — *unknown*

397 DISEASES OF OTHER ENDOCARDIAL STRUCTURES

This rubric includes chronic rheumatic heart diseases of the tricuspid, pulmonary, and unspecified heart valves. Note that diseases of the tricuspid valve are presumed to be of rheumatic etiology, but diseases of the pulmonary or unspecified heart valves must be stated as due to a late effect of rheumatic heart disease.

Diseases of the tricuspid valve are classified to codes in the 397.0 subclassification, and report insufficiency, obstruction, regurgitation, and stenosis of the tricuspid valve. Tricuspid regurgitation may occur secondary to right ventricular pressure overload from left-sided lesions. It also may occur as a result of primary rheumatic heart disease of the tricuspid valve itself. Tricuspid stenosis serves as a mechanical obstruction blocking the return of blood to the right ventricle of the heart. All diseases of the of the tricuspid valve not specifically directed to other code categories in the ICD-9-CM index are included in 397.0.

↙5th   Needs fifth-digit   **OK**   Valid three-digit code

Rheumatic diseases of pulmonary valves (397.1) include valve insufficiency and stenosis. Pulmonary valve insufficiency is a reflux of blood back into the right ventricle through an incompetent pulmonary valve and may be associated with pulmonary hypertension. Pulmonary valve stenosis is an obstruction of the blood through the pulmonary valve. This subclassification, 397.1, includes all diseases of the pulmonary valve specified as due to a late effect of rheumatic heart disease not directed to other code categories in the ICD-9-CM index.

397.0   Diseases of tricuspid valve — *including insufficiency, obstruction, regurgitation, stenosis*

397.1   Rheumatic diseases of pulmonary valve — *including insufficiency, obstruction, regurgitation, stenosis*

397.9   Rheumatic diseases of endocardium, valve unspecified — *unknown valve*

398 OTHER RHEUMATIC HEART DISEASE

This rubric includes rare occurrences of chronic rheumatic heart disease not involving the heart valves. Chronic inflammation of the muscular walls of the heart (myocarditis) specified as due to or a late effect of rheumatic heart disease is reported with 398.0. Code this condition in addition to rheumatic valve disease when indicated. Congestive rheumatic heart failure is reported with 398.91 and includes left heart failure and congestive heart failure due to rheumatic heart disease. Left and congestive heart failure, common in the rheumatic valvular diseases described in rubrics 394-396, may be coded in addition to rheumatic valvular disease when indicated.

398.0   Rheumatic myocarditis — *myocardium*

398.90   Unspecified rheumatic heart disease — *unknown*

398.91   Rheumatic heart failure (congestive) — *left ventricular failure*

398.99   Other and unspecified rheumatic heart diseases — *not otherwise specified, including inactive pancarditis with rheumatic fever*

401-405 Hypertensive Disease

Hypertensive disease is a condition in which the diastolic pressure exceeds 100 mm Hg in persons 60 years old or greater or 90-mm Hg in persons less than 60 years old. The World Health Organization (WHO) defines hypertension as pressures exceeding 160/90 mm Hg, but studies have shown that increased morbidity and mortality are associated with diastolic pressures of just 85 mm Hg. It is generally asymptomatic until complications develop. Complications may include retinal changes, loud aortic sounds and early systolic ejection click heard on auscultation, headache, tinnitus, and palpitations.

Excluded from this rubric is transient hypertension, reported with 796.2; in pregnancy, reported with a code from the series 642.0-642.9; or hypertensive disease involving coronary vessels (414.00-410.9).

Rubrics 401-404 include primary (essential) hypertension of no known cause and account for approximately 90 percent of the population. The remaining 10 percent of the population have secondary hypertension classifiable to 405, due to definitive and diagnosable disease such as Cushing's syndrome. Use the hypertension table in the ICD-9-CM index to distinguish between primary and secondary hypertension and assign the correct code.

Use the fourth digits in categories 401-405 to specify the course of hypertensive disease as malignant, benign, or unspecified. Malignant hypertension is said to exist when the

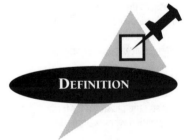

DEFINITION

Hypertension crisis: emergency requiring immediate treatment in which blood pressure is severely elevated to 200/120 Hg or greater. Symptoms may include headache, malaise, chest pain, or palpitations. Hypertension crisis is classified according to the type and nature of the hypertension, with additional codes used to identify associated conditions.

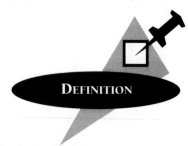

DEFINITION

Benign hypertension: considered relatively mild and chronic, with likely slow progression of disease.

Controlled hypertension: high blood pressure that is mitigated by medications. This is not an axis of ICD-9 code selection, but is often seen in documentation.

Malignant hypertension: considered severe and difficult to treat, with likely quick progression of the disease.

Transient hypertension: elevated blood pressure when no diagnosis of hypertension has been made.

Uncontrolled hypertension: high blood pressure that cannot be regulated by medication or other treatment. This is not an axis of ICD-9 code selection, but is often seen in documentation.

Unspecified hypertension: that has not been documented as malignant or benign (consult the physician for further information whenever possible).

Blood pressure has two measurements: the diastolic pressure and the systolic pressure.

Diastole: relaxation of the heart muscles in the heartbeat cycle.

Systole: contraction of the heart muscles in the heartbeat cycle.

diastolic pressure exceeds 140 mm Hg or is measurably unstable. However, do not try to make the distinction between benign and malignant without first obtaining physician verification for coding and classification purposes.

401 ESSENTIAL HYPERTENSION

Use rubric 401 to report all primary forms of hypertension without mention of heart or renal disease, including arterial, idiopathic, systemic, and vascular hypertension.

401.0	Essential hypertension, malignant — *severe high arterial blood pressure without apparent organic cause*
401.1	Essential hypertension, benign — *mild elevation in arterial blood pressure without apparent organic cause*
401.9	Unspecified essential hypertension — *unknown*

402 HYPERTENSIVE HEART DISEASE

Use rubric 402 to report heart disease due to the effects of systemic hypertension. It is characterized by concentric hypertrophy of the left ventricle that in time can lead to left ventricular failure. Rubric 402 includes heart disease caused by hypertension classifiable to codes 428.0-428.9, 429.0-429.3, 429.8 and 429.9. Note that there must be a stated or implied cause and effect relationship between the heart disease and the hypertension. For example, the statement "benign hypertension with congestive heart failure" is coded to 401.1 and 428.0; but the statement "benign hypertensive heart disease with congestive heart failure" is reported with 402.11.

402.00	Malignant hypertensive heart disease without congestive heart failure — *severe high blood pressure causing heart complications*
402.01	Malignant hypertensive heart disease with congestive heart failure — *severe high blood pressure causing heart complications*
402.10	Benign hypertensive heart disease without congestive heart failure — *mild elevation in blood pressure causing heart complications*
402.11	Benign hypertensive heart disease with congestive heart failure — *mild elevation in blood pressure causing heart complications*
402.90	Unspecified hypertensive heart disease without congestive heart failure — *high blood pressure of unknown degree causing heart complications*
402.91	Unspecified hypertensive heart disease with congestive heart failure — *high blood pressure of unknown degree causing heart complications*

403 HYPERTENSIVE RENAL DISEASE

Hypertensive renal disease is a condition also known as arteriolar nephrosclerosis, and is reported with codes from rubric 403. It is characterized by intimal thickening of the afferent arteriole of the glomerulus and due to long-standing or poorly controlled hypertension. In severe nephrosclerosis, the nephron is deprived of its blood supply, and areas of infarction occur with subsequent scar formation. Renal insufficiency occurs when the kidney is scarred and contracted. In most cases, the patient will eventually develop renal failure.

This rubric reports chronic renal failure associated with hypertensive renal disease due to progressive and irreversible destruction of the nephrons and should not be confused with acute renal failure. Acute renal failure is classified to rubric 584 and describes failure of the kidneys to perform their essential function due to trauma, impaired blood flow, toxic substances, bacterial infection, or obstruction of the urinary tract.

Both diabetes mellitus and hypertension have associated renal manifestations such as renal failure. In cases where the diagnostic statement indicates hypertensive renal failure due to diabetes mellitus, report the diabetes with renal manifestations from the series 250.4 and 403.91 to indicate the renal failure due to hypertension. If the diagnostic statement indicates diabetes with chronic renal failure and hypertension secondary to hypervolemia, report codes from the series 250.4, and rubrics 405 and 585.

For coding and classification purposes, any condition classifiable to categories 585-587 with hypertension is presumed due to hypertension, so no cause and effect relationship need be stated or implied in the diagnostic statement.

403.0 ✔5th Hypertensive renal disease, malignant — *severe high blood pressure causing kidney malfunctions*

403.1 ✔5th Hypertensive renal disease, benign — *mild high blood pressure causing kidney malfunctions*

403.9 ✔5th Unspecified hypertensive renal disease — *high blood pressure of unknown degree causing kidney malfunctions*

404 HYPERTENSIVE HEART AND RENAL DISEASE

This category is used for combined forms of heart and renal disease as classified in categories 402 and 403. For coding and classification purposes, the heart disease must be stated or implied as due to hypertension, but the renal disease may be presumed. For example, the statement "hypertensive congestive heart failure and chronic renal failure" would be coded 404.93 even though hypertension is not the stated cause of the chronic renal failure.

404.0 ✔5th Hypertensive heart and renal disease, malignant — *severe high blood pressure causing kidney and heart malfunctions*

404.1 ✔5th Hypertensive heart and renal disease, benign — *mild high blood pressure causing kidney and heart malfunctions*

404.9 ✔5th Unspecified hypertensive heart and renal disease — *high blood pressure of unknown degree causing kidney and heart malfunctions*

405 SECONDARY HYPERTENSION

Secondary hypertension is a condition caused by renovascular or other diseases. Renovascular hypertension is the obstruction of renal blood flow at the level of the renal artery. The obstruction stimulates the renin-angiotensin system causing an increase in systemic angiotensin, which in turn causes the retention of sodium and water resulting in hypertension. Surgical reconstruction of the renal artery or percutaneous transluminal angioplasty may be performed to relieve the obstruction. Other causes of secondary hypertension include renal parenchymal diseases, oral contraceptives, primary aldosteronism, Cushing's syndrome, pheochromocytoma, hyperparathyroidism, hyperthyroidism, and acromegaly.

ICD-9-CM separates only renovascular hypertension from all other etiologies at the fifth-digit level. Renal parenchymal diseases are conditions that reduce kidney function by affecting the kidney's ability to excrete water and sodium and are not the same as renovascular hypertension. Do not code renal parenchymal disease to the neovascular fifth-digit 1.

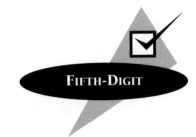

FIFTH-DIGIT

The following fifth-digit subclassification is for use with category 403:

0 without mention of renal failure

1 with renal failure

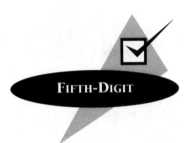

FIFTH-DIGIT

The following fifth-digit subclassification is for use with category 404:

0 without mention of congestive heart failure or renal failure

1 with congestive heart failure

2 with renal failure

3 with congestive heart failure and renal failure

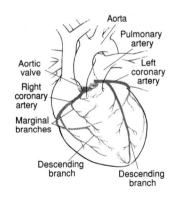

405.01	Secondary renovascular hypertension, malignant — *severe high blood pressure as a result of an underlying disease or condition*
405.09	Other secondary hypertension, malignant — *severe high blood pressure as a result of an underlying disease or condition*
405.11	Secondary renovascular hypertension, benign — *mild high blood pressure as a result of an underlying disease or condition*
405.19	Other secondary hypertension, benign — *mild high blood pressure as a result of an underlying disease or condition*
405.91	Secondary renovascular hypertension, unspecified — *high blood pressure of unknown degree as a result of an underlying disease or condition*
405.99	Other secondary hypertension, unspecified — *high blood pressure of unknown degree as a result of an underlying disease or condition*

410-414 Ischemic Heart Disease

Ischemic heart disease is an inadequate flow of blood through the coronary arteries to the tissue of the heart. The predominant etiology of the ischemia is arteriosclerosis. Partially obstructed coronary artery blood flow can manifest in angina pectoris; complete obstruction results in an infarction of the myocardium. Use an additional code to identify presence of hypertension (401.0-405.9) with ischemic heart disease.

410 ACUTE MYOCARDIAL INFARCTION

Rubric 410 reports sudden partial or total reduction in the supply of blood to the heart, which results in necrosis of the myocardium. Occlusion of one of the coronary arteries due to thrombosis is believed to be the most common etiology. Other possible precipitating conditions include prolonged coronary artery spasm, subintimal hemorrhage at the site of atheromatous narrowing and nonocclusive etiologies such as postoperative or traumatic shock, gastrointestinal bleeding with acute blood loss anemia, hypotension, and dehydration.

The fourth digits for rubric 410 identify the site of the acute myocardial infarction as identified on an EKG. One exception to this is the fourth digit 7, which is for subendocardial and nontransmural infarctions regardless of site. A subendocardial infarction is one that involves the pericardium and not the endocardium; a nontransmural infarction is one that fails to extend from the endocardium to the epicardium. "Non-Q-wave" infarctions also are classified here. In some instances, the diagnostic statement will include the term "subendocardial" or "nontransmural" along with a specific site for the infarction.

Acute myocardial infarction is classified as an initial episode of care when the history does not mention a previous infarction. A myocardial infarction of greater than eight weeks duration with persistent symptoms is classified to 414.8.

410.0 ✓5th	Acute myocardial infarction of anterolateral wall — *including coronary artery embolism, occlusion, rupture, thrombosis*
410.1 ✓5th	Acute myocardial infarction of other anterior wall
410.2 ✓5th	Acute myocardial infarction of inferolateral wall — *including coronary artery embolism, occlusion, rupture, thrombosis*
410.3 ✓5th	Acute myocardial infarction of inferoposterior wall — *including coronary artery embolism, occlusion, rupture, thrombosis*
410.4 ✓5th	Acute myocardial infarction of other inferior wall — *diaphragmatic wall or inferior wall, not othweise specificed; including coronary artery embolism, occlusion, rupture, thrombosis*

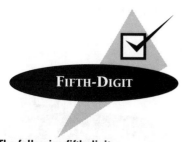

FIFTH-DIGIT

The following fifth-digit subclassification is for use with category 410:

0 episode of care unspecified

Use when the source document does not contain sufficient information for the assignment of fifth digit 1 or 2.

1 initial episode of care

Use fifth digit 1 to designate the first episode of care (regardless of facility site) for a newly diagnosed myocardial infarction. The fifth digit 1 is assigned regardless of the number of times a patient may be transferred during the initial episode of care.

2 subsequent episode of care

Use fifth-digit 2 to designate an episode of care following the initial episode when the patient is admitted for further observation, evaluation, or treatment for a myocardial infarction that has received initial treatment, but is still less than eight weeks old.

✓5th   Needs fifth-digit   **OK** Valid three-digit code

410.5 ☑5th Acute myocardial infarction of other lateral wall — *apical-lateral, basal-lateral, high lateral, posterolateral; including coronary artery embolism, occlusion, rupture, thrombosis*

410.6 ☑5th Acute myocardial infarction, true posterior wall infarction — *posterobasal, strictly posterior; including coronary artery embolism, occlusion, rupture, thrombosis*

410.7 ☑5th Acute myocardial infarction, subendocardial infarction — *nontransmural; including coronary artery embolism, occlusion, rupture, thrombosis*

410.8 ☑5th Acute myocardial infarction of other specified sites — *not otherwise specified, including atrium, papillary muscle, septum alone; including coronary artery embolism, occlusion, rupture, thrombosis*

410.9 ☑5th Acute myocardial infarction, unspecified site — *unknown site; including coronary artery embolism, occlusion, rupture, thrombosis*

411 OTHER ACUTE AND SUBACUTE FORMS OF ISCHEMIC HEART DISEASE

This rubric includes all acute and subacute forms of ischemic heart disease excluding acute myocardial infarction. Acute forms of ischemia include conditions with a relatively short and severe course, and subacute forms of ischemia denote a course of ischemic disease that falls in between acute and chronic disease.

Postmyocardial infarction syndrome is reported with 411.0 and is a complication occurring several days to several weeks following an acute myocardial infarction. Also known as Dressler's syndrome, this condition is believed to be due to an antibody antigen reaction that takes place in the myocardial tissue during the healing phase of an infarction. Some patients will continue to experience unstable angina pectoris their recent myocardial infarction because of persistent coronary artery disease. Do not confuse angina due to ischemic heart disease (coronary artery disease) following a myocardial infarction with postmyocardial infarction syndrome. Code postmyocardial angina due to myocardial ischemia to 413.9 or 411.1. Code Dressler's syndrome and postmyocardial angina due to postmyocardial infarction syndrome to 411.0.

Intermediate coronary syndrome is reported with 411.1 and is an intermediate state between angina pectoris of effort and acute myocardial infarction. Since the mortality rate for myocardial infarction is greatest within the first few hours, unstable angina with its increased likelihood of impeding myocardial infarction is a medical emergency and requires acute care hospitalization. The term "class III' and "class IV" describing the functional classification of patients with heart disease may be used in conjunction with unstable angina. However, do not assume every patient with class III or class IV angina or heart disease has unstable angina. Code 411.1 cannot be assigned when the condition evolves into a myocardial infarction for which a code from rubric 410 will be assigned.

Coronary occlusion without myocardial infarction is reported with 411.81. This code classifies patients with an acute or subacute, complete or incomplete, occlusion of the coronary artery, not associated with acute myocardial infarction. The occlusion may be embolic, thrombotic, other or unspecified and will usually be associated with some form of angina. This code may be used in conjunction with a diagnosis of stable or unstable angina.

411.0	Postmyocardial infarction syndrome — *fever, pain, and inflammation within six weeks of MI; Dressler's syndrome*
411.1	Intermediate coronary syndrome — *impending infarction, preinfarction angina, unstable angina*
411.81	Coronary occlusion without mycocardial infarction — *interruption of blood flow without death of heart tissue*
411.89	Other acute and subacute form of ischemic heart disease — *coronary insufficiency, subendocardial ischemia*

412 OLD MYOCARDIAL INFARCTION OK

This rubric includes diagnoses with a history of myocardial infarction. These patients usually demonstrate EKG changes but currently present no symptoms and warrant no clinical intervention. Patients can have both an acute myocardial infarction and an old myocardial infarction in different sites during the same episode of care. Code both conditions. Also, it is possible that an old myocardial infarction may "reinfarct," extending the degree of necrosis at the site of the old myocardial infarction. In this case, code only the acute myocardial infarction.

413 ANGINA PECTORIS

Angina pectoris is a clinical syndrome due to myocardial ischemia caused by atherosclerotic heart disease, but may be due to coronary artery spasm, severe aortic stenosis or insufficiency, syphilitic aortitis, vasculitis, marked anemia, paroxysmal tachycardia with rapid ventricular rates or any disease or disorder that markedly increases metabolic demands. Angina decubitus is a form of angina occurring at night or when the patient is resting quietly. Prinzmetal angina is a variant characterized by chest pain at rest and by sinus tachycardia (ST) segment elevation, rather than depression, during the attack. Report 413.9 for angina not specified or classified elsewhere, including stable angina pectoris. Angina described with class I or class II heart disease is often classified to, 413.9, but coders are cautioned not to equate these functional classifications of heart disease as synonymous for stable angina.

Assignment of a code from rubric 413 cannot be made in addition to a code from rubric 410 for the same episode of care.

413.0	Angina decubitus — *nocturnal angina; occurs only when lying down*
413.1	Prinzmetal angina — *occurs only when lying down; associatred with ST-segment elevations; variant angina pectoris*
413.9	Other and unspecified angina pectoris — *including Herberden's, Likoff's, X syndromes; syncope anginosa, stenocardia*

414 OTHER FORMS OF CHRONIC ISCHEMIC HEART DISEASE

This rubric classifies obstruction of blood flow to the heart, usually due to a mechanical obstruction of one or more of the coronary arteries. Obliterative atherosclerosis of the coronary arteries is by far the most common form of ischemic heart disease. In time, the accumulations may calcify throughout the cardiovascular system, leading to the condition colloquially known as "hardening of the arteries."

Coronary atherosclerosis is localized, subintimal accumulations of fatty and fibrous tissue caused by proliferation of smooth muscle cells in combination with a disorder of lipid metabolism. Atherosclerotic heart disease eventually leads to acute and subacute forms of ischemic heart disease such as unstable angina and myocardial infarction.

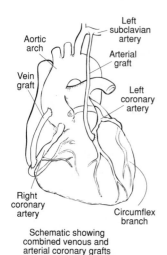

Aortic arch
Left subclavian artery
Arterial graft
Vein graft
Left coronary artery
Right coronary artery
Circumflex branch

Schematic showing combined venous and arterial coronary grafts

⤶5th Needs fifth-digit   OK Valid three-digit code

Aneurysm of the heart is a dilatation, stretching, weakening or bulging of the tissue of the heart or of the coronary arteries. An aneurysm of the heart wall is an aneurysm of heart muscle, known as a cardiac, mural, or ventricular wall aneurysm, which is usually a consequence of myocardial infarction. Aneurysm of the coronary vessels is a circumscribed dilation of a coronary artery or a blood-containing tumor connecting directly with the lumen of a coronary artery.

Report 414.11 for abnormal communication between a coronary artery and vein resulting in the formation of an arteriovenous aneurysm, usually resulting from myocardial infarction. Report 414.19 for an arteriovenous fistula of the coronary vessels.

414.00	Coronary atherosclerosis of unspecified type of vessel, native or graft — *unknown*
414.01	Coronary atherosclerosis of native coronary artery — *including ASHD, arteriosclerosis, arteritis, atheroma, sclerosis, stricture in natural heart vessels*
414.02	Coronary atherosclerosis of autologous vein bypass graft — *plaque deposit in grafted vein originating within patient*
414.03	Coronary atherosclerosis of nonautologous biological bypass graft — *plaque deposit in grafted vessel originating outside patient*
414.04	Coronary atherosclerosis of artery bypass graft — *plaque deposit in grafted artery originating within patient*
414.05	Coronary atherosclerosis of unspecified type of bypass graft — *plaque deposit in vessel of unknown origin*
414.10	Aneurysm of heart (wall) — *dilation of a wall in the heart*
414.11	Aneurysm of coronary vessels — *dilation of a wall of a coronary vessel*
414.19	Other aneurysm of heart — *acquired arteriovenous fistula*
414.8	Other specified forms of chronic ischemic heart disease — *including chronic coronary insufficiency, chronic myocardial ischemia*
414.9	Unspecified chronic ischemic heart disease — *unknown or not otherwise specified*

415-417 Diseases of Pulmonary Circulation

Diseases of the pulmonary circulation include acute pulmonary heart disease (415), chronic pulmonary heart disease (416), and other diseases of the pulmonary circulation (417).

415 ACUTE PULMONARY HEART DISEASE

Acute cor pulmonale is a dilation and failure of the right side of the heart due to pulmonary embolism. The condition is usually reversible. Pulmonary embolism and infarction is a condition that occurs when a thrombus, usually forming in the veins of the lower extremities or pelvis but may be secondary to atrial fibrillation or flutter, travels through the right-sided circulation, and becomes lodged in the pulmonary artery. Pulmonary infarction is the consequential hemorrhagic consolidation and necrosis of the lung parenchyma.

415.0	Acute cor pulmonale
415.11	Iatrogenic pulmonary embolism and infarction — *death of lung tissue doe to blocked vessels from medical treatment*
415.19	Other pulmonary embolism and infarction — *not otherwise specified*

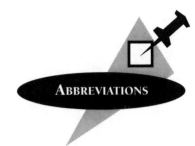

ABBREVIATIONS

AEB: atrial ectopic beat

CAD: coronary artery disease

CVL: central venous line

CVP: central venous pressure

EF: ejection fraction (stroke volume related to end-diastolic volume)

HOCM: hypertrophic obstructive cardiomyopathy

LVEDP: left ventricular end-diastolic pressure

MAST: medical antishock trousers

MVP: mitral valve prolapse

PAWP: pulmonary artery wedge pressure

PTCA: percutaneous transluminal coronary angioplasty

RV: right ventricular

ST: sinus tachycardia

SVC: superior vena cava

416 CHRONIC PULMONARY HEART DISEASE

Chronic pulmonary heart disease is a rare increase in pulmonary circulation, often resulting in right ventricular failure or fatal syncope.

Primary pulmonary hypertension is a condition characterized by pulmonary hypertension and raised pulmonary vascular resistance in the lungs in the absence of any other disease of the lungs or heart. It is marked by diffuse narrowing of the pulmonary arterioles and, in moderate to severe cases, formation of pulmonary thrombi and emboli. The clinical picture is similar to pulmonary hypertension from any other cause, and has a poor prognosis with patients developing severe right heart failure within two years to three years.

Kyphoscoliotic heart disease arises from a forward and lateral deformity of the spine. It is characterized by difficult breathing, respiratory alkalosis, pulmonary hypertension and, in severe cases, congestive heart failure. It is a form of chronic secondary pulmonary hypertension.

Report 416.8 in cases of pulmonary hypertension secondary to a known etiology (excluding kyphoscoliosis), such as chronic bronchitis, chronic obstructive pulmonary disease, obesity-hypoventilation syndrome, chronic mountain sickness, obstructive sleep apnea, and neuromuscular disease.

416.0	Primary pulmonary hypertension — *including idiopathic pulmonary arteriosclerosis, pulmonary hyptertension, Arrillaga-Ayerza and Cardiacos negros syndromes*
416.1	Kyphoscoliotic heart disease — *high blood pressure within the lungs as a result of curvature of the spine*
416.8	Other chronic pulmonary heart diseases — *including pulmonary hypertension, secondary*
416.9	Unspecified chronic pulmonary heart disease — *unknown*

417 OTHER DISEASES OF PULMONARY CIRCULATION

Arteriovenous fistula of the pulmonary vessels is an abnormal communication between a pulmonary artery and vein that may result in embolization or ischemia. It may occur as a result of previous pulmonary infarction. Aneurysm of pulmonary artery is a dilation of the pulmonary artery or a blood-containing tumor within the lumen of the pulmonary artery. Both true and false (pseudo-) aneurysms are reported with 417.1

417.0	Arteriovenous fistula of pulmonary vessels — *abnormal communication between blood vessels within the lung*
417.1	Aneurysm of pulmonary artery — *dilation of the wall of the main artery in the lung*
417.8	Other specified disease of pulmonary circulation — *including arteritis; rupture or stricture of pulmonary vessel, endarteritis*
417.9	Unspecified disease of pulmonary circulation — *unknown*

420-429 Other Forms of Heart Disease

This section covers inflammatory conditions of the pericardium, endocardium, and myocardium, as well as heart valve disorders, cardiomyopathies, and nerve conduction disorders of the heart.

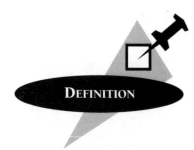

DEFINITION

Conduction: the electrical system of the heart is composed of the following: sinoatrial (SA) node; atrioventricular (AV) node; and bundle of HIS, at the atrioventricular junction; the left bundle branch; right bundle branch; and Purkinje's network and fibers. Electrical conduction allows both sides of the heart to synchronize action, even though they function independently.

🖙5th   Needs fifth-digit   **OK**   Valid three-digit code

420 ACUTE PERICARDITIS

Acute pericarditis is inflammation of the fibroserous membrane that surrounds the heart. The inflammation may be described as fibrinous, serous, sanguineous, hemorrhagic, or purulent. Etiologies for acute pericarditis include myocardial infarction, Dressler's syndrome, viral and bacterial infections, collagen vascular disease, adverse reaction to drugs (such as procainamide, hydralazine and isoniazid), metastatic disease, and uremia.

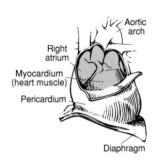

Rubric 420.0 reports acute pericarditis in diseases classified elsewhere. Report the etiology first, then the manifestation.

Unspecified acute pericarditis, including cases in which the specific infective organism is unknown, or in which the etiology is unknown, is reported with 420.90. This code may also be used to report acute pericarditis due to a malignant neoplasm. Acute idiopathic pericarditis, a benign, nonspecific or viral pericarditis that often follows upper respiratory infections, is reported with 420.91. Use this code only when other etiologies have been ruled out.

Report 420.99 for acute pericarditis caused by bacterial infection or when the acute pericarditis has no known etiology.

420.0	Acute pericarditis in diseases classified elsewhere — (Code first underlying disease, as: 017.9, 039.8, 066.8, 585) — *secondary to disease*
420.90	Unspecified acute pericarditis — *unknown cause*
420.91	Acute idiopathic pericarditis — *inflammation of heart lining, cause unknown*
420.99	Other acute pericarditis — *including pneumococcal, purulent, staphylococcal, streptococcal, pneumopyopericardium, pyopericardium*

421 ACUTE AND SUBACUTE ENDOCARDITIS

Use this rubric for diseases in which the endocardium is inflamed, usually due to bacterial infection. A variety of organisms may cause endocarditis, but *Staphylococcus aureus* is the most common pathogen. Infection of previously damaged valves is due to *Viridans streptococci* or other organisms comprising normal oral flora and may be secondary to a dental procedure. Infection of a prosthetic valve usually is due to *Staphylococci* within the first two months of surgery, and *Streptococci* more than two months after surgery. Infection of normal valves is rare and usually associated with intravenous drug abuse.

Acute endocarditis due to fungal infection is excluded from this rubric, and classified to rubrics 112 and 115.

421.0	Acute and subacute bacterial endocarditis — (Use additional code to identify infectious organism) — *including bacterial, infective, lenta, malignant, purulent, septic, ulcerative, vegetative, SBE*
421.1	Acute and subacute infective endocarditis in diseases classified elsewhere — (Code first underlying disease, as: 002.0, 083.0, 116.0) — *sudden, severe inflammation of lining of the heart secondary to other disease*
421.9	Unspecified acute endocarditis — *unknown cause*

422 ACUTE MYOCARDITIS

This rubric reports focal or diffuse inflammation of the myocardium that may be due to toxins, adverse reactions to drugs, or viral, bacterial, rickettsial, fungal, or parasitic disease. Excluded from this rubric are myocarditis due rheumatic fever (391.2) to Coxsackie virus

(074.23), diphtheritic infection (032.82), meningococcal infection (036.43), syphilis (093.82), and toxoplasmosis (130.3).

In myocarditis in disease classified elsewhere, code first the underlying disease, as in influenza (487.8) or tuberculosis (017.9).

For acute myocarditis secondary to metastatic disease, report 422.99.

422.0	Acute myocarditis in diseases classified elsewhere — (Code first underlying disease, as: 017.9, 487.8) — *sudden severe inflammation of muscle of the heart secondary to other disease*
422.90	Unspecified acute myocarditis — *cause unknown*
422.91	Idiopathic myocarditis — *giant cell, isolated, nonspecific, Fiedler's myocarditis*
422.92	Septic myocarditis — (Use additional code to identify infectious organism) — *caused by bacteria, including pneumococcal and staphylococcal*
422.93	Toxic myocarditis — *as a reaction to a toxic substance*
422.99	Other acute myocarditis — *not otherwise specified*

423 OTHER DISEASES OF PERICARDIUM

Hemopericardium is the presence of blood in the pericardial sac. It includes cardiac tamponade due to hemoperitoneum. Emergency pericardiocentesis is usually performed. Excluded from this rubric is hemopericardium due to trauma, classified as an internal injury of the chest in rubric 860.

Report adhesive pericarditis for adhesions between the two-pericardial layers, between the heart and the pericardium, or between the pericardium and other contiguous structures in the chest.

Constrictive pericarditis is a diffuse thickening of the pericardium as a late effect of inflammation. Cardiac output is limited due to the reduced distensibility of the cardiac chambers, and filling pressures are increased in response to the external constrictive force placed on the heart by the pericardium. This condition may be associated with congestive heart failure.

Reserve 423.8 for diseases of the pericardium not reported elsewhere in this rubric, including calcified pericardium, diverticula of pericardium, cyst of pericardium, and fistula of pericardium. Code 423.9 is usually reserved for cardiac tamponade due to nontraumatic pericardial effusion, not specified as hemorrhagic or due to hemopericardium, pericardial compression scarring, and pneumohemopericardium.

423.0	Hemopericardium — *escape of blood into the lining of the heart*
423.1	Adhesive pericarditis — *adherent, fibrosis, milk spots, obliterative*
423.2	Constrictive pericarditis — *loss of elasticity; including Concato's or Pick's disease, Gouley's syndrome*
423.8	Other specified diseases of pericardium — *not elsewhere specified; calcification, fistula, acquired diverticula, cholesterol pericarditis, cyst*
423.9	Unspecified disease of pericardium — *unknown*

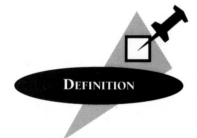

DEFINITION

Milk spots: also called Soldier's patches, white patches of fibrous tissue on the lining of the heart causing inflammation.

Tamponade heart (Rose's): an accumulation of fluid in the pericardium that causes pressure and restricts the blood flowing into the heart.

5th   Needs fifth-digit   **OK**   Valid three-digit code

424 OTHER DISEASES OF ENDOCARDIUM

This rubric includes disease of the heart valves that are specified or presumed to be non-rheumatic in origin, classified to categories 394-397.

Syphilitic endocarditis is excluded from 424.91 *Endocarditis in disease classified elsewhere.* For this code, sequence first the underlying disease, for example, tuberculosis (017.9) or disseminated lupus erythematosus (710.0).

424.0	Mitral valve disorders — *incompetence, insufficiency, regurgitation, prolapse; including ballooning posterior leaflet syndrome, Barlow's syndrome*
424.1	Aortic valve disorders — *incompetence, insufficiency, regurgitation, stenosis, nonrheumatic*
424.2	Tricuspid valve disorders, specified as nonrheumatic — *incompetence, insufficiency, regurgitation, stenosis, nonrheumatic*
424.3	Pulmonary valve disorders — *incompetence, insufficiency, regurgitation, stenosis, nonrheumatic*
424.90	Endocarditis, valve unspecified, unspecified cause — *incompetence, insufficiency, regurgitation, stenosis, endocardial tag, nonrheumatic, unknown cause*
424.91	Endocarditis in diseases classified elsewhere — (Code first underlying disease, as: 017.9, 710.0) — *secondary to underlying disease*
424.99	Other endocarditis, valve unspecified — *incompetence, insufficiency, regurgitation, stenosis, nonrheumatic, with specified cause*

425 CARDIOMYOPATHY

Cardiomyopathy is a complex and heterogenous group of diseases of the heart muscle. Rubric 425 includes diseases of the heart muscle itself that are classified to specific etiologies. Note that the term "cardiomyopathy" often is used for a disease or disorder that should be classified elsewhere. For example, the term, "ischemic cardiomyopathy" should be interpreted as ischemic heart disease and classified to the series 414.8.

Endomyocardial fibrosis is a thickening of the ventricular endocardium due to fibrosis. Occasionally, the tricuspid and mitral valves may be involved and there is thrombus formation. Endomyocardial fibrosis is reported with 425.0.

Hypertrophic obstructive cardiomyopathy, idiopathic hypertrophic subaortic stenosis, and asymmetrical septal hypertrophy are reported with 425.1. The etiology is believed to be an autosomal dominant genetic disorder and is characterized by an excessively hypertrophied interventricular septum. Left ventricular outflow obstruction results when the septum mechanically obstructs the anterior leaflet of the mitral valve.

Idiopathic cardiomegaly, idiopathic mural endomyocardial disease, Becker's disease and South African cardiomyopathy are all types of obscure cardiomyopathy of Africa, reported with 425.2. These conditions are thought to be late effects of an infectious myocarditis, and are rarely encountered in the United States.

Endocardial fibroelastosis (425.3) is a congenital condition characterized by thickening of the endocardium and subendocardium, with malformation of the cardiac valves, hypertrophy of the heart, and proliferation of elastic tissue in the myocardium. It is also called elastomyofibrosis. Many patients with this condition do not survive infancy.

Report 425.4 for unspecified cardiomyopathy and cardiomyopathy of unknown or obscure etiology. Both obstructive cardiomyopathy and hypertrophic cardiomyopathy may be

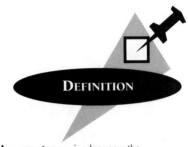

DEFINITION

Incompetence: inadequacy; the insufficiency of heart or venous valves when closing.

Regurgitation: when blood flows backward due to a heart valve not functioning properly.

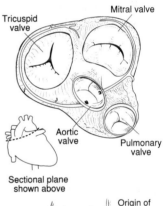

Tricuspid valve · Mitral valve · Aortic valve · Pulmonary valve

Sectional plane shown above

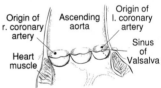

Origin of r. coronary artery · Ascending aorta · Origin of l. coronary artery · Sinus of Valsalva · Heart muscle

Depiction of opened aortic root showing semilunar cusps

classified to 425.4, but the combined form of hypertrophic obstructive cardiomyopathy is reported with 425.1.

For cardiomyopathy due to underlying disease, code first the underlying disease, then the myopathy with 435.7 or 435.8. Some examples of underlying disease include amyloidosis (277.3); beriberi (265.0); cardiac glycogenesis (271.0); mucopolysaccharidosis (277.5); thyrotoxicosis (242.0-242.9); Friedreich's ataxia (334.0); myotonia atrophica (359.1) and sarcoidosis (135). Subclassification 435.7 excludes gouty tophi of heart, reported with 274.82, and subclassification 437.8 excludes cardiomyopathy in Chagas' disease (086.0).

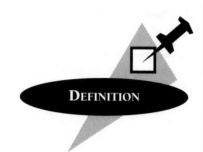

Becker's disease: disease of the heart muscle that leads to congestive heart failure and spreads to the inner heart tissue, originated in South Africa.

425.0	Endomyocardial fibrosis — *fibrous tissue invading the muscle of the heart*
425.1	Hypertrophic obstructive cardiomyopathy — *abnormal growth of the left ventricle wall causing obstructed blood flow; idiopathic hypertrophic subaortic stenosis*
425.2	Obscure cardiomyopathy of Africa — *including Becker's disease, South African cardiomyopathy syndrome, idiopathic mural endomyocardial disease*
425.3	Endocardial fibroelastosis — *increased elastic tissue production with enlarged left ventricle wall; elastomyofibrosis*
425.4	Other primary cardiomyopathies — *congestive, restrictive, familial, hypertrophic, idiopathic, nonobstructive, obstructive, restrictive, cardiovascular collagenosis*
425.5	Alcoholic cardiomyopathy — *heart disease resulting from excessive alcohol consumption*
425.7	Nutritional and metabolic cardiomyopathy — (Code first underlying disease, as: 242.00–242.91, 265.0, 271.0, 277.3, 277.5) — *secondary to specific underlying disease*
425.8	Cardiomyopathy in other diseases classified elsewhere — (Code first underlying disease, as: 135, 334.0, 359.1, 359.2) — *secondary to specific underlying disease*
425.9	Unspecified secondary cardiomyopathy

426 CONDUCTION DISORDERS

Nerve conduction disorders include a group of conditions in which the transmission of cardiac electrical impulses controlling heart rhythm is abnormal, slowed, or interrupted.

Complete atrioventricular block is the most advanced form of heart block. Usually, there is a lesion distal to the bundle of His and is associated with bilateral bundle branch block. Some patients may go through periods of transition between partial and complete heart block.

426.0	Atrioventricular block, complete — *including third degree atrioventricular block, Lev's and Rytand-Lipsitch syndrome*
426.10	Unspecified atrioventricular block — *AV block, incomplete or partial*
426.11	First degree atrioventricular block — *first degree incomplete AV block; prolonged P-R interval not specified elsewhere*
426.12	Mobitz (type) II atrioventricular block — *incomplete AV block, Mobitz type II, second degree*
426.13	Other second degree atrioventricular block — *incomplete AV block, Mobitz, type I, second degree; Wenckebach's phenomenon*
426.2	Left bundle branch hemiblock — *left anterior or posterior fascicular block*
426.3	Other left bundle branch block — *complete, main stem, anterior fascicular with posterior fascicular, not otherwise specified*
426.4	Right bundle branch block

✔5th   Needs fifth-digit   **OK**   Valid three-digit code

426.50	Unspecified bundle branch block — *unknown*
426.51	Right bundle branch block and left posterior fascicular block
426.52	Right bundle branch block and left anterior fascicular block
426.53	Other bilateral bundle branch block — *including bifascicular block not otherwise specified; right bundle ranch with left bundle brand block*
426.54	Trifascicular block
426.6	Other heart block — *intraventricular, diffuse, myofibrillar, sinoatrial, sinoauricular block*
426.7	Anomalous atrioventricular excitation — *accelerated, accessory, pre-excitation; including bundle of Kent syndrome, Wolff-Parkinson-White syndrome*
426.81	Lown-Ganong-Levine syndrome — *short P-R interval, normal QRS complexes, and supraventricular tachycardias*
426.89	Other specified conduction disorder — *AV, interference, isorhythmic dissociation, nonparoxysmal AV nodal tachycardia*
426.9	Unspecified conduction disorder — *unknown*

427 CARDIAC DYSRHYTHMIAS

Cardiac dysrhythmias are disturbances in cardiac rate and rhythm, including abnormalities in the rate, regularity, and sequence of atrial and/or ventricular contractions. Cardiac dysrhythmias can take many forms; the clinical significance of each depends on the extent to which they lower blood pressure and reduce cardiac output with resulting hypoperfusion of vital organs such as the brain, kidneys, and the heart. Cardiac dysrhythmias may be benign or malignant depending on the severity of the dysrhythmia and the patient's ability to tolerate it.

The etiology of cardiac dysrhythmia may be idiopathic, due to heart disease such as arteriosclerosis and rheumatic heart disease or due to other noncardiac etiologies such as thyrotoxicosis, alcoholism, trauma, and intravenous drug abuse. Many cardiac dysrhythmias are chronic, but acute dysrhythmias also can occur in cases of acute infection or digitalis toxicity. Symptoms may include fatigue, light-headedness, decreased exercise tolerance, or syncope, but often, there are no symptoms.

427.0	Paroxysmal supraventricular tachycardia — *very rapid atrial rhythm; including PAT, AV, junctional, nodal*
427.1	Paroxysmal ventricular tachycardia — *very rapid ventricular rhythm*
427.2	Unspecified paroxysmal tachycardia — *including Bouveret-Hoffmann syndrome, essential paroxysmal tachycardia*
427.31	Atrial fibrillation — *irregular, rapid atrial contractions*
427.32	Atrial flutter — *regular, rapid atrial contractions*
427.41	Ventricular fibrillation — *irregular, rapid ventricular contractions*
427.42	Ventricular flutter — *regular, rapid ventricular contractions*
427.5	Cardiac arrest — *heart stops and atrial blood pressure flattens*
427.60	Unspecified premature beats — *ectopic beats, extrasystolic arrhythmia, premature contractions; unknown site*
427.61	Supraventricular premature beats — *ectopic beats, extrasystolic arrhythmia, premature contractions; atrial*
427.69	Other premature beats — *ectopic beats, extrasystolic arrhythmia, premature contractions, site not otherwise specified*
427.81	Sinoatrial node dysfunction — *persistent or severe sinus bradycardia; including sick sinus syndrome*
427.89	Other specified cardiac dysrhythmias — *not otherwise specified, including bigeminy, trigeminy, split heart sounds, wandering pacemaker, gallop rhythm*
427.9	Unspecified cardiac dysrhythmia — *unknown*

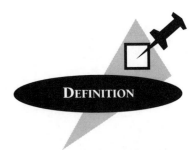

DEFINITION

Paroxysmal ventricular tachycardia: rare arrhythmia with rapid ventricular impulses revealing a rate of 160 beats to 240 beats per minute.

Atrial fibrillation: common cardiac arrhythmia characterized by rapid (400 to 600 per minute) irregular impulses of the atria. The ventricular response is also irregular, with rates of 80 beats to 160 beats per minute in the untreated state.

Atrial flutter: uncommon atrial dysrhythmia characterized by rapid regular atrial contractions of 250 to 400 per minute. The ventricular rate is usually half of the atrial rate.

Ventricular fibrillation: malignant arrhythmia characterized by rapid, irregular and chaotic ventricular rate, often seen following myocardial infarction; constitutes a medical emergency.

Ventricular flutter: ventricular tachycardia with rapid, regular pattern of ventricular contractions.

Cardiac arrest: cessation of effective circulatory performance following loss of cardiac function.

Premature beats: premature depolarization, premature contractions and similarly described conditions involving extrasystolic or ectopic beats of atria or ventricles, characterized by depolarization of either the atria, ventricles, or both, prior to the next expected sinus beat.

Bigeminy: an incident of a pair of heart beats.

Sick sinus syndrome: a slowing of the heartbeat alternating with repeating ectopic heart beats followed by a quickening of the heart beat.

Trigeminy: triple heart beats, usually a sinus beat succeeded by two extra systoles.

428 HEART FAILURE

Congestive heart failure is a mechanical inability of the heart to pump blood efficiently, thus compromising circulation and causing systemic complications due to congestion and edema of fluids in the tissues. Etiologies fall into three groups: disorders that decrease contractile function; disorders than increase myocardial overload; and abnormalities in myocardial preload.

Contractile function of the heart decreases when the myocardium has been damaged as in myocardial infarction, thus reducing the ventricles' ability to contract forcefully.

Increased myocardial afterload refers to the increased force that the myocardium must generate to contract the ventricles. For example, in acute and severe systemic hypertension, the force exerted upon the ventricle by increased blood pressure exceeds the force the ventricle must generate to contract, leading to pulmonary congestion.

Myocardial preload refers to the stretching of the myocardial fibers prior to myocardial contraction. Although this stretching increases the force-generating capabilities of the ventricles, eventually pulmonary congestion occurs when the ventricular filling pressure concomitantly increases.

In ICD-9-CM, congestive heart failure also is defined as right ventricular failure or right ventricular failure due to left ventricular failure. Right ventricular failure is most frequently due to failure of the left ventricle, but may occur independently of left ventricular failure. Chronic obstructive pulmonary disease can produce a pressure overload in the right ventricle independent of any failure on the left side.

Documentation of an impaired heart muscle or left ventricular dysfunction does not indicate heart failure unless symptoms of fatigue, shortness of breath, and fluid retention are documented. Documentation indicating impaired heart muscle implies definitive causes, such as virus or drug abuse. Documentation of idiopathic or dilated congested cardiomyopathy indicates only that there is four-chamber enlargement of the heart, which may occur without heart failure. Classify compensated and decompensated heart failure to 428.0.

428.0   Congestive heart failure — *right heart failure; decreased efficiency of heart output causing fluid collection in lungs, hypertension, and congestion of the vessels*

428.1   Left heart failure — *decreased efficiency of the left ventricle of the heart causing fluid in lungs*

428.9   Unspecified heart failure — *unknown whether right or left*

429 ILL-DEFINED DESCRIPTIONS AND COMPLICATIONS OF HEART DISEASE

429.0   Unspecified myocarditis — (Use additional code to identify presence of arteriosclerosis) — *inflammation, cause unknown, but not rheumatic*

429.1   Myocardial degeneration — (Use additional code to identify presence of arteriosclerosis) — *including Beau's syndrome, softening, fatty, mural, muscular disease*

429.2   Unspecified cardiovascular disease — (Use additional code to identify presence of arteriosclerosis) — *ASCVD, specifics unknown*

429.3   Cardiomegaly — *enlargement of the heart; dilation, hypertrophy, dilatation*

429.4   Functional disturbances following cardiac surgery — *or due to prosthesis*

429.5   Rupture of chordae tendineae — *torn tissue between heart valves and papillary muscles*

⮡5th   Needs fifth-digit   **OK**   Valid three-digit code

429.6 Rupture of papillary muscle — *torn muscle between chordae tendineae and heart wall*

429.71 Acquired cardiac septal defect — (Use additional code to identify associated (condition) 410.00–410.92, 414.8)

429.79 Other certain sequelae of myocardial infarction, not elsewhere classified — (Use additional code to identify associated (condition) 410.00–410.92, 414.8) — *mural thrombus following MI, not otherwise specified*

429.81 Other disorders of papillary muscle — *atrophy, degeneration, dysfunction, incompetence, incoordination, scarring*

429.82 Hyperkinetic heart disease — *abnormally increased motor function of the heart*

429.89 Other ill-defined heart disease — *not specified elsewhere, including carditis, hemorrhage of heart, ventricular asynergy, ventricular dyssnergia*

429.9 Unspecified heart disease — *unknown type or site*

430-438 Cerebrovascular Disease

This section of ICD-9-CM classifies the acute, organic conditions of the cerebrovascular system. Conditions coded to this section are nontraumatic in origin and include hemorrhages, thromboses, embolisms, transient cerebral ischemia, other ill-defined cerebrovascular diseases and the late effects of cerebrovascular disease.

These classifications include cardiovascular disease with mention of hypertension (conditions classifiable to 401-405). Use an additional code to identify the presence of hypertension, excluding 430-434, 436, 437, and 674.0.

430 SUBARACHNOID HEMORRHAGE OK

A subarachnoid hemorrhage is an extravasation of blood into the subarachnoid space. The episodes usually are sudden in nature and account for five percent to 10 percent of all cerebrovascular accidents. The etiology may be secondary to head trauma and classified to the Injury chapter, or due to primary disease such as arteriosclerotic aneurysm, arteriovenous malformation, or hemorrhagic diathesis. This rubric excludes syphilitic ruptured cerebral aneurysm (094.87).

431 INTRACEREBRAL HEMORRHAGE OK

An intracerebral hemorrhage is a spontaneous extravasation of blood within the brain. Etiologies include hypertension with microaneurysmal formation, bleeding diathesis (leukemia, thrombocytopenia, hemophilia), disseminated intravascular coagulation, anticoagulant therapy, liver disease, cerebral amyloid angiopathy, AV malformation, and brain neoplasms.

432 OTHER AND UNSPECIFIED INTRACRANIAL HEMORRHAGE

This rubric classifies nontraumatic extradural (epidural) and subdural hemorrhage of the cerebrovascular system. Excluded from this rubric is extradural and subdural hemorrhage as a spinal cord vascular disease.

432.0 Nontraumatic extradural hemorrhage — *bleeding between the skull and the lining of the brain*

432.1 Subdural hemorrhage — *bleeding between the outermost and other layers of the lining of the brain*

432.9 Unspecified intracranial hemorrhage — *unknown site*

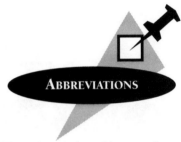

ABBREVIATIONS

CVA: cerebrovascular accident, a stroke

ICH: intracerebral /cranial hemorrhage/hematoma

SAH: subarachnoid hemorrhage/hematoma

SDH: subdural hemorrhage/hematoma

TIA: transient ischemic attack, vascular insufficiency to the brain causing a sudden neurological impairment

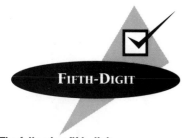

The following fifth-digit subclassification is for use with categories 433 and 434:

0 without mention of cerebral infarction

1 with cerebral infarction

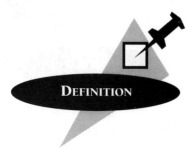

Subclavian steal syndrome: cerebrovascular insufficiency due to subclavian artery obstruction proximal to the origin of the vertebral artery. In subclavian steal, blood flow through the vertebral artery is reversed; thus the subclavian artery steals cerebral blood, causing a hypoperfusion of the tissue normally perfused by the vertebral artery.

Hypertensive encephalopathy: hypertensive crisis is medical emergency in which the patient develops a greatly elevated blood pressure (often 250/150 or higher), cerebral involvement may cause stroke due to thrombosis or sudden hemorrhage from small penetrating intracranial arteries.

Moyamoya/Moya Moya: mental retardation, seizure disorders, and hemiplegia are common sequela of this condition of unknown etiology that most commonly affects young patients of Japanese ancestry.

Verbiest's syndrome: also claudication intermittens spinalis, symptoms in a moving limb including pain, tension, and weakness but absent at rest. Caused by occlusive arterial diseases of the limbs.

433 OCCLUSION AND STENOSIS OF PRECEREBRAL ARTERIES

433.0 ✓5th Occlusion and stenosis of basilar artery — *embolism, narrowing, obstruction, thrombosis*

433.1 ✓5th Occlusion and stenosis of carotid artery — *embolism, narrowing, obstruction, thrombosis*

433.2 ✓5th Occlusion and stenosis of vertebral artery — *embolism, narrowing, obstruction, thrombosis*

433.3 ✓5th Occlusion and stenosis of multiple and bilateral precerebral arteries — *embolism, narrowing, obstruction, thrombosis*

433.8 ✓5th Occlusion and stenosis of other specified precerebral artery — *pontine, meningeal, hypophyseal, communicating posterior, choroidal, cerebellar, internal auditory, anterior spinal artery; embolism, narrowing, obstruction, thrombosis*

433.9 ✓5th Occlusion and stenosis of unspecified precerebral artery — *embolism, narrowing, obstruction, thrombosis; unknown site*

434 OCCLUSION OF CEREBRAL ARTERIES

Cerebrovascular accident (CVA) is a vague term often used to describe a condition best classified to this category. However, do not classify CVA to this category without obtaining physician verification, since the term can also describe other acute cerebrovascular conditions that would be properly classified elsewhere.

434.0 ✓5th Cerebral thrombosis — *blood clot*

434.1 ✓5th Cerebral embolism — *complete blockage*

434.9 ✓5th Unspecified cerebral artery occlusion — *extent unknown*

435 TRANSIENT CEREBRAL ISCHEMIA

Transient cerebral ischemia describes episodes of focal neurological symptoms. Its most common form is known as a transient ischemic attack (TIA). A typical TIA lasts between two minutes and 15 minutes and always resolves within 24 hours. Commonly the etiology of the TIA is embolization due to cardiac causes such as rheumatic heart disease, cardiac dysrhythmias, mitral valve disease, infective endocarditis, mural thrombi complicating myocardial infarction, and myxoma.

This rubric includes reversible ischemic neurological deficits (RIND), if the patient's neurological deficits are associated with TIA and abate within 24 hours. RIND also may be associated with other conditions in rubrics 430-437 and should be coded to the underlying condition causing the deficits. RIND may require a second code to classify the specific neurological deficit and the appropriate code from categories 430-437.

435.0　Basilar artery syndrome

435.1　Vertebral artery syndrome — *including Verbiest's syndrome*

435.2　Subclavian steal syndrome

435.3　Vertebrobasilar artery syndrome

435.8　Other specified transient cerebral ischemias — *including carotid artery insufficiency*

435.9　Unspecified transient cerebral ischemia — *unknown; including TIA, Alvarez syndrome, impending cerebrovascular accident*

436 ACUTE, BUT ILL-DEFINED, CEREBROVASCULAR DISEASE ⓄⓀ

Wallenberg syndrome is characterized by difficulty in swallowing and hoarseness due to paralysis of the ipsilateral vocal cord and, in some cases, partial lost of the sense of taste due to associated affects on the tongue. The glossopharyngeal (IX) & vagus (X) are the primary cranial nerves involved in this syndrome. Occlusion of the posterior inferior cerebellar artery (PICA) leads to damage to the posterior region of the medulla, which explains the name 'lateral medullary plate syndrome' often used to refer to this disorder.

This rubric excludes any condition classifiable to categories 430-435.

437 OTHER AND ILL-DEFINED CEREBROVASCULAR DISEASE

437.0	Cerebral atherosclerosis — *deposits narrowing arteries that branch into the brain*
437.1	Other generalized ischemic cerebrovascular disease — *chronic cerebral ischemia, acute cerebrovascular insufficiency not otherwise specified*
437.2	Hypertensive encephalopathy — *brain disease caused by high blood pressure*
437.3	Cerebral aneurysm, nonruptured — *dilation of artery in the brain*
437.4	Cerebral arteritis — *inflammation of artery within the brain*
437.5	Moyamoya disease — *tiny neovacularizations in patients with ischemia*
437.6	Nonpyogenic thrombosis of intracranial venous sinus
437.7	Transient global amnesia — *temporary memory loss not due to psychological factors*
437.8	Other ill-defined cerebrovascular disease — *including cerebral hyperemia, hypertensive paralysis, necrotic brain, mollities, cortical or cerebral quadriplegia*
437.9	Unspecified cerebrovascular disease — *unknown*

438 LATE EFFECTS OF CEREBROVASCULAR DISEASE

This rubric classifies conditions in categories 430-437 as the cause of a late effect. ICD-9-CM classifies late effects of cerebrovascular disease according to the neurological deficit. Excluded from this rubric is history of cerebrovascular disease when no neurological deficit is present as a late effect. The appropriate code in that case would be V12.59 Personal history of other disease of the circulatory system.

Assign a code from rubric 438 in addition to a code from 430-437 if the patient has a current CVA in addition to deficits from the old CVA.

438.0	Cognitive deficits — *thought, memory, perception*
438.10	Speech and language deficit, unspecified — *unknown*
438.11	Aphasia — *speech loss or deficit*
438.12	Dysphasia — *inability to organize words in their appropriate order*
438.19	Other speech and language deficits — *not otherwise specified*
438.20	Hemiplegia affecting unspecified side
438.21	Hemiplegia affecting dominant side
438.22	Hemiplegia affecting nondominant side
438.30	Monoplegia of upper limb affecting unspecified side
438.31	Monoplegia of upper limb affecting dominant side
438.32	Monoplegia of upper limb affecting nondominant side
438.40	Monoplegia of lower limb affecting unspecified side
438.41	Monoplegia of lower limb affecting dominant side
438.42	Monoplegia of lower limb affecting nondominant side
438.50	Other paralytic syndrome affecting unspecified side
438.51	Other paralytic syndrome affecting dominant side

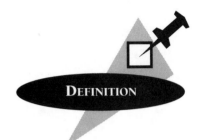

DEFINITION

Transient global amnesia: sudden loss of memory and inability to record new memories in a transient condition associated with migraine headaches, vertebrobasilar ischemia, seizures, medication reactions, or head trauma. The condition lasts several hours.

Beck's Syndrome: occlusion of the spinal artery as result of injury, disk damage, or cardiovascular disease.

Cestan-Raymond Syndrome: quadriplegia, anesthesia, and nystagmus caused by obstruction of twigs of the basilar artery and lesions in the pontine region.

Hyperemia: an abnormal quantity of blood in an organ.

Mollities: a softening of the consistency of an organ.

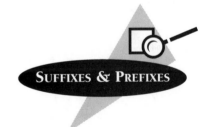

SUFFIXES & PREFIXES

-asia: pertaining to speech

-phagia: pertaining to swallowing

Aph-: absence of

Dys-: difficulty

438.52	Other paralytic syndrome affecting nondominant side
438.53	Other paralytic syndrome, bilateral
438.81	Apraxia — *inability to properly use an object or carry out normal tasks*
438.82	Dysphagia — *difficulty in swallowing*
438.89	Other late effects of cerebrovascular disease — (Use additional code to identify the late effect) — *not specified elsewhere*
438.9	Unspecified late effects of cerebrovascular disease — *unknown*

440-448 Diseases of Arteries, Arterioles, and Capillaries

This section includes conditions affecting the arteries, arterioles, and capillaries, including atherosclerosis, aneurysm, peripheral vascular disease, embolism and thrombosis, arteritis, and stricture.

440 ATHEROSCLEROSIS

Atherosclerosis is a form of arteriosclerosis characterized by irregularly distributed atheromas accumulating within the tunica intima of arteries. The deposits are associated with calcification and fibrosis, reducing the size of the arterial lumen and resulting in obstructive ischemia.

440.0	Atherosclerosis of aorta — *includes atheroma, degeneration, endarteritis,*
440.1	Atherosclerosis of renal artery — *includes atheroma, degeneration, endarteritis*
440.20	Atherosclerosis of native arteries of the extremities, unspecified — *unknown manifestations*
440.21	Atherosclerosis of native arteries of the extremities with intermittent claudication — *including Charcot's due to atherosclerosis*
440.22	Atherosclerosis of native arteries of the extremities with rest pain
440.23	Atherosclerosis of native arteries of the extremities with ulceration — (Use additional code for any associated ulceration: 707.10-707.9)
440.24	Atherosclerosis of native arteries of the extremities with gangrene
440.29	Other atherosclerosis of native arteries of the extremities — *not otherwise specified*
440.30	Atheroslerosis of unspecified bypass graft of extremities — *graft origin unknown*
440.31	Atheroslerosis of autologous vein bypass graft of extremities — *graft from patient*
440.32	Atheroslerosis of nonautologous biological bypass graft of extremities — *graft other than from patient*
440.8	Atherosclerosis of other specified arteries — *not otherwise specified; including arteriosclerotic retinitis*
440.9	Generalized and unspecified atherosclerosis — *unknown or disseminated*

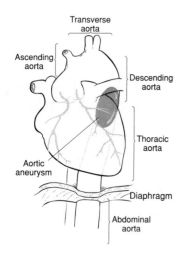

Transverse aorta

Ascending aorta

Descending aorta

Thoracic aorta

Aortic aneurysm

Diaphragm

Abdominal aorta

441 AORTIC ANEURYSM AND DISSECTION

Aortic aneurysms are circumscribed dilations of the aorta or a blood-containing tumor connecting directly within the lumen of the aorta. Generally, an aneurysm is considered clinically significant if its diameter is twice that of the normal artery. A dissecting aneurysm is characterized by blood entering through a split or tear in the intima of the artery wall or by interstitial hemorrhage. Dissecting aortic aneurysms may rupture, constituting a medical emergency. This condition is most frequently seen in men between 40 and 60 years of age.

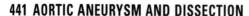

✍5th Needs fifth-digit   **OK** Valid three-digit code

441.00 Dissecting aortic aneurysm (any part), unspecified site — *dilation and split of aorta lining, site unknown*

441.01 Dissecting aortic aneurysm (any part), thoracic — *dilation and split of aorta lining in the chest cavity*

441.02 Dissecting aortic aneurysm (any part), abdominal — *dilation and split of aorta lining in the abdomen*

441.03 Dissecting aortic aneurysm (any part), thoracoabdominal — *dilation and split of aorta lining in chest and abdomen*

441.1 Thoracic aneurysm, ruptured — *dilation and tear in aorta in chest*

441.2 Thoracic aneurysm without mention of rupture — *dilation in aorta in chest*

441.3 Abdominal aneurysm, ruptured — *dilation and tear of aorta in abdomen*

441.4 Abdominal aneurysm without mention of rupture — *dilation of aorta in abdomen*

441.5 Aortic aneurysm of unspecified site, ruptured — *dilation and tear of aorta in unknown site*

441.6 Thoracoabdominal aneurysm, ruptured — *dilation and tear of aorta in abdomen and chest*

441.7 Thoracoabdominal aneurysm without mention of rupture — *dilation of aorta in abdomen and chest*

441.9 Aortic aneurysm of unspecified site without mention of rupture — *dilation of aorta, site and rupture status unknown*

442 OTHER ANEURYSM

442.0 Aneurysm of artery of upper extremity — *dilation; brachial, radial, interosseous, ulnar, superficial palmar arch*

442.1 Aneurysm of renal artery — *dilation*

442.2 Aneurysm of iliac artery — *dilation*

442.3 Aneurysm of artery of lower extremity — *dilation; femoral, popliteal artery, medial plantar, posterior tibial, anterior tibial*

442.81 Aneurysm of artery of neck — *dilation; internal, external, common carotid*

442.82 Aneurysm of subclavian artery — *dilation*

442.83 Aneurysm of splenic artery — *dilation*

442.84 Aneurysm of other visceral artery — *dilation; celiac, gastroduodenal, hepatic, pancreaticoduodenal, superior mesenteric, gastroepiploic*

442.89 Aneurysm of other specified artery — *dilation; mediastinal, spinal artery*

442.9 Other aneurysm of unspecified site — *unknown site*

443 OTHER PERIPHERAL VASCULAR DISEASE

443.0 Raynaud's syndrome — (Use additional code to identify associated (condition) 785.4) — *construction of arteries of the digits caused by cold or stress*

443.1 Thromboangiitis obliterans (Buerger's disease) — *inflammation and swelling in distal arteries, causing occlusions*

443.81 Peripheral angiopathy in diseases classified elsewhere — (Code first underlying disease, as: 250.7) — *secondary to underlying disease*

443.89 Other peripheral vascular disease — *not otherwise specified, including Crocq's, Gerhardt's, Weir Mitchell's disease, acrocyanosis, erythrocyanosis, Schultz's acroparesthesia, Nothnagel's vasomotor acroparesthesia, erythromelalgia*

443.9 Unspecified peripheral vascular disease — *unknown*

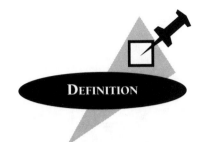

DEFINITION

Charcot's syndrome: symptoms in a moving limb including pain, tension, and weakness but absent at rest. Caused by occlusive arterial diseases of the limbs.

Crocq's: acrocyanosis, a lack of oxygen in the blood of the extremities causing a bluish appearance.

Gerhardt's disease: erythromelalgia, a burning sensation in the extremities that take on a red appearance.

Weir Mitchell's: also erythromelalgia.

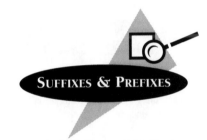

SUFFIXES & PREFIXES

-cyanosis: lack of oxygen in the blood causing a bluish appearance

-melalgia: a burning pain in the lower extremities

-paresthesia: tingling feeling or sensation

Acro-: extremity or the point

Erythro-: redness

The hallmark feature of Raynaud's syndrome is fingertips that become purple from constricted arteries, particularly during cold and times of stress

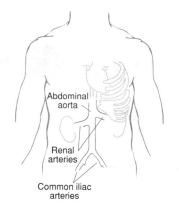

Abdominal aorta

Renal arteries

Common iliac arteries

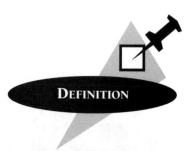

DEFINITION

Bagratuni's syndrome: also Horton's disease, temporal arteritis.

Churg-Strauss syndrome: allergic reaction characterized by multiple granulomas.

Kawasaki disease: also mucocutaneous lymph node syndrome, a childhood disease characterized by an erythematous fever. Conjunctivitis, cervical lymphadenopathy, vasculitis, and pharyngitis often accompany this disease.

Martorell-Fabere: also Raeder-Harbitz syndrome, ischemia, transient blindness, facial atrophy, and many other symptoms. Progressive obliteration of the brachiocephalic trunk and the left subclavian and common carotid arteries above their source in the aortic arch.

444 ARTERIAL EMBOLISM AND THROMBOSIS

An arterial embolism is a partial or complete obstruction of an artery due to the migration of a blood clot or other foreign material. An arterial thrombosis is the formation of a blood clot within the lumen of an artery. In each case, infarction of the tissues perfused by the artery is a potential complication.

444.0 Embolism and thrombosis of abdominal aorta — *aortic bifurcation and Leriche's syndromes, saddle embolus, aortoiliac obstruction*

444.1 Embolism and thrombosis of thoracic aorta — *embolism of thrombosis of thoracic aorta*

444.21 Embolism and thrombosis of arteries of upper extremity — *brachial, radial, interosseous, ulnar, superficial palmar arch*

444.22 Embolism and thrombosis of arteries of lower extremity — *femoral, popliteal artery, medial plantar, posterior tibial, anterior tibial*

444.81 Embolism and thrombosis of iliac artery

444.89 Embolism and thrombosis of other specified artery — *including hepatic and splenic arteries*

444.9 Embolism and thrombosis of unspecified artery — *unknown*

446 POLYARTERITIS NODOSA AND ALLIED CONDITIONS

Polyarteritis nodosa is a systemic disease characterized by segmental inflammation with infiltration and necrosis of medium-sized or small arteries. It is most common in males and produces symptoms related to involvement of arteries in the kidneys, muscles, gastrointestinal tract, and heart, and is reported with 446.0.

446.0 Polyarteritis nodosa — *inflammation of small and medium size arteries causing tissue death; disseminated necrotizing periarteritis, necrotizing angiitis, Harkavy's syndrome*

446.1 Acute febrile mucocutaneous lymph node syndrome (MCLS) — *inflammatory disease causing fever, skin eruptions, and edema; including Kawasaki disease*

446.20 Unspecified hypersensitivity angiitis — *unknown inflammatory disease of vessels caused by antigen sensitivity*

446.21 Goodpasture's syndrome — *antiglomerular basement membrane antibody-mediated nephritis with pulmonary hemorrhage*

446.29 Other specified hypersensitivity angiitis — *not otherwise specified*

446.3 Lethal midline granuloma — *tumor that begins midface and leads to death; malignant granuloma of face*

446.4 Wegener's granulomatosis — *necrotizing granulomatous inflammation of vessels of respiratory tract; Churg-Strauss syndrome*

446.5 Giant cell arteritis — *giant cells and inflammation in large artery, leading to occlusion; including cranial arteritis, Horton's disease, Bagratuni's syndrome*

446.6 Thrombotic microangiopathy — *blockages in the smallest arteries and arterioles; including Moschcowitz's syndrome, Baehr-Schiffrin disease*

446.7 Takayasu's disease — *progressive inflammation of brachiocephalic truck and left common carotid arteries above source in aortic arch; including Martorell-Fabre, Raeder-Harbitz, young female syndromes, pulseless disease*

447 OTHER DISORDERS OF ARTERIES AND ARTERIOLES

447.0 Arteriovenous fistula, acquired — *communication between an artery and vein caused by error in healing*

447.1 Stricture of artery — *structurally narrow section of an artery*

447.2 Rupture of artery — *tearing of artery with bleeding, not associated with aneurysm, but caused by erosion, (not arteriovenous) fistula or ulcer*

✔5th   Needs fifth-digit   **OK**   Valid three-digit code

447.3 Hyperplasia of renal artery — *overgrowth of cells in the muscular lining of the renal artery*
447.4 Celiac artery compression syndrome — *compression of the celiac artery by the median arcuate ligament; celiac axis, Marable's, medial arcuate ligament syndromes*
447.5 Necrosis of artery — *death of arterial tissue*
447.6 Unspecified arteritis — *unknown*
447.8 Other specified disorders of arteries and arterioles — *not otherwise specified; including fibromuscular hyperplasia of nonrenal artery; Dego's, Wright's, or popliteal artery entrapment syndromes; dilation, hyperabduction, hypertrophy, papulosis*
447.9 Unspecified disorders of arteries and arterioles — *unknown*

448 DISEASE OF CAPILLARIES

448.0 Hereditary hemorrhagic telangiectasia
448.1 Nevus, non-neoplastic — *araneus, senile, spider, stellar*
448.9 Other and unspecified capillary diseases — *not otherwise specified, or unknown; including thrombosis, rupture, hemorrhage, hyperpermeability, telangiectasia*

451-459 Diseases of Veins and Lymphatics, and Other Diseases of Circulatory System

451 PHLEBITIS AND THROMBOPHLEBITIS

Phlebitis is inflammation of a vein. Thrombophlebitis is a partial or complete obstruction of a vein with secondary inflammatory reaction in the wall of the vein. Classify phlebitis and thrombophlebitis according to the vessel. Use an additional E code to identify the drug, if the condition is drug induced.

This rubric excludes thrombophlebitis that is due to or following implant or catheter device (996.61-996.62) or infusion, perfusion, or transfusion (999.2).

451.0 Phlebitis and thrombophlebitis of superficial vessels of lower extremities — (Use additional E code to identify drug, if drug induced) — *inflammation and formation of a blood clot in the superficial veins of the legs and feet; including greater and lesser saphenous veins*
451.11 Phlebitis and thrombophlebitis of femoral vein (deep) (superficial) — *inflammation and formation of a femoral blood clot*
451.19 Phlebitis and thrombophlebitis of other deep vessels of lower extremities — *inflammation and formation of a blood clot in the femoropopliteal, tibia, popliteal veins; blue phlebitis*
451.2 Phlebitis and thrombophlebitis of lower extremities, unspecified — (Use additional E code to identify drug, if drug induced) — *unknown*
451.81 Phlebitis and thrombophlebitis of iliac vein — -- *inflammation and formation of a blood clot*
451.82 Phlebitis and thrombophlebitis of superficial veins of upper extremities — *inflammation and formation of a blood clot in the antecubital, basilic, cephalic veins*
451.83 Phlebitis and thrombophlebitis of deep veins of upper extremities — *inflammation and formation of a blood clot in the brachial, radial, ulnar veins*
451.84 Phlebitis and thrombophlebitis of upper extremities, unspecified — *unknown*
451.89 Phlebitis and thrombophlebitis of other site — *not otherwise specified, including axillary, jugular, subclavian, hepatic, umbilical veins*
451.9 Phlebitis and thrombophlebitis of unspecified site

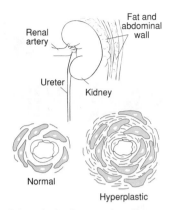

Schematic showing normal renal lumen and one depicting concentric proliferation of smooth muscle cells in the vessel walls

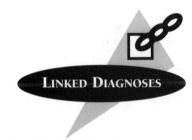

LINKED DIAGNOSES

Classification of Vessels

Deep vein:
Lower extremity: femoral, femoropopliteal, popliteal, tibial

Upper extremity: brachial, radial, ulnar

Superficial vein:
Lower extremity: greater saphenous, lesser saphenous

Upper extremity: antecubital, basilic, cephalic

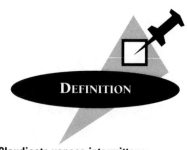

Claudicate venosa intermittens:
stenosis of the arteries causing ischemic muscles, most often in the lower extremities.

Paget-Schroetter syndrome: stress thrombosis of subclavian or axillary vein.

Trousseau's syndrome: spontaneous development of thromboses in extremities as a result of visceral neoplasm.

Phlebectasia varix: venous vasodilation.

Stasis dermatitis: erythema and inflammation of the skin of the lower extremities due to impaired blood flow.

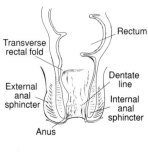

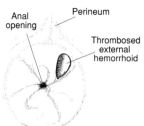

452 PORTAL VEIN THROMBOSIS `OK`

This type of thrombosis describes inflammation and blood clot in the main vein of the liver. The classification excludes hepatic vein thrombosis (453.0) and phlebitis of portal vein (572.1).

453 OTHER VENOUS EMBOLISM AND THROMBOSIS

Deep vein thrombosis may be associated with inflammation, phlebitis and thrombophlebitis. If the documentation states that the thrombus is not associated with inflammation, assign the appropriate code from rubric 453. If the signs and symptoms associated with inflammation (swelling, erythema, pain, induration) are documented, query the physician as to whether the condition is deep vein thrombophlebitis and, if it is, assign a code from rubric 451 instead.

453.0	Budd-Chiari syndrome — *hepatic vein thrombosis with liver enlargement and severe hypertension*
453.1	Thrombophlebitis migrans — *spontaneous, recurring inflammation of veins with blood clots; including Trousseau's and carcinogenic thrombophlebitis syndromes*
453.2	Embolism and thrombosis of vena cava — *blockage and clotting of vena cava*
453.3	Embolism and thrombosis of renal vein — *blockage and clotting of major kidney vein*
453.8	Embolism and thrombosis of other specified veins — *not otherwise specified; including iliac, femoral axillary veins; Paget-Schroetter syndrome*
453.9	Embolism and thrombosis of unspecified site — *unknown*

454 VARICOSE VEINS OF LOWER EXTREMITIES

Varicose veins are dilated, elongated, and tortuous networks in the subcutaneous venous system resulting from valvular incompetence. Other etiologies include congenital or acquired arteriovenous fistulas and valve damage following deep venous thrombophlebitis. The condition develops predominantly in the lower extremities. Most commonly, the long saphenous vein and its tributaries are involved, but the short saphenous vein also may be affected. Symptoms include night cramps, localized pain, edema, inflammation, or hemorrhage and a dull aching or fatigue exacerbated by standing in place.

454.0	Varicose veins of lower extremities with ulcer — *incompetent vein valves allow reversed blood flow and erosion of tissue*
454.1	Varicose veins of lower extremities with inflammation — *incompetent vein valves allow reversed blood flow and inflammation*
454.2	Varicose veins of lower extremities with ulcer and inflammation — *incompetent vein valves allow reversed blood flow, erosion of tissue, and inflammation*
454.9	Varicose veins of lower extremities without mention of ulcer or inflammation — *incompetent vein valves allow reversed blood flow, without complication*

455 HEMORRHOIDS

Hemorrhoids are dilated veins of the hemorrhoidal plexus in the lower rectum. External hemorrhoids are on the outer side of the external sphincter, covered by skin of the anal canal. Internal hemorrhoids are within the external sphincter, covered with rectal mucosa.

Internal hemorrhoids may be classified as first, second, third, or fourth degree. Fourth-degree hemorrhoids are the most severe and are a characterized as both incarcerated and prolapsed; third-degree hemorrhoids are prolapsed. Both third- and fourth-degree hemorrhoids should be classified as complicated.

455.0	Internal hemorrhoids without mention of complication — *reversed blow flow and dilation of vein; contained within rectum*
455.1	Internal thrombosed hemorrhoids — *reversed blow flow and clotted blood in vein; contained within rectum*
455.2	Internal hemorrhoids with other complication — *reversed blow flow with strangulation, ulcer, prolapse, or bleeding; contained within rectum*
455.3	External hemorrhoids without mention of complication — *reversed blow flow and dilation of vein; extending beyond anus*
455.4	External thrombosed hemorrhoids — *reversed blow flow and clotted blood in vein; extending beyond anus*
455.5	External hemorrhoids with other complication — *reversed blow flow with strangulation, ulcer, prolapse, or bleeding; extending beyond anus*
455.6	Unspecified hemorrhoids without mention of complication — *reversed blow flow and dilation of vein; unknown site*
455.7	Unspecified thrombosed hemorrhoids — *reversed blow flow and clotted blood in vein; unknown site*
455.8	Unspecified hemorrhoids with other complication — *reversed blow flow with strangulation, ulcer, prolapse, or bleeding; unknown site*
455.9	Residual hemorrhoidal skin tags — *redundant tissue remains in anus or rectum following treatment of hemorrhoids*

456 VARICOSE VEINS OF OTHER SITES

Varicose veins may occur at sites other than the lower extremities. Esophageal varices are the most clinically significant and comprise longitudinal venous varices located in the distal end of the esophagus. They are almost always due to portal hypertension (456.2). Code the portal hypertension first, followed by 456.20, if bleeding is present, or 456.21, without bleeding.

456.0	Esophageal varices with bleeding — *distended, tortuous veins of the esophagus, with leaking of blood*
456.1	Esophageal varices without mention of bleeding — *distended, tortuous veins of the esophagus, without bleeding*
456.20	Esophageal varices with bleeding in diseases classified elsewhere — (Code first underlying cause, as: 571.0–571.9, 572.3) — *secondary to underlying disease*
456.21	Esophageal varices without mention of bleeding in diseases classified elsewhere — (Code first underlying cause, as: 571.0–571.9, 572.3) — *secondary to underlying disease*
456.3	Sublingual varices — *distended, tortuous veins beneath the tongue*
456.4	Scrotal varices — *distended, tortuous veins of the scrotum*
456.5	Pelvic varices — *distended, tortuous veins within the pelvic region*
456.6	Vulval varices — *distended, tortuous veins of the external female genitalia*
456.8	Varices of other sites — *distended, tortuous veins of sites not otherwise specified, including orbit, pharynx, renal papilla, spine, spleen, urethra, vocal cord, nasal septum*

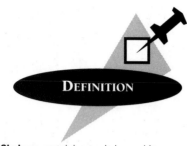

DEFINITION

Chylous: pertaining to chyle, a white or yellowish fluid transferred into the lymphatic system from the intestines as a part of the digestion process.

Elephantiasis: enlargement or swelling of the skin and subcutaneous tissue.

Lymphangiectasis: dilation of the lymphatic system channels.

Phleboliths: a stone-shaped substance consisting of lime and calcium deposited in a vein.

Stasis dermatitis: erythema and inflammation of the skin of the lower extremities due to impaired blood flow.

Vena cava syndrome: an obstruction of the vena cava.

457 NONINFECTIOUS DISORDERS OF LYMPHATIC CHANNELS

Postmastectomy syndrome is a form of lymphedema due to excision of the axillary lymphatic structures during mastectomy.

457.0	Postmastectomy lymphedema syndrome — *edema in arms and hands caused by pooling in interstitial fluids, due to reduced lymphatic circulation*
457.1	Other noninfectious lymphedema — *other retention of fluids due to reduced lymphatic circulation; including elephantiasis, lymphedema*
457.2	Lymphangitis — *subacute or chronic inflammation of the lymph glands*
457.8	Other noninfectious disorders of lymphatic channels — *not otherwise specified, including sclerotic lymph gland, chylocele, or lymph node fistula, cyst infarction, or rupture*
457.9	Unspecified noninfectious disorder of lymphatic channels — *unknown*

458 HYPOTENSION

Orthostatic hypotension is an excessive fall in blood pressure when assuming an erect position. Severe orthostatic hypotension can be associated with a neuropathic disorder known as Shy-Drager syndrome or idiopathic orthostatic hypotension, classified to 333.0. It may also be due to volume depletion.

Iatrogenic hypotension or postoperative hypotension is classified to 458.2. This code fully describes postoperative hypotension and does not require an additional code to indicate complication of surgical or medical care.

Use code 458.8 to code postmyocardial infarction hypotension. Sequence the myocardial infarction code first.

458.0	Orthostatic hypotension — *abnormally low blood pressure worsened when the seated patient stands*
458.1	Chronic hypotension — *persistent abnormally low blood pressure*
458.2	Iatrogenic hypotension — *abnormally low blood pressure as a result of medical treatment*
458.8	Other specified hypotension — *not otherwise specified*
458.9	Unspecified hypotension — *unknown*

459 OTHER DISORDERS OF CIRCULATORY SYSTEM

Excluded from this rubric are cases of hemorrhage due to trauma. Postphlebitic syndrome is a complex of symptoms due to venous hypertension as a consequence of postphlebitic incompetence of communicating veins.

459.0	Unspecified hemorrhage — *spontaneous rupture of blood vessel, not otherwise specified*
459.1	Postphlebitic syndrome — *complex symptoms including deep vein thrombosis with edema, pain, purpura, increased cutaneous pigmentation and eczema*
459.2	Compression of vein — *stricture of vein; vena cava syndrome*
459.81	Unspecified venous (peripheral) insufficiency — (Use additional code for any associated ulceration: 707.10-707.9) — *unknown*
459.89	Other specified circulatory system disorders — *not otherwise specified*
459.9	Unspecified circulatory system disorder — *unknown site and unknown disorder*

✔5th Needs fifth-digit   **OK** Valid three-digit code

Chapter 8

460-519
Diseases of the Respiratory System

This chapter classifies diseases and disorders of the nose (external, nasal cavity), sinuses (frontal, ethmoid, sphenoid, maxillary), pharynx (nasopharynx, oropharynx), larynx (true and false vocal cords, glottis), trachea, bronchi (left, right, main, carina), and lungs (intrapulmonary bronchi, bronchioli, lobes, alveoli, pleura).

This complex of organs is responsible for pulmonary ventilation and the exchange of oxygen and carbon dioxide between the lungs and ambient air. The organs of the respiratory system also perform nonrespiratory functions such as warming and moisturizing the air passing into the lungs, providing airflow for the larynx and vocal cords for speech, and releasing excess body heat in the process of thermoregulation for homeostasis. The lung also performs important metabolic and embolic filtering functions.

Pneumonia is found in this chapter and is classified according to the infective agent. For bronchitis and other infection, code first the infection, and report the infective agent, classified to Chapter 1 Infectious and Parasitic Diseases, secondarily.

460-466 Acute Respiratory Infections

Pneumonia and influenza are excluded from this section and can be found in rubrics 480-487.8.

460 ACUTE NASOPHARYNGITIS [COMMON COLD] OK

This rubric classifies nasopharyngitis, rhinitis, coryza, or nasal catarrh of an acute nature. Chronic nasopharyngitis is reported with 472.2. Acute nasopharyngitis is the most common of the upper respiratory infections, and is characterized by edema of the nasal mucous membrane, discharge, and obstruction.

461 ACUTE SINUSITIS

This rubric classifies sinusitis that is sudden and severe, according to the site of infection: frontal, maxillary, ethmoidal, sphenoidal, or multiple sites. Included in the definition of acute sinusitis are abscess, empyema, and suppuration. Acute sinusitis is usually preceded by an acute respiratory infection. A second code from Chapter 1 Infectious and Parasitic Diseases can be reported to identify the infectious agent, which most commonly is *streptococci*, *pneumococci*, *H. influenzae*, or *staphylococci*. In the case of immunocompromised patients, the infectious agents are more likely to be *aspergillosis*, *candidiasis*, or fungal infections of the order *Mucorales*.

Chronic sinusitis is excluded from this rubric and is reported with 473.0-473.9.

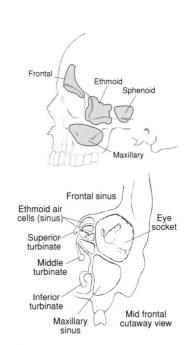

461.0	Acute maxillary sinusitis — *behind cheekbones*
461.1	Acute frontal sinusitis — *above the eyes*
461.2	Acute ethmoidal sinusitis — *between the eyes on either side of the nose*
461.3	Acute sphenoidal sinusitis — *behind the eyes on either side of the nose*
461.8	Other acute sinusitis — *pansinusitis*
461.9	Acute sinusitis, unspecified — *unknown*

462 ACUTE PHARYNGITIS OK

Acute pharyngitis is an acute inflammatory disorder of the throat, which may be caused by a virus or bacteria. Frequently, coryza or other communicable disease precedes acute pharyngitis. A code from Chapter 1 Infectious and Parasitic Diseases of ICD-9 can be reported secondarily to identify the infective agent in pharyngitis. The most common causes are the infectious agent *streptococci*, *mycoplasma pneumoniae*, *Chlamydia pneumoniae*, or a virus.

Signs and symptoms of acute pharyngitis include history of tobacco or alcohol abuse, sore throat, dysphagia, fever, headache, and muscle and joint pain.

Therapies include warm saline gargles and analgesics such as aspirin to relieve throat discomfort, bed rest, IV hydration in severe cases, and antibiotics for suspected bacterial acute pharyngitis. Associated conditions include dehydration, sinusitis, and allergies.

Do not use this code to report chronic pharyngitis (472.1), abscess of the peritonsillar region (475), pharynx (478.29), or retropharynx (478.24). Also excluded is acute pharyngitis due to Coxsackie virus (074.0), gonococcus (098.6), herpes simplex (054.79), flu (487.1), or streptococcus (034.0). Septic pharyngitis is reported with 034.0.

463 ACUTE TONSILLITIS OK

A sudden severe inflammation of the palatine tonsil is classified to this rubric. The infective agent is most commonly streptococcal or viral. Tonsillitis may be accompanied by throat pain, high fever, and in some cases, vomiting.

Excluded from this rubric are chronic tonsillitis (474.0), hypertrophy of tonsil (474.1), streptococcal tonsillitis (034.0), and sore throat not otherwise specified (462).

464 ACUTE LARYNGITIS AND TRACHEITIS

Sudden and severe inflammation of the larynx, trachea, and epiglottis associated with infection are classified to this rubric, with obstruction of the airway being an axis for code choice. Laryngitis and tracheitis usually follow an upper respiratory infection, but may occur during the course of pneumonia, bronchitis, flu, or measles. Excluded from this rubric are cases associated with the flu (487.1) or strep infection (034.0). For chronic laryngitis, see rubric 476; for chronic tracheitis, report 491.8.

If inflammation of the larynx is combined with inflammation of the trachea, report codes from the subclassification 464.2 Acute laryngotracheitis.

The definition of acute epiglottitis is acute inflammation of the epiglottis. Acute epiglottitis usually is due to an infection by *Haemophilus influenzae*, pneumococci or group A *streptococci* and can develop into a laryngeal airway obstruction. Signs and symptoms of

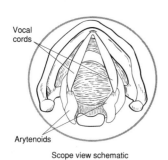

Vocal cords

Arytenoids

Scope view schematic of vocal cords

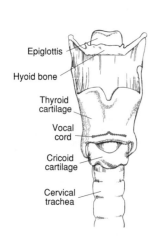

Epiglottis

Hyoid bone

Thyroid cartilage

Vocal cord

Cricoid cartilage

Cervical trachea

✔5th	Needs fifth-digit	OK	Valid three-digit code

acute epiglottitis include history of upper respiratory infection or chronic lung disease, high fever, sore throat, dysphagia, stridor, and respiratory distress.

Diagnostic tests/reports/findings include throat exam to reveal enlarged, edematous epiglottis. Laryngoscopy or lateral neck x-rays reveal inflammatory changes and signs of obstruction. Therapies include endotracheal intubation for obstruction, IV hydration to prevent dehydration, antibiotics (parenteral), oxygen therapy, and blood gas monitoring for hypoxia and hypercapnia.

Croup is an acute laryngotracheobronchitis usually seen early childhood and characterized by stridor, respiratory distress, and swelling. Parainfluenza virus is usually the infective agent, although respiratory syncytial virus can also cause croup.

464.0	Acute laryngitis — *septic, H. influenzae, pneumococcal, suppurative, ulcerative*
464.10	Acute tracheitis without mention of obstruction — *sudden, severe inflammation of vocal cords*
464.11	Acute tracheitis with obstruction — *sudden, severe inflammation of vocal cords w/ obstruction*
464.20	Acute laryngotracheitis without mention of obstruction — *sudden, severe inflammation of trachea and vocal cords*
464.21	Acute laryngotracheitis with obstruction — *sudden, severe inflammation of trachea and vocal cords w/ obstruction*
464.30	Acute epiglottitis without mention of obstruction — *sudden, severe inflammation of epiglottis*
464.31	Acute epiglottitis with obstruction — *sudden, severe inflammation of epiglottis w/ obstruction*
464.4	Croup — *barking cough with inflammation of larynx*

465 ACUTE UPPER RESPIRATORY INFECTIONS OF MULTIPLE OR UNSPECIFIED SITES

This rubric is reserved for acute infections of multiple sites or when the site is not otherwise specified. Excluded from this rubric are upper respiratory infections due to flu (487.1) or strep (034.0).

465.0	Acute laryngopharyngitis — *sudden, severe inflammation of vocal cords and pharynx*
465.8	Acute upper respiratory infections of other multiple sites — *multiple URI*
465.9	Acute upper respiratory infections of unspecified site — *unknown site, URI*

466 ACUTE BRONCHITIS AND BRONCHIOLITIS

Acute bronchitis is sudden and severe inflammation of the tracheobronchial tree. Acute bronchitis may have an infectious or irritative etiology.

Signs and symptoms of acute bronchitis include history of upper respiratory infection or exposure to irritants such as dust or fumes, cough, malaise, fever, and pain in back and chest. Therapies include bed rest and antibiotics such as oral tetracycline when purulent sputum is present. For patients with chronic respiratory disease, therapy includes antipyretics for fever, bronchodilators for bronchial asthma, and monitoring of arterial blood gases (ABGs) in cases of significant underlying chronic respiratory disease.

Associated conditions include underlying chronic lung disease such as chronic obstructive bronchitis or COPD, pneumonia or bronchopneumonia, or allergies. Excluded from this rubric are acute bronchitis with asthma (493), bronchiectasis (494.1), and COPD (491.21).

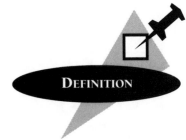

DEFINITION

Dyspnea: symptom of perceived difficulty in breathing.

Orthopnea: respiratory discomfort upon reclining, forcing the patient to sit up.

Cyanosis: bluish skin color resulting from a decrease in the oxygen level in the blood.

Croupous bronchitis: inflammatory process of the bronchial membrane in which a fibrinous drainage hardens forming a shell around the inside of the bronchial tree which obstructs the flow of air.

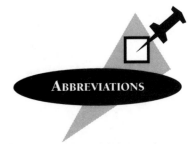

ABBREVIATIONS

RSV: respiratory syncytial virus, a minor respiratory infection in adults with symptoms of a cough and nasal drainage and can be a severe infection in children causing bronchitis and bronchopneumonia

URI: upper respiratory tract infection

466.0	Acute bronchitis — *sudden, severe inflammation of bronchial tree main branches*
466.11	Acute bronchiolitis due to respiratory syncytial virus (RSV) — *bronchiolitis, capillary pneumonia due to RSV*
466.19	Acute bronchiolitis due to other infectious organisms — *bronchiolitis, capillary pneumonia, other infectious agent*

470-478 Other Diseases of the Upper Respiratory Tract

Included in this rubric are many chronic inflammatory diseases of the upper respiratory tract.

470 DEVIATED NASAL SEPTUM OK

Deviated nasal septum is a common disorder that often requires no treatment. However, in some cases, the deviation in the septum, the result of past trauma, causes obstructions in the nasal passages that lead to chronic conditions like sinusitis or epistaxis. If the deviation predisposes the patient to chronic problems, the condition may be treated surgically. When coding, sequence the code for sinusitis or epistaxis first, and the deviation secondarily.

Excluded from this rubric is congenital deviated septum, which is reported with 754.0.

471 NASAL POLYPS

Nasal polyps are a natural reaction to chronic sinusitis due to infection or allergy. Polyps most commonly form around the ostia of the maxillary sinus, and are classified according to site. Polyps may be asymptomatic, or they may block the nasal airways or promote chronic sinus infection.

Excluded from this rubric is adenomatous polyps (212.0).

471.0	Polyp of nasal cavity — *choanal, nasopharyngeal*
471.1	Polypoid sinus degeneration — *Woakes' syndrome or ethmoiditis*
471.8	Other polyp of sinus — *accessory, ethmoidal, maxillary, sphenoidal, frontal, turbinate, mucous membrane*
471.9	Unspecified nasal polyp — *nasal polyp*

472 CHRONIC PHARYNGITIS AND NASOPHARYNGITIS

Persistent inflammation of the pharynx and nasopharynx can be the result of an infective agent or due to an allergy or exposure to an irritant. Allergic rhinitis (477) is excluded from this rubric, as are all acute forms of pharyngitis or nasopharyngitis.

472.0	Chronic rhinitis — *persistent ozena, atrophic, granulomatous, purulent, ulcerative*
472.1	Chronic pharyngitis — *persistent sore throat, atrophic, hypertrophic*
472.2	Chronic nasopharyngitis — *persistent inflammation from the nares to the pharynx*

473 CHRONIC SINUSITIS

Chronic sinusitis includes any persistent abscess, empyema, or infection of the nasal sinuses. It can be caused by an infective agent or by exposure to an allergic agent or irritant. Code selection is based on site: maxillary, frontal, ethmoidal, sphenoidal, or multiple sites. Excluded from this rubric is acute sinusitis, which is classified to rubric 461.

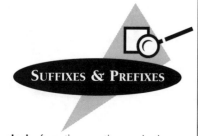

SUFFIXES & PREFIXES

-plasia: formation, creation, production

-trophic: nourishment

A-: absence of

Hyper-: above, more than, over

5th — Needs fifth-digit   OK Valid three-digit code

473.0	Chronic maxillary sinusitis — *persistent inflammation of the sinus cavities behind the cheekbone; cloudy antrum*
473.1	Chronic frontal sinusitis — *persistent inflammation of the sinus cavities above the eyes*
473.2	Chronic ethmoidal sinusitis — *persistent inflammation of the sinus cavities between the eyes on either side of the nose*
473.3	Chronic sphenoidal sinusitis — *persistent inflammation of the sinus cavities behind the eyes on either side of the nose*
473.8	Other chronic sinusitis — *persistent pansinusitis*
473.9	Unspecified sinusitis (chronic) — *persistent sinusitis, unknown site*

474 CHRONIC DISEASE OF TONSILS AND ADENOIDS
Excluded from this rubric is acute or unspecified tonsillitis, which is classified to 463.

474.00	Chronic tonsillitis — *persistent inflammation, tonsil*
474.01	Chronic adenoiditis — *persistent inflammation, adenoid*
474.02	Chronic tonsillitis and adenoiditis — *persistent inflammation tonsil and adenoid*
474.10	Hypertrophy of tonsil with adenoids — *enlargement, tonsil and adenoid*
474.11	Hypertrophy of tonsils alone — *enlargement, tonsil*
474.12	Hypertrophy of adenoids alone — *enlargement, adenoid*
474.2	Adenoid vegetations — *fungus-like growth*
474.8	Other chronic disease of tonsils and adenoids — *including amygdalolith, calculus, cicatrix, tag, ulcer, cyst, plica, necrosis*
474.9	Unspecified chronic disease of tonsils and adenoids — *unknown*

475 PERITONSILLAR ABSCESS OK
Use this code to report an abscess of the tonsil, peritonsillar cellulitis, or Quinsy. In peritonsillar abscess, tonsillitis extends beyond tonsillar tissue to include soft palate or the space between the tonsillar pillars. Excluded from this rubric are chronic tonsillitis (474.0) and acute tonsillitis (463).

476 CHRONIC LARYNGITIS AND LARYNGOTRACHEITIS
Chronic laryngitis and laryngotracheitis are related to allergic reactions, inhalation of irritants, gastroesophageal reflux, or voice overuse. The voice is compromised, hoarse, or absent. Excluded from this rubric are chronic inflammations of the trachea (491.8) and acute laryngitis or tracheitis, classified to 464.0-464.4.

476.0	Chronic laryngitis — *persistent inflammation, vocal cords*
476.1	Chronic laryngotracheitis — *persistent inflammation, vocal cords and trachea*

477 ALLERGIC RHINITIS
477.0	Allergic rhinitis due to pollen — *pollinosis*
477.1	Allergic rhinitis, due to food — *allergic rhinitis*
477.8	Allergic rhinitis due to other allergen — *nonfood*
477.9	Allergic rhinitis, cause unspecified — *unknown*

478 OTHER DISEASES OF UPPER RESPIRATORY TRACT
Tornwaldt's cyst is a superficial nasopharyngeal cyst that causes purulent exudate and drainage, sore throat, and eustachian tube complications. It is reported with 478.26.

478.0	Hypertrophy of nasal turbinates — *overgrowth of nasal cavity bones*
478.1	Other diseases of nasal cavity and sinuses — *including abscess, necrosis, ulcer, cyst, mucocele, rhinolith*

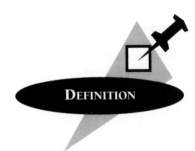

DEFINITION

Reinke's space: subepithelial space in the vocal cords in which fluid accumulates to cause laryngitis.

Pyocele: a sac-like pus accumulation.

Vacuum: a space void of air and gas; empty.

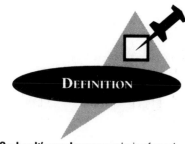

Gerhardt's syndrome: paralysis of vocal cords causing inspiratory dyspnea.

Millar's asthma: asthma caused by inhaling flour allergens.

Singer's nodes: nodules on the vocal cords.

Thornwaldt's bursitis: also Tornwaldt's, a chronic pharyngeal infection, symptoms include nasal discharge, headache, and cervical muscle stiffness.

478.20	Unspecified disease of pharynx — *unknown*
478.21	Cellulitis of pharynx or nasopharynx — *inflammation of deep, soft tissues*
478.22	Parapharyngeal abscess — *pocket of pus*
478.24	Retropharyngeal abscess — *pocket of pus*
478.25	Edema of pharynx or nasopharynx — *fluid retention*
478.26	Cyst of pharynx or nasopharynx — *fluid-filled sac*
478.29	Other disease of pharynx or nasopharynx — *including abscess, hyperactive gag reflex, polyp, Tornwaldt's bursitis, ulcer, perforation, spontaneous rupture*
478.30	Unspecified paralysis of vocal cords or larynx — *unknown side*
478.31	Unilateral partial paralysis of vocal cords or larynx — *one side*
478.32	Unilateral complete paralysis of vocal cords or larynx — *one side*
478.33	Bilateral partial paralysis of vocal cords or larynx — *both sides*
478.34	Bilateral complete paralysis of vocal cords or larynx — *both sides*
478.4	Polyp of vocal cord or larynx — *growth of benign tissue*
478.5	Other diseases of vocal cords — *including abscess, cellulitis, granuloma, leukoplakia, chorditis, singer's nodes*
478.6	Edema of larynx — *fluid retention*
478.70	Unspecified disease of larynx — *unknown*
478.71	Cellulitis and perichondritis of larynx — *inflammation of deep soft tissue*
478.74	Stenosis of larynx — *narrowing of the diameter of larynx*
478.75	Laryngeal spasm — *involuntary muscle contraction; laryngismus, Millar's asthma*
478.79	Other diseases of larynx — *including abscess, necrosis, obstruction, pachyderma, ulcer, nodule, ossification, sclerosis*
478.8	Upper respiratory tract hypersensitivity reaction, site unspecified — *site unknown*
478.9	Other and unspecified diseases of upper respiratory tract — *including abscess and cicatrix of trachea, not otherwise specified*

480-487 Pneumonia and Influenza

Pneumonia and influenza are inflammations in the alveolar parenchyma of the lung caused by microbial infection, irradiation, or physicochemical agents. Microbial agents include viral, bacterial, fungal, protozoal, mycobacterial, mycoplasmal, or rickettsial pathogens. Physicochemical agents may be inhaled or reach the lung via the bloodstream. Inhaled agents include toxic gases, irritant particles or irritant fluids such as gastric juice. Bleomycin is an example of a blood-borne anticancer agent that can cause pneumonia.

The terms "pneumonia" and "pneumonitis" describe two clinical patterns of inflammatory reaction in the lung. The unqualified term "pneumonia" generally refers to pneumonia with exudation in the air spaces. Inflammatory exudate fills the lung alveoli, which are then rendered airless and solid, in a process called consolidation. The terms "pneumonitis" and "interstitial pneumonia" commonly refer to pneumonia with interstitial exudate.

Signs and symptoms of pneumonia and influenza vary according to etiology (for example, with bacterial pneumonia, coughing, sputum production, pleuritic chest pain, shaking chills, fever; with aspiration pneumonia, chest rales, dyspnea, cyanosis, hypotension, and tachycardia).

In pneumonia, chest x-ray shows infiltration or consolidation. Blood work may show normal, slightly elevated or markedly elevated white blood cell count (WBC), depending on etiology. Smears, cultures, and gram stains of sputum and/or pleural fluid isolate and identify bacteria. Percutaneous aspiration of lung tissue, endoscopic or open lung, biopsy identifies difficult nonbacterial agents such as cytomegalovirus.

➤5th   Needs fifth-digit   **OK**   Valid three-digit code

Therapies include antibiotics for confirmed and suspected bacterial pneumonia, oxygen therapy, complete bed rest, and intubation and ventilatory support for critically ill patients developing respiratory failure. In addition, there is respiratory therapy, which involves suctioning, coughing, and deep breathing exercises.

Associated conditions include pleural effusion, respiratory failure, empyema, atelectasis, and underlying chronic lung disease such as COPD.

To ensure proper code assignment, first refer to the ICD-9-CM index under the main terms "Pneumonia" and "Pneumonitis." Many forms of pneumonia are classified to other chapters of ICD-9-CM because of etiology. For example, candidal pneumonia is classified to code 112.4, and congenital toxoplasmosis pneumonitis is classified to codes 771.2 and 484.8.

480 VIRAL PNEUMONIA

480.0	Pneumonia due to adenovirus — *viral infection of lung*
480.1	Pneumonia due to respiratory syncytial virus — *viral infection of lung*
480.2	Pneumonia due to parainfluenza virus — *viral infection of lung*
480.8	Pneumonia due to other virus not elsewhere classified — *viral infection of lung*
480.9	Unspecified viral pneumonia — *viral infection of lung, unknown virus*

481 PNEUMOCOCCAL PNEUMONIA (STREPTOCOCCUS PNEUMONIAE PNEUMONIA) OK

482 OTHER BACTERIAL PNEUMONIA

482.0	Pneumonia due to Klebsiella pneumoniae — *bacterial infection of lung*
482.1	Pneumonia due to Pseudomonas — *bacterial infection of lung*
482.2	Pneumonia due to Hemophilus influenzae (H. influenzae) — *bacterial infection of lung*

482.3 Pneumonia due to Streptococcus
This rubric excludes pneumonia due to Streptococcus pneumoniae (481).

482.30	Pneumonia due to unspecified Streptococcus — *strep infection of lung, unknown variety*
482.31	Pneumonia due to Streptococcus, group A — *strep infection of lung*
482.32	Pneumonia due to Streptococcus, group B — *strep infection of lung*
482.39	Pneumonia due to other Streptococcus — *strep infection of lung, not otherwise specified*
482.40	Pneumonia due to Staphylococcus, unspecified — *staph infection of lung, unknown variety*
482.41	Pneumonia due to Staphylococcus aureus — *staph infection of lung*
482.49	Other Staphylococcus pneumonia — *staph infection of lung, unknown variety*
482.81	Pneumonia due to anaerobes — *bacteroides, gram-negative anaerobes*
482.82	Pneumonia due to escherichia coli (E. coli)
482.83	Pneumonia due to other gram-negative bacteria — *proteus, Serratia marcescens, gram-negative not otherwise specified*
482.84	Legionnaires' disease
482.89	Pneumonia due to other specified bacteria — *not elsewhere classified*
482.9	Unspecified bacterial pneumonia — *bacterial pneumonia, unknown*

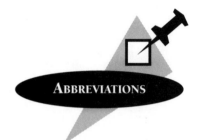

ABBREVIATIONS

CMV: cytomegalovirus

PPLO: pleuropneumonia-like organism

RSV: respiratory syncytial virus

E. coli: escherichia coli

H. influenzae: hemophilus influenzae

Staph: staphylococcus

Strep: streptococcus

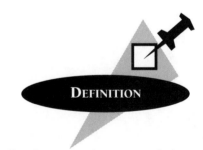

DEFINITION

Eaton's agent: a primary pneumonia that becomes systemic, caused by *Mycoplasma pneumoniae.*

Pneumatocele: a gas-filled swelling or cavity formed in the lung. Occurs often with staphylococcus pneumonia.

Serratia marcescens: a gram-negative bacteria found in food, water and insects.

483 PNEUMONIA DUE TO OTHER SPECIFIED ORGANISM

483.0 Pneumonia due to Mycoplasma pneumoniae — *Eaton's agent, pleuropneumonia-like organism [PPLO]*

Mycoplasma pneumoniae is also known as Eaton agent pneumonia.

Signs and symptoms of pneumonia due to *mycoplasma pneumoniae* include history of recent upper respiratory infection or bronchitis, headache, fever, severe and minimally productive cough, harsh or diminished breath sounds, earache, and cervical lymphadenopathy.

Diagnostic tests include gram stain and culture of sputum or throat washing to reveal polymorphonuclear leukocytes with no dominant organism. Other lab work demonstrates fourfold or greater rise in complement-fixing antibodies and elevated cold agglutinins (IgM antibodies binding to the erythrocyte I antigen). Chest x-ray shows pulmonary infiltrates resembling bacterial or viral pneumonia.

Therapies include antibiotics such as erythromycin or tetracycline, bed rest, and high protein diet.

Associated conditions include cold agglutinin induced hemolytic anemia, arthralgia and polyarthritis, skin rashes, Stevens-Johnson syndrome, transverse myelitis, meningoencephalitis, and myocarditis.

483.1 Pneumonia due to Chlamydia
483.8 Pneumonia due to other specified organism — *not elsewhere classified*

484 PNEUMONIA IN INFECTIOUS DISEASES CLASSIFIED ELSEWHERE

484.1 Pneumonia in cytomegalic inclusion disease — (Code first underlying disease 078.5) — *infection of lung*
484.3 Pneumonia in whooping cough — (Code first underlying disease 033.0–033.9) — *infection of lung*
484.5 Pneumonia in anthrax — (Code first underlying disease 022.1) — *infection of lung*
484.6 Pneumonia in aspergillosis — (Code first underlying disease 117.3) — *infection of lung*
484.7 Pneumonia in other systemic mycoses — (Code first underlying disease) — *infection of lung*
484.8 Pneumonia in other infectious diseases classified elsewhere — (Code first underlying disease, as: 002.0, 083.0) — *infection of lung*

485 BRONCHOPNEUMONIA, ORGANISM UNSPECIFIED `OK`

486 PNEUMONIA, ORGANISM UNSPECIFIED `OK`

487 INFLUENZA

Influenza is an acute respiratory infection due to orthomyxoviruses characterized by the abrupt onset of acute tracheobronchitis. The severity of the disease varies from a mild upper respiratory infection to an extensive pneumonia that can be fatal.

✔5th Needs fifth-digit   `OK` Valid three-digit code

Influenza virus types A is the most common and causes epidemics of varying severity. Influenza virus type B is associated with more limited epidemics and has been linked to Reye's syndrome. Influenza virus type C is an uncommon strain that causes very mild upper respiratory symptoms.

Signs and symptoms of influenza include fever, chills, malaise, cough, muscle aches, and excessive catarrh.

Diagnostic tests/reports/findings include blood work that may show leukopenia and proteinuria. Inoculation of embryonated eggs or cell cultures of throat washing isolate the virus. Chest x-ray may show pneumonia, commonly due to secondary pneumococcal or staphylococcal pneumonia.

Therapies include bed rest, antibiotics for secondary bacterial pneumonia, antipyretics for fever, and aerosol ribavirin for influenza type A or B.

Associated conditions include Reye's syndrome, secondary pneumococcal or staphylococcal pneumonia, acute sinusitis, otitis media, and, rarely, circulatory system complications such as pericarditis, myocarditis, and thrombophlebitis.

487.0	Influenza with pneumonia — *flu with any form of pneumonia or bronchopneumonia*
487.1	Influenza with other respiratory manifestations — *flu with upper respiratory infection [URI], except pneumonia or bronchopneumonia*
487.8	Influenza with other manifestations — *including encephalopathy*

490-496 Chronic Obstructive Pulmonary Disease and Allied Conditions

490 BRONCHITIS, NOT SPECIFIED AS ACUTE OR CHRONIC OK

Excluded from this rubric is bronchitis due to allergy (493.9), fumes and vapors (506.0), or with asthma (493.9).

491 CHRONIC BRONCHITIS

491.0	Simple chronic bronchitis — *persistent, catarrhal, smoker's cough*
491.1	Mucopurulent chronic bronchitis — *persistent, purulent, recurrent*

491.2 Obstructive chronic bronchitis

Obstructive chronic bronchitis is chronic bronchitis combined with obstructive lung disease. Chronic bronchitis is defined as a persistent cough with sputum production occurring on most days for at least three months of the year for at least two years. Obstructive lung disease is defined as a chronic or recurrent reduction in expiratory airflow within the lung. Obstructive chronic bronchitis is characterized by an increased mass of mucous glands in the lung, resulting in an increase in the thickness of the bronchial mucosa. Its most common etiology is cigarette smoking, but it also may be caused by environmental pollution or inhalation of irritant chemicals.

Signs and symptoms of obstructive chronic bronchitis include history of cigarette smoking or other respiratory irritants, sputum productive cough, exertional dyspnea, weight gain due to edema, cyanosis, tachypnea, rhonchi, wheezing with prolonged expiratory time, use of accessory muscles of respiration, jugular or neck vein distention, and pedal edema.

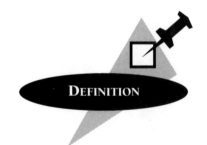

DEFINITION

Blue bloater: a term used to identify patients with a severe bronchial disorder in which hypercapnia and hypoxemia set in early in the disease process.

Pink puffer: also Swyer-James and MacLeod's, acquired unilateral hyperlucent lung with severe airway obstruction during expiration, oligemia, and a small hilum. Also, a term used to identify patients with severe emphysema but a normal ventilation effort. Hypercapnia and hypoxemia usually doesn't appear until later stages in the disease process.

Diagnostic tests include chest x-ray that may show hyperinflation with increased bronchovascular markings. Pulmonary function tests show increased residual volume, decreased vital capacity, and forced expiratory volumes, normal static compliance, and diffusing capacity; ABGs reveal decreased pO_2 and normal or increased pCO_2. Culture of sputum reveals many neutrophils and varied organisms.

Therapies include oxygen therapy for hypoxia, antibiotics for concomitant respiratory infections, bronchodilators such as aminophylline to control bronchospasm and promote mucociliary expectoration, diuretics for edema, and ultrasonic or mechanical nebulizer treatments to loosen and help mobilize secretions.

Associated conditions include respiratory failure, atrial arrhythmias, and acute respiratory infections.

Assign a fifth digit 0 to indicate obstructive chronic bronchitis without mention of acute exacerbation and fifth digit 1 for obstructive chronic bronchitis with acute exacerbation. Acute exacerbation of chronic obstructive bronchitis is not the same as acute bronchitis (code 466.0), so do not assign code 466.0 as an additional code or substitute code for 491.21. However, when the condition causing the acute exacerbation is known, it may be listed as an additional code (principal diagnosis if appropriate). For example, the diagnosis of acute exacerbation of chronic bronchitis due to acute influenzal upper respiratory infection is coded as 487.1 and 491.21.

491.20	Obstructive chronic bronchitis without mention of acute exacerbation — *persistent, with asthma, emphysema*
491.21	Obstructive chronic bronchitis with acute exacerbation — *persistent, with asthma, emphysema, with sudden worsening of condition*
491.8	Other chronic bronchitis — *including tracheitis or tracheobronchitis*
491.9	Unspecified chronic bronchitis — *unknown type*

492 EMPHYSEMA

Emphysema refers to any condition in which air is present in a small area of an organ or tissue, for example, in the interstices of the conjunctival tissue. Emphysema classified to category 492 refers to pulmonary emphysema only.

492.0 Emphysematous bleb — *tension pneumatocele, vanishing lung, giant bullous emphysema*

The definition of emphysematous bleb is a disease characterized by the formation of subpleural, air-filled cystlike structures that are greater than one centimeter in diameter. Also known as emphysematous bullae, they can be found in association with other forms of pulmonary emphysema or can occur alone, especially in younger patients. Apical bullae are the most common cause of spontaneous pneumothorax in young patients.

492.8 Other emphysema — *including pink puffer, MacLeod's syndrome, Swyer-James syndrome*

Other emphysema is abnormal irreversible enlargement of the air spaces distal to the terminal bronchioli accompanied by destruction of alveolar walls. The condition results in a reduction of the alveolar surface necessary for gas exchange. There are two major types of pulmonary emphysema: centroacinar and panacinar.

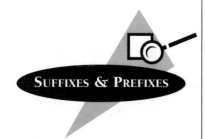

SUFFIXES & PREFIXES

-capnia: also -carbia, denotes carbon dioxide

-oxemia: combined suffixes meaning oxygen in the blood

Hyper-: above, more than, over

Hypo-: below, less than, under

⌐5th Needs fifth-digit   **OK** Valid three-digit code

Centroacinar, or centrilobar, emphysema affects the central parts of the lung acini and destroys the respiratory bronchioli. It often is associated with chronic bronchitis and smoking.

Panacinar, or pan lobar, emphysema destroys the alveolar walls and is distributed uniformly among the lung acini. The disease is more diffuse than centroacinar emphysema. Like centroacinar emphysema, panacinar emphysema occurs in cigarette smokers, but is also found in young adults with a familial history of emphysema.

Signs and symptoms of other emphysema include history of cigarette smoking, barrel-chested appearance, shortness of breath, anorexia, weight loss, breathing abnormalities such as the use of accessory muscles, prolonged expiration, grunting, pursed lip breathing, tachypnea, peripheral cyanosis, and digital clubbing.

Associated conditions include recurrent respiratory infections, cor pulmonale, and respiratory failure.

Other forms of pulmonary emphysema classified to this subcategory are distal acinar or paraseptal emphysema, irregular or paracicatricial emphysema, mixed emphysema, and unclassified forms of emphysema.

When chronic (obstructive) bronchitis is coupled with a diagnosis of centroacinar or panacinar emphysema, assign a code from 491.2.

493 ASTHMA

Asthma is the narrowing of the airways due to increased responsiveness of the trachea and bronchi to various stimuli. Asthma is reversible, changing in severity either spontaneously or as a result of treatment. Asthma is associated with bronchospasm and pathologic features such as increased mucous secretion, mucosal edema and hyperemia, hypertrophy of bronchial smooth muscle, and acute inflammation.

Signs and symptoms of asthma include recurrent or chronic episodes of wheezing, dyspnea, cough, chest tightness, chest pain, tachycardia, tachypnea, increased accessory muscle respiration, and history of familial allergy.

Diagnostic tests include blood work that may show increased WBC during acute attack and eosinophilia. ABGs may show hypoxemia and respiratory alkalosis. Gross exam of sputum demonstrates viscidity, while microscopic exam of sputum reveals mucus casts, eosinophils, and elongated rhomboid crystals. Pulmonary function tests show typical abnormalities of obstructive dysfunction. Chest x-ray may show hyperinflated lungs and skin tests and inhalation bronchial challenge tests identify and evaluate clinical significance of allergens.

Therapies include bronchodilators such as epinephrine, aminophylline, albuterol; other medications such as cromolyn sodium, anticholinergics, corticosteroids, hyposensitization or "allergy" shots; oxygen therapy; and intubation and ventilation therapy for severe attacks of asthma.

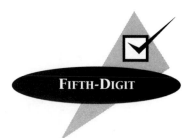

The following fifth-digit subclassification is for use with category 493:

0 without mention of status asthmaticus

1 with status asthmaticus

2 with acute exacerbation

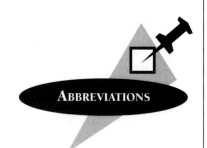

ABBREVIATIONS

ERV: expiratory reserve volume

FRC: functional residual capacity

FVC: forced vital capacity

MEP: maximal expiratory pressure

MIP: maximal inspiratory pressure

MVV: maximal voluntary ventilation

PEF: peak expiratory flow

PFT: pulmonary function testing

PND: paroxysmal nocturnal dyspnea

RV: residual volume

TLC: total lung capacity

VC: vital capacity

Associated conditions include respiratory failure, eosinophilia, pneumothorax, acute cor pulmonale, and atelectasis.

Triad asthma is a syndrome that occurs in patients with three conditions that can be coded: intrinsic asthma (subclassification 493.0), aspirin sensitivity (apply codes according to ICD-9-CM coding rules regarding adverse reaction), and nasal polyposis (rubric 471).

In ICD-9, asthma is classified as extrinsic, intrinsic, or unspecified. Extrinsic asthma is asthma due to allergenic exposure to substances such as pollen, house dust, animal dander, molds, food or beverages, vapors, or drugs. Most prevalent in children, this condition is associated with abnormally high levels of IgE immunoglobulins, indicating an allergic reaction.

Intrinsic asthma is asthma due to nonallergenic factors such as emotional stresses, fatigue, endocrine changes, irritants (nonallergenic) such as dust and chemicals, and acute respiratory infection. More prevalent in adults, intrinsic asthma is associated with normal IgE immunoglobulin levels, indicating a nonallergic reaction.

This differentiation between extrinsic or intrinsic is considered archaic by many clinicians because manifestations of both extrinsic and intrinsic diseases commonly occur in the same patient. It is recommended that hospitals and physician offices develop coding policies for patients diagnosed with both intrinsic and extrinsic asthmatic conditions.

493.0 ✔5th Extrinsic asthma — *caused by environmental factor (allergy)*
493.1 ✔5th Intrinsic asthma — *caused by body's response to infection or other factor*
493.2 ✔5th Chronic obstructive asthma — *persistent restriction of airflow and labored breathing*
493.9 ✔5th Unspecified asthma — *unknown type*

494 BRONCHIECTASIS

Bronchiectasis is dilation of bronchi with mucus production and persistent cough. Mounier-Kuhn syndrome is a form of bronchiectasis. Code choice is determined by whether the patient also presents with acute bronchitis (acute exacerbation).

Excluded from this rubric is bronchiectasis as a congenital disorder (748.61) and bronchiectasis in active tuberculosis (011.5).

494.0 Bronchiectasis without acute exacerbation — *dilation of bronchi, mucous production, cough*
494.1 Bronchiectasis with acute exacerbation — *dilation of bronchi, mucous production, cough, with sudden worsening of condition*

495 EXTRINSIC ALLERGIC ALVEOLITIS

Codes in this rubric report inflammation of the alveoli of the lung due to allergic reaction to the environment, including inhaled organic dust particles of fungal, thermophilic actinomycete, or other origin.

495.0 Farmers' lung — *antigen: Micropolyspora faeni or Thermoactinomyces vulgaris in moldy hay*
495.1 Bagassosis — *antigen: Micropolyspora faeni or Thermoactinomyces vulgaris in sugarcane waste*
495.2 Bird-fanciers' lung — *antigen: bird droppings from parakeets, pigeons and chickens*

✔5th   Needs fifth-digit   **OK**   Valid three-digit code

495.3	Suberosis — *antigen: moldy cork dust; "cork-handler's lung"*
495.4	Malt workers' lung — *antigen: Aspergillus clavatus or Aspergillus fumigatus in moldy barley or malt*
495.5	Mushroom workers' lung — *antigen: Micropolyspora faeni or Thermoactinomyces vulgaris in mushroom compost*
495.6	Maple bark-strippers' lung — *antigen: Cryptostroma corticale in infected maple bark*
495.7	"Ventilation" pneumonitis — *antigen: any of numerous organisms growing in ventilation systems*
495.8	Other specified allergic alveolitis and pneumonitis — *including wood asthma, coffee workers' lung, fish meal workers' lung, furrier's lung*
495.9	Unspecified allergic alveolitis and pneumonitis — *unknown extrinsic alveolitis*

496 CHRONIC AIRWAY OBSTRUCTION, NOT ELSEWHERE CLASSIFIED OK

Chronic airway obstruction is a nonspecific condition characterized by a chronic or recurrent reduction in expiratory airflow within the lung. Chronic obstructive pulmonary disease (COPD) and chronic obstructive lung disease (COLD) are the two most common descriptive diagnostic terms assigned to this code category.

Signs and symptoms of chronic airway obstruction, not elsewhere classified, include history of cigarette smoking and frequent respiratory infections, dyspnea on exertion with reduced exercise tolerance, sputum-productive cough, rhonchi, decreased intensity of breath sounds, and prolonged expiration. Therapies include bronchodilators such as theophylline, corticosteroids such as prednisone, oxygen therapy and chest physiotherapy, and antibiotics for superimposed acute respiratory infections. Associated conditions include cor pulmonale (chronic pulmonary hypertension), sinus tachycardia, supraventricular arrhythmias, secondary polycythemia, acute bronchitis, pneumonia, left ventricular failure, pulmonary embolism, and acute respiratory insufficiency or failure.

Do not assign code 496 with any code from categories 491 through 493.

500-508 Pneumoconioses and Other Lung Diseases Due to External Agents

500 COAL WORKERS' PNEUMOCONIOSIS OK

501 ASBESTOSIS OK

502 PNEUMOCONIOSIS DUE TO OTHER SILICA OR SILICATES OK

503 PNEUMOCONIOSIS DUE TO OTHER INORGANIC DUST OK

504 PNEUMONOPATHY DUE TO INHALATION OF OTHER DUST OK

505 UNSPECIFIED PNEUMOCONIOSIS OK

506 RESPIRATORY CONDITIONS DUE TO CHEMICAL FUMES AND VAPORS

| 506.0 | Bronchitis and pneumonitis due to fumes and vapors — (Use additional E code to identify cause) — *sudden, severe chemical bronchitis* |
| 506.1 | Acute pulmonary edema due to fumes and vapors — (Use additional E code to identify cause) — *sudden, severe edema* |

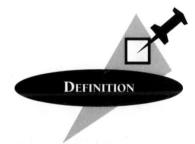

DEFINITION

Anthracosilicosis: inflammation and fibrosis of the lungs caused by inhalation of coal dust.

Berylliosis: granulomatous fibrosis of the lungs caused by chronic inhalation of beryllium.

Byssinosis: disease of the lungs caused by inhalation of cotton, flax or hemp dust particles, usually exhibited by wheezing and coughing.

Cannabinols: disease of the lungs caused by inhalation of dust particles of cannabis.

Pneumoconiosis: inflammation of the lungs caused by inhalation of dust particles, may lead to fibrosis of the lungs.

Shaver's syndrome: pulmonary emphysema and pneumothorax caused by inhalation of bauxite fumes and aluminum dust particles.

506.2   Upper respiratory inflammation due to fumes and vapors — (Use additional E code to identify cause) — *upper respiratory infection [URI] other than what is specified*

506.3   Other acute and subacute respiratory conditions due to fumes and vapors — (Use additional E code to identify cause) — *not specified elsewhere*

506.4   Chronic respiratory conditions due to fumes and vapors — (Use additional E code to identify cause) — *emphysema, obliterative bronchiolitis, pulmonary fibrosis*

506.9   Unspecified respiratory conditions due to fumes and vapors — (Use additional E code to identify cause) — *unknown*

507 PNEUMONITIS DUE TO SOLIDS AND LIQUIDS

Pneumonitis due to solids and liquids is pneumonitis and pneumonia due to aspiration of foreign material into the tracheobronchial tree. Aspiration of inert material such as drinking water may cause asphyxia (category 934), but rarely results in pneumonia or pneumonitis. Aspiration of gastric contents or toxic materials such as petroleum distillates often causes pneumonia or pneumonitis due to an inflammatory response in the lungs and lung parenchyma.

Pneumonitis due to inhalation of food or vomitus is pneumonitis and pneumonia due to inhalation or aspiration of food or gastric contents into the lung. "Cafe coronary syndrome" is an acute condition characterized by obstruction of the trachea or bronchi due to large particulate material such as meat and often results in a necrotizing pneumonitis. Signs and symptoms of pneumonitis due to inhalation of food or vomitus include history of feeding disorder, convulsive disorder, marked debility or disturbance of consciousness, drug or alcohol intoxication, rales, dyspnea, cyanosis, hypotension, and tachycardia.

Diagnostic tests include chest x-ray to locate areas of multilobar infiltrates. ABGs suggest hypoxemia and gross exam may show blood-tinged sputum. Culture of sputum may reveal gram-positive and gram-negative organisms if infective nasopharyngeal organisms have been aspirated. Associated conditions include dehydration, concomitant bacterial pneumonia, bronchiectasis, pulmonary fibrosis, and acute respiratory failure.

Aspiration of gastric acid with a pH of less than 2.5, which can result in a life-threatening pneumonitis, may be referred to as "chemical pneumonitis." Although chemical pneumonitis usually is classified to rubric 506, when chemical pneumonitis is due to aspiration, assign 507.0.

Aspiration pneumonia or pneumonitis due to — or resulting from the presence of — a nasogastric tube, endotracheal tube, or tracheostomy is classified as a postoperative complication (997.3). The code for aspiration pneumonia may be used as a secondary code to further explain the nature of the respiratory complication. Note that, in the case of aspiration pneumonia or pneumonitis following anesthesia, the proper cause and effect relationship needs to be determined. For example, if the aspiration pneumonia or pneumonitis is due to the induction of anesthesia (endotracheal intubation and aspiration, including Mendelson's syndrome), assign 997.3. If the aspiration pneumonia or pneumonitis is due to the anesthetic agent, follow ICD-9-CM coding rules regarding adverse reactions to drugs and chemicals.

Subcategory 507.1 includes lipid (or "lipoid") pneumonia when due to an exogenous source. Lipid pneumonia is a chronic syndrome due to the repeated aspiration of oil-

✔5th   Needs fifth-digit   **OK**   Valid three-digit code

containing substances such as mineral oil, cod liver oil, and oily nose drops. This code excludes endogenous lipid pneumonia, which is caused by retention of lipids in the lung parenchyma released during the breakdown of tissue. Endogenous lipid pneumonia is reported with 516.8.

Subcategory 507.8 includes hydrocarbon pneumonitis and pneumonia due to inhalation or aspiration of solids and liquids. It excludes hydrocarbon pneumonitis and pneumonia due to fumes and vapors, which are classified in rubric 506.

507.0   Pneumonitis due to inhalation of food or vomitus — *aspiration pneumonia from food, saliva, vomit, not otherwise specified*

507.1   Pneumonitis due to inhalation of oils and essences — *exogenous lipoid pneumonia*

507.8   Pneumonitis due to other solids and liquids — *including detergent asthma*

508 RESPIRATORY CONDITIONS DUE TO OTHER AND UNSPECIFIED EXTERNAL AGENTS

508.0   Acute pulmonary manifestations due to radiation — (Use additional E code to identify cause) — *radiation pneumonitis*

508.1   Chronic and other pulmonary manifestations due to radiation — (Use additional E code to identify cause) — *fibrosis of lung following radiation*

508.8   Respiratory conditions due to other specified external agents — (Use additional E code to identify cause) — *not elsewhere specified*

508.9   Respiratory conditions due to unspecified external agent — (Use additional E code to identify cause) — *unknown*

510-519 Other Diseases of Respiratory System

510 EMPYEMA

Empyema is an infection in the pleural space. It is frequently accompanied by chest pain, shortness of breath, weakness, fever, and hemoptysis. A code for the infective agent in empyema can be found in Chapter 1 Infectious and Parasitic Diseases, and should be reported secondarily. Empyema is classified according to whether a fistula is present.

510.0   Empyema with fistula — (Use additional code to identify infectious organism 041.00–041.9) — *including thoracic, pleural, mediastinal, hepatopleural, bronchopleural, bronchocutaneous*

510.9   Empyema without mention of fistula — (Use additional code to identify infectious organism 041.00–041.9) — *with abscess, pyothorax, pyopneumothorax, empyema, fibrinopurulent pleurisy*

511 PLEURISY

511.0   Pleurisy without mention of effusion or current tuberculosis — *with adhesion, calcification, thickening of pleura*

511.1   Pleurisy with effusion, with mention of bacterial cause other than tuberculosis — *including pneumococcal, staphylococcal, streptococcal*

511.8   Pleurisy with other specified forms of effusion, except tuberculous — *including encysted pleurisy, hemopneumothorax, hemothorax, hydropneumothorax, pleurorrhea, hydrothorax*

511.9   Unspecified pleural effusion — *unknown*

The definition of unspecified pleural effusion is abnormal accumulation of fluid in the pleural space, unspecified as to etiology. Included are transudative and exudative pleurisy and pleural effusions without further

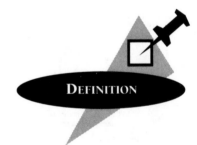

DEFINITION

Hydrothorax: Serous effusion in the pleura.

Chylothorax: Fatty lymphatic effusion in the pleura.

Hemothorax: Bloody effusion in the pleura.

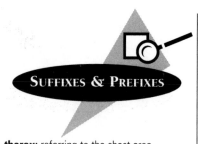

SUFFIXES & PREFIXES

-thorax: referring to the chest area

Hemo-: relating to blood

Hydro-: relating to fluid, water, or hydrogen

specification. Pleural effusion is a common manifestation of both systemic and intrathoracic diseases.

Signs and symptoms of unspecified pleural effusion include pleuritic chest pain, dyspnea, decreased tactile fremitus, pleural friction rub, dullness to percussion, egophony, and distant breath sounds. Therapies include thoracentesis (percutaneous) to remove excess fluid and relieve pain, tube thoracostomy for continuous drainage, and pleurodesis or pleurectomy for malignant pleural effusion.

Malignant pleural effusion (197.2) and pleurisy with tuberculosis (012.0) are excluded from the rubric.

512 PNEUMOTHORAX

Pneumothorax is air or other gas in the pleural space. This gas displaces lung capacity, and is commonly referred to as a "collapsed lung" because of the reduction in lung volume.

An iatrogenic pneumothorax occurs as the result of air introduced into the pleural space, or lung puncture during a medical procedure. Most commonly, iatrogenic pneumothorax will occur during thoracentesis, catheter placement, arteriography, or intercostal nerve block.

Spontaneous pneumothorax is most common in adult males, and has a high incidence of occurrence among patients with Marfan's syndrome. Nearly a third of patients with spontaneous pneumothorax have underlying chronic pulmonary disease.

Tension pneumothorax occurs when pressure in the pleural space is not sufficient to displace the mediastinum to the opposite side. Because this compromises venous return, tension pneumothorax is considered a medical emergency.

Trachea and mediastinum shift away from pneumothorax

Defect in chest wall

Chest wall

Pleural space fills with air

Open pneumothorax during inhalation

Trachea and mediastinum shift toward side of defect

Air has entered the pleural space and collapsed the lung

Exhalation

512.0	Spontaneous tension pneumothorax — *air leaking from the lung, and trapped in the lung lining*	
512.1	Iatrogenic pneumothroax — *air leaking from the lung, following surgery*	
512.8	Other spontaneous pneumothorax — *including spontaneous or sucking pneumothorax, or pneumothorax not otherwise specified*	

513 ABSCESS OF LUNG AND MEDIASTINUM

513.0	Abscess of lung — *abscess, necrosis, or gangrene*
513.1	Abscess of mediastinum — *pocket of pus in the tissue between the organs behind the sternum*

514 PULMONARY CONGESTION AND HYPOSTASIS **OK**

515 POSTINFLAMMATORY PULMONARY FIBROSIS **OK**

516 OTHER ALVEOLAR AND PARIETOALVEOLAR PNEUMONOPATHY

516.0	Pulmonary alveolar proteinosis — *chronic proteinaceous deposits in alveoli; Rosen-Castleman-Liebow syndrome*
516.1	Idiopathic pulmonary hemosiderosis — (Code first underlying disease 275.0) — *essential brown induration of lung*
516.2	Pulmonary alveolar microlithiasis — *minute concretions in alveoli*

↙5th   Needs fifth-digit   **OK**   Valid three-digit code

516.3	Idiopathic fibrosing alveolitis — *including alveolar capillary block, diffuse pulmonary, Hamman-Rich syndrome*
516.8	Other specified alveolar and parietoalveolar pneumonopathies — *not otherwise classified, including endogenous lipoid pneumonia*
516.9	Unspecified alveolar and parietoalveolar pneumonopathy — *unknown*

517 LUNG INVOLVEMENT IN CONDITIONS CLASSIFIED ELSEWHERE

Codes in this rubric should not be used as the principal or primary diagnosis. Code first the underlying disease.

517.1	Rheumatic pneumonia — (Code first underlying disease 390)
517.2	Lung involvement in systemic sclerosis — (Code first underlying disease 710.1)
517.8	Lung involvement in other diseases classified elsewhere — (Code first underlying disease, as: 135, 277.3, 710.0, 710.2, 710.4) — *not otherwise specified*

518 OTHER DISEASES OF LUNG

518.0 Pulmonary collapse — *no air in a part of the lung; atelectasis, Brock's syndrome, middle lobe syndrome*

Pulmonary collapse is incomplete expansion of lobules (clusters of alveoli) or lung segments. Also called atelectasis, this condition may result in partial or complete lung collapse, which impairs gas exchange, resulting in hypoxia. Pulmonary collapse may be due to obstructions, such as mucous plugs, neoplasms and foreign bodies, or to external compression of the lungs from conditions such as pleural effusion, enlarged thoracic lymph nodes, and pneumothorax.

Signs and symptoms of pulmonary collapse include asymptomatic with slowly developing or minor atelectasis, decreased breath sounds, dull chest percussions with rapidly developing or massive atelectasis, sudden dyspnea, cyanosis, hypotension, tachycardia, elevated temperature, peripheral circulatory collapse or shock, diaphoresis, and substernal or intercostal retraction. Associated conditions include bronchiectasis, pulmonary fibrosis, infective pneumonitis, pleural effusion, enlarged thoracic lymph nodes, and pneumothorax.

518.1	Interstitial emphysema — *air trapped inappropriately in tissue outside bronchi, alveoli, or bronchioli; mediastinal emphysema or Hamman's syndrome*
518.2	Compensatory emphysema — *overdistension of lung tissue into a void created when adjacent tissue was excised or damaged*
518.3	Pulmonary eosinophilia — *transient infiltrations of lungs by eosinophilia; Löffler's syndrome, PIE syndrome, Weingarten's syndrome*
518.4	Unspecified acute edema of lung — *Severe, sudden fluid retention within the lung, including postoperative*
518.5	Pulmonary insufficiency following trauma and surgery — *adult respiratory distress syndrome [ARDS], Woillez's disease*
518.6	Allergic bronchopulmonary aspergillosis

518.8 Acute respiratory failure

Respiratory failure is failure of oxygenation and/or ventilation that is severe enough to impair or threaten the functioning of vital organs. With failure of oxygenation, the tissues of the lung are not functioning properly. An example of failure of oxygenation would be an

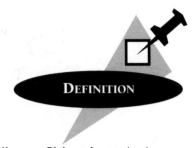

DEFINITION

Hamman-Rich syndrome: chronic inflammation, progressive fibrosis of the pulmonary alveolar walls, and progressive dyspnea leading to death by oxygen deprivation or right heart failure.

Rosen-Castleman-Liebow syndrome: chronic disease of lungs marked by chest pain, weakness, hemoptysis, dyspnea, and productive cough. Ventilation of affected areas is prevented by a proteinaceous material.

Honeycomb lung: fibrosis and dilation of the bronchioles that gives the lung a honeycomb appearance. Occurs as a result of many diseases, including eosinophilia and sarcoidosis.

Pneumatocele: a gas-filled swelling or cavity formed in the lung. Occurs often with *staphylococcus pneumonia*.

Shock lung: collapse of the alveoli due to diminished perfusion and edema of the alveoli as a result of shock.

Atelectasis: the failure of a lung to expand or a collapse of a lung causing a lack of air in all or part of the lung.

Middle lobe syndrome: also Brock's syndrome, incomplete expansion of the right middle lobe of a lung with chronic pneumonitis.

acute exacerbation of bronchial asthma in a patient with emphysema. With failure of ventilation, airflow in and out of the lungs is impaired, for example, by compression of the trachea caused by metastatic carcinoma of the thoracic lymph nodes.

Signs and symptoms of respiratory failure include headache, cyanosis, dyspnea, impaired motor function, restlessness, confusion, anxiety, delirium, and occasionally symptoms of depressed consciousness, tachypnea, tachycardia, and tremor. Associated conditions include chronic obstructive lung disease such as chronic obstructive bronchitis, emphysema, cystic fibrosis, acute obstructive lung disease such as asthma, pneumonia, and acute bronchitis.

Diagnosis of respiratory failure based on ABG values is not absolute and may be adjusted according to the patient's baseline blood gas levels. Since some COPD patients have chronically abnormal values, the diagnosis of respiratory failure is made based on further decompensation from the patient's baseline.

518.81	Acute respiratory failure — *not otherwise specified*
518.82	Other pulmonary insufficiency, not elsewhere classified — *including acute respiratory distress not elsewhere classified*
518.83	Chronic respiratory failure — *persistent*
518.84	Acute and chronic respiratory failure — *sudden, severe*
518.89	Other diseases of lung, not elsewhere classified — *including cyst, degeneration, scarring, pulmolithiasis, calcification, broncholithiasis, or occlusion*

519 OTHER DISEASES OF RESPIRATORY SYSTEM

This nonspecific code should be used only as a last resort when no other diagnosis can be made.

519.00	Unspecified tracheostomy complication — *unknown*
519.01	Infection of tracheostomy
519.02	Mechanical complication of tracheostomy — *tracheal stenosis*
519.09	Other tracheostomy complications — *including hemorrhage, fistula*
519.1	Other diseases of trachea and bronchus, not elsewhere classified — *including calcification, stenosis, ulcer*
519.2	Mediastinitis — *inflammation of the tissue between the organs behind the sternum*
519.3	Other diseases of mediastinum, not elsewhere classified — *fibrosis, hernia, retraction*
519.4	Disorders of diaphragm — *including diaphragmitis, paralysis, relation*
519.8	Other diseases of respiratory system, not elsewhere classified — *including cyst of pleura*
519.9	Unspecified disease of respiratory system — *unknown, but including chronic respiratory disease not otherwise specified*

✔5th Needs fifth-digit   **OK** Valid three-digit code

Chapter 9

520-579
Diseases of the Digestive System

This chapter classifies diseases and disorders of all of the organs along the alimentary (digestive) tract — the long, muscular tube begins at the mouth and ends at the anus. The major digestive organs include the pharynx, esophagus, stomach, and intestines. Accessory, or secondary, organs include the salivary and parotid glands, jaw, teeth and the supporting structures of teeth, tongue, liver, gallbladder and biliary tract, pancreas, and peritoneum.

The primary function of the digestive system is to mechanically break down and chemically dissolve foodstuffs to provide the body with essential vitamins, proteins, minerals, and water. Diseases and disorders that interfere with this function are classified here, along with diseases and disorders that affect the organs of the digestive tract although they may have no direct affect on digestion. For example, dental caries have a direct effect on digestion because they interfere with mastication, the mechanical breakdown of food by chewing. Portal hypertension does not directly affect digestion, but is included here because it represents a disease of a digestive system organ. Portal hypertension would have no discernible effect on the digestive process until the disease has progressed to the point that the liver can no longer perform its function as a digestive organ.

520-529 Diseases of Oral Cavity, Salivary Glands, and Jaws

This category includes diseases and disorders of the jaw, salivary and parotid glands, teeth, gingiva and periodontium, lips, oral mucosa, and tongue.

520 DISORDERS OF TOOTH DEVELOPMENT AND ERUPTION

This rubric includes disorders of tooth development and eruption in all patients regardless of age. It is one of the few categories in ICD-9-CM that classifies congenital anomalies and hereditary disturbances outside of Chapter 14 Congenital Anomalies (740-759).

520.0   Anodontia — *complete absence of teeth*

520.1   Supernumerary teeth — *distomolar, fourth molar, mesiodens, paramolar*

520.2   Abnormalities of size and form of teeth — *including fusion, concrescence, gemination, macrodontia, microdontia, dens evaginates, dens in dente, taurodontism, tuberculum paramolar*

520.3   Mottled teeth — *including dental fluorosis, enamel opacities, mottling of enamel*

Excessive use of fluoride can cause mottled bleaching of the enamel. The problem can be particularly evident in communities with drinking water containing greater than two parts per million, which can cause dental fluorosis. The signs are whitish flecks or spots, particularly on the front teeth, or dark spots or stripes in more severe cases. While tooth-whitening products can approve appearance in most cases, discoloration of enamel

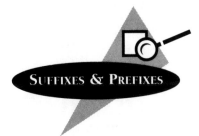

SUFFIXES & PREFIXES

-dontia: referring to the teeth

Hypo-: below, less than, under

Macro-: meaning oversized, large

Micro-: small

Oligo-: indicates few

can also be a structural problem that requires proper diagnosis and treatment

520.4   Disturbances of tooth formation — *including aplasia and hypoplasia of cementum, dilaceration of tooth, enamel hypoplasia, Horner's or Turners tooth, hypocalcification*

520.5   Hereditary disturbances in tooth structure, not elsewhere classified — *including amelogenesis, dentinogenesis, odontogenesis, dentinal dysplasia, shell teeth*

520.6   Disturbances in tooth eruption — *including embedded, impacted, obstructed, premature eruption, premature shedding of deciduous tooth*

520.7   Teething syndrome

520.8   Other specified disorders of tooth development and eruption — *not otherwise specified, including pre-eruptive color change*

520.9   Unspecified disorder of tooth development and eruption — *unknown*

521 DISEASES OF HARD TISSUES OF TEETH

This rubric includes the crown, dentin, enamel, and cementum of the tooth. Note that the pulp of the tooth is not a hard tissue and is classified to category 522, but certain conditions such as internal granuloma of the pulp may be classified here (code 521.4).

521.0   Dental caries — *including in cementum, dentin, enamel*

This rubric includes caries of the cementum, dentin, enamel, as well as infantile melanodontia and white spot lesions of the teeth.

Dental caries are a demineralization of a tooth's enamel caused by acids produced by bacteria, particularly Streptococcus mutans. The first sign of demineralization is a small "white spot" (initial caries, incipient caries). It is not yet a cavity, the surface is still hard. It is not calculated as decayed, according to criteria of WHO. Variations in intraoral mechanical forces such as chewing or grinding of the teeth determine the continued formation of bacteria on the teeth and the plaque that can lead to dental caries. Other causes are related to feeding behaviors, such a baby bottle tooth decay in infants, in addition to craniofacial problems, neurologic abnormalities, or impaired cognitive abilities that can interfere with proper dental care.

The bacteria that cause caries are microflora that are present not only in the oral cavity but also in the gastrointestinal tract and other parts of the body, increasing the risk of many disease states and changes in health status due to oral diseases. For example, poorly controlled diabetes (characterized by hyperglycemia and increased salivary glucose) is associated with an increased risk of several dental diseases and conditions.

Diagnosis of dental caries generally involves the use of a sharp explorer, a viewing mirror, and an artificial light source as well as the drying of tooth surfaces to improve visibility. Radiographs or fiberoptic illumination may reveal smaller caries on the hidden surfaces between adjacent teeth. Four major types of primary prevention are fluoride therapy, fissure-sealant therapy, dietary counselling, and oral-hygiene measures.

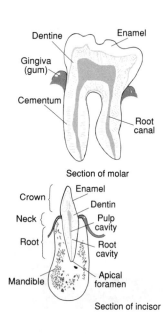

Dentine
Enamel
Gingiva (gum)
Cementum
Root canal

Section of molar

Crown
Enamel
Neck
Dentin
Root
Pulp cavity
Root cavity
Apical foramen
Mandible

Section of incisor

⌙5th   Needs fifth-digit   **OK**   Valid three-digit code

521.1   Excessive attrition of teeth — *including approximal wear, occlusal wear*

521.2   Abrasion of teeth — *including dentifrice, habitual, occupational, ritual, traditional*

521.3   Erosion of teeth — *including idiopathic, occupational, or due to medicine or persistent vomiting*

521.4   Pathological resorption of teeth — *including internal granuloma of pulp, resorption of tooth or root*

521.5   Hypercementosis — *excessive deposits of cementum on the root of the tooth; including cementation hyperplasia*

521.6   Ankylosis of teeth — *abnormal union of tooth to surrounding bone*

521.7   Posteruptive color changes of teeth — *staining due to drugs, metal, pulpal bleeding, or not otherwise specified*

521.8   Other specified diseases of hard tissues of teeth — *not otherwise specified, including irradiated enamel, sensitive dentin*

521.9   Unspecified disease of hard tissues of teeth — *unknown*

522 DISEASES OF PULP AND PERIAPICAL TISSUES

522.0   Pulpitis — *including abscess, polyp; acute or chronic*

522.1   Necrosis of dental pulp — *death of pulp tissue; including pulp gangrene*

522.2   Dental pulp degeneration — *including denticles, pulp calcifications, pulp stones*

522.3   Abnormal hard tissue formation in dental pulp — *including secondary or irregular dentin*

522.4   Acute apical periodontitis of pulpal origin — *severe inflammation of periodontal ligament, resulting from pulpal inflammation or necrosis*

An advanced bacterial infection of the pulp can, if untreated, spread to the root. If the root of the tooth dies, the toothache may stop, but the infection remains active and continues to spread and destroy tissue.

Signs and symptoms of acute apical periodontitis include swollen and red gum that may drain thick purulent material and often a throbbing pain that tends to radiate along the jaw. There is sensitivity of the teeth to hot or cold, possible fever and swollen glands of the neck, and a swollen area of the jaw in very serious cases. Biting or closing the mouth tightly also increases pain. The presence of an abscess, which is a collection of pus, requires immediate dental attention and antibiotics to control the infection, often prior to surgical intervention (e.g., root canal or, in extreme cases, an apicoectomy to drain the abscess prior to a root canal).

522.5   Periapical abscess without sinus — *dental or dentoalveolar*

522.6   Chronic apical periodontitis — *persistent inflammation of periodontal ligament, from granuloma or not elsewhere specified*

522.7   Periapical abscess with sinus — *including dental or alveolar process fistula*

522.8   Radicular cyst of dental pulp — *including apical, periapical, radiculodental, periodontal cyst*

522.9   Other and unspecified diseases of pulp and periapical tissues — *not specified elsewhere or unknown*

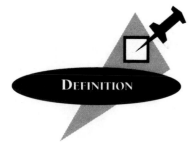

DEFINITION

Pericementitis: inflammation of the tissue that surrounds the teeth, due to bacterial plaque on the bordering teeth.

Periodontal pocket: a pocket created from a gingival detachment from the tooth.

523 GINGIVAL AND PERIODONTAL DISEASES

Gingival and periodontal diseases include acute and chronic gingivitis, gingival recession, acute and chronic periodontitis, accretions on teeth, as well as other specified periodontal diseases such as gingival polyps and peripheral giant cell granuloma. Excluded from this category are acute necrotizing ulcerative gingivitis (101); herpetic gingivostomatitis (054.2); acute apical periodontitis (522.4); chronic apical periodontitis (522.6); periapical abscess (522.5, 522.7); and leukoplakia of gingiva (528.6).

Gingivitis is defined as the inflammation or swelling of the gum tissues. Gingivitis and periodontitis can be considered one disease complex caused by bacteria that incorporates into the dental plaque. Gingivitis often goes unnoticed in the early stages but once advanced it spreads to the bony tissues, which lie under the gums and support the teeth. This is called periodontitis. In later stages of periodontitis, the teeth can become loose and severely infected with pus oozing from around the sockets. In very advanced periodontitis, the teeth can actually fall out or may have to be removed because of infection.

There are no symptoms in the early stages of gingivitis. Signs and symptoms of advanced gingivitis and periodontitis include blood on the tooth brush when brushing the teeth, swollen and red gums, tenderness when the gums are touched, pus around the teeth, bad taste in the mouth, and visible deposits of tartar or calculus on the teeth. A diagnosis of advanced gingivitis and periodontitis is by examination, gum probing, and dental x-rays. If untreated, gingivitis and periodontitis can lead to the loss of the teeth and infection of advanced periodontal disease can spread to other parts of the body, including the heart. Depending on the stage of the disease, treatment can range anywhere from simple cleaning, called prophylaxis, and home care to complex periodontal surgery. In advanced cases, some or all the teeth may have to be extracted.

523.0	Acute gingivitis — *severe inflammation of the gingiva*
523.1	Chronic gingivitis — *persistent inflammation of the gingiva*
523.2	Gingival recession — *generalized, localized, postinfective, postoperative*
523.3	Acute periodontitis — *severe inflammation of the tissues that surround and support the teeth*
523.4	Chronic periodontitis — *persistent inflammation of the tissues that surround and support the teeth*
523.5	Periodontosis — *inflammation of the tissues that surround and support the teeth*
523.6	Accretions on teeth — *foreign material on surface of teeth, usually plaque or calculus*
523.8	Other specified periodontal diseases — *including cysts, hemorrhage, occlusion, pocket, ulcer, pain, fibromatosis, lesions, giant cell granuloma*
523.9	Unspecified gingival and periodontal disease — *unknown*

524 DENTOFACIAL ANOMALIES, INCLUDING MALOCCLUSION

Malocclusion is defined as an abnormal alignment of teeth and the way that the upper and lower teeth fit together (bite). It is often hereditary and may cause problems with biting and chewing but can usually be corrected with a brace on the teeth and proper orthodontic care.

Dentofacial anomalies classified in this chapter may be acquired or due to congenital anomalies not classified to Chapter 14. Look in the ICD-9-CM index under both the condition and the main term "Anomaly, anomalous" to ensure proper code assignment.

✔5th Needs fifth-digit   **OK** Valid three-digit code

524.0 Major anomalies of jaw size

This subcategory classifies conditions affecting the size of the jaw, including hyperplasia, hypoplasia, macrogenia, and microgenia.

524.00 Unspecified major anomaly of jaw size — *unknown*
524.01 Maxillary hyperplasia — *overgrowth or overdevelopment of maxillary bone*
524.02 Mandibular hyperplasia — *overgrowth or overdevelopment of jaw bone*
524.03 Maxillary hypoplasia — *incomplete or underdevelopment of maxillary bone*
524.04 Mandibular hypoplasia — *incomplete or underdevelopment of jaw bone*
524.05 Macrogenia — *abnormal largeness of the chin*
524.06 Microgenia — *abnormal smallness of the chin*
524.09 Other specified major anomaly of jaw size — *not otherwise specified*

524.1 Anomalies of relationship of jaw to cranial base

This subcategory classifies inequality in the size or shape of one side of the maxilla and/or mandible compared with the other, or a difference in placement or arrangement of one of the jawbones about the craniofacial axis. These anomalies include prognathism, retrognathism, and maxillary asymmetry. Prognathism is anterior protrusion of the mandible or maxilla beyond the projection of the forehead. Retrognathism is the location of the maxilla or mandible behind the frontal plane of the forehead; it also is used as a general term meaning underdevelopment of the maxilla or mandible.

524.10 Unspecified anomaly of relationship of jaw to cranial base — *unspecified, including prognathism and retrognathism*
524.11 Maxillary asymmetry — *unequal development*
524.12 Other jaw asymmetry — *including unequal development of mandible*
524.19 Other specified anomaly of relationship of jaw to cranial base — *not otherwise specified*
524.2 Anomalies of dental arch relationship — *including crossbite, overjet, soft tissue impingement, midline deviation, overbite, disto-occlusion, mesio-occlusion*
524.3 Anomalies of tooth position — *including normal or impacted tooth with crowding, diastema, displacement, rotation, abnormal spacing, transposition*
524.4 Unspecified malocclusion
524.5 Dentofacial functional abnormalities — *including abnormal jaw closure, malocclusion due to mouth breathing, tongue, lip or finger habits, or abnormal swallowing*
524.60 Unspecified temporomandibular joint disorders — *TMJ syndrome; including Costen's syndrome*
524.61 Adhesions and ankylosis (bony or fibrous) of temporomandibular joint — *a union or stiffening of the TMJ due to bony or fibrous union across the joint*
524.62 Arthralgia of temporomandibular joint — *pain of TMJ, not inflammatory in nature*
524.63 Articular disc disorder (reducing or non-reducing) of temporomandibular joint
524.69 Other specified temporomandibular joint disorders — *not otherwise specified, including snapping jaw*

524.7 Dental alveolar anomalies

This subcategory classifies anomalies of the dental alveoli and alveolar ridge, including hyperplasia and hypoplasia. Dental alveoli are the tooth sockets of the maxilla and mandible. The alveolar ridge is the bony process of the maxilla or mandible that contains the tooth sockets. Hyperplasia of the alveoli is an overgrowth or overdevelopment of bone, and hypoplasia of the alveoli is an underdevelopment or agenesis of bone.

524.70 Unspecified alveolar anomaly — *unknown*

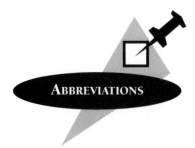

TMJ: temporomandibular joint-pain-dysfunction syndrome, headache, dizziness, tinnitus, and other symptoms resulting from dysfunction of the mandibular joint

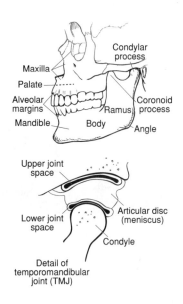

Condylar process
Maxilla
Palate
Alveolar margins
Coronoid process
Ramus
Mandible
Body
Angle

Upper joint space
Lower joint space
Articular disc (meniscus)
Condyle

Detail of temporomandibular joint (TMJ)

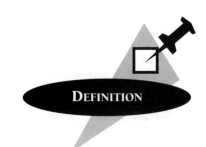

DEFINITION

Costen's syndrome: otalgia, dizziness, headache, tinnitus or loss of hearing, and burning sensation of throat, tongue, and side of the nose originally thought to be dysfunction of mandibular joint, but now thought to be worsened by other causes as well.

524.71 Alveolar maxillary hyperplasia — *overgrowth or underdevelopment of alveolar tissue of the maxillary bones*

524.72 Alveolar mandibular hyperplasia — *overgrowth or underdevelopment of alveolar tissue of the mandibular bones*

524.73 Alveolar maxillary hypoplasia — *incomplete or underdevelopment of alveolar tissue of the maxillary bones*

524.74 Alveolar mandibular hypoplasia — *incomplete or underdevelopment of alveolar tissue of the mandibular bones*

524.79 Other specified alveolar anomaly — *not otherwise specified*

524.8 Other specified dentofacial anomalies — *not otherwise specified, including narrowing palate*

524.9 Unspecified dentofacial anomalies — *unknown*

525 OTHER DISEASES AND CONDITIONS OF THE TEETH AND SUPPORTING STRUCTURES

525.0 Exfoliation of teeth due to systemic causes — *loss of teeth due to underlying condition*

525.1 Loss of teeth due to accident, extraction, or local periodontal disease — *acquired absence of teeth*

525.2 Atrophy of edentulous alveolar ridge — *wasting away or death of toothless supportive tissue*

525.3 Retained dental root

525.8 Other specified disorders of the teeth and supporting structures — *not otherwise specified, including cicatrix, cleft, hemorrhage, lesion, or enlargement of alveolar process or tissue; loose tooth; obliteration of vestibule*

525.9 Unspecified disorder of the teeth and supporting structures — *unknown cause of pain or other symptom*

526 DISEASES OF THE JAWS

526.0 Developmental odontogenic cysts — *including dentigerous, eruption, follicular, lateral development, keratocyst, primordial cyst*

Odontogenic cysts are developmental cysts arising from the enamel organ of teeth and include about 90 percent of all jaw cysts. While it is sometimes difficult to distinguish which type of odontogenic cyst is present, some have distinguishing features.

The radicular cyst is the most common of the odontogenic cysts, associated with a nonvital tooth; present at the apex of the root of a tooth or teeth. Other odontogenic cysts include residual cysts associated with the removal of teeth and primordial cysts associated with undeveloped teeth. Globulomaxillary cysts are located in the anterior region of the upper jaw and dentigerous cysts that form in association with an unerupted permanent tooth, although they can occasionally surround a primary tooth, due to fluid accumulation.

Dentigerous cysts are found in children and adolescents. Adults can have dentigerous cysts associated with unerupted third molars. These cysts may expand, causing displacement or resorption of adjacent teeth. In a radiograph, dentigerous cysts appear as a dark area around the crown of the tooth.

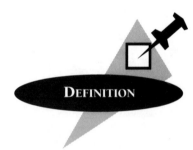

DEFINITION

Cherubism: abnormal fibrous tissue development of the jaws that causes the jaws to enlarge giving a cherub look to the face of children.

Dry socket: also alveoalgia, a complication after tooth removal in which the blood clots in the socket disintegrates. The result is a painful, inflammation of the empty socket.

Keratocyst: a cyst formed from tissue from the dental lamina during the process of tooth formation.

Sequestrum: necrotic tissue or bone that has detached from the adjoining healthy tissue or bone.

✔5th Needs fifth-digit　　**OK** Valid three-digit code

Treatment for the dentigerous cyst includes removal and microscopic examination of the cyst wall since the cyst lining may have a neoplastic change, such as ameloblastoma, squamous cell carcinoma, or mucoepidermoid carcinoma. Marsupialization is a second method of treatment that involves removing the overlying soft tissue and bone, allowing discharge of matter.

526.1   Fissural cysts of jaw — *including globulomaxillary, incisor canal, median anterior maxillary, medial palatal, nasopalatine*

526.2   Other cysts of jaws — *including aneurysmal, hemorrhagic, traumatic*

526.3   Central giant cell (reparative) granuloma

526.4   Inflammatory conditions of jaw — *including abscess, osteitis, sequestrum of jawbone, periostitis*

526.5   Alveolitis of jaw — *inflammation of alveoli or tooth socket of jaw; including dry socket; alveolar osteitis*

526.81   Exostosis of jaw — *bony projection that develops from cartilage of jaw*

526.89   Other specified disease of the jaws — *not otherwise specified, including cherubism, fibrous dysplasia, latent bone cyst, fistula, perforation, unilateral condylar hyper- or hypoplasia of mandible*

526.9   Unspecified disease of the jaws — *unknown cause of pain or other symptom*

527 DISEASES OF THE SALIVARY GLANDS

Atrophy (527.0) in the diseases of the salivary glands is defined as a wasting away or death of tissue, while hypertrophy (527.1) is overgrowth or overdevelopment of tissue of salivary glands. Sialoadenitis (527.2) is the inflammation of a salivary gland and sialolithiasis (527.5) is the formation or presence of a salivary calculus.

527.0   Atrophy of salivary gland — *wasting away or death of tissue*

527.1   Hypertrophy of salivary gland — *overgrowth or over development of tissue; Mikulicz's syndrome*

527.2   Sialoadenitis — *inflammation*

527.3   Abscess of salivary gland — *pocket of pus*

527.4   Fistula of salivary gland — *abnormal sinus tract communicating between salivary gland and another site*

527.5   Sialolithiasis — *formation or presence of salivary calculus; stone, sialodocholithiasis*

527.6   Mucocele of salivary gland — *dilated salivary gland filled with accumulation of mucous*

527.7   Disturbance of salivary secretion — *including hyposecretion, ptyalism, sialorrhea, xerostomia, Zagari's disease*

527.8   Other specified diseases of the salivary glands — *not otherwise specified, including stenosis, stricture or obstruction of salivary duct; pneumoparotid; sialosis; obstruction of Stensen's or submaxillary duct; sialectasia*

527.9   Unspecified disease of the salivary glands — *unknown disorder*

528 DISEASES OF THE ORAL SOFT TISSUES, EXCLUDING LESIONS SPECIFIC FOR GINGIVA AND TONGUE

528.0   Stomatitis — *inflammation of the mucous membrane of mouth*

528.1   Cancrum oris — *gangrenous, ulcerative, inflammatory lesion of mouth*

Cancrum oris, or noma, is sudden, rapidly progressive tissue destruction. The mucus membranes (e.g., gums, lining of the cheeks) become inflamed and develop ulcers. The infection spreads from the mucus membranes to the skin. The tissues in the lips and cheeks die. Rapid, painless tissue

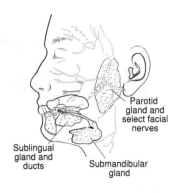

Parotid gland and select facial nerves

Sublingual gland and ducts

Submandibular gland

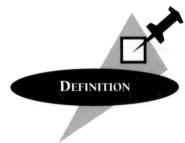

DEFINITION

Aerophagia: excessive swallowing of air, leading to gastrointestinal symptoms of distention and belching.

Achalasia: esophageal spasm, impairing peristalsis and causing dysphagia.

Dyspepsia: indigestion and gaseousness in the upper abdomen.

Dysphagia: difficulty in swallowing. Dysphagia may be pre-esophageal, meaning the patient has difficulty moving matter from the oral pharynx into the esophagus; or esophageal, meaning the food has difficulty progressing through the esophagus.

Globus hystericus: subjective sensation of having a lump in the throat; often associated with grief or anxiety.

Odynophagia: pain during swallowing.

Mikulicz's syndrome: complex of lacrimal and salivary gland swelling, which may include enlargement associated with other syndromes, such as Sjögren's.

Ranula: a cyst on the bottom of the tongue or the floor of the mouth.

Xerostomia: disorder of the salivary glands causing dry mouth.

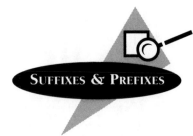

SUFFIXES & PREFIXES

-edema: excess amount or accumulation of fluid in tissues or cavities

-keratosis: a lesion characterized by an excess of growth of the horny layer

-plakia: plaque

Leuko-: white

Melano-: black, pigmented, or dark colored

breakdown continues and this gangrenous process can destroy the soft tissue and bone. Noma can also affect the mucus membranes of the genitals, spreading to the genital skin (this is sometimes called noma pudendi). Risk factors include Kwashiorkor and other forms of severe malnutrition, poor sanitation and poor cleanliness, disorders such as measles or leukemia, and living in an underdeveloped country.

Signs and symptoms include red and tender gums and inner cheeks, ulcers that develop a foul-smelling drainage, and eventual destruction of the bones around the mouth cause deformity and loss of teeth. A physical exam shows inflamed areas of the mucus membranes, mouth ulcers, and skin ulcers, and other signs of malnutrition. Noma can be fatal if left untreated or heal over time even without treatment. However, it can cause massive tissue destruction before healing. Treatment with penicillin and improving nutrition halts progression of the disease. Skin lesions eventually heal even without treatment, but severe scarring and deformity can develop.

528.2   Oral aphthae — *including canker sore, aphthous stomatitis, periadenitis mucosa necrotica recurrens*

528.3   Cellulitis and abscess of oral soft tissues — *including oral fistula, Ludwig's angina*

528.4   Cysts of oral soft tissues — *including dermoid, epidermoid, Epstein's pearl, nasolabial, nasoalveolar, lymphoepithelial*

528.5   Diseases of lips — *including abscess, cellulitis, fistula, hypertrophy; cheilitis, celiodynia, cheilosis*

528.6   Leukoplakia of oral mucosa, including tongue — *white patch on oral mucosa which cannot be attributed to a specific disease; lip, tongue, mucosa, gingiva*

528.7   Other disturbances of oral epithelium, including tongue — *including erythroplakia, focal epithelial hyperplasia, leukoedema, leukokeratosis nicotina palati*

528.8   Oral submucosal fibrosis, including of tongue

528.9   Other and unspecified diseases of the oral soft tissues — *including cheek/lip biting; denture sore mouth; denture stomatitis, melanoplakia; buccal lesion; fistula in soft palate; redundant uvula; melanoplakia*

529 DISEASES AND OTHER CONDITIONS OF THE TONGUE

529.0   Glossitis — *abscess or traumatic ulceration of tongue; including Riga-Fede disease*

529.1   Geographic tongue — *including benign migratory glossitis; glossitis areata exfoliativa*

Geographic tongue is described as a common and harmless condition in which one or more irregularly shaped patches appear on the tongue, in a design that may resemble a map of a country. The center area is redder than the rest of the tongue and the edges of the patch are whitish in color. The etiology is unknown, although a viral infection is assumed and it may be associated with a variety of inflammatory or allergic conditions as well. Geographic tongue often goes away without treatment, but can be treated with topical steroids such as topical Lidex gel.

529.2   Median rhomboid glossitis — *asymptomatic lesion of dorsum of tongue due to Candida albicans infection*

✓5th   Needs fifth-digit   **OK**   Valid three-digit code

529.3	Hypertrophy of tongue papillae — *including black hairy tongue; coated tongue, lingua villosa nigra, hypertrophy of foliate papillae*
529.4	Atrophy of tongue papillae — *including bald tongue, glazed tongue, Hunter's or Moeller's glossitis, glossodynia exfoliativa, smooth atrophic tongue*
529.5	Plicated tongue — *fissured, furrowed, scrotal*
529.6	Glossodynia — *including painful tongue; glossopyrosis*
529.8	Other specified conditions of the tongue — *not otherwise specified, including cicatrix, hemorrhage, paralysis, glossoncus, glossoplegia, atrophy, crenated, enlargement, hypertrophy, hemiatrophy, glossocele, glossoptosis*
529.9	Unspecified condition of the tongue — *unknown*

530-537 Diseases of Esophagus, Stomach, and Duodenum

530   Diseases of esophagus

This category includes diseases and disorders of the esophagus, a muscular, tubular structure that serves as a conduit for the passage of food and water from the pharynx to the stomach. It functions by transporting food and fluids from the mouth to the stomach (and sometimes in the reverse direction) by a combination of gravity and peristaltic waves. The esophagus is equipped with two sphincters. The first is the pharyngeal-esophageal sphincter located at the level of the cricoid cartilage; the second is the gastroesophageal sphincter (also known as the lower esophageal sphincter) located at the level of the esophageal hiatus of the diaphragm.

530.0   Achalasia and cardiospasm — *failure of the esophagogastric sphincter to relax; aperistalsis of esophagus; megaesophagus*

This subcategory classifies neuromuscular disorder characterized by an absence of peristalsis, dilation of the body of the esophagus, and a conically narrowed cardioesophageal junction. The dominant symptom is dysphagia. Vigorous achalasia is a variant form characterized by recurring esophageal spasms.

530.1 Esophagitis

This subcategory classifies inflammation of the esophagus due to reflux, chemicals and infection. Reflux esophagitis, sometimes referred to as peptic or regurgitant esophagitis, is the most common form of esophagitis and is caused by the reflux of acid and pepsin from the stomach into the esophagus. Normally, the gastroesophageal sphincter prevents the reflux of gastric juice into the esophagus, but a variety of conditions can compromise the sphincter's competency. Frequently, hiatal hernia is an underlying cause of sphincter incompetence. Other causes are pregnancy, certain drugs (anticholinergic agents, calcium channel blockers, beta-adrenergic agonists), scleroderma, obesity, placement of nasogastric tubes and surgical vagotomy.

Chemical (corrosive) esophagitis is a chemical burn caused by ingestion (and regurgitation) of caustic liquids or solids. The caustic agent may result in sloughing of the mucous membrane, edema and inflammation of the submucosa, thrombosis of the esophageal vessels, secondary infection, perforation and mediastinitis. Chemical esophagitis can cause severe damage and may constitute a medical emergency depending on the strength of the chemical and the length of time the chemical remains in the esophagus.

Esophagitis due to infection is relatively rare.

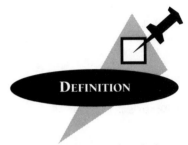

DEFINITION

Barrett's syndrome: gastrointestinal reflux in the esophagus, associated heartburn, and regurgitation caused by a stricture constructed of epithelium

Barsony-Polgar syndrome: also Barsony-Teschendorf, strong, uncoordinated contraction of the esophagus evoked by swallowing in the elderly. Appears as a series of concentric narrows or as spiral on an x-ray

Boerhaave's syndrome: spontaneous rupture of esophagus either as result of defect or in response to stress

Mallory-Weiss syndrome: a gastrointestinal hemorrhage originating from a tear in the esophagus caused by vomiting, dry heaving or hiccups

Zenker's diverticulum: the mucosa of the pharynx protrudes through the cricopharyngeal muscle

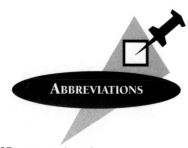

GE: gastroesophageal

GERD: gastroesophageal reflux disease, backing up of the contents of the stomach into the esophagus

GI: gastrointestinal

PUD: peptic ulcer disease

Signs and symptoms of esophagitis include heartburn after eating or while resting in recumbent position, chest pain sometimes masquerading as angina pectoris, regurgitation (water brash) and dysphagia due to inflammatory edema or stricture in distal esophagus, and, in patients with chemical esophagitis, history of ingesting caustic liquids or solids, intense pain and chemical burns of lips, buccal cavity, tongue.

Esophagoscopy and biopsy may be performed to assess severity of the esophagitis and rule out associated conditions such as strictures, ulcers, and carcinoma. Esophageal manometry may be performed to assess competency of the gastroesophageal sphincter. Acid perfusion test, also known as the Bernstein test, may be done to reproduce the pain associated with reflux and an acid reflux test may be performed to monitor the intraesophageal pH after instillation of hydrochloric acid into the stomach. Barium swallow and upper GI series are of limited diagnostic importance except in the most severe cases.

Therapies include alterations in diet and mealtimes, antacids, drugs to increase gastroesophageal sphincter tone such as bethanechol and metoclopramide, and avoidance of drugs known to decrease gastroesophageal sphincter pressure (anticholinergic agents, beta-adrenergic drugs). Surgical intervention includes antireflux surgery such as Nissen fundoplication, Belsey fundoplication, placement of Angelchik ring (prosthesis) around distal esophagus, and replacement of esophagus with segments of stomach, jejunum, or colon in cases of severe damage.

Associated conditions include perforation and bleeding, ulcer formation, secondary infection, mediastinitis, tracheoesophageal fistulas, strictures, hiatal hernia, aspiration pneumonia, carcinoma.

Assign code 530.10 for unspecified esophagitis, 530.11 for reflux esophagitis and 530.19 for other specified types of esophagitis.

530.10	Unspecified esophagitis — (Use additional E code to identify cause, if induced by chemical or drug) — *unknown*
530.11	Reflux esophagitis — (Use additional E code to identify cause, if induced by chemical or drug) — *inflammation of the lower esophagus from regurgitation of acid gastric contents*
530.19	Other esophagitis — (Use additional E code to identify cause, if induced by chemical or drug) — *not otherwise specified, including chemical burn, abscess, postoperative esophagitis*
530.2	Ulcer of esophagus — (Use additional E code to identify cause, if induced by chemical or drug) — *fungal, peptic, due to ingestion of aspirin, chemicals, medicine; including Barrett's syndrome*
530.3	Stricture and stenosis of esophagus — *compression, obstruction*
530.4	Perforation of esophagus — *rupture; including Boerhaave's syndrome*
530.5	Dyskinesia of esophagus — *curling, corkscrew, spasm; including Barsony-Polgar or Barsony-Teschendorf syndromes*
530.6	Diverticulum of esophagus, acquired — *herniated pouch or sac opening within the esophagus; epiphrenic, pharyngoesophageal, subdiaphragmatic, hypopharyngeal; esophagocele; traction, pulsion, pouch*
530.7	Gastroesophageal laceration-hemorrhage syndrome — *Mallory-Weiss syndrome*
	This subcategory classifies mucosal laceration (or vertical tear) of the esophagus or cardioesophageal junction. More commonly known as

✔5th   Needs fifth-digit   **OK**   Valid three-digit code

Mallory-Weiss syndrome, this condition follows prolonged or forceful vomiting.

530.81 Esophageal reflux — *regurgitation of contents of stomach into the esophagus, without inflammation*

530.82 Esophageal hemorrhage — *bleeding, except for varices*

530.83 Esophageal leukoplakia — *white patch in the esophagus which cannot be attributed to a specific disease*

530.84 Tracheoesophageal fistula — *acquired communication between trachea and esophagus*

530.89 Other specified disorder of the esophagus — *not otherwise specified, including cyst, deviation, erosion, fistula, pain, necrosis, relaxation, insufficiency*

530.9 Unspecified disorder of esophagus — *unknown*

531 GASTRIC ULCER

This rubric classifies a condition formed by discreet tissue destruction within the lumen of the stomach. The destruction is due to the action of hydrochloric (gastric) acid and pepsin on areas of gastric mucosa having a decreased resistance to ulceration.

Signs and symptoms of gastric ulcer include pain exacerbated by eating, weight loss, repeated vomiting, which is a sign of possible gastric outlet obstruction, vomiting of frank red blood or "coffee ground" material, black and tarry stools or heme positive stools if the ulcer is bleeding.

Lab work may show hypochromic blood loss anemia; gastric analysis shows acid pH after administration of histamine or pentagastrin with usual finding of low to normal secretion of gastric acid; upper GI series may be performed; upper endoscopy with biopsy may be performed to determine ulcer's benign or malignant status.

Therapies include antacids, diet modification, H2 receptor antagonist drugs such as cimetidine and ranitidine, and other therapeutic agents (sucralfate, carbenoxolone, bismuth, certain prostaglandins, tricyclic antidepressants such as doxepin). In addition, gastric irradiation may be performed to reduce acid production temporarily in patients who cannot tolerate drugs or surgery. Other therapies include distal subtotal gastrectomy, subtotal gastrectomy with wedge resection of gastric ulcer, vagotomy with drainage, and vagotomy with antrectomy.

Associated conditions include acute and/or chronic blood loss anemia and gastric outlet obstruction. A common factor in peptic ulcer is the presence of *Helicobacter pylori*, which is treated with bismuth salicylate and oral amoxicillin. The *H. pylori* should be reported secondarily with 041.86.

531.0 ✔5th Acute gastric ulcer with hemorrhage — *sudden, severe; prepyloric, pylorus, stomach; with bleeding*

531.1 ✔5th Acute gastric ulcer with perforation — *sudden, severe; prepyloric, pylorus, stomach; with leaking stomach contents*

531.2 ✔5th Acute gastric ulcer with hemorrhage and perforation — *sudden, severe; prepyloric, pylorus, stomach; with bleeding and leaking stomach contents*

531.3 ✔5th Acute gastric ulcer without mention of hemorrhage or perforation — *sudden, severe; prepyloric, pylorus, stomach; without bleeding or leaking stomach contents*

531.4 ✔5th Chronic or unspecified gastric ulcer with hemorrhage — *persistent; prepyloric, pylorus, stomach; with bleeding*

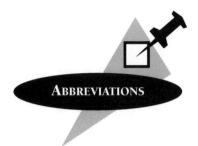

ABBREVIATIONS

BAD: basal acid output

DU: duodenal ulcer

GER: gastroesophageal reflux

GI: gastrointestinal

GU: gastric ulcer

IBS: irritable bowel syndrome

MAO: maximal acid output

PAO: peak acid output (same as MAO)

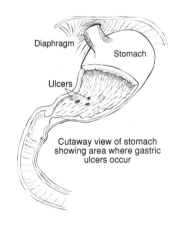

Cutaway view of stomach showing area where gastric ulcers occur

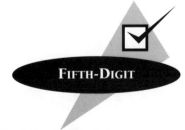

FIFTH-DIGIT

The following fifth-digit subclassification is for use with categories 531-535:

0 without mention of obstruction

1 with obstruction

531.5 ✓5th Chronic or unspecified gastric ulcer with perforation — *persistent; prepyloric, pylorus, stomach; with leaking stomach contents*

531.6 ✓5th Chronic or unspecified gastric ulcer with hemorrhage and perforation — *persistent; prepyloric, pylorus, stomach; with bleeding and leaking stomach contents*

531.7 ✓5th Chronic gastric ulcer without mention of hemorrhage or perforation — *persistent; prepyloric, pylorus, stomach; without bleeding or leaking stomach contents*

531.9 ✓5th Gastric ulcer, unspecified as acute or chronic, without mention of hemorrhage or perforation — *unknown whether sudden or persistent; prepyloric, pylorus, stomach; unknown status of bleeding or leaking stomach contents*

532 DUODENAL ULCER

Duodenal ulcers are ulcers formed in the duodenum by discreet tissue destruction due to the actions of hydrochloric (gastric) acid and pepsin on areas of the mucosa having a decreased resistance to ulceration. Duodenal ulcers occur about five times more frequently than gastric ulcers. About 95 percent occur in the area of the duodenal bulb or cap.

Signs and symptoms of duodenal ulcer include pain with cramps, burning, gnawing, heartburn, vomiting of highly acidic fluid with no retained food, deep epigastric tenderness, voluntary muscle guarding, unilateral rectus spasm over duodenal bulb, and melena and occult blood in stools in chronic ulcers. Pain diminishes by eating, but recurs two hours to three hours later.

Gastric analysis shows acid in all cases and a basal and maximal gastric hypersecretion of hydrochloric acid in some patients. Lab work may show hypochromic blood loss anemia. Radiographs demonstrate ulcer crater formation when the ulcer is not obscured by duodenal bulb formation. Esophagogastroduodenoscopy proves duodenal ulcer in cases not demonstrated radiographically.

Therapies include antacids, diet modification, H2 receptor antagonist drugs such as cimetidine and ranitidine, and other therapeutic agents (sucralfate, carbenoxolone, bismuth, certain prostaglandins, tricyclic antidepressants such as doxepin). Surgical interventions include subtotal gastrectomy, vagotomy, antrectomy, gastrojejunostomy, and total gastrectomy.

532.0 ✓5th Acute duodenal ulcer with hemorrhage — *sudden, severe; duodenum, postpyloric; with bleeding*

532.1 ✓5th Acute duodenal ulcer with perforation — *sudden, severe; duodenum, postpyloric; with leaking stomach contents*

532.2 ✓5th Acute duodenal ulcer with hemorrhage and perforation — *sudden, severe; duodenum, postpyloric; with bleeding and leaking stomach contents*

532.3 ✓5th Acute duodenal ulcer without mention of hemorrhage or perforation — *sudden, severe; duodenum, postpyloric; without bleeding or leaking stomach contents*

532.4 ✓5th Chronic or unspecified duodenal ulcer with hemorrhage — *persistent; duodenum, postpyloric; with bleeding*

532.5 ✓5th Chronic or unspecified duodenal ulcer with perforation — *persistent; duodenum, postpyloric; with leaking stomach contents*

532.6 ✓5th Chronic or unspecified duodenal ulcer with hemorrhage and perforation — *persistent; duodenum, postpyloric; with bleeding and leaking stomach contents*

532.7 ✓5th Chronic duodenal ulcer without mention of hemorrhage or perforation — *persistent; duodenum, postpyloric; without bleeding or leaking stomach contents*

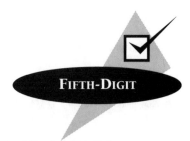

FIFTH-DIGIT

The following fifth-digit subclassification is for use with categories 531-535:

0 without mention of obstruction

1 with obstruction

✓5th Needs fifth-digit   **OK** Valid three-digit code

532.9 ✔5th Duodenal ulcer, unspecified as acute or chronic, without mention of hemorrhage or perforation — *unknown whether sudden or persistent; duodenum, postpyloric; unknown status of bleeding or leaking stomach contents*

533 PEPTIC ULCER, SITE UNSPECIFIED

This rubric classifies acute or chronic benign ulcer occurring in a portion of the digestive tract accessible to gastric secretions. Peptic ulcers result from the corrosive action of acid gastric juice on a vulnerable epithelium.

This rubric includes only peptic ulcers for which no site has been specified. Peptic ulcers may occur in the esophagus (code 530.2), stomach (code category 531), duodenum (code category 532), jejunum and gastrojejunal (code category 534), and ileum (code 569.82).

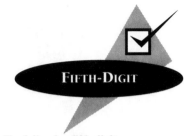

The following fifth-digit subclassification is for use with categories 531-535:

0 without mention of obstruction

1 with obstruction

533.0 ✔5th Acute peptic ulcer, unspecified site, with hemorrhage — *sudden, severe; site unknown; with bleeding*

533.1 ✔5th Acute peptic ulcer, unspecified site, with perforation — *sudden, severe; site unknown; with leaking stomach contents*

533.2 ✔5th Acute peptic ulcer, unspecified site, with hemorrhage and perforation — *sudden, severe; site unknown; with bleeding and leaking stomach contents*

533.3 ✔5th Acute peptic ulcer, unspecified site, without mention of hemorrhage and perforation — *sudden, severe; site unknown; without bleeding or leaking stomach contents*

533.4 ✔5th Chronic or unspecified peptic ulcer, unspecified site, with hemorrhage — *persistent; site unknown; with bleeding*

533.5 ✔5th Chronic or unspecified peptic ulcer, unspecified site, with perforation — *persistent; site unknown; with leaking stomach contents*

533.6 ✔5th Chronic or unspecified peptic ulcer, unspecified site, with hemorrhage and perforation — *persistent; site unknown; with bleeding and leaking stomach contents*

533.7 ✔5th Chronic peptic ulcer, unspecified site, without mention of hemorrhage or perforation — *persistent; site unknown; without bleeding or leaking stomach contents*

533.9 ✔5th Peptic ulcer, unspecified site, unspecified as acute or chronic, without mention of hemorrhage or perforation — *unknown whether sudden or persistent; site unknown; unknown status of bleeding or leaking stomach contents*

534 GASTROJEJUNAL ULCER

This rubric classifies ulcer formation at or proximal to the junction of a previous gastrojejunal anastomosis. The signs and symptoms, diagnostics, therapies and associated conditions are virtually the same as for gastric or duodenal ulcers.

534.0 ✔5th Acute gastrojejunal ulcer with hemorrhage — *sudden, severe; jejunal, gastrocolic, gastrointestinal, marginal, stomal, anastomotic; with bleeding*

534.1 ✔5th Acute gastrojejunal ulcer with perforation — *sudden, severe; jejunal, gastrocolic, gastrointestinal, marginal, stomal, anastomotic; with leaking stomach contents*

534.2 ✔5th Acute gastrojejunal ulcer with hemorrhage and perforation — *sudden, severe; jejunal, gastrocolic, gastrointestinal, marginal, stomal, anastomotic; with bleeding and leaking stomach contents*

534.3 ✔5th Acute gastrojejunal ulcer without mention of hemorrhage or perforation — *sudden, severe; jejunal, gastrocolic, gastrointestinal, marginal, stomal, anastomotic; without bleeding or leaking stomach contents*

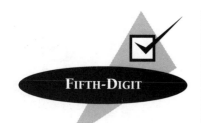

FIFTH-DIGIT

The following fifth-digit subclassification is for use with categories 531-535:

0 without mention of obstruction

1 with obstruction

SUFFIXES & PREFIXES

-acidity: the acid quantity in a fluid

-chlorhydria: hydrochloric acid (in stomach)

-motility: motion or movement

-tonicity: normal tension or pressure between tissues

Hyper-: above, more than, over

Hypo-: below, less than, under

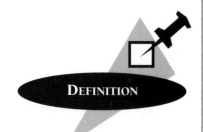

DEFINITION

Hematochezia: Frank blood in the stool.

Hematemesis: Vomiting of blood.

Maldigestion: Impaired digestion.

Melena: Dark, pitched blood in the stool.

Steatorrhea: Excessive fat in the stool.

Potain's syndrome: dilation of stomach with indigestion.

534.4 ✔5th Chronic or unspecified gastrojejunal ulcer with hemorrhage — *persistent; jejunal, gastrocolic, gastrointestinal, marginal, stomal, anastomotic; with bleeding*

534.5 ✔5th Chronic or unspecified gastrojejunal ulcer with perforation — *persistent; jejunal, gastrocolic, gastrointestinal, marginal, stomal, anastomotic; with leaking stomach contents*

534.6 ✔5th Chronic or unspecified gastrojejunal ulcer with hemorrhage and perforation — *persistent; jejunal, gastrocolic, gastrointestinal, marginal, stomal, anastomotic; with bleeding and leaking stomach contents*

534.7 ✔5th Chronic gastrojejunal ulcer without mention of hemorrhage or perforation — *persistent; jejunal, gastrocolic, gastrointestinal, marginal, stomal, anastomotic; without bleeding or leaking stomach contents*

534.9 ✔5th Gastrojejunal ulcer, unspecified as acute or chronic, without mention of hemorrhage or perforation — *unknown whether sudden or persistent; jejunal, gastrocolic, gastrointestinal, marginal, stomal, anastomotic; unknown status of bleeding or leaking stomach contents*

535 GASTRITIS AND DUODENITIS

This rubric classifies self-limiting illnesses characterized by nausea, vomiting, anorexia, epigastric pain, and some systemic symptoms. Manifestations may be variable but anorexia is a consistent feature.

535.0 ✔5th Acute gastritis — *severe inflammation of stomach*

535.1 ✔5th Atrophic gastritis — *inflammation of the stomach with atrophy of the mucous membrane and destruction of the peptic glands*

535.2 ✔5th Gastric mucosal hypertrophy — *increase in size and number of cells in tissue of gastric mucosa; Menetrier's syndrome*

535.3 ✔5th Alcoholic gastritis

535.4 ✔5th Other specified gastritis — *including allergic, bile-induced, irritant, superficial, toxic*

535.5 ✔5th Unspecified gastritis and gastroduodenitis — *unknown type*

535.6 ✔5th Duodenitis — *inflammation of the intestine between the pylorus and the jejunum*

536 DISORDERS OF FUNCTION OF STOMACH

536.0 Achlorhydria — *the absence of stomach acid, usually the result of atrophy of gastric mucosa; gastric anacidity*

536.1 Acute dilatation of stomach — *acute distention; Potain's syndrome*

536.2 Persistent vomiting — *habit, uncontrollable, Leyden's disease; not associated with pregnancy*

536.3 Gastroparesis — *a slight degree of paralysis within the muscular coat of the stomach*

536.40 Unspecified gastrostomy complication — *unknown type*

536.41 Infection of gastrostomy — (Use additional code to specify type of infection, such as: 682.2, 038.0–038.9) (Use additional code to identify organism: 041.00–041.9)

536.42 Mechanical complication of gastrostomy

536.49 Other gastrostomy complications — *not otherwise specified*

536.8 Dyspepsia and other specified disorders of function of stomach — *including hypermotility, hourglass contraction, hyperacidity, indigestion, pain, hypertonicity, Reichmann's syndrome, spasms, hypochlorhydria, hyperchlorhydria, Rossbach's disease*

536.9 Unspecified functional disorder of stomach — *unknown disorder or disturbance*

✔5th Needs fifth-digit   **OK** Valid three-digit code

537 OTHER DISORDERS OF STOMACH AND DUODENUM

537.0 Acquired hypertrophic pyloric stenosis — *construction, obstruction, stricture*

537.1 Gastric diverticulum — *herniated pouch or sac opening within the stomach or duodenum*

537.2 Chronic duodenal ileus — *persistent obstruction between the pylorus and jejunum*

537.3 Other obstruction of duodenum — *including cicatrix, stenosis, stricture, volvulus*

537.4 Fistula of stomach or duodenum — *including gastrocolic, gastrojejunocolic*

537.5 Gastroptosis — *downward displacement of the stomach*

537.6 Hourglass stricture or stenosis of stomach — *cascade stomach*

537.81 Pylorospasm — *spasmodic contraction of the distal aperture of the stomach*

537.82 Angiodysplasia of stomach and duodenum (without mention of hemorrhage) — *vascular abnormalities of stomach and duodenum, without bleeding*

537.83 Angiodysplasia of stomach and duodenum with hemorrhage — *vascular abnormalities of stomach and duodenum, with bleeding*

537.89 Other specified disorder of stomach and duodenum — *not otherwise specified, including prolapse, rupture, intestinal metaplasia of gastric mucosa, lesion, necrosis, gastrolith, hypertony, obstruction, volvulus, efferent loop syndrome, passive congestion, mechanical difficulty of gastroduodenal stoma*

537.9 Unspecified disorder of stomach and duodenum

540-543 Appendicitis

Appendicitis is inflammation of the vermiform appendix. It is usually initiated by obstruction of the appendiceal lumen by a fecalith, inflammation, neoplasm, or foreign body. The obstruction is followed by infection, edema, and, frequently, infarction of the appendiceal wall. Intraluminal tension develops rapidly and tends to cause mural necrosis and perforation.

Signs and symptoms of appendicitis include abdominal pain, usually beginning with epigastric or periumbilical pain associated with one or two episodes of vomiting. The abdominal may shift during the next 12 hours to the right lower quadrant (McBurney's point) where it persists as steady soreness aggravated by walking or coughing, anorexia, moderate malaise, slight to moderate fever, constipation (or occasionally diarrhea), rebound tenderness, and spasm.

Blood work may show moderate increase in white blood cells to 10,000/cu mm to 20,000/cu mm with an increase in neutrophils. Urinalysis may show presence of microscopic hematuria and pyuria and barium enema may be used to visualize the entire appendix in uncertain cases.

Therapies include antibiotic therapy, nasogastric intubation, rehydration, and appendectomy with few exceptions.

Appendicitis is the most common nonobstetrical complication of pregnancy.

540 ACUTE APPENDICITIS

540.0 Acute appendicitis with generalized peritonitis — *fulminating, gangrenous, obstructive; with perforation, rupture*

540.1 Acute appendicitis with peritoneal abscess — *generalized peritonitis; pocket of pus*

540.9 Acute appendicitis without mention of peritonitis — *without rupture, perforation, peritonitis*

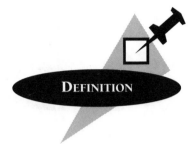

DEFINITION

Appendiclausis: withering or blockage of the appendix.

Fulminating: quickly increasing in severity.

Intussusception: when one part of an organ introverts into another part.

Reichmann's syndrome: excessive secretion of gastric juice either constantly or during digestion only.

Stercolith: a stone-like mass consisting of hardened feces.

Vascular splanchnic syndrome: visceral circulation syndrome.

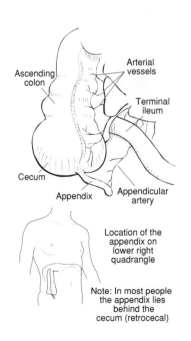

Ascending colon

Arterial vessels

Terminal ileum

Cecum

Appendix

Appendicular artery

Location of the appendix on lower right quadrangle

Note: In most people the appendix lies behind the cecum (retrocecal)

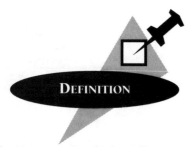

DEFINITION

Bezoar: aggregation of hair, seeds, or concretions in the digestive tract. A trichobezoar is formed from hair, and a phytobezoar is formed from vegetable matter. Bezoars can create obstructions or symptoms that are classified to this chapter. Bezoars are classified according to their site: stomach, 935.2; intestine, 936; other site in the digestive system, 938.

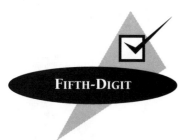

FIFTH-DIGIT

The following fifth-digit subclassification is for use with category 550:

0 unilateral or unspecified (not specified as recurrent)

1 unilateral or unspecified, recurrent

2 bilateral (not specified as recurrent)

3 bilateral, recurrent

541 APPENDICITIS, UNQUALIFIED **OK**

542 OTHER APPENDICITIS **OK**

543 OTHER DISEASES OF APPENDIX

543.0   Hyperplasia of appendix (lymphoid) — *increase in size and number of cells of appendix*

543.9   Other and unspecified diseases of appendix — *not otherwise specified, including adhesion, cyst, mucocele, stercolith, fecalith, fistula, sloughing, strangulation, atrophy, intussusception, diverticulum, concretion*

550-553 Hernia of Abdominal Cavity

The definition of hernia of abdominal cavity is protrusion of tissue, organ or part of an organ through an abnormal opening in the wall of the body cavity in which it is normally confined. The majority of hernias are abdominal resulting from herniation of abdominal contents through the internal or external inguinal rings, femoral rings or defects in the abdominal wall resulting from trauma or improper healing after a surgical procedure.

550 INGUINAL HERNIA

An inguinal hernia is defined as a condition in which a loop of intestine enters the inguinal canal, a tubular passage through the lower layers of the abdominal wall. A hernia occurs when part of an organ protrudes through a weak point or tear in the thin muscular wall that holds the abdominal organs in place. A direct inguinal hernia creates a bulge in the groin area, and an indirect hernia descends into the scrotum. Inguinal hernias occur less often in women than men.

Hernias are caused by congenital (defects at birth) or age-related weaknesses in the abdominal walls. In males, they are congenital and caused by an improper closure of the abdominal cavity. They can also be caused by an increase in pressure within the abdominal cavity due to heavy lifting, straining, violent coughing, obesity, or pregnancy.

Signs and symptoms include a protrusion in the groin area between the pubis and the top of the leg in the area known as the inguinal region of the abdomen or pain during urination or a bowel movement or when lifting a heavy object. The pain can be sharp and immediate. There may be a dull aching sensation, nausea or constipation; these feelings typically get worse toward the end of the day or after standing for long periods of time and may disappear when lying down.

A hernia that can be pushed back into the abdominal cavity (called a reducible hernia) is not considered an immediate health threat, though it does require surgery to repair the hernia. A hernia that cannot be pushed back in (called a nonreducible hernia) may lead to dangerous complications such as the obstruction of the flow of the intestinal contents or intestinal blood supply (strangulation), leading to tissue death, and requires immediate surgery.

550.0 ✔5th Inguinal hernia, with gangrene — *direct, double, indirect, oblique, sliding hernia; incarceration, irreducibility, strangulation*

550.1 ✔5th Inguinal hernia, with obstruction, without mention of gangrene — *direct, double, indirect, oblique, sliding hernia; incarceration, irreducibility, strangulation*

550.9 ✔5th Inguinal hernia, without mention of obstruction or gangrene — *direct, double, indirect, oblique, sliding hernia*

✔5th   Needs fifth-digit   **OK**   Valid three-digit code

551 OTHER HERNIA OF ABDOMINAL CAVITY, WITH GANGRENE

551.0 ✓5th Femoral hernia with gangrene — *abnormal protrusion of tissue into the femoral canal*

551.1 Umbilical hernia with gangrene — *abnormal protrusion of the intestine at the umbilicus*

551.20 Unspecified ventral hernia with gangrene — *abnormal protrusion of tissue through the abdominal wall, cause unknown*

551.21 Incisional ventral hernia, with gangrene — *abnormal protrusion of tissue through the abdominal wall, postoperative*

551.29 Other ventral hernia with gangrene — *abnormal protrusion of tissue through the abdominal wall, not otherwise specified*

551.3 Diaphragmatic hernia with gangrene — *hiatal, paraesophageal, thoracic stomach*

551.8 Hernia of other specified sites, with gangrene — *including Gruber's, Hesselbach's Rieux's; ischiorectal, lumbar, obturator, sciatic, retroperitoneal*

551.9 Hernia of unspecified site, with gangrene — *including enterocele, epiplocele, interstitial, intestinal, intraabdominal, sacroepiplocele*

552 OTHER HERNIA OF ABDOMINAL CAVITY, WITH OBSTRUCTION, BUT WITHOUT MENTION OF GANGRENE

552.0 ✓5th Femoral hernia with obstruction — *abnormal protrusion of tissue into the femoral canal; incarcerated, irreducible, strangulated*

552.1 Umbilical hernia with obstruction — *abnormal protrusion of the intestine of the umbilicus; incarcerated, irreducible, strangulated*

552.20 Unspecified ventral hernia with obstruction — *abnormal protrusion of tissue through the abdominal wall, cause unknown; incarcerated, irreducible, strangulated*

552.21 Incisional hernia with obstruction — *abnormal protrusion of tissue through the abdominal wall, postoperative; incarcerated, irreducible, strangulated*

552.29 Other ventral hernia with obstruction — *abnormal protrusion of tissue through the abdominal wall, not otherwise specified; incarcerated, irreducible, strangulated*

552.3 Diaphragmatic hernia with obstruction — *hiatal, esophageal, paraesophageal, thoracic stomach; incarcerated, irreducible, strangulated*

552.8 Hernia of other specified site, with obstruction — *other sites including Gruber's, Hesselbach's Rieux's; Treitz's, ischiorectal, lumbar, obturator, retroperitoneal; incarcerated, irreducible, strangulated*

552.9 Hernia of unspecified site, with obstruction — *unknown site*

553 OTHER HERNIA OF ABDOMINAL CAVITY WITHOUT MENTION OF OBSTRUCTION OR GANGRENE

553.0 ✓5th Femoral hernia without mention of obstruction or gangrene — *abnormal protrusion of tissue into the femoral canal*

553.1 Umbilical hernia without mention of obstruction or gangrene — *abnormal protrusion of the intestine at the umbilicus; paraumbilical*

553.20 Unspecified ventral hernia without mention of obstruction or gangrene — *abnormal protrusion of tissue through the abdominal wall; cause unknown*

553.21 Incisional hernia without mention of obstruction or gangrene — *abnormal protrusion of tissue through the abdominal wall; postoperative*

553.29 Other ventral hernia without mention of obstruction or gangrene — *not otherwise specified; including epigastric, spigelian*

553.3 Diaphragmatic hernia without mention of obstruction or gangrene — *hiatal, paraesophageal, thoracic stomach*

Use this code to report protrusion of part of the stomach through the esophageal hiatus of the diaphragm. The esophageal hiatus is the opening

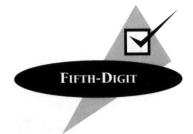

FIFTH-DIGIT

The following fifth-digit subclassification is for use with categories 551.0, 552.0, and 553.0:

0 unilateral or unspecified (not specified as recurrent)

1 unilateral or unspecified, recurrent

2 bilateral (not specified as recurrent)

3 bilateral, recurrent

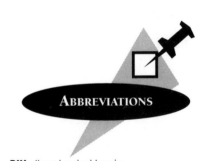

ABBREVIATIONS

DIH: direct inguinal hernia

HH: hiatal hernia, bulging of the stomach through the esophageal hiatus of the diaphragm

RIH: recurrent inguinal hernia

VH: ventral hernia

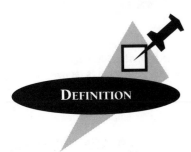

DEFINITION

Cooper's: a femoral hernia with two protrusions.

Hesselbach's: a hernia of the diverticula through the fascia that covers the upper thigh.

Holthouse's: a hernia of the intestine along the ligamentum inguinale.

Petit's disease: a hernia occurring in trigonum lumbale, an area of the abdominal wall.

Richter's: a hernia of the intestinal wall.

Treitz's: a duodenojejunal hernia.

in the diaphragm between the central tendon and the hiatus aorticus where the esophagus and the two vagus nerves pass. Clinicians recognize two different types of esophageal hiatal hernias: paraesophageal and sliding (by far the more common type of hiatal hernia).

The paraesophageal hiatal hernia is characterized by all or part of the stomach herniating into the thorax immediately adjacent and to the left of a nondisplaced gastroesophageal junction. Reflux of the gastric contents does not occur because the gastroesophageal sphincter functions normal. Although this type of hiatal hernia is usually asymptomatic, complications can include hemorrhage, incarceration, obstruction, and strangulation.

With a sliding hiatal hernia, the upper stomach, along with the cardioesophageal junction, herniates upward into the posterior mediastinum. The stomach displacement may be stationary, or it may actually slide in and out of the thorax with movement, after a large meal or with alterations of the pressure in the abdominal and thoracic cavities. Esophageal reflux and esophagitis are characteristic and due to abnormalities in the esophageal sphincter. Sliding hiatal hernia may be complicated by development of ulcers or structure formation. Carcinoma is occasionally associated with sliding hiatal hernia.

Signs and symptoms of diaphragmatic hernia without mention of obstruction or gangrene include dysphagia and retrosternal and epigastric burning for sliding hiatal hernia with reflux esophagitis, and is asymptomatic until complications develop.

Diagnostic tests include x-ray examination and fluoroscopy with or without contrast to demonstrate protrusion of stomach through esophageal hiatus. Esophagoscopy and biopsy assess the severity of any esophagitis and rule out associated conditions such as strictures, polyps, ulcers, and carcinomas. Esophageal motility studies assess the competency of the esophageal sphincter and prolonged monitoring of the patient's pH in the lower esophagus establishes presence of abnormal reflux.

Therapies include diet and antacids for esophagitis. There is no intervention for asymptomatic hiatal hernias. Surgery (for about 15 percent of patients with persistent and severe symptoms) includes Nissen fundoplication, Belsey fundoplication, and placement of doughnut shaped silicone prosthesis around the intraabdominal esophagus (Angelchik procedure) for uncomplicated hernias. The Collis procedure or Collis-Nissen operation may be performed when hernia is associated with acquired short esophagus. Other treatments include vagotomy, antrectomy, or a Roux-en-Y gastrojejunostomy when scar tissue around gastroesophageal junction from previous surgery prevents a fundoplication.

✔5th   Needs fifth-digit   **OK**   Valid three-digit code

Associated conditions include reflux esophagitis, esophageal stricture, polyps, ulcer formation with or without bleeding, carcinoma, and Saint's triad (hiatal hernia, gallbladder disease, and colon diverticulosis).

553.8   Hernia of other specified sites of abdominal cavity without mention of obstruction or gangrene — *including appendix, obturator, pudendal, retroperitoneal, sciatic, lumbar, ischiatic, ischiorectal, duodenojejunal, mesenteric, mesocolon, omental*

553.9   Hernia of unspecified site of abdominal cavity without mention of obstruction or gangrene — *unknown*

555-558 Noninfectious Enteritis and Colitis

555 REGIONAL ENTERITIS

Regional enteritis is a form of inflammatory bowel disease characterized by a chronic granulomatous disease. Also known as Crohn's disease, regional enteritis most often affects the large intestines but may occur anywhere in the gastrointestinal tract (e.g., mouth, esophagus, stomach, duodenum, large intestine, appendix, and anus). The disease often results in multiple bowel resections.

Associated conditions include multiple strictures, bacterial overgrowth, and malabsorption.

555.0   Regional enteritis of small intestine — *Crohn's disease, granulomatous enteritis; duodenum, ileum, jejunum*

555.1   Regional enteritis of large intestine — *Crohn's disease, granulomatous enteritis; colon, large bowel, rectum*

555.2   Regional enteritis of small intestine with large intestine — *Crohn's disease, granulomatous enteritis; regional ileocolitis*

555.9   Regional enteritis of unspecified site — *unknown*

556 ULCERATIVE COLITIS

Ulcerative colitis is a disease that causes inflammation and ulcers in the top layers of the lining of the large intestine. The inflammation usually occurs in the rectum and lower part of the colon, but it may affect the entire colon and makes the colon empty frequently, causing diarrhea. Ulcers form in places where the inflammation has killed colon cells; the ulcers bleed and produce pus and mucus.

Ulcerative colitis rarely affects the small intestine except for the lower section, called the ileum. The disease can be difficult to diagnose because its symptoms are similar to other intestinal disorders such as irritable bowel syndrome and Crohn's disease, which usually occurs in the small intestine but may occur anywhere in the GI tract.

The most common symptoms of ulcerative colitis are abdominal pain and bloody diarrhea. Patients also may experience fatigue, weight loss, and rectal bleeding.

Blood tests may be performed to check for anemia, which could indicate bleeding in the colon or rectum. Blood tests may also reveal a high white blood cell count. A stool sample indicates whether there is bleeding or infection in the colon or rectum. A colonoscopy visualizes the inside of the colon and rectum. A barium enema x-ray of the colon allows a clear view of the colon, including any ulcers or other abnormalities. Treatment for ulcerative colitis depends on the seriousness of the disease. Most people are treated with

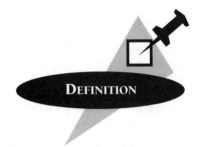

DEFINITION

Gangrene: necrosis due to infarction, may be dry or wet (with a bacterial infection causing cellulitis in the bordering tissue).

Infarction: insufficiency or blockage of blood flow due to an embolus, thrombus, or other type of blockage or pressure on vessel.

Ischemia: an lack of blood flow to affected area.

Necrosis: irreversible damage to tissue causing a death of the cells.

Vascular splanchnic syndrome: visceral circulation syndrome.

Wilkie's syndrome: complete of partial block of the superior mesenteric artery with symptoms of vomiting, pain, blood in the stool, and distended abdomen. Results in bowel infarction.

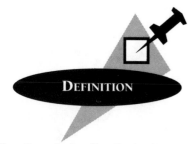

DEFINITION

Grey Turner's sign: Blue discoloration, a bruising, of the skin of the loin seen in acute hemorrhagic pancreatitis.

Cullen's sign: Blue discoloration, a bruising, of the skin around the umbilicus seen in hemorrhagic abdominal disease.

Psoas sign: Pain on hyperextension of the hip, often seen in appendicitis.

Rovsing's sign: Pain upon palpation pressure in the right lower quadrant, often associated with appendicitis.

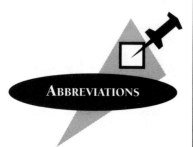

ABBREVIATIONS

CD: Crohn's disease, an inflammation of the distal ileum and colon and sometimes part of the gastrointestinal tract

GE: gastroenteritis

UC: ulcerative colitis

medication, although in severe cases, a patient may need surgery to remove the diseased colon.

556.0	Ulcerative (chronic) enterocolitis — *persistent inflammation of the mucous membrane of small and large intestines*
556.1	Ulcerative (chronic) ileocolitis — *persistent inflammation of the mucous membrane of ileum and colon*
556.2	Ulcerative (chronic) proctitis — *persistent inflammation of the mucous membrane of the rectum*
556.3	Ulcerative (chronic) proctosigmoiditis — *persistent inflammation of the mucous membrane of the sigmoid colon and rectum*
556.4	Pseudopolyposis of colon
556.5	Left sided ulcerative (chronic) colitis
556.6	Universal ulcerative (chronic) colitis — *persistent inflammation of the mucous membrane of the entire colon*
556.8	Other ulcerative colitis
556.9	Unspecified ulcerative colitis

557 VASCULAR INSUFFICIENCY OF INTESTINE

557.0	Acute vascular insufficiency of intestine — *infarction, necrosis, hemorrhage, gangrene, thrombosis, embolism*
557.1	Chronic vascular insufficiency of intestine — *abdominal angina, ischemic colitis or enteritis, stricture, artery syndrome, vascular insufficiency, Wilkie's syndrome*
557.9	Unspecified vascular insufficiency of intestine — *unknown*

558 OTHER NONINFECTIOUS GASTROENTERITIS AND COLITIS

558.1	Gastroenteritis and colitis due to radiation — *radiation enterocolitis*
558.2	Toxic gastroenteritis and colitis
558.3	Gastroenteritis and colitis, allergic
558.9	Other and unspecified noninfectious gastroenteritis and colitis — *including dietetic, noninfectious*

Other and unspecified noninfectious gastroenteritis and colitis include gastroenteritis and colitis that do not have an infectious or presumed infectious origin. The three most common forms are enteritis, gastroenteritis, and diarrhea not otherwise specified.

Often, enteritis, gastroenteritis and diarrhea, when specified as due to an underlying condition, should be classified to a different category. Infectious disease is the most frequent cause of gastritis and gastroenteritis and is classified to Chapter 1 Infectious and Parasitic Diseases (001-139).

Commonly caused by infection, diarrhea may also be caused by chronic bowel disease, malabsorption states, food poisoning, adverse reactions to medications, and dietary factors such as malnutrition and food allergy. Diarrhea also may be the result of cholestatic syndromes, pancreatic disease, metabolic disease, neurological disease, psychogenic disorders, heavy metal poisoning, laxative abuse, reflex from other viscera, and immunodeficiency disease.

✒5th   Needs fifth-digit   **OK**   Valid three-digit code

560-569 Other Diseases of Intestines and Peritoneum

560 INTESTINAL OBSTRUCTION WITHOUT MENTION OF HERNIA

560.0   Intussusception — *prolapse of one section of bowel into an immediate adjacent section; invagination*

560.1   Paralytic ileus — *adynamic, paralysis*

Use this code to report functional obstruction of the intestines, usually the colon. Also known as adynamic ileus, this condition represents a neurogenic impairment of peristalsis that can lead to complete intestinal obstruction. The intraabdominal etiologies for paralytic ileus include gastrointestinal surgery (997.4), peritoneal irritations (such as intraabdominal hemorrhage, ruptured viscus, pancreatitis or peritonitis), or anoxic organic obstruction. Other etiologies include drugs with anticholinergic properties, renal colic, vertebral fractures, spinal cord injuries, uremia, severe infection, diabetic coma, and electrolyte imbalances.

Signs and symptoms of paralytic ileus include continuous mild to moderate abdominal pain, vomiting, constipation, and abdominal distention. There may be absent borborygmus, minimal to absent bowel sounds, and signs of dehydration. Lab work may show hemoconcentration and electrolyte imbalances. Leukocytosis, anemia, elevated serum amylase may be present depending on the initiating condition. X-ray of the abdomen shows distended gas-filled loops of bowel and may show air-fluid levels in the distended bowel.

Therapies include bed rest, restriction of oral intake, rehydration, and gastrointestinal suctioning. Surgical decompression via enterostomy or cecostomy may be performed in severe cases. Associated conditions include dehydration and other electrolyte imbalances.

When assigning this code, coders also should classify any initiating diseases or disorders such as those outlined in the definition.

560.2   Volvulus — *knotting, strangulation, torsion, twists*

560.30   Unspecified impaction of intestine — *unknown type*

560.31   Gallstone ileus — *obstruction by gallstone*

560.39   Other impaction of intestine — *fecal reservoir syndrome, fecal impaction, enterolith, concretion*

560.81   Intestinal or peritoneal adhesions with obstruction (postoperative) (postinfection) — *abnormal joining of separate tissue in the peritoneum or intestine*

560.89   Other specified intestinal obstruction — *including mural thickening causing obstruction, sympathicotonic obstruction, Ogilvie's syndrome*

560.9   Unspecified intestinal obstruction — *unknown*

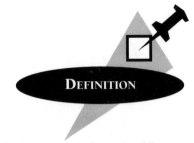

DEFINITION

Borborygmus: gurgling and rumbling sounds that are caused by the movement of gas through the intestines.

562 DIVERTICULA OF INTESTINE

Report any associated peritonitis with an additional code (567.0-567.9). Excluded from this rubric are congenital diverticulum of the colon (751.5); diverticulum of the appendix (543.9); and Meckel's diverticulum (751.0).

562.00	Diverticulosis of small intestine (without mention of hemorrhage) — (Use additional code to identify any associated condition, as: 567.0–567.9) — *sac-like herniations of the mucosal lining; duodenum, ileum, jejunum*
562.01	Diverticulitis of small intestine (without mention of hemorrhage) — (Use additional code to identify any associated condition, as: 567.0–567.9) — *inflammation of sac-like herniations of mucosal lining; duodenum, ileum, jejunum*
562.02	Diverticulosis of small intestine with hemorrhage — (Use additional code to identify any associated condition, as: 567.0–567.9) — *sac-like herniations of the mucosal lining; duodenum, ileum, jejunum; bleeding*
562.03	Divertulitis of small intestine with hemorrhage — (Use additional code to identify any associated condition, as: 567.0–567.9) — *inflammation of sac-like herniations of mucosal lining; duodenum, ileum, jejunum; bleeding*

562.1 Diverticula of colon

Use this subclassification to report formation of a pouch or sac in the colon due to pressure from within the colon. Diverticula and diverticulosis tend to occur in higher-pressure areas such as the sigmoid colon and dissect along the course of nutrient vessels. They consist of a mucosal coat and serosa and usually herniate through the muscularis of the colon.

Signs and symptoms of diverticula of colon include left lower quadrant pain, either steady or severe lasting for days or cramping and intermittent and relieved by bowel movement, and constipation (or occasionally diarrhea). Guaiac testing shows occult blood in 20 percent of patients with diverticulosis. X-ray reveals diverticula and in some cases colonic spasm and interhaustral thickening or narrowing of the colonic lumen. Endoscopic exam with or without biopsy is performed when bleeding occurs to rule out other pathology. Therapies include increased bulk and fiber in diet, anticholinergic medications to control sigmoid colon spasm, and antibiotics for diverticulitis. Surgical resection of involved portion of bowel may be performed when there are recurrent bouts of diverticulitis or to treat complications such as hemorrhage, perforation, and abscess formation.

True diverticula contain all layers of the bowel and are rare in the colon. False diverticula consist of mucous and submucosa that have herniated through the muscularis. For coding purposes, the terms "true" and "false" have no significance and should be treated as nonessential modifiers.

Diverticula of the colon are considered pulsion type because they are pushed out by intraluminal pressure. In the ICD-9-CM index, the term "pulsion" is an essential modifier under the main term "Diverticula, diverticulosis, diverticulum," leading to code 530.6 for diverticula of the esophagus. Do not assign this code for a pulsion diverticula when it refers to other anatomic sites such as the colon.

562.10	Diverticulosis of colon (without mention of hemorrhage) — (Use additional code to identify any associated condition, as: 567.0–567.9) — *sac-like herniations of the mucosal lining*
562.11	Diverticulitis of colon (without mention of hemorrhage) — (Use additional code to identify any associated condition, as: 567.0–567.9) — *inflammation of sac-like herniations of mucosal lining*

✔5th Needs fifth-digit **OK** Valid three-digit code

562.12   Diverticulosis of colon with hemorrhage — (Use additional code to identify any associated condition, as: 567.0–567.9) — *sac-like herniations of the mucosal lining; bleeding*

562.13   Diverticulitis of colon with hemorrhage — (Use additional code to identify any associated condition, as: 567.0–567.9) — *inflammation of sac-like herniations of mucosal lining; bleeding*

564 FUNCTIONAL DIGESTIVE DISORDERS, NOT ELSEWHERE CLASSIFIED

Excluded from this rubric are functional disorders of the stomach (536.0-536.9) and digestive disorders that have been specified as psychogenic (306.4).

564.0   Constipation — *infrequent or incomplete bowel movement*

564.1   Irritable bowel syndrome — *IBS, irritable bowel*

564.2   Postgastric surgery syndromes — *dumping, jejunal, postgastrectomy, postvagotomy syndromes*

564.3   Vomiting following gastrointestinal surgery

564.4   Other postoperative functional disorders — *including diarrhea*

564.5   Functional diarrhea — *diarrhea with no detectable organic cause*

564.6   Anal spasm — *proctalgia fugax*

564.7   Megacolon, other than Hirschsprung's — *dilatation of colon; faulty bowel habit syndrome*

564.81   Neurogenic bowel

564.89   Other functional disorders of intestine — *including atony of colon*

564.9   Unspecified functional disorder of intestine — *unknown*

565 ANAL FISSURE AND FISTULA

Excluded from this rubric are traumatic fissures (863.89, 863.99), and fistulas of the rectum to internal organs. Refer to the index of ICD-9 to accurately classify fistulas of the rectum to internal organs.

565.0   Anal fissure — *nontraumatic tear*

565.1   Anal fistula — *anorectal, rectum to skin*

567 PERITONITIS

Use this rubric to report acute or chronic inflammation of the peritoneum. It may be in response to agents such as bacteria, viruses, bile, hydrochloric acid, and chemicals such as continuous ambulatory peritoneal dialysis (CAPD) fluid. Other causative agents include parasites, fungi, and foreign bodies such as barium sulfate used in diagnostic roentgenographic studies. Ruptured viscus and surgical procedures are two common underlying factors in secondary peritonitis. Chronic peritonitis can lead to dense, widespread abdominal adhesions.

Excluded from this rubric are peritonitis defined as benign paroxysmal (277.3); female pelvic (614.5, 614.7); periodic familial (277.3); puerperal (670); or in cases of abortion (rubrics 634-638); appendicitis (540.0-540.1); or ectopic/molar pregnancy (639.0).

567.0   Peritonitis in infectious diseases classified elsewhere — (Code first underlying disease) — *secondary to underlying disease*

567.1   Pneumococcal peritonitis — *inflammation of peritoneal*

567.2   Other suppurative peritonitis — *abdominopelvic, mesenteric, omentum, peritoneum, retrocecal, retroperitoneal, subdiaphragmatic, subhepatic, subphrenic*

567.8   Other specified peritonitis — *not otherwise specified, including fat necrosis, peritonitis due to bile or urine*

567.9   Unspecified peritonitis — *unknown*

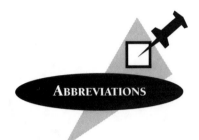

ABBREVIATIONS

BS: bowel sounds

IBS: irritable bowel syndrome, also spastic colon, and a gastrointestinal disorder of motility. Symptoms can be diarrhea, constipation, pain and abdominal distention and can be exacerbated by food ingestion or stress

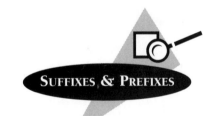

SUFFIXES & PREFIXES

Peri-: around, encircling, surrounding

Retro-: in back of, behind

Sub-: beneath, less than, below, under

568 OTHER DISORDERS OF PERITONEUM

568.0   Peritoneal adhesions (postoperative) (postinfection) — *abdominal wall, diaphragm, intestine, male pelvis, mesenteric, omentum, stomach, adhesive bands*

568.81   Hemoperitoneum (nontraumatic) — *blood in the peritoneal cavity*

568.82   Peritoneal effusion (chronic) — *persistent escape of fluid within the peritoneal cavity*

568.89   Other specified disorder of peritoneum — *not otherwise specified, including acquired deforming, hemorrhage, rupture, degeneration, cyst, granuloma, pneumatosis*

568.9   Unspecified disorder of peritoneum — *unknown*

569 OTHER DISORDERS OF INTESTINE

569.0   Anal and rectal polyp — *not otherwise specified*

569.1   Rectal prolapse — *procidentia; anus, rectum*

569.2   Stenosis of rectum and anus — *stricture*

569.3   Hemorrhage of rectum and anus — *bleeding*

569.41   Ulcer of anus and rectum — *solitary, stercoral*

569.42   Anal or rectal pain — *proctalgia*

569.49   Other specified disorder of rectum and anus — *not otherwise specified, including hypertrophy of anal papillae; granuloma, rupture, male proctocele/rectocele, relaxation, paralysis, cicatrix*

569.5   Abscess of intestine — *pocket of pus*

569.60   Unspecified complication of colostomy or enterostomy — *unknown*

569.61   Infection of colostomy or enterostomy — (Use additional code to specify type of infection, such as: 682.2, 038.0–038.9)

569.62   Mechanical complication of colostomy and enterostomy — *malfunction*

569.69   Other complication of colostomy or enterostomy — *not otherwise specified, including fistula, hernia, stenosis, prolapse*

569.81   Fistula of intestine, excluding rectum and anus — *abnormal communication between intestine and other internal organ or site*

569.82   Ulceration of intestine

569.83   Perforation of intestine — *hole through the intestinal wall*

569.84   Angiodysplasia of intestine (without mention of hemorrhage) — *degenerative dilation of vasculature of intestine, without bleeding*

569.85   Angiodysplasia of intestine with hemorrhage — *degenerative dilation of vasculature of intestine, with bleeding*

569.89   Other specified disorder of intestines — *not otherwise specified, including enteroptosis, granuloma, prolapse, acquired deformity, sacculation, Lane's, Glenard's, or Payr's disease*

569.9   Unspecified disorder of intestine — *unknown*

570-579 Other Diseases of Digestive System

570 ACUTE AND SUBACUTE NECROSIS OF LIVER `OK`

Excluded from this rubric are icterus gravis of newborn (773.0-773.2); serum hepatitis (070.2-070.3); necrosis in viral hepatitis (070.0-070.9); and necrosis with abortion, ectopic pregnancy, molar pregnancy, childbirth, pregnancy, or the puerperium (see Chapter 11).

571 CHRONIC LIVER DISEASE AND CIRRHOSIS

Use this rubric to report chronic liver disease and cirrhosis not due to infection. The liver is the largest gland in the body and serves many metabolic purposes including secretion of bile. Chronic alcohol use leads to three similar forms of liver disease: steatosis (fatty liver),

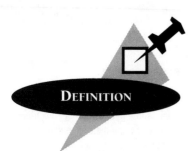

DEFINITION

Glenard's syndrome: also Payr's syndrome, bloating, gas, pain, and fullness experienced in left upper abdominal quadrant with pain sometimes radiating up into left chest. Downward displacement of viscera may cause bulging of abdomen and other symptoms.

✎5th   Needs fifth-digit   `OK`   Valid three-digit code

hepatitis, and cirrhosis. The conditions have many overlapping features and each may occur without involvement of alcohol. Alcoholic cirrhosis accounts for about 60 percent of all cirrhosis cases and the risk appears to rise with the amount of alcohol consumed daily. The liver tends to shrink and become fibrotic.

Hepatitis is defined as inflammation of the liver, which is usually due to viral infection classified elsewhere or to toxic agents such as alcohol or drugs. Cirrhosis of the liver is a chronic, progressive disease characterized by damage to the hepatic parenchymal cells and nodular regeneration, fibrosis formation, and disturbance of the normal architecture. Two different types of cirrhosis have been described based on the amount of regenerative activity in the liver: chronic sclerosing cirrhosis in which the liver is small and hard, and nodular cirrhosis in which the liver may be quite enlarged initially.

571.0	Alcoholic fatty liver
571.1	Acute alcoholic hepatitis — *severe inflammation of the liver due to alcoholic liver disease; Zieve's syndrome*
571.2	Alcoholic cirrhosis of liver — *fibrosis and dysfunction of the liver due to alcoholic liver disease; Laennec's cirrhosis*
571.3	Unspecified alcoholic liver damage — *unknown*
571.40	Unspecified chronic hepatitis — *unknown*
571.41	Chronic persistent hepatitis — *persistent*
571.49	Other chronic hepatitis — *not otherwise specified, including Bearn-Kunkel-Slater syndrome, Wadenstrom's hepatitis*
571.5	Cirrhosis of liver without mention of alcohol — *fibrosis and dysfunction of the liver not due to alcohol consumption; cryptogenic, macronodular, micronodular; posthepatic, postnecrotic; Cruveilhier-Baumgarten cirrhosis*
571.6	Biliary cirrhosis — *fibrosis and dysfunction of the liver due to obstruction or infection of bile ducts; cholangitic, cholestatic*
571.8	Other chronic nonalcoholic liver disease — *not otherwise specified, including fatty liver without alcohol, hardening liver, chronic yellow atrophy*
571.9	Unspecified chronic liver disease without mention of alcohol — *unknown disease of liver*

572 LIVER ABSCESS OF SEQUELAE OF CHRONIC LIVER DISEASE

Excluded from this rubric is amebic liver abscess (006.3) and hepatorenal syndrome following delivery (674.8).

572.0	Abscess of liver — *pocket of pus*
572.1	Portal pyemia — *inflammation of portal vein or its branches; phlebitis, thrombophlebitis, pylephlebitis*
572.2	Hepatic coma — *portal-systemic encephalopathy*
572.3	Portal hypertension — *abnormally high blood pressure in the portal vein*
572.4	Hepatorenal syndrome — *kidney failure associated with liver disease; Heyd's syndrome*
572.8	Other sequelae of chronic liver disease — *not elsewhere specified, including adhesion, granuloma*

573 OTHER DISORDERS OF LIVER

Excluded from this rubric are amyloid or lardaceous degeneration of liver (277.3); congenital cystic liver disease (751.62); glycogen infiltration of liver (271.0); hepatomegaly not otherwise specified (789.1); and portal vein obstruction (452).

Code first underlying disease as appropriate.

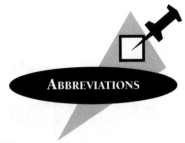

ABBREVIATIONS

ADH: alcohol dehydrogenase

FFA: Free fatty acids

MCV: mean corpuscular volume

MEOS: microsomal ethanol oxidizing system

NADH: nicotinamide adenine dinucleotide

PBC: primary biliary cirrhosis

PSC: primary sclerosing cholangitis

CLD: chronic liver disease

FFA: free fatty acids, when these accumulate in the liver it is a disorder called fatty liver or steatosis. This is a common result of the liver to injury and alcohol damage

PBC: primary biliary cirrhosis, cirrhosis due to biliary obstruction that is identified by a chronic diminished or blocked flow of bile

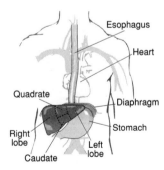

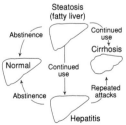

Interelationships among alcoholic steatosis, hepatitis, and cirrhosis

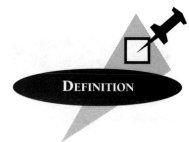

DEFINITION

Bearn-Kunkel-Slater syndrome: chronic hepatitis with autoimmune manifestations.

Glisson's cirrhosis: chronic thickening of the liver which results in a shriveled and deformed organ.

Laennec's cirrhosis: also portal cirrhosis, usually caused by alcoholism, a type of cirrhosis in which small nodules replace the healthy liver lobules.

Rokitansky's disease: a wasting of the liver causing a yellowish color.

Zieve's syndrome: acute hepatitis or cirrhosis of the liver associated with alcoholism.

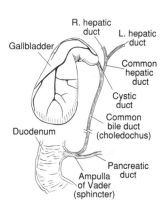

573.0   Chronic passive congestion of liver — *persistent accumulation of escaped blood in liver tissue*

573.1   Hepatitis in viral diseases classified elsewhere — (Code first underlying disease, as: 074.8, 075, 078.5) — *secondary to underlying disease*

573.2   Hepatitis in other infectious diseases classified elsewhere — (Code first underlying disease, as: 084.9) — *secondary to underlying disease*

573.3   Unspecified hepatitis — (Use additional E code to identify cause) — *unknown*

573.4   Hepatic infarction — *area of dead liver tissue due to an interruption in circulation in that area*

573.8   Other specified disorders of liver — *including hepatoptosis, hypertrophy, hemorrhage, obstruction, induration, lesion, prolapse, nontraumatic rupture*

573.9   Unspecified disorder of liver — *unknown, including distention, palpable or torpid liver*

574 CHOLELITHIASIS

Use this rubric to report the presence or formation of concretions (calculi or "gallstones") in the gallbladder. The concretions contain cholesterol, calcium carbonate, or calcium bilirubinate either in pure forms or in various combinations. Many factors contribute to concretion formation, but they generally can be grouped into three categories: abnormal composition of bile, abnormal contractility of the gallbladder, and abnormal epithelial secretions. The disease is rare in children, and the rate of incidence is greater in people of Native American ancestry and in women.

Choledocholithiasis is the presence or formation of concretions in any of the bile ducts. Common duct stones usually originate in the gallbladder, but may form spontaneously in the common duct following cholecystectomy. Features, in addition to those of cholecystitis, that suggest choledocholithiasis include Charcot's triad and cholangitis. Charcot's triad is a symptom complex consisting of frequently recurring attacks of severe, persistent, right upper quadrant pain lasting for hours; chills and fever associated with severe colic; and a history of jaundice chronologically associated with abdominal pain. Secondary pancreatitis, biliary cirrhosis, and hypoprothrombinemia may complicate choledocholithiasis.

Signs and symptoms of cholelithiasis include cramps or severe epigastric pain, nausea and vomiting, heartburn, eructation, flatulence, sensation of dullness in stomach, jaundice, distention of gallbladder, and pain on palpation of gallbladder. It is asymptomatic in many patients. X-rays of abdomen may show cholelithiasis, but most concretions are made up of cholesterol, which is radiolucent and cannot be visualized. Gallbladder ultrasound, HIDA scanning (a form of radionuclide excretion scan involving the intravenous injection of iminodiacetic acid), oral cholecystography confirm the diagnosis. Lab work reveals cholesterol crystal formation in bile, and granules of calcium bilirubinate in duodenal aspirate; with acute cholecystitis. Lab work may reveal increased white blood cell count and serum bilirubin.

Therapies include administration of chenodeoxycholic acid for one year to two years to dissolve concretions in asymptomatic patients; in asymptomatic diabetic patients, cholecystectomy is performed to avoid serious future complications. For acute cholecystitis, cholecystectomy (by open incision, laparoscopy, or endoscopically) is performed at the time of the acute cholecystitis, or electively four weeks to six weeks after recovery in uncomplicated cases. A cholangiogram detects concretions blocking common bile duct. If

✔5th   Needs fifth-digit   **OK**   Valid three-digit code

concretions are found, there is common bile duct exploration or insertion of T-tube with infusion of mono-octanoin to dissolve the stones.

Associated conditions include acute cholecystitis (including its major complications of empyema, perforations, pericholecystic abscess, bile peritonitis, and cholecystenteric fistulas), chronic cholecystitis, biliary adhesions, secondary pancreatitis, postcholecystectomy syndrome, Crohn's disease, liver damage, and obesity.

574.0 ✔5th Calculus of gallbladder with acute cholecystitis — *severe inflammation due to gallstone(s); cholelithiasis,*

574.1 ✔5th Calculus of gallbladder with other cholecystitis — *inflammation, persistent or unspecified, due to gallstone(s); cholelithiasis*

574.2 ✔5th Calculus of gallbladder without mention of cholecystitis — *presence of gallstone(s) without inflammation*

574.3 ✔5th Calculus of bile duct with acute cholecystitis — *severe inflammation of gallbladder due to stone(s) in bile duct*

574.4 ✔5th Calculus of bile duct with other cholecystitis — *inflammation, persistent and unspecified, of gallbladder due to stone(s) in bile duct*

574.5 ✔5th Calculus of bile duct without mention of cholecystitis — *presence of bile duct stone(s) without inflammation of gallbladder*

574.6 ✔5th Calculus of gallbladder and bile duct with acute cholecystitis — *presence of bile duct and gallbladder stones with severe inflammation*

574.7 ✔5th Calculus of gallbladder and bile duct with other cholecystitis — *presence of bile duct and gallbladders stones, inflammation persistent and unspecified*

574.8 ✔5th Calculus of gallbladder and bile duct with acute and chronic cholecystitis — *severe and persistent inflammation of gallbladder with stones of gallbladder and bile duct*

574.9 ✔5th Calculus of gallbladder and bile duct without cholecystitis — *stones of gallbladder and bile duct without inflammation*

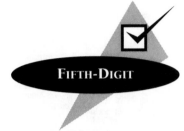

The following fifth-digit subclassification is for use with category 574:
0 without mention of obstruction

1 with obstruction

575 OTHER DISORDERS OF GALLBLADDER
Excluded from this rubric is cholelithiasis (rubric 574).

575.0 Acute cholecystitis — *severe inflammation gallbladder, no stones*

Acute cholecystitis is acute inflammation of the gall bladder without mention of cholelithiasis (calculi or "gallstones" of the gallbladder or bile ducts). This condition may be caused by obstruction of the cystic duct by another process (such as a malignant tumor), bile stasis ("sludge" formation, which is a precipitant of calcium bilirubinate calculi formation), or infection due to organisms such as *Escherichia coli*, *E. clostridia*, or *Salmonella typhi*.

About 95 percent of acute cholecystitis is due to obstruction of the cystic duct by a gallstone impacted in Hartmann's pouch and classified to category 574.

575.1 Other cholecystitis
Use this subclassification to report cholecystitis not otherwise specified and chronic cholecystitis without mention of cholelithiasis (calculi or "gallstones" of the gallbladder or bile ducts). Chronic cholecystitis rarely occurs in the absence of lithiasis but can occur in conditions such as cholesterolosis and adenomatous hyperplasia.

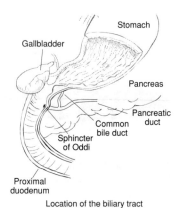

Location of the biliary tract

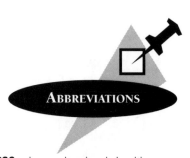

ABBREVIATIONS

PSC: primary sclerosing cholangitis, a chronic syndrome in which the bile ducts are inflamed and fibrous

TPN cholestasis: total parenteral nutrition cholestasis, a blocked or diminished flow of bile due to a long duration of TPN therapy

575.10	Cholecystitis, unspecified — *inflammation of gallbladder of unknown type, no stones*
575.11	Chronic cholecystitis — *persistent inflammation of gallbladder, no stones*
575.12	Acute and chronic cholecystitis — *occlusion, stenosis, stricture, without stones*
575.2	Obstruction of gallbladder — *including occlusion, stenosis, and stricture of cystic duct or gallbladder without mention of calculus*
575.3	Hydrops of gallbladder — *abnormal collection of fluid, gallbladder*
575.4	Perforation of gallbladder — *hole in gallbladder wall*
575.5	Fistula of gallbladder — *abnormal communication between gallbladder and other tissue*
575.6	Cholesterolosis of gallbladder — *abnormal deposits of cholesterol in tissue of gallbladder*
575.8	Other specified disorder of gallbladder — *including adhesions, atrophy, cyst, hypertrophy, ulcer, calcification, infarct, sepsis, torsion, Hartmann's pouch, Rokitansky-Aschoff sinuses*
575.9	Unspecified disorder of gallbladder — *pain in gallbladder for unknown cause*

576 OTHER DISORDERS OF BILIARY TRACT

Excluded from this rubric are disorders of the biliary tract involving the cystic duct or gallbladder (575.0-575.9).

576.0	Postcholecystectomy syndrome — *jaundice or abnormal pain following cholecystectomy*
576.1	Cholangitis — *inflammation of bile duct; recurrent, secondary, chronic, primary, acute, suppurative, sclerosing*
576.2	Obstruction of bile duct — *occlusion, stenosis, stricture; Mirizzi's syndrome*
576.3	Perforation of bile duct — *hole in the wall of bile duct*
576.4	Fistula of bile duct — *abnormal communication between bile duct and other tissue*
576.5	Spasm of sphincter of Oddi — *abnormal contraction in muscle of the threshold between bile duct and duodenum*
576.8	Other specified disorders of biliary tract — *including adhesions, atrophy, cyst, hypertrophy, stasis, ulcer, cicatrix, obliteration, torsion of bile duct; abscess or inflammation of hepatic duct*
576.9	Unspecified disorder of biliary tract — *unknown*

577 DISEASES OF PANCREAS

Excluded from this rubric are mumps pancreatitis (072.3); islet cell tumor of pancreas (211.7); and pancreatic steatorrhea (579.4).

Signs and symptoms of diseases of pancreas include abdominal pain, weakness, dizziness, somnolence, grossly bloody or "coffee ground" vomitus, grossly bloody or black and tarry stools, and a history of bleeding diathesis. Other signs and symptoms include chronic conditions such as diverticulosis, fall in blood pressure of more than 10 mm Hg or rise in pulse rate of more than 20 beats per minute between supine and standing positions, altered level of consciousness, pallor, diaphoresis, and peripheral vasoconstriction.

577.0	Acute pancreatitis — *severe inflammation; necrotic, acute, hemorrhagic, subacute, suppurative, infective; including Fitz's syndrome*
577.1	Chronic pancreatitis — *persistent inflammation; infectious, interstitial, painless, recurrent, relapsing*
577.2	Cyst and pseudocyst of pancreas

✔5th   Needs fifth-digit   **OK**   Valid three-digit code

577.8   Other specified disease of pancreas — *including atrophy, calculus, cirrhosis, fibrosis, necrosis, fistula, hyperfunction, insufficiency, sclerosis, nontraumatic rupture, duct obstruction; Hadfield-Clarke or Burke's syndrome*

577.9   Unspecified disease of pancreas — *unknown*

578 GASTROINTESTINAL HEMORRHAGE

Use this rubric to report bleeding of the stomach, ileum, jejunum, duodenum, and/or colon. The condition may be described as acute or chronic and involve a grossly bloody (visible) appearance or be detected by laboratory examination only (occult bleeding). GI bleeding is classified as either hematemesis (vomiting of blood), blood in stool which includes melena (partially digested blood showing as dark tarry stools) and hematochezia (passage of red blood in stools), and GI bleeding not specified as hematemesis or blood in stool.

Diagnostic tests may include a CBC to reveal normal hematocrit and hemoglobin for first six hours of acute bleeding (the body can compensate for acute blood loss by vasoconstriction, delaying the intravascular fluids from entering the bloodstream). Peripheral blood smear in acute hemorrhage greater than six hours often demonstrates normochromic and normocytic blood loss anemia. In chronic GI hemorrhage (acute exacerbation of chronic GI hemorrhage), peripheral blood smear is characteristic of chronic blood loss showing microcytic, hypochromic anemia with marked increase in reticulocyte count. Abnormal BUN and creatinine levels suggest bleeding in upper GI tract, and elevated liver enzymes indicate hypoperfusion of the liver following a bleeding episode. Nasogastric aspiration may be performed to confirm upper GI bleed and upper or lower endoscopy identifies exact site and pathology of the bleeding. Upper GI series or barium enema locates site when bleeding is inactive at the time of the test and a nuclear bleeding scan, such as technetium-labeled red cell scan and technetium sulfur-colloid scan, locates site in the lower GI tract when bleeding is minimal. Angiography may be performed for both upper and lower GI bleeding and is often performed in anticipation of surgery.

Therapies include gastric lavage for upper GI bleeding confined to stomach and medical management for lower GI bleeding unless the bleeding becomes life threatening. There also is therapeutic angiography using selective intraarterial vasopressin or selective embolization of a bleeding vessel to control GI hemorrhage. Use of endoscopic laser or heat probe induces coagulation, while surgery is directed at the etiology when bleeding is severe (e.g., gastrectomy and Billroth I reconstruction for GI bleeding due to perforated gastric ulcer or hemicolectomy for extensive diverticulosis of the colon).

Associated conditions include acute and/or chronic blood loss anemia, dehydration, gastritis, diverticulitis, neoplasms, arteriovenous malformations, chronic renal failure, diabetes mellitus, chronic obstructive lung disease, colitis, bleeding diathesis, chronic liver disease, Osler-Weber-Rendu syndrome, and valvular heart disease.

This category excludes bleeding of the anus and rectum for classification purposes. The terms "upper" and "lower" have no value as modifiers for classification of GI bleeding. GI bleeding must be assigned to code 578.9 (hemorrhage of gastrointestinal tract, unspecified) when not further defined as hematemesis or blood in stool. Since upper GI bleeding may present not only as hematemesis but also as melena and even hematochezia in some cases. Thus, the codes are distinguished by the presentation of the GI bleeding, not the site.

Excluded from this rubric are gastrointestinal hemorrhage with angiodysplasia of stomach and duodenum (537.83); angiodysplasia of intestine (537.85); diverticulitis and diverticulosis (rubric 562); gastritis and duodenitis (535.0-535.6); and duodenal, gastric, gastrojejunal, or peptic ulcer (531.00-534.91).

578.0   Hematemesis — *vomiting blood*

Use this subclassification to report vomiting of frank red or partially digested blood. Hematemesis usually is indicative of bleeding of the upper gastrointestinal tract. Occult bleeding can be detected by analysis of vomitus or nasogastric tube aspiration. Gastric and gastroduodenal ulcers, gastritis, arteriovenous malformations, and neoplasms are the most common etiologies for hematemesis.

Certain conditions such as epistaxis may cause the patient to swallow and then vomit blood. Such vomiting of swallowed blood sometimes masquerades as hematemesis due to gastrointestinal hemorrhage.

578.1   Blood in stool — *melena*

Use this subclassification to report passage of frank red or partially digested blood in the stools which may be due to a condition in the upper or lower GI tract.

The general term "rectal bleeding" is used by clinicians to describe GI hemorrhage (classified here) or bleeding from sites within the rectum or anus classified to code 569.3. If the etiology of the rectal bleeding is a condition of the gastrointestinal tract excluding the anus and rectum, assign this code. Occult bleeding may be detected by performing a guaiac test on a stool sample. A positive guaiac test without further documentation of GI bleeding is classified to code 792.1, nonspecific abnormal findings in stool contents.

578.9   Unspecified, hemorrhage of gastrointestinal tract — *not otherwise specified*

579 INTESTINAL MALABSORPTION

579.0   Celiac disease — *crisis, rickets, gluten enteropathy, nontropical spur*

Celiac disease (also called coeliac, nontropical sprue, celiac sprue, gluten intolerant enteropathy, or gluten sensitive enteropathy) is a condition in which there is a chronic reaction to certain proteins, commonly referred to as glutens, found in some cereal grains. This reaction destroys the villi in the small intestine, with resulting malabsorption of nutrients.

The disease affects both sexes, and it can begin at any age, from infancy (as soon as cereal grains are introduced) to later life (even though the individual has consumed cereal grains all along). The onset of the disease seems to require genetic predisposition and some kind of trigger, such as overexposure to wheat, a pregnancy, an operation, or a viral infection.

579.1   Tropical sprue — diarrhea associated with enteric infection and nutritional deficiency

579.2   Blind loop syndrome

579.3   Other and unspecified postsurgical nonabsorption

⌐5th   Needs fifth-digit   **OK**   Valid three-digit code

579.4   Pancreatic steatorrhea — passage of large amounts of fat in the feces due
              to absence of pancreatic juice from intestine
579.8   Other specified intestinal malabsorption
579.9   Unspecified intestinal malabsorption

Chapter 10

580-629
Diseases of the Genitourinary System

This chapter classifies diseases and disorders of the kidney, ureter, bladder, urethra, prostate, male genital organs, female and male breast, and female genital organs.

Excluded from this chapter is hypertensive renal disease, found in rubric 403. Signs and symptoms of genitourinary system disorders that may describe the emerging nature of the patient's condition are found in rubric 788, which includes codes specific to incontinence of urine, painful or frequent urination, and kidney pain. Also, some genitourinary diseases are familial linked. Family history can be found in rubrics V16-V19.

580-589 Nephritis, Nephrotic Syndrome, and Nephrosis

The kidneys are behind the parietal peritoneum at the back of the abdominal cavity. They are located on either side of the vertebral column from the level of the 12th thoracic vertebra to the 3rd lumbar vertebra. The left kidney is often slightly larger than the right, and usually slightly higher in position, presumably because of the space taken by the liver. They kidneys are encased in heavy cushions of fat, which, with the renal fasciae connective tissue, anchors them in place. The average kidney is about 11 centimeters by 7 centimeters by 3 centimeters and roughly oval with a medial indentation (bean-shaped). The concave notch at this indentation is called the hilum, and is where structures enter and leave the kidney. Tough, white, fibrous connective tissue encapsulates each kidney.

The outer region of the kidney is the cortex. The medulla is the inner region, consisting of about a dozen distinct triangular wedges of tissue called the renal pyramids. The papilla (points) of the pyramids face inward and jut into cuplike structures, called calyces, where urine is collected for transport via the renal pelvis out of the kidney and into the ureter. The functional units of the kidney are the nephrons. Nephrons are microscopic units which process blood and form urine by filtration, reabsorption and secretion. There are over a million nephrons in each kidney, which make up the bulk of the organ's tissue.

580 ACUTE GLOMERULONEPHRITIS

Acute glomerulonephritis is acute inflammation in the glomeruli of the kidneys. Also known as acute hemorrhagic glomerulonephritis and acute nephritis, this condition frequently is a late complication of pharyngitis or skin infection.

Signs and symptoms of acute glomerulonephritis include history of infection, usually streptococcal, history of concurrent systemic vasculitis or hypersensitivity reaction, malaise, headache, anorexia, low-grade fever, mild generalized edema, and retinal hemorrhages.

In acute glomerulonephritis, urinalysis reveals hematuria (may be microscopic or grossly bloody or coffee colored) and urine sediment containing protein, hyaline and granular casts

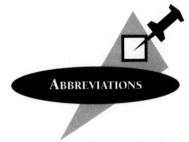

ABBREVIATIONS

ADPKD: autosomal dominant polycystic kidney disease

ARF: acute renal failure

ARPKD: autosomal recessive polycystic kidney disease

BUN: blood urea nitrogen

CAPD: continuous ambulatory peritoneal dialysis

CAVH: continuous arteriovenous hemodialysis

CCPD: continuous cycling peritoneal dialysis

CRF: chronic renal failure

ECM: extracellular material

EPD: equilibrium peritoneal dialysis

ERSD: end stage renal disease

GBM: glomerular basement membrane

GFR: glomerular filtration rate

IPD: (manual) intermittent peritoneal dialysis

IRD: immune renal disease

ISD: Intrinsic (urethral) sphincter deficiency

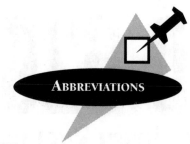

IVU: intravenous urography (urogram)

KUB: kidney, ureter, bladder

MCD: minimal change disease

MPGN: membranoproliferative glomerulonephritis

NDI: nephrogenic diabetes insipidus

NS: nephrotic syndrome

PIGN: postinfectious glomerulonephritis

PSGN: poststreptococcal glomerulonephritis

RBC: red blood cell

RBF: renal blood flow

RPGN: rapidly progressive glomerulonephritis

RTA: renal tubular acidosis

RVT: renal vein thrombosis

SCUF: slow continuous ultrafiltration

TN: tubulointerstitial nephritis

UTI: urinary tract infection

WBC: white blood cell

in large numbers, and erythrocyte casts. Blood work reveals elevated BUN and creatinine, rapid sedimentation rate, and mild normochromic anemia. Therapies include antibiotics to eradicate underlying infection (e.g., streptococcal pharyngitis), symptomatic treatment to prevent overhydration and hypertension, and dietary restriction of protein and sodium. Associated conditions include hypertension, hypertensive encephalopathy, congestive heart failure, infection (e.g., streptococcal pharyngitis, skin cellulitis), and retinal hemorrhage.

When acute glomerulonephritis does not heal within one year to two years, or when it progresses to chronic renal failure or chronic renal insufficiency, it is designated as chronic glomerulonephritis. For this reason, it is rare that a patient will carry codes from both categories 580 and 582 during the same episode of care. Acute exacerbation of chronic glomerulonephritis is classified to chronic glomerulonephritis (582) alone when the exacerbation refers to a progressive deterioration or worsening of symptoms of chronic glomerulonephritis. When the cause of the exacerbation is known, such as an intercurrent infection (e.g., streptococcal septicemia, 038.0), report the infection along with a code from category 582.

580.0   Acute glomerulonephritis with lesion of proliferative glomerulonephritis — *including acute nephritis*

Acute glomerulonephritis with lesion of proliferative glomerulonephritis is characterized by hypercellularity of the glomeruli. The condition is due to proliferation of endothelial and/or mesangial cells and infiltration of the tissues with neutrophils and monocytes.

580.4   Acute glomerulonephritis with lesion of rapidly progressive glomerulonephritis — *including acute nephritis with lesion of necrotizing glomerulitis*

Acute glomerulonephritis with lesion of rapidly progressive glomerulonephritis is acute glomerulonephritis with lesion characterized by rapid deterioration of kidney function, usually a few weeks to two months. Most patients who survive this condition, which is also known as acute crescentic glomerulonephritis, develop chronic renal failure within two years.

580.81   Acute glomerulonephritis with other specified pathological lesion in kidney in disease classified elsewhere — (Code first underlying disease, as: 002.0, 070.0–070.9, 072.79, 421.0) — *code infectious hepatitis, mumps, or typhoid fever first*

580.89   Other acute glomerulonephritis with other specified pathological lesion in kidney — *including acute glomerulonephritis with lesion of exudative nephritis*

580.9   Acute glomerulonephritis with unspecified pathological lesion in kidney — *hemorrhagic glomerulonephritis specified as acute*

581 NEPHROTIC SYNDROME

Nephrotic syndrome is a condition characterized by proteinuria more than 3.5 g/100 ml, hypoalbuminemia less than 3 g/100 ml, hyperlipemia (cholesterol greater than 300 mg/100 ml), and massive edema. Usually due to some form of glomerulonephritis, nephrotic syndrome may result in chronic renal failure.

581.0   Nephrotic syndrome with lesion of proliferative glomerulonephritis

Nephrotic syndrome with lesion of proliferative glomerulonephritis is nephrotic syndrome with lesion characterized by hypercellularity of the glomeruli. The condition is due to proliferating endothelial and/or mesangial cells, and infiltration of the tissues with neutrophils and monocytes as a result of acute or membranoproliferative glomerulonephritis.

581.1   Nephrotic syndrome with lesion of membranous glomerulonephritis — *including epimembranous nephritis; idiopathic membranous glomerular disease*

Nephrotic syndrome with lesion of membranous glomerulonephritis is nephrotic syndrome with lesion characterized by insidious onset of proteinuria. It is the result of protein deposits and diffuse thickening of the capillary basement membrane of the glomeruli.

581.2   Nephrotic syndrome with lesion of membranoproliferative glomerulonephritis — *including nephrotic syndrome with lesion of lobular glomerulonephritis; nephrotic syndrome with lesion of mesangiocapillary glomerulonephritis*

Nephrotic syndrome with lesion of membranoproliferative glomerulonephritis is nephrotic syndrome with lesion characterized by infiltration of inflammatory cells, proliferating intrinsic glomerular cells, and altered structure and function of the basement membrane of the glomeruli.

581.3   Nephrotic syndrome with lesion of minimal change glomerulonephritis — *including foot process disease; lipoid necrosis; minimal change nephrotic syndrome*

581.81   Nephrotic syndrome with other specified pathological lesion in kidney in diseases classified elsewhere — (Code first underlying disease, as: 084.9, 250.4, 277.3, 446.0, 710.0) — *code amyloidosis, diabetes mellitus, polyarteritis first*

581.89   Other nephrotic syndrome with specified pathological lesion in kidney — *including glomerulonephritis with edema and lesion of exudative nephritis*

581.9   Nephrotic syndrome with unspecified pathological lesion in kidney — *including nephritis, nephrotic NOS; nephritis with edema NOS*

582 CHRONIC GLOMERULONEPHRITIS

Chronic glomerulonephritis is a slowly progressing disease (up to 30 years in some cases) characterized by chronic inflammation of the glomeruli, which results in sclerosis, scarring and eventual chronic renal failure. Etiologies for chronic glomerulonephritis include primary renal disorders (classified to categories 580 and 581) and systemic diseases such as Goodpasture's syndrome, systemic lupus erythematosus, amyloidosis, and hemolytic-uremic syndrome.

Signs and symptoms of chronic glomerulonephritis include azotemia, nausea, vomiting, fatigue, malaise, pruritus, dyspnea, hematuria, and hypertension. Urinalysis reveals hematuria (may be microscopic or grossly bloody or coffee colored) and urine sediment containing protein, cylindruria (granular tube casts), and erythrocyte casts. Blood work reveals elevated BUN and creatinine, rapid sedimentation rate, mild normochromic anemia. X-ray or renal ultrasound shows bilateral smaller kidneys and renal biopsy identifies underlying disease.

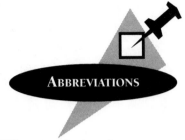

ABBREVIATIONS

ANS: acute nephrotic syndrome

MPGN: membranoproliferative glomerulonephritis

PIGN: postinfectious glomerulonephritis

PSGN: poststreptococcal glomerulonephritis

RPGN: rapidly progressing glomerulonephritis

Therapies include antibiotics to treat any intercurrent infections, drugs such as diuretics to control hypertension, IV hydration, and fluid restriction or diuresis to correct fluid and electrolyte imbalances. There are dietary restrictions of sodium and protein and renal dialysis or renal transplant for patients with ESRD (end stage renal disease or chronic renal failure).

Associated conditions include congestive heart failure, and fluid, electrolyte, and acid-base imbalances. There may be hypertension, hypertensive encephalopathy, intercurrent infection, and underlying disease (e.g., systemic lupus erythematosus).

Refer to the ICD-9-CM index under "Glomerulonephritis, due to or associated with" for a list of underlying (etiologic) conditions that can cause glomerulonephritis. Note that the index will refer you to codes in categories 580-583 in slanted brackets, indicating a manifestation code. Modify these suggested manifestation codes according to the amount of specificity in the physician's diagnostic statement. For example, for glomerulonephritis due to or associated with tuberculosis, the ICD-9-CM index lists codes 016.0 to classify the underlying disease of tuberculosis (add the appropriate fifth digit) and 583.81 for the manifestation of glomerulonephritis not specified as acute or chronic in diseases classified elsewhere. If the diagnostic statement specifies that the patient has chronic glomerulonephritis due to tuberculosis, the proper codes would be 016.0 and 582.81 for chronic glomerulonephritis in diseases classified elsewhere.

582.0   Chronic glomerulonephritis with lesion of proliferative glomerulonephritis — *including chronic (diffuse) proliferative glomerulonephritis*

Chronic glomerulonephritis with lesion of proliferative glomerulonephritis is chronic glomerulonephritis with lesion characterized by hypercellularity of the glomeruli due to proliferation of endothelial and/or mesangial cells and infiltration of the tissues with neutrophils and monocytes as a result of repeated attacks of acute inflammation.

582.1   Chronic glomerulonephritis with lesion of membranous glomerulonephritis — *including focal glomerulonephritis; segmental hyalinosis*

Chronic glomerulonephritis with lesion of membranous glomerulonephritis is chronic glomerulonephritis with lesion characterized by the insidious onset of proteinuria. It is the result of protein deposits and diffuse thickening of the capillary basement membrane of the glomeruli.

582.2   Chronic glomerulonephritis with lesion of membranoproliferative glomerulonephritis — *including chronic endothelial glomerulonephritis; chronic mesangiocapillary glomerulonephritis*

Chronic glomerulonephritis with lesion of membranoproliferative glomerulonephritis is chronic glomerulonephritis with lesion characterized by infiltration of inflammatory cells, proliferation of intrinsic glomerular cells, and altered structure and function of the basement membrane of the glomeruli.

582.4   Chronic glomerulonephritis with lesion of rapidly progressive glomerulonephritis — *chronic nephritis with lesion of necrotizing glomerulitis*

Chronic glomerulonephritis with lesion of rapidly progressive glomerulonephritis is chronic glomerulonephritis with lesion characterized by rapid deterioration of kidney function, usually a few weeks to two months. Most patients with this condition, also known as chronic crescentic glomerulonephritis, develop chronic renal failure within one year to two years.

582.81 Chronic glomerulonephritis with other specified pathological lesion in kidney in diseases classified elsewhere — (Code first underlying disease, as: 277.3, 710.0) — *code amyloidosis and systemic lupus erythematosus first*

582.89 Other chronic glomerulonephritis with specified pathological lesion in kidney — *chronic glomerulonephritis with lesion of exudative nephritis*

582.9 Chronic glomerulonephritis with unspecified pathological lesion in kidney — *including chronic hemorrhagic glomerulonephritis; small white kidney*

583 NEPHRITIS AND NEPHROPATHY, NOT SPECIFIED AS ACUTE OR CHRONIC

583.0 Nephritis and nephropathy, not specified as acute or chronic, with lesion of proliferative glomerulonephritis — *including proliferative nephritis NOS; proliferative nephropathy NOS*

Nephritis and nephropathy, not specific as acute or chronic, with lesion of proliferative glomerulonephritis are diseases with lesion characterized by hypercellularity of the glomeruli due to proliferating endothelial and/or mesangial cells, and infiltration of the tissues with neutrophils and monocytes as a result of acute inflammation.

583.1 Nephritis and nephropathy, not specified as acute or chronic, with lesion of membranous glomerulonephritis — *including membranous glomerulonephritis NOS; membranous nephropathy NOS*

Nephritis and nephropathy, not specified as acute or chronic, with lesion of membranous glomerulonephritis are diseases with lesion characterized by the insidious onset of proteinuria and unspecified nephritis or nephropathy. They are the result of protein deposits and diffuse thickening of the capillary basement membrane of the glomeruli.

583.2 Nephritis and nephropathy, not specified as acute or chronic, with lesion of membranoproliferative glomerulonephritis — *including membranoproliferative nephropathy NOS; nephritis NOS, with lesion of hypocomplementemic, lobular, or mesangiocapillary glomerulonephritis*

Nephritis and nephropathy, not specified as acute or chronic, with lesion of membranoproliferative glomerulonephritis are diseases with lesion characterized by infiltration of inflammatory cells, proliferation of intrinsic glomerular cells and alteration of the structure and function of the basement membrane of the glomeruli.

583.4 Nephritis and nephropathy, not specified as acute or chronic, with lesion of rapidly progressive glomerulonephritis — *including necrotizing or rapidly progressive nephritis NOS; nephritis, unspecified, with lesion of necrotizing glomerulitis*

Nephritis and nephropathy, not specified as acute or chronic, with lesion of rapidly progressive glomerulonephritis are severe forms of glomerulonephritis with lesion characterized by rapid deterioration of

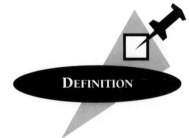

DEFINITION

Anasarca: edema with pleural effusion.

Anuria: little or no urinary output; daily urine volume of less than 100 ml.

Dysuria: painful urination.

Enuresis: bed-wetting.

Micturition: urination.

Polyuria: high urinary output; daily urine volume of more than 2500 ml.

Oliguria: low urinary output; daily urine volume of less than 500 ml.

Tenesmus: painful straining in urination.

IgA nephropathy: also Berger's disease, a disorder characterized by hematuria and proteinuria and possibly advancing to renal failure.

IgM nephropathy: also mesangial proliferative glomerulonephritis, a nephrotic syndrome in which there is an increase in the cells of the glomerulus, main symptom is proteinuria.

kidney function, usually a few weeks to two months. Most patients with these diseases, also known as crescentic glomerulonephritis, develop chronic renal failure within one year to two years.

583.6   Nephritis and nephropathy, not specified as acute or chronic, with lesion of renal cortical necrosis — *including nephritis NOS; renal cortical necrosis NOS*

583.7   Nephritis and nephropathy, not specified as acute or chronic, with lesion of renal medullary necrosis — *including nephritis NOS with (renal) medullary [papillary] necrosis*

583.81   Nephritis and nephropathy, not specified as acute or chronic, with other specified pathological lesion in kidney, in diseases classified elsewhere — (Code first underlying disease, as: 016.0, 098.19, 250.4, 277.3, 446.21, 710.0) — *code first amyloidosis, Goodpasture's syndrome*

583.89   Other nephritis and nephropathy, not specified as acute or chronic, with specified pathological lesion in kidney — *including glomerulitis with lesion of exudative nephritis; renal disease with lesion of interstitial nephritis*

583.9   Nephritis and nephropathy, not specified as acute or chronic, with unspecified pathological lesion in kidney — *including glomerulitis NOS; nephritis NOS*

584 ACUTE RENAL FAILURE

Acute renal failure is sudden interruption of renal function following any one of a variety of conditions that insult the normal kidney. Although usually reversible with treatment, acute renal failure may progress to chronic renal insufficiency and chronic renal failure or death. Recovery from acute renal failure is marked by a conversion from an oliguric phase to a diuretic phase within a few days to six weeks.

The causes of acute renal failure are classified to prerenal, intrinsic (renal) or postrenal. Prerenal failure is due to diminished blood flow to the kidneys caused by conditions such as dehydration, shock, embolism, cardiac failure, hepatic failure, or sepsis. Intrinsic failure results from diseases and disorders of the kidneys. Acute tubular necrosis is the most common cause, and results from conditions such as systemic lupus, erythematosus, sickle cell disease, nephrotoxins, renal ischemia, acute pyelonephritis, and acute poststreptococcal glomerulonephritis. Postrenal failure is caused by bilateral obstruction of urinary outflow, as seen with ureteral calculi, blood clots, neoplasms, benign prostatic hypertrophy, and urethral strictures.

Signs and symptoms of acute renal failure include, in early stages, oliguria, sometimes anuria, azotemia, hypotension, electrolyte imbalances, fever and chills (indicating infection), anorexia, nausea, vomiting, diarrhea or constipation, uremic breath, headache, mental changes, pruritus, pallor, purpura, fluid overload, edema, and Kussmaul respirations. Blood work shows elevated BUN, serum creatinine, potassium; decreased serum calcium, arterial pH, bicarbonate. Urinalysis reveals urine specific gravity of approximately 1.010 (indicating isosthenuria) and sometimes protein, and, cellular debris. Radiology such as kidney ultrasound, intravenous pyelography, retrograde pyelography, and nephrotomography identify pathology such as outflow obstruction or hydronephrosis. Therapies include dietary management and restriction of fluid intake with careful monitoring of electrolytes, peritoneal dialysis, or hemodialysis to control uremia.

Excluded from this rubric are acute renal failure following labor and delivery (669.3); posttraumatic (958.5); and that complicating abortion (rubrics 634-638); or ectopic/molar pregnancy (639.3).

✔5th   Needs fifth-digit   **OK**   Valid three-digit code

584.5   Acute renal failure with lesion of tubular necrosis — *sudden onset of renal failure, compared to chronic, due to lower nephron necrosis; acute tubular necrosis*

584.6   Acute renal failure with lesion of renal cortical necrosis — *severe decline in kidney function due to destruction of kidney filtering tissue, sudden onset*

584.7   Acute renal failure with lesion of renal medullary (papillary) necrosis — *including necrotizing renal papillitis*

584.8   Acute renal failure with other specified pathological lesion in kidney — *including acute renal failure with pathological lesion in kidney NEC*

584.9   Unspecified acute renal failure — *unspecified*

585 CHRONIC RENAL FAILURE ⬛🅚

Chronic renal failure is multisystem disease due to a progressive loss of renal function. It usually develops gradually as a consequence of a wide spectrum of diseases such as primary and secondary glomerular disease, diabetes mellitus, and hereditary renal disease such as polycystic kidneys, hypertension, obstructive uropathy, chronic infection, and interstitial nephritis. When the loss of renal function is incomplete, the term "chronic renal insufficiency" (593.9) often is used. When the loss of renal function is complete, the term "end-stage renal disease" or "chronic uremia" may be used. Because chronic renal failure causes major changes in all body systems, signs and symptoms may be widespread and varied.

Signs and symptoms of chronic renal failure includes weakness, fatigue, peripheral edema, headaches, pallor, thirst, anorexia, weight loss, nausea, vomiting, pruritus, polyuria (early stages), oliguria (late stages), nocturia, mental changes, and is asymptomatic until more than 75 percent of renal failure is lost. Blood work shows elevated BUN, serum creatinine, potassium. Decreased serum calcium, arterial pH, bicarbonate; normochromic, normocytic anemia. Urinalysis reveals urine specific gravity of approximately 1.010 (indicating isosthenuria) and sometimes protein, glucose, WBCs, RBCs, waxy and granular casts; chest x-ray may show cardiac enlargement, interstitial edema, lung edema, frank pulmonary congestion. Other radiology, such as x-rays of kidney-ureter-bladder, intravenous pyelography, renal arteriography, renal scans such as selected radionuclide studies, ultrasound, may aid in diagnosis and treatment; kidney biopsy and histological examination identify underlying pathology.

Therapies include dietary management such as protein restriction, iron and/or folate supplements, and restriction of fluid intake with careful monitoring of urine volume and electrolytes. Other therapies includes transfusion of blood or blood products to treat anemia, peritoneal dialysis or hemodialysis to control uremia in patients with ESRD, and renal transplant for patients with ESRD.

Associated conditions include normochromic, normocytic anemia, electrolyte imbalances, underlying disease (e.g., diabetes mellitus, hypertension), cardiovascular complications (congestive heart failure, dysrhythmias, uremic pericarditis, pericardial effusion), respiratory complications (Kussmaul respirations due to acidosis, uremic pleuritis, uremic pneumonitis, pleural effusion), renal osteodystrophy (bone disease), and gastrointestinal complications (gastritis, pancreatitis, duodenal ulcer, uremic colitis).

Excluded from this code is chronic renal failure with any condition classifiable to 401 (403.0-403.9 with fifth-digit 1).

586 RENAL FAILURE, UNSPECIFIED OK
Excluded from this rubric are renal failure following labor and delivery (669.3); posttraumatic (958.5); that complicating abortion (rubrics 634-638) or ectopic/molar pregnancy (639.3); extrarenal or prerenal uremia (788.9); or renal failure with any condition classifiable to 401 (403.0-403.9 with fifth-digit 1).

587 RENAL SCLEROSIS, UNSPECIFIED OK
Excluded from this rubric is arteriolar or arteriosclerotic nephrosclerosis (403.00-403.92).

588 DISORDERS RESULTING FROM IMPAIRED RENAL FUNCTION
588.0   Renal osteodystrophy — *including azotemic osteodystrophy; renal dwarfism; renal rickets*

588.1   Nephrogenic diabetes insipidus — *kidneys fail to resorb filtered fluids, leading to extreme thirst and frequent urination*

588.8   Other specified disorder resulting from impaired renal function — *including Lightwood's disease; renal acidosis*

588.9   Unspecified disorder resulting from impaired renal function — *disorder NOS due to impaired renal function*

589 SMALL KIDNEY OF UNKNOWN CAUSE
These codes are considered nonspecific codes and should be used only when a more specific diagnosis of acquired or congenital small kidney cannot be determined.

589.0   Unilateral small kidney

589.1   Bilateral small kidneys

589.9   Unspecified small kidney — *of unknown cause*

590-599 Other Diseases of Urinary System

590 INFECTIONS OF KIDNEY
Use an additional code to identify infective agents, such as *Escherichia coli* (041.4).

590.00   Chronic pyelonephritis without lesion of renal medullary necrosis — (Code first the associated condition 593.70, 593.71, 593.72, 593.73) — *chronic pyelitis, or pyonephrosis, without lesion of renal medullary necrosis*

590.01   Chronic pyelonephritis with lesion of renal medullary necrosis — (Code first the associated condition 593.70, 593.71, 593.72, 593.73) — *chronic pyelitis or pyonephrosis with lesion of renal medullary necrosis*

590.10   Acute pyelonephritis without lesion of renal medullary necrosis — (Use additional code to identify organism) — *acute pyelitis or acute pyonephrosis without lesion of renal medullary necrosis*

590.11   Acute pyelonephritis with lesion of renal medullary necrosis — (Use additional code to identify organism) — *acute pyelitis or acute pyonephrosis with lesion of renal medullary necrosis*

590.2   Renal and perinephric abscess — (Use additional code to identify organism) — *including nephritic abscess; perirenal abscess*

590.3   Pyeloureteritis cystica — (Use additional code to identify organism) — *including ureteritis cystica; infection of renal pelvis and ureter*

590.80   Unspecified pyelonephritis — (Use additional code to identify organism) — *including pyelonephritis NOS*

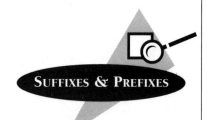

SUFFIXES & PREFIXES

-itis: inflammation

-osis: a condition

Hydro-: relating to fluid, water, or hydrogen

Pyelo-: relating to the pelvis

Pyo-: relating to pus

✔5th   Needs fifth-digit   **OK**   Valid three-digit code

590.81 Pyelitis or pyelonephritis in diseases classified elsewhere — (Code first underlying disease, as: 016.0) — *in disease classified elsewhere, code tuberculosis first*

590.9 Unspecified infection of kidney — (Use additional code to identify organism)

591 HYDRONEPHROSIS OK

Use this code to report dilation of the renal pelvis and calyces due to the obstruction of the flow of urine. Obstruction occurring at the ureteropelvic junction is sometimes referred to as primary hydronephrosis, and obstruction at any point distal to the ureteropelvic junction is sometimes referred to as secondary hydronephrosis.

Signs and symptoms of hydronephrosis include history of condition causing urinary obstruction, colicky pain in acute hydronephrosis, dull and aching flank pain in chronic hydronephrosis, and hematuria. Blood work may show azotemia (excess urea and other nitrogenous byproducts). Urinalysis may reveal red blood cells and pyuria if a concomitant urinary infection is present. Radiology, such as intravenous pyelography, cystoureterography, and kidney ultrasound, identify the site of obstruction and confirms the diagnosis.

Therapies include cystoscopy to correct conditions such as benign prostatic hypertrophy and ureteral calculus (basket extraction of calculus or stent insertion), extracorporeal shock wave lithotripsy to break up calculi in kidney or ureter, nephrostomy for severe obstructions, and surgery to correct conditions such as strictures, neoplasms, congenital malformations.

Associated conditions include urinary tract infection, urinary calculus formation, benign prostatic hypertrophy or prostate cancer, urinary stricture formation, and congenital abnormalities.

Excluded from this code are congenital hydronephrosis (753.29) and hydroureter (593.5).

592 CALCULUS OF KIDNEY AND URETER

Use this rubric to report stones of the kidney and ureter. Most stones are composed of calcium salts or magnesium/ammonium phosphate; most are idiopathic. Other stones may be composed of cystine or uric acid, and are a result of a defect in urinary acidification.

Nausea, infection, severe pain, and hematuria usually accompany kidney stones, if the stone is obstructing flow of urine. If there is no obstruction, there may be no symptoms.

Ureteral calculi have migrated to the ureter from the kidney, and obstruction can compromise renal function. Symptoms are the same as for renal calculi.

Excluded from this rubric is nephrocalcinosis (275.4).

592.0 Calculus of kidney — *including renal calculus or stone; staghorn calculus*
592.1 Calculus of ureter — *including ureteric stone; ureterolithiasis*
592.9 Unspecified urinary calculus — *renal or ureteral calculus NOS*

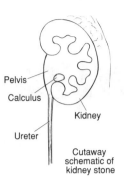

Pelvis
Calculus
Kidney
Ureter
Cutaway schematic of kidney stone

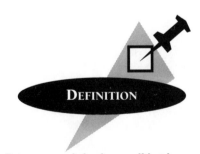

DEFINITION

Extracorporeal shock wave lithotripsy (ESWL): In ESWL, shock waves are focused onto the site of the stone, and the stone is fragmented and passed spontaneously through the urinary system within a few days. ESWL is effective against calcium, uric acid, and magnesium stones, but not on cystine stones.

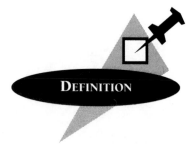

DEFINITION

Hyposthenuria: a disorder of the kidney tubules in which they lack they ability to generate a undiluted urine.

Ormond's syndrome: retroperitoneal structures involving and often obstructing ureters sometimes following certain types of chemical treatment; there is no identified cause.

Thorn's syndrome: also salt-losing nephritis, damage to the renal tubulus that results in a renal loss of abnormal amounts of sodium chloride. May be characterized by hyponatremia, dehydration, acidosis, and azotemia.

593 OTHER DISORDERS OF KIDNEY AND URETER

The ureter is the tube leading from the kidney to the urinary bladder. It is approximately 28 centimeters long and is composed of three layers of tissue. The inner layer is a mucous lining. The smooth, muscular middle layer propels the urine from the kidney to the bladder by peristalsis. The outer layer is fibrous connective tissue. Each ureter leaves the kidney from the hilum, a concave notch on the middle surface, and enters the bladder through narrow valvelike orifice that prevents backflow of urine to the kidney.

593.0	Nephroptosis — *including floating kidney; mobile kidney*
593.1	Hypertrophy of kidney — *enlargement of kidney*
593.2	Acquired cyst of kidney — *peripelvic (lymphatic) cyst*
593.3	Stricture or kinking of ureter — *stricture of pelviureteric junction*
593.4	Other ureteric obstruction — *including idiopathic retroperitoneal fibrosis; occlusion NOS of ureter*
593.5	Hydroureter — *dilation of ureter due to obstructed urinary flow*
593.6	Postural proteinuria — *including benign postural proteinuria; orthostatic proteinuria*
593.70	Vesicoureteral reflux, unspecified or without reflex nephropathy — *backflow of urine from bladder into ureter*
593.71	Vesicoureteral reflux with reflux nephropathy, unilateral — *one-sided backflow of urine into ureter, causing renal scarring*
593.72	Vesicoureteral reflux with reflux nephropathy, bilateral — *backflow of urine into ureters on both sides, causing renal scarring*
593.73	Vesicoureteral reflux with reflux nephropathy, NOS — *backflow of urine into ureters, causing renal scarring*
593.81	Vascular disorders of kidney — *including renal artery embolism; renal artery hemorrhage; renal artery thrombosis; renal infarction*
593.82	Ureteral fistula — *including intestinoureteral fistula*
593.89	Other specified disorder of kidney and ureter — *including adhesions, kidney or ureter; periureteritis; ureteral polyp; ureterocele*
593.9	Unspecified disorder of kidney and ureter — *including renal disease NOS; salt-losing nephritis or syndrome; Thorn's syndrome*

Use this code for kidney and ureter disorders that are not further specified as acute or chronic or are lacking a stated pathology or cause. Also classified to this code are syndromes of low salt, salt-losing, or salt depletion not further specified, as well as salt-losing or salt-wasting nephritis, nephropathy, or renopathy not further specified.

594 CALCULUS OF LOWER URINARY TRACT

594.0	Calculus in diverticulum of bladder — *stone in pouch of bladder wall*
594.1	Other calculus in bladder — *urinary bladder stone*
594.2	Calculus in urethra — *urinary stone in urethra*
594.8	Other lower urinary tract calculus — *suburethral urinary stone*
594.9	Unspecified calculus of lower urinary tract

595 CYSTITIS

This rubric reports infections and inflammations of the bladder. An additional code should be reported to identify the infectious agent, as in *E. coli* 041.4. If the bladder inflammation or infection is due to a disease classified elsewhere, code first the underlying disease.

The urinary bladder is an expandable and collapsible bag located behind the symphysis pubis (pubic bone) and below the parietal peritoneum. This protective membrane covers

✏5th   Needs fifth-digit   **OK**   Valid three-digit code

only the top of the bladder. The bladder has a strong, specialized muscular layer called the detrusor muscle, a network of muscle bundles that run in all directions. The lining of the bladder is a mucous transitional epithelium that forms folds called rugae. These specialized tissue layers allow for the distension of the bladder as it fills with urine from the kidneys.

There are three openings in the floor of the bladder. The two ureters enter at the back of the bladder, guarded by the valvelike narrow regions that prevent backflow up to the kidneys. The opening into the urethra is in the front lower corner of the bladder. The bladder has two major functions: it stores urine before it leaves the body; and, by means of the urethra, expels urine from the body.

Cystitis is a common complication of catheterization. When this occurs, report a cystitis code from this rubric, 996.64 Infection and inflammatory reaction due to indwelling urinary catheter, and a cystitis code from this rubric.

Excluded from this rubric are prostatocystitis, reported with 601.3; cystitis in diphtheria (032.84); gonococcal cystitis (098.11, 098.31); monilial cystitis (112.2); trichomonal cystitis (131.09); and tuberculous cystitis (subclassification 016.1).

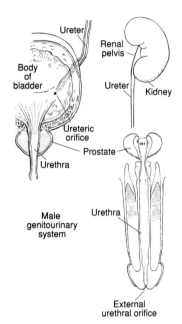

595.0	Acute cystitis — (Use additional code to identify organism) — *acute infection of bladder*
595.1	Chronic interstitial cystitis — (Use additional code to identify organism) — *Hunner's ulcer; panmural fibrosis of bladder; submucous cystitis*
595.2	Other chronic cystitis — (Use additional code to identify organism) — *chronic cystitis NOS; subacute cystitis*
595.3	Trigonitis — (Use additional code to identify organism) — *follicular cystitis; acute or chronic trigonitis; urethrotrigonitis*
595.4	Cystitis in diseases classified elsewhere — (Code first underlying disease, as: 006.8, 039.8, 120.0–120.9, 122.3, 122.6) — *code actinomycosis, amebiasis, echinococcus infections first*
595.81	Cystitis cystica — (Use additional code to identify organism) — *bladder inflammation due to multiple cysts*
595.82	Irradiation cystitis — (Use additional code to identify organism) — *bladder inflammation due to radiation*
595.89	Other specified types of cystitis — (Use additional code to identify organism) — *including bladder abscess; emphysematous cystitis*
595.9	Unspecified cystitis

596 OTHER DISORDERS OF BLADDER

Use an additional code to report any urinary incontinence (625.6, 788.30-788.39).

596.0 Bladder neck obstruction — (Use additional code to identify associated (condition) 625.6, 788.30–788.39) — *contracture of bladder neck or other vesicoureteral orifice*

Use this subclassification to report a condition, also known as bladder outlet obstruction or vesicourethral obstruction, which occurs mostly in males and usually as a consequence of benign prostatic hypertrophy or prostatic cancer. It also may occur in either sex due to strictures (formed following radiation therapy, cystoscopy, catheterization injury, or infection), blood clots, bladder cancer, impacted calculi, extrinsic tumors, or disease compressing the bladder neck.

Bladder neck obstruction is associated with complications such as hydronephrosis, hydroureteronephrosis, or ureteronephrosis. The obstruction also may be due to bladder thickening and hypertrophy, trabeculation or diverticula; hypertrophy and subsequent dilatation and atony of the renal pelvis; or renal parenchymal compression and ischemic atrophy.

Congenital bladder neck obstruction is excluded from this subclassification and should be reported with 753.6.

596.1 Intestinovesical fistula — (Use additional code to identify associated (condition) 625.6, 788.30–788.39) — *including enterovesical fistula; vesicorectal fistula*

596.2 Vesical fistula, not elsewhere classified — (Use additional code to identify associated (condition) 625.6, 788.30–788.39) — *including urethrovesical fistula; vesicocutaneous fistula*

596.3 Diverticulum of bladder — (Use additional code to identify associated (condition) 625.6, 788.30–788.39) — *including bladder diverticulitis*

596.4 Atony of bladder — (Use additional code to identify associated (condition) 625.6, 788.30–788.39) — *including hypotonicity of bladder; bladder inertia*

596.5 Other functional disorders of bladder

Use this subclassification to report functional disorders of the bladder, the musculomembranous sac that serves as a reservoir for urine received from the kidneys through the ureters and as a contractile organ actively expelling its contents into the urethra. Functional disorders prevent the bladder from performing either or both of these functions. Included are hypertonicity, low bladder compliance, paralysis, neurogenic bladder, and detrusor sphincter dyssynergia.

Hypertonicity refers to excessive muscle tonus or tension. In the bladder, it usually refers to prolonged detrusor (bladder) muscle spasms, and hypersensitivity or hyperreflexia of the detrusor muscle.

Low bladder compliance refers to the relative change in bladder volume when measured against bladder (detrusor muscle) pressure. Compliance can be measured by inflow cystometry. If the cystometry demonstrates a large bladder volume with little pressure change in the bladder, the patient is said to have a bladder of high compliance; if the cystometry reveals a tense, firm bladder with high pressure, the bladder is said to be of low compliance.

Paralysis of the bladder is a general term meaning loss of the ability of the detrusor muscles to contract. Such paralysis may have a variety of etiologies such as trauma, drugs, disease, or other structural or functional disorders in the bladder muscle or nerves.

Neurogenic bladder is due to a nervous system lesion. Terms used to describe neurogenic bladder are spastic bladder, reflex bladder, and flaccid bladder.

Detrusor sphincter dyssynergia, also known as bladder neck dyssynergia, is a condition in which urinary outflow is obstructed because the bladder neck fails to relax or tightens when the detrusor muscle contracts during micturition. The condition is rarely observed in females.

596.51   Hypertonicity of bladder — (Use additional code to identify associated (condition) 625.6, 788.30–788.39) — *including hyperactivity of bladder; overactivity of bladder*

596.52   Low bladder compliance — (Use additional code to identify associated (condition) 625.6, 788.30–788.39) — *small or sensitive bladder that requires frequent emptying*

596.53   Paralysis of bladder — (Use additional code to identify associated (condition) 625.6, 788.30–788.39) — *bladder unable to contract*

596.54   Neurogenic bladder, NOS — (Use additional code to identify associated (condition) 625.6, 788.30–788.39) — *loss of bladder control most often due to spinal nerve damage from injury or neurological disease*

596.55   Detrusor sphincter dyssynergia — (Use additional code to identify associated (condition) 625.6, 788.30–788.39) — *loss of coordination between bladder emptying nerves and external urethral sphincter*

596.59   Other functional disorder of bladder — (Use additional code to identify associated (condition) 625.6, 788.30–788.39) — *including detrusor instability*

596.6   Nontraumatic rupture of bladder — (Use additional code to identify associated (condition) 625.6, 788.30–788.39) — *spontaneous tear in bladder wall*

596.7   Hemorrhage into bladder wall — (Use additional code to identify associated (condition) 625.6, 788.30–788.39) — *including hyperemia of bladder*

596.8   Other specified disorder of bladder — (Use additional code to identify associated (condition) 625.6, 788.30–788.39) — *including calcified bladder; bladder hypertrophy*

596.9   Unspecified disorder of bladder — (Use additional code to identify associated (condition) 625.6, 788.30–788.39) — *including bladder disease NOS*

597 URETHRITIS, NOT SEXUALLY TRANSMITTED, AND URETHRAL SYNDROME

Excluded from this rubric is nonspecific urethritis, so stated, reported with 099.4.

597.0   Urethral abscess — *including periurethral abscess; bulbourethral gland abscess*

597.80   Unspecified urethritis — *including urethritis NOS*

597.81   Urethral syndrome NOS — *unspecified*

597.89   Other urethritis — *including Cowperitis (males); urethral ulcer; para-urethritis; littritis (males); adenitis, Skene's glands (females)*

598 URETHRAL STRICTURE

A urethral stricture is a narrowing of the urethra. The urethra is a small tube lined with mucous membrane that leads from the bladder to the exterior of the body. In the male, it is approximately 20 centimeters long and passes through the prostate gland just below the bladder, where it joins the ejaculatory ducts. The tube extends forward and down to enter the base of the penis, and travels centrally through the length of the penis to end as a urinary meatus at the tip. In the female, the urethra lies directly behind the symphysis pubis and in front of the vagina, and is only about 3 centimeters long.

The function of the urethra in the female is to void urine from the bladder reservoir. In the male, the urethra is part of two different systems: in addition to voiding urine, the urethra also serves as the pathway for semen (fluid containing sperm) as it is ejaculated out of the body through the penis. Urine is prevented from mixing with semen during ejaculation by the reflex closure of the sphincter muscles guarding the opening into the bladder.

Use an additional code to identify urinary incontinence (625.6; 788.30-788.39). Code first underlying disease, as appropriate.

598.00 Urethral stricture due to unspecified infection — (Use additional code to identify associated (condition) 625.6, 788.30–788.39) — *urethral stricture due to infection NOS*

598.01 Urethral stricture due to infective diseases classified elsewhere — (Code first underlying disease, as: 095.8, 098.2, 120.0–120.9, 625.6, 788.30–788.39) — *code gonococcal infection or schistosomiasis first*

598.1 Traumatic urethral stricture — (Use additional code to identify associated (condition) 625.6, 788.30–788.39) — *including postobstetric urethral stricture*

598.2 Postoperative urethral stricture — (Use additional code to identify associated (condition) 625.6, 788.30–788.39) — *including postcatheterization stricture of urethra*

598.8 Other specified causes of urethral stricture — (Use additional code to identify associated (condition) 625.6, 788.30–788.39) — *other specified cause of urethral stricture NEC*

598.9 Unspecified urethral stricture — (Use additional code to identify associated (condition) 625.6, 788.30–788.39) — *including pinhole meatus; ankylurethria*

599 OTHER DISORDERS OF URETHRA AND URINARY TRACT

Excluded from this rubric is candidiasis of urinary tract (112.2). Use an additional code to identify the infective agent, as in *E. coli* (041.4).

599.0 Urinary tract infection, site not specified — (Use additional code to identify organism) — *including bacteriuria; pyuria*

The definition of urinary tract infection, site not specified, is a wide variety of clinical conditions characterized by a significant number of microorganisms in an unspecified part of the urinary tract. Predisposing factors for urinary tract infection include, but are not limited to, calculi or other urinary tract obstruction, foreign bodies such as stents or catheters, congenital urinary anomalies, pregnancy, diabetes mellitus, neurogenic bladder, immunosuppression (such as following renal transplant), and vesicovaginal or intestinal fistulas. Many urinary tract infections recur due to bacterial persistence or reinfection from new organisms outside the urinary tract. Women are approximately 10 times more likely to develop a urinary tract infection than men.

Signs and symptoms of urinary tract infection, site not specified, include history of recurrent urinary tract infections, burning pain on urination, polyuria, suprapubic or abdominal pain, fever, and turbid, foul-smelling, dark urine. Urinalysis shows significant bacteriuria, often accompanied by proteinuria, hematuria and pyuria, and urine culture reveals growth of more than 100,000 colonies of single organism. Blood work may reveal neutrophilic leukocytosis and positive blood culture, especially if infection involves upper urinary tract. Radiology, such as intravenous urography or pyelography, voiding cystography, and renal ultrasound, may demonstrate complicating factors such as calculi, abscess formation, hydronephrosis, and congenital anomalies. Cystoscopy and ureteral catheterization to obtain differential urine specimens localize the infection site.

DEFINITION

Albuminuria: excess serum protein in the urine (proteinuria).

Bacteriuria: bacteria in the urine.

Chyluria/Galacturia: chyle in the urine.

Hematuria: blood in the urine.

Pneumaturia: gas in the urine, usually indicative of a fistula between the bowel and the urinary tract.

Proteinuria: excess serum protein in the urine.

Pyuria: pus in the urine.

Uremia: buildup of protein metabolism byproducts in the blood.

✔5th   Needs fifth-digit   **OK**   Valid three-digit code

Therapies include antibiotics such as ampicillin, gentamicin, tetracycline, and tobramycin. Surgery can correct complications due to urinary tract infections (such as ureteral strictures) and conditions that predispose the patient to chronic or recurrent urinary tract infections (such as ureteral calculi or congenital abnormalities).

Associated conditions include urosepsis (septicemia), diabetes mellitus, pregnancy (complicated), urinary tract obstruction (e.g., calculi, fibrosis), neurogenic bladder, congenital urinary tract anomalies, benign prostatic hypertrophy, prostatitis, infected diverticula, foreign bodies, vesicovaginal and intestinal fistulas, ureteral stump following nephrectomy, papillary necrosis, and urachal cyst.

Infections of the prostate, vagina, epididymis and testis are classified elsewhere but may be swept into the nonspecific diagnosis of urinary tract infection by some clinicians.

Urinalysis and the urine culture are the most important indicators for urinary tract infection. However, two important points need to be made about these tests. Urine specimens, including the so-called "clean-catch" midstream specimen, are subject to contamination during collection from microorganisms surrounding the external urethra or by improper handling and storage. Thus, the presence of three or more species of microorganisms growing in large numbers suggests contamination, except in patients who have had an indwelling catheter for a long time. Also, patients who have received antibiotic therapy for any reason prior to testing may present false negative test results.

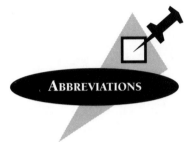

ABBREVIATIONS

BPH: benign prostatic hypertrophy

SI: stress (urinary) incontinence

UTI: urinary tract infection

599.1	Urethral fistula — *including urinary fistula NOS*
599.2	Urethral diverticulum — *pouch in urethral wall*
599.3	Urethral caruncle — *urethral polyp*
599.4	Urethral false passage — *passage without opening at urethral meatus*
599.5	Prolapsed urethral mucosa — *including urethrocele*
599.6	Unspecified urinary obstruction — (Use additional code to identify associated (condition) 625.6, 788.30–788.39) — *obstructive uropathy NOS*
599.7	Hematuria — *including benign hematuria; essential hematuria*

This subclassification reports a condition in which blood appears in the urine. Also known as hemuresis, hematuria may present as gross, visible blood in the urine or as RBCs visible only under microscopy (microscopic hematuria). Hematuria may be due to a urethral infection, bladder neoplasms or radiation injury, ureteral calculus, or kidney conditions such as polycystic disease, renal artery thrombosis, or trauma. Hematuria also can be caused by systemic disorders such as hemophilia, sickle cell crisis, thrombocytopenia, anaphylactoid purpura with renal involvement, and adverse effect of anticoagulant therapy.

Often the presentation of the hematuria gives clues as to the source of the bleeding. When blood appears only during the first fraction of voided urine (initial hematuria), the source is likely the anterior urethra or prostate gland. When blood appears during the terminal fraction of voided urine (terminal hematuria), the source is likely in the posterior urethra, vesicle neck or trigone. Blood mixed in with the total urine volume (total hematuria) is from the kidneys, ureters, or bladder. Painful hematuria usually indicates infection, calculi, trauma, or foreign body in the lower urinary tract. Painless hematuria is often associated with a neoplasm or vascular disorder.

599.8 Other specified disorders of urethra and urinary tract

The definition of other specified disorders of urethra and urinary tract is disorders of the urethra and urinary tract not elsewhere classifiable, such as urethral hypermobility, intrinsic (urethral) sphincter deficiency, and urethral instability.

Urethral hypermobility refers to inferior and posterior motion of the urethra into the potential space of the vagina and is due to a loss of urethral supporting and backing structures of the pelvis and pelvic floor. Urethral hypermobility is associated with pathologies such as vaginal prolapse and cystoceles and is commonly seen in females with urinary stress incontinence.

Intrinsic (urethral) sphincter deficiency (ISD) is due to intrinsic sphincteric damage in which the urethra is usually well supported but there is a posterior rotation and opening of the bladder neck and posterior urethra during straining.

Urethral instability is a reflex relaxation of the urethral muscle with or without detrusor muscle contraction resulting in incontinence. The condition commonly is associated with females who have multiple sclerosis.

599.81	Urethral hypermobility — (Use additional code to identify associated (condition) 625.6, 788.30–788.39) — *hypermobility*
599.82	Intrinsic (urethral) sphincter deficiency (ISD) — (Use additional code to identify associated (condition) 625.6, 788.30–788.39) — *deficiency*
599.83	Urethral instability — (Use additional code to identify associated (condition) 625.6, 788.30–788.39) — *instability*
599.84	Other specified disorders of urethra — (Use additional code to identify associated (condition) 625.6, 788.30–788.39) — including *nontraumatic rupture of urethra; urethral cyst; malacoplakia of urethra*
599.89	Other specified disorders of urinary tract — (Use additional code to identify associated (condition) 625.6, 788.30–788.39) — including *hymeno-urethral fusion; suburethral cyst*
599.9	Unspecified disorder of urethra and urinary tract — *unspecified*

600-608 Diseases of Male Genital Organs

The male reproductive system includes the two testes that produce spermatozoa (sperm) and male hormones. The system of ducts convey sperm to the exterior of the body (including the epididymis and vas deferens), the seminal vesicles (glands which contribute secretions to semen), and the external genitalia, the scrotum, and penis. The prime function of the male genital system is sexual intercourse and propagation of the species.

600 HYPERPLASIA OF PROSTATE

This rubric classifies a condition believed to arise as fibrostromal proliferation in the periurethral glands. The etiology is unknown, but a relationship between aging and prostate enlargement is well documented. Most theories regarding the cause of benign prostatic

✔5th   Needs fifth-digit   **OK**   Valid three-digit code

hypertrophy focus on possible hormonal imbalances occurring in the male after age 50. The disease usually becomes symptomatic after age 60 and is due to median and/or lateral lobe (inner gland) enlargement. The outer prostate glands are pushed against the prostate capsule, resulting in a thick pseudocapsule referred to as the surgical capsule. As the enlargement continues and intracapsular pressure increases, urinary outflow is obstructed due to impingement of the urethra. Frequently, the typical signs and symptoms of benign prostatic hypertrophy are referred to as "prostatism."

Signs and symptoms of hyperplasia of prostate include reduced urinary stream caliber and force, urinary hesitancy, feelings of incomplete voiding, nocturia, straining to initiate urination, severe urgency, suprapubic pain, bladder distention when in urinary retention, hematuria, increased urine residual, and prostate enlargement palpable with rectal exam. Urinalysis may reveal concomitant infection; blood work may show elevated serum creatinine and BUN with prolonged obstruction. Excretory urograms reveal ureteral dilation, hydronephrosis or hydroureteronephrosis, or post voiding urinary retention. Pelvic ultrasound may be used to calculate exact amounts of residual urine. Cystoscopy shows enlargement of periurethral prostate glands and demonstrates secondary bladder wall changes such as trabeculation, vesicle calculi, acute and/or chronic inflammation due to infection, and bladder diverticula.

Therapies include sexual stimulation and prostatic massage and catheterization for acute urine retention, which may result in a return to adequate voiding function. Other therapies include alpha-adrenergic drugs, such as terazosin and prazosin, to relax the external sphincter and prevent contractions of prostatic capsule, prostatectomy (transurethral, retropubic, suprapubic, or peroneal) for patients with moderate to severe obstruction, and cryosurgery or transurethral balloon urethroplasty for patients who are poor surgical risks.

Use an additional code to identify urinary incontinence (788.30-788.39). Excluded from this rubric are benign neoplasm of the prostate (222.2) and malignant neoplasm of the prostate (185).

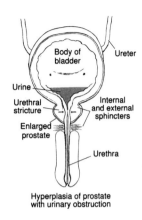

Hyperplasia of prostate with urinary obstruction

600.0	Hypertrophy (benign) of prostate — *including benign prostatic hypertrophy*
600.1	Nodular prostate — *including multinodular prostate*
600.2	Benign localized hyperplasia of prostate — *including adenofibromatous hypertrophy of prostate; fibroadenoma of prostate*
600.3	Cyst of prostate — *prostatic cyst*
600.9	Hyperplasia of prostate, unspecified — *including median bar; prostatic obstruction, unspecified*

601 INFLAMMATORY DISEASES OF PROSTATE
Use an additional code to identify the infective agent, such as *Staphylococcus* (041.1) or *Streptococcus* (041.0). For prostatitis in diseases classified elsewhere, code first the underlying disease. Excluded from this rubric are gonococcal prostatitis (098.12, 098.32); monilial prostatitis (112.2); and trichomonal prostatitis (131.03).

601.0	Acute prostatitis — (Use additional code to identify organism) — *sudden onset of inflammation of prostate*
601.1	Chronic prostatitis — (Use additional code to identify organism) — *persistent inflammation of prostate*
601.2	Abscess of prostate — (Use additional code to identify organism) — *pus pocket in wall of prostate*

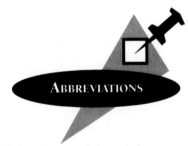

ABBREVIATIONS

BPH: benign prostatic hyperplasia

BUN: blood urea nitrogen

PSA: prostate specific antigen

TURP: transurethral resection of prostate

601.3   Prostatocystitis — (Use additional code to identify organism) — *inflammation of both prostate and bladder*

601.4   Prostatitis in diseases classified elsewhere — (Code first underlying disease, as: 016.5, 039.8, 095.8, 116.0) — *code actinomycosis, syphilis, or tuberculosis first*

601.8   Other specified inflammatory disease of prostate — (Use additional code to identify organism) — *including cavitary prostatitis; granulomatous prostatitis*

601.9   Unspecified prostatitis — (Use additional code to identify organism) — *including prostatitis NOS*

602 OTHER DISORDERS OF PROSTATE

602.0   Calculus of prostate — *prostatic stone*

602.1   Congestion or hemorrhage of prostate — *bleeding or collection of fluid in prostate*

602.2   Atrophy of prostate — *loss of prostatic tissue*

602.8   Other specified disorder of prostate — *including prostatic fistula; prostatic infarction; periprostatic adhesions; prostatorrhea*

602.9   Unspecified disorder of prostate — *palpable prostate*

603 HYDROCELE

Included in this rubric is a hydrocele of the spermatic cord, testis, or tunica vaginalis. The tunica vaginalis is the double-layer membrane that surrounds each testis; it consists of an outer parietal layer and an inner visceral serous layer. In the embryo, the tunica vaginalis is an extension of the peritoneum, the membrane in the abdominal cavity. If, after it separates, the closure is not complete, and fluid collects above the testes in a painless swelling called a hydrocele. Excluded from this rubric is a congenital hydrocele, reported with 778.6.

603.0   Encysted hydrocele — *encysted*

603.1   Infected hydrocele — (Use additional code to identify organism) — *infection in fluid-filled sac in testicular membrane*

603.8   Other specified type of hydrocele — *other specified hydrocele NEC*

603.9   Unspecified hydrocele — *hydrocele NOS*

604 ORCHITIS AND EPIDIDYMITIS

The testes are two small oval glands contained in the scrotum. The left testis is usually about one centimeter lower in the scrotal sac than the right. Both are suspended in the pouch by scrotal tissue and the spermatic cords; they are separated by a central partition. Dense fibrous tissue, the tunica albuginea, encases each testis, enters the gland, and divides the glandular tissue into some 200 or 300 lobules. Each lobule contains coiled seminiferous tubules that produce sperm and which converge into about 20 small ducts that pass through the tunica albuginea and enter the epididymis.

The testes have two main functions: the production of sperm (spermatogenesis) and the secretion of hormones, mostly testosterone, which is responsible for the development of sexual characteristics in adolescent males and for the functioning of the male reproductive system.

Each epididymis lies along the top and back of the testis. It consists of a single, tightly coiled tube, enclosed in fibrous connective tissue casing. The epididymis tube is extremely small in diameter, but about six meters long. It forms a comma-shaped structure, with the blunt head at the top, a central body, and a tapered tail, which connects to the vas deferens.

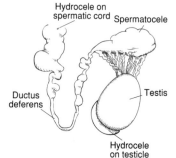

Hydrocele on spermatic cord   Spermatocele

Ductus deferens

Testis

Hydrocele on testicle

Examples of hydroceles of the testes and spermatic cord as well as a cyst of the epididymis (spermatocele)

The epididymis has three main functions, serving as one of the ducts through which the sperm pass, as a storage reservoir for maturing sperm, and as a contributor to seminal fluid.

Use an additional code to identify the infective agent, such as *E. coli* (041.4); *Staphylococcus* (041.1); or *Streptococcus* (041.0). For orchitis and epididymitis in diseases classified elsewhere, code first the underlying disease. Excluded from this rubric are gonococcal orchitis (098.13, 098.33); mumps (072.0); tuberculous orchitis (016.5); and tuberculous epididymitis (016.4).

604.0	Orchitis, epididymitis, and epididymo-orchitis, with abscess — *testicular abscess*
604.90	Unspecified orchitis and epididymitis — *orchitis and epididymitis NOS*
604.91	Orchitis and epididymitis in disease classified elsewhere — (Code first underlying disease, as: 032.89, 095.8, 125.0–125.9) — *code diphtheria, syphilis and filariasis first*
604.99	Other orchitis, epididymitis, and epididymo-orchitis, without mention of abscess — *including orchitis, epididymitis and epididymo-orchitis, without mention of abscess NOS*

605 REDUNDANT PREPUCE AND PHIMOSIS ☑️

606 INFERTILITY, MALE

From 30 percent to 50 percent of infertility in couples is attributable to the male.

To report sperm count for fertility testing, see V26.21 *Fertility testing*, or V26.22 *Aftercare following sterilization reversal.*

606.0	Azoospermia — *including Sertoli cell syndrome; Del Castillo's syndrome; infertility due to germinal cell aplasia*
606.1	Oligospermia — *due to germinal cell desquamation; hypospermatogenesis*
606.8	Infertility due to extratesticular causes — *due to drug therapy, infection, radiation*
606.9	Unspecified male infertility

607 DISORDERS OF PENIS

The penis is the organ of copulation and is shaped like an inverted pyramid. It lies under the bladder, with the apex pointing downwards and composed of three cylindrical layers of tissue, which are enclosed in fibrous connective tissue, with an outer layer of skin. The smaller, lower cylinder is called the corpus spongiosum, through which the urethra passes to the external urinary meatus. The two upper and larger cylinders are the corpora cavernosa. At the end of the penis, the corpus spongiosum overlaps the ends of the corpora cavernosa, forming the bulging structure of the glans penis. Over this is a double fold of retractable skin called the prepuce, or foreskin. Surgical removal of foreskin is called circumcision.

The functions of the penis are copulation and to provide transport through the urethra of semen. Urine from the bladder is also excreted via the urethra.

Excluded from this rubric is phimosis (605).

607.0	Leukoplakia of penis — *kraurosis*
607.1	Balanoposthitis — *balanitis*
607.2	Other inflammatory disorders of penis — *boil of corpus cavernosum*

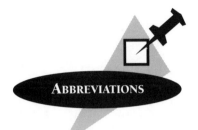

ABBREVIATIONS

AI: artificial insemination

AIH: artificial insemination, husband's sperm

GIFT: gamete intrafallopian transfer

IVF: in vitro fertilization

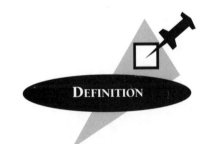

DEFINITION

Dell Castillo's syndrome: also Sertoli-cell-only, sterility due to an absence of living spermatozoa in the semen.

Peyronie's disease: also van Buren's disease, the corpus cavernosum of the penis is surrounded by fibrous material which causes pain during erection.

607.3	Priapism — *painful erection*
607.81	Balanitis xerotica obliterans — *including induratio penis plastica*
607.82	Vascular disorders of penis — *including embolism of corpus cavernosum; hemorrhage of corpus cavernosum*
607.83	Edema of penis — *edema*
607.84	Impotence of organic origin — *impotence, organic*
607.89	Other specified disorder of penis — *including atrophy of corpus cavernosum; cicatrix; phagedena*
607.9	Unspecified disorder of penis — *disorder NOS*

608 OTHER DISORDERS OF MALE GENITAL ORGANS

Use an additional code to identify the infective agent in infections and inflammatory disorders. In disorders of male genital organs in disease classified elsewhere, code first the underlying disease.

608.0	Seminal vesiculitis — *including abscess of seminal vesicle; vesiculitis (seminal)*
608.1	Spermatocele — *epididymal cyst filled with sperm-containing fluid*
608.2	Torsion of testis — *including spermatic cord torsion; testicular torsion*
608.3	Atrophy of testis — *wasting of testicular tissue*
608.4	Other inflammatory disorder of male genital organs — *including scrotal boil; cellulitis of testicle*
608.81	Specified disorder of male genital organs in diseases classified elsewhere — (Code first underlying disease, as: 016.5, 125.0–125.9) — *code filariasis and tuberculosis first*
608.83	Specified vascular disorder of male genital organs — *including testicular hematoma; hematocele, NOS, male*
608.84	Chylocele of tunica vaginalis — *chylocele*
608.85	Stricture of male genital organs — *stricture of vas deferens*
608.86	Edema of male genital organs — *fluid retention in male reproductive structure*
608.89	Other specified disorder of male genital organs — *specified disorders NEC*
608.9	Unspecified disorder of male genital organs — *including neuralgia; pain*

610-611 Disorders of Breast

The breasts are located in the subcutaneous tissue of the front thorax, forming elevations. The mammary glands, accessory organs of the female reproductive system, are contained within these elevations.

Each breast contains 15 lobes to 20 lobes of glandular tissue consisting of smaller lobuli of alveoli (secreting cells) and ducts. The smaller ducts unite into a single milk-carrying duct for each lobe and these converge toward the nipple. The glandular tissue is contained within dense connective tissue that attaches to the pectoral muscle, and with suspensory ligaments, which extend from the skin to the pectoral muscle to provide support.

The nipple is located near the tip of each breast surrounded by a circular area of pigmented and irregular surfaced skin called the areola.

The function of the mammary gland is lactation, which is the secretion of colostrum and subsequently milk for the nourishment of newborn infants. Successful lactation relies on pre- and post-natal production of hormones including progesterone, estrogen, prolactin, and oxytocin.

5th Needs fifth-digit   **OK** Valid three-digit code

610 BENIGN MAMMARY DYSPLASIAS

610.0 Solitary cyst of breast — *cyst (solitary)*

610.1 Diffuse cystic mastopathy — *cysts scattered throughout*

610.2 Fibroadenosis of breast — *including cystic fibroadenosis of breast; diffuse fibroadenosis*

610.3 Fibrosclerosis of breast — *fibrosclerosis*

610.4 Mammary duct ectasia — *including periductal mastitis*

610.8 Other specified benign mammary dysplasias — *including mazoplasia; sebaceous cyst*

610.9 Unspecified benign mammary dysplasia — *benign NOS*

611 OTHER DISORDERS OF BREAST

611.0 Inflammatory disease of breast — *including acute or chronic abscess of areola; mammillary fistula; acute or subacute mastitis*

611.1 Hypertrophy of breast — *massive pubertal hypertrophy*

611.2 Fissure of nipple — *crack in nipple*

611.3 Fat necrosis of breast — *fat necrosis (segmental)*

611.4 Atrophy of breast — *wasting of breast tissue*

611.5 Galactocele

611.6 Galactorrhea not associated with childbirth — *flow of milk*

611.71 Mastodynia — *pain*

611.72 Lump or mass in breast — *lump*

611.79 Other sign and symptom in breast — *induration; inversion of nipple; thickening*

611.8 Other specified disorder of breast — *including hematoma, (nontraumatic); infarction; pendulous*

611.9 Unspecified breast disorder — *disorder NOS*

614-616 Inflammatory Disease of Female Pelvic Organs

614 INFLAMMATORY DISEASE OF OVARY, FALLOPIAN TUBE, PELVIC CELLULAR TISSUE, AND PERITONEUM

614.0 Acute salpingitis and oophoritis — *any condition classifiable to 614.2, specified as acute or subacute*

614.1 Chronic salpingitis and oophoritis — *including hydrosalpinx; salpingitis follicularis*

614.2 Salpingitis and oophoritis not specified as acute, subacute, or chronic — *including pyosalpinx; tubo-ovarian inflammatory disease*

614.3 Acute parametritis and pelvic cellulitis — *including acute inflammatory pelvic disease*

614.4 Chronic or unspecified parametritis and pelvic cellulitis — *including chronic inflammatory pelvic disease; abscess of broad ligament; pelvic cellulitis*

614.5 Acute or unspecified pelvic peritonitis, female — *including metroperitonitis*

614.6 Pelvic peritoneal adhesions, female (postoperative) (postinfection) — (Use additional code to identify any associated (condition) 628.2) — *including peritubal adhesions, tubo-ovarian adhesions*

614.7 Other chronic pelvic peritonitis, female

614.8 Other specified inflammatory disease of female pelvic organs and tissues — *specified inflammatory disease of female pelvic organs and tissues NEC*

614.9 Unspecified inflammatory disease of female pelvic organs and tissues — *including pelvic infection or inflammation, female NOS*

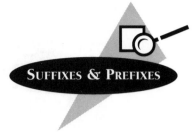

SUFFIXES & PREFIXES

-adenosis: a disease of the glands

-sclerosis: rigid, solid or hard, or the process of becoming so

-trophy: nourishment, food, or sustenance

Fibro-: referring to fiber

Hyper-: above, more than, over

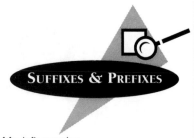

SUFFIXES & PREFIXES

-itis: inflammation

Endo-: within, inside, internal

Oophor-: referring to the ovary

Peri-: around, encircling, surrounding

Salping-: referring to the fallopian tube

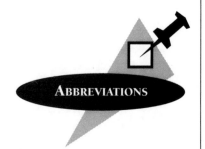

ABBREVIATIONS

DUB: dysfunctional uterine bleeding

PID: pelvic inflammatory disease

PMS: premenstrual syndrome

OC: oral contraceptive

615 INFLAMMATORY DISEASES OF UTERUS, EXCEPT CERVIX

615.0 Acute inflammatory disease of uterus, except cervix — *any condition classifiable to 615.9, specified as acute or subacute*

615.1 Chronic inflammatory disease of uterus, except cervix — *any condition classifiable to 615.9, specified as chronic*

615.9 Unspecified inflammatory disease of uterus — *including endometritis; endomyometritis; perimetritis; pyometra*

616 INFLAMMATORY DISEASE OF CERVIX, VAGINA, AND VULVA

616.0 Cervicitis and endocervicitis — *including cervicitis with or without mention of erosion or ectropion; Nabothian (gland) cyst of follicle*

616.10 Unspecified vaginitis and vulvovaginitis — *including postirradiation vaginitis; vaginitis NOS*

616.11 Vaginitis and vulvovaginitis in diseases classified elsewhere — (Code first underlying disease, as: 127.4) — *code first underlying disease such as pinworm vaginitis*

616.2 Cyst of Bartholin's gland — *fluid-filled sac within one of the paired glands*

616.3 Abscess of Bartholin's gland — *pocket of pus within one of the paired glands*

616.4 Other abscess of vulva — *including vulvar carbuncle; vulvar boil*

616.50 Unspecified ulceration of vulva — *ulcer NOS of vulva*

616.51 Ulceration of vulva in disease classified elsewhere — (Code first underlying disease, as: 016.70–016.76, 136.1) — *code Behcet's syndrome and tuberculosis first*

616.8 Other specified inflammatory disease of cervix, vagina, and vulva — *including caruncle of vagina or labium*

616.9 Unspecified inflammatory disease of cervix, vagina, and vulva — *vaginal disorder NOS*

617-629 Other Disorders of Female Genital Tract

617 ENDOMETRIOSIS

Endometriosis is the presence of endometrial tissue (functioning endometrial glands and stoma) outside of its normal location (lining the uterine cavity). The etiology is unknown, though previous uterine surgery or heredity may be predisposing factors.

Signs and symptoms of endometriosis include acquired dysmenorrhea characterized by pain (that usually begins five to seven days before menstruation and lasts two to three days) in lower abdomen, vagina, posterior pelvis, or back; bleeding from vagina, rectum or bladder depending on site involved; dyspareunia, or cramps. Pelvic exam may locate sites of endometriosis, while laparoscopy confirms diagnosis and stage of disease. Diagnostic radiology such as barium enema may rule out malignancy or inflammatory bowel disease.

Therapies include drugs such as progestins, danazol (a testosterone derivative), oral contraceptives, surgery ranging from local excision of endometrial tissue and preservation of pelvic organs (for women who wish to bear children) to total abdominal hysterectomy with bilateral salpingo-oophorectomy (for older women and those with extensive disease).

Associated conditions include infertility, spontaneous abortion, and pelvic adhesions.

617.0 Endometriosis of uterus — *including adenomyosis; cervical endometriosis*

617.1 Endometriosis of ovary — *including chocolate cyst of ovary; endometrial cystoma of ovary*

✔5th Needs fifth-digit   **OK** Valid three-digit code

617.2 Endometriosis of fallopian tube — *aberrant uterine mucosal tissue inflaming tissues of fallopian tube*

617.3 Endometriosis of pelvic peritoneum — *aberrant uterine mucosal tissue inflaming tissues of peritoneum*

617.4 Endometriosis of rectovaginal septum and vagina — *aberrant uterine mucosal tissue inflaming tissues behind or in vagina*

617.5 Endometriosis of intestine — *including endometriosis of appendix, colon or rectum*

617.6 Endometriosis in scar of skin — *aberrant uterine mucosal tissue inflaming scar tissues*

617.8 Endometriosis of other specified sites — *including endometriosis of bladder, lung, umbilicus, vulva*

617.9 Endometriosis, site unspecified — *endometriosis NOS*

618 GENITAL PROLAPSE

618.0 Prolapse of vaginal walls without mention of uterine prolapse — (Use additional code to identify associated (condition) 625.6, 788.31, 788.33–788.39) — *including cystocele; cystourethrocele*

618.1 Uterine prolapse without mention of vaginal wall prolapse — (Use additional code to identify associated (condition) 625.6, 788.31, 788.33–788.39) — *including descensus uteri; complete uterine prolapse*

618.2 Uterovaginal prolapse, incomplete — (Use additional code to identify associated (condition) 625.6, 788.31, 788.33–788.39) — *downward displacement of uterus into vagina*

618.3 Uterovaginal prolapse, complete — (Use additional code to identify associated (condition) 625.6, 788.31, 788.33–788.39) — *downward displacement and exposure of uterus within external genitalia*

618.4 Uterovaginal prolapse, unspecified — (Use additional code to identify associated (condition) 625.6, 788.31, 788.33–788.39) — *uterine prolapse NOS*

618.5 Prolapse of vaginal vault after hysterectomy — (Use additional code to identify associated (condition) 625.6, 788.31, 788.33–788.39) — *posthysterectomy vaginal vault prolapse*

618.6 Vaginal enterocele, congenital or acquired — (Use additional code to identify associated (condition) 625.6, 788.31, 788.33–788.39) — *including pelvic enterocele, congenital or acquired*

618.7 Genital prolapse, old laceration of muscles of pelvic floor — (Use additional code to identify associated (condition) 625.6, 788.31, 788.33–788.39)

618.8 Other specified genital prolapse — (Use additional code to identify associated (condition) 625.6, 788.31, 788.33–788.39) — *including incompetence or weakening of pelvic fundus; prolapsed perineum*

618.9 Unspecified genital prolapse — (Use additional code to identify associated (condition) 625.6, 788.31, 788.33–788.39) — *including prolapsus*

619 FISTULA INVOLVING FEMALE GENITAL TRACT

619.0 Urinary-genital tract fistula, female — *including cervicovesical, ureterovaginal, urethrovesicovaginal fistula*

619.1 Digestive-genital tract fistula, female — *including intestinouterine, rectovulvar, uterorectal fistula*

619.2 Genital tract-skin fistula, female — *including vaginoperineal fistula*

619.8 Other specified fistula involving female genital tract — *including cervical, vaginal fistula*

619.9 Unspecified fistula involving female genital tract — *genital tract fistula NOS*

620 NONINFLAMMATORY DISORDERS OF OVARY, FALLOPIAN TUBE, AND BROAD LIGAMENT

620.0 Follicular cyst of ovary — *including cyst of graafian follicle*

620.1 Corpus luteum cyst or hematoma — *including lutein cyst*

620.2 Other and unspecified ovarian cyst — *including corpus albicans cyst of ovary; retention cyst NOS of ovary*

620.3 Acquired atrophy of ovary and fallopian tube — *including senile involution of ovary*

620.4 Prolapse or hernia of ovary and fallopian tube — *including displacement of ovary and fallopian tube; salpingocele*

620.5 Torsion of ovary, ovarian pedicle, or fallopian tube — *including torsion of accessory tube; torsion of hydatid of Morgagni*

620.6 Broad ligament laceration syndrome — *including Masters-Allen syndrome*

620.7 Hematoma of broad ligament — *including hematocele, broad ligament*

620.8 Other noninflammatory disorder of ovary, fallopian tube, and broad ligament — *including cyst of broad ligament; infarction of ovary or fallopian tube; ovarian remnant syndrome; spastic fallopian tube*

620.9 Unspecified noninflammatory disorder of ovary, fallopian tube, and broad ligament — *broad ligament disorder NOS*

621 DISORDERS OF UTERUS, NOT ELSEWHERE CLASSIFIED

621.0 Polyp of corpus uteri — *including endometrial polyp*

621.1 Chronic subinvolution of uterus

621.2 Hypertrophy of uterus — *bulky uterus*

621.3 Endometrial cystic hyperplasia — *including adenomatous hyperplasia*

621.4 Hematometra — *including hemometra*

621.5 Intrauterine synechiae — *including adhesions of uterus; Asherman's syndrome*

621.6 Malposition of uterus — *including anteversion of uterus; retroflexion of uterus*

621.7 Chronic inversion of uterus — *uterus is turned inside out*

621.8 Other specified disorders of uterus, not elsewhere classified — *including boggy uterus; sclerotic endometrium*

621.9 Unspecified disorder of uterus — *uterine disorder NOS*

622 NONINFLAMMATORY DISORDERS OF CERVIX

622.0 Erosion and ectropion of cervix — *including ulcer of cervix*

622.1 Dysplasia of cervix (uteri)

622.2 Leukoplakia of cervix (uteri)

622.3 Old laceration of cervix — *including adhesions of cervix*

622.4 Stricture and stenosis of cervix — *including atresia (acquired) of cervix; cervical contracture*

622.5 Incompetence of cervix — *cervical incompetence*

622.6 Hypertrophic elongation of cervix — *overgrowth of cervix extends downward into vagina*

622.7 Mucous polyp of cervix — *polyp NOS of cervix*

622.8 Other specified noninflammatory disorder of cervix — *including (senile) atrophy of cervix; fibrosis of cervix*

622.9 Unspecified noninflammatory disorder of cervix — *noninflammatory NOS*

623 NONINFLAMMATORY DISORDERS OF VAGINA

623.0 Dysplasia of vagina — *abnormal cells*

623.1 Leukoplakia of vagina — *thickened white patches*

623.2 Stricture or atresia of vagina

623.3 Tight hymenal ring — *including rigid hymen, acquired or congenital; tight introitus*

✔5th Needs fifth-digit   **OK** Valid three-digit code

623.4	Old vaginal laceration — *scarring*
623.5	Leukorrhea, not specified as infective — *thick, white discharge*
623.6	Vaginal hematoma — *blood pocket*
623.7	Polyp of vagina — *mucosal growth*
623.8	Other specified noninflammatory disorder of vagina — *kraurosis*
623.9	Unspecified noninflammatory disorder of vagina — *noninflammatory disease NOS*

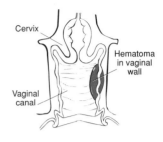

624 NONINFLAMMATORY DISORDERS OF VULVA AND PERINEUM

624.0	Dystrophy of vulva — *kraurosis; leukoplakia*
624.1	Atrophy of vulva — *wasting of external genitalia*
624.2	Hypertrophy of clitoris — *overgrowth of erectile body at anterior cleft of vulva*
624.3	Hypertrophy of labia — *vulvar hypertrophy NOS*
624.4	Old laceration or scarring of vulva
624.5	Hematoma of vulva — *pocket of blood in tussue*
624.6	Polyp of labia and vulva — *mucosal growth*
624.8	Other specified noninflammatory disorder of vulva and perineum — *including cyst; edema; vitiligo*
624.9	Unspecified noninflammatory disorder of vulva and perineum — *unspecified*

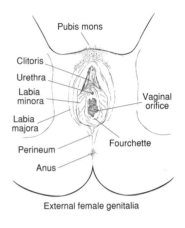

External female genitalia

625 PAIN AND OTHER SYMPTOMS ASSOCIATED WITH FEMALE GENITAL ORGANS

625.0	Dyspareunia — *pain during sexual intercourse*
625.1	Vaginismus — *including colpospasm; vulvismus*
625.2	Mittelschmerz — *ovulation pain*
625.3	Dysmenorrhea — *painful menstruation*
625.4	Premenstrual tension syndromes — *including premenstrual syndrome; menstrual migraine*
625.5	Pelvic congestion syndrome — *including congestion-fibrosis syndrome*
625.6	Female stress incontinence — *involuntary escape of urine during coughing, laughing or sneezing*
625.8	Other specified symptom associated with female genital organs — *including palpable uterus; perineal swelling; vicarious (nasal) menstruation*
625.9	Unspecified symptom associated with female genital organs — *including pain in broad ligament, ovary, round ligament*

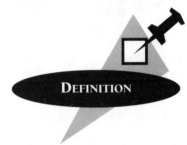

DEFINITION

626 DISORDERS OF MENSTRUATION AND OTHER ABNORMAL BLEEDING FROM FEMALE GENITAL TRACT

626.0	Absence of menstruation — *including amenorrhea (primary) (secondary)*
626.1	Scanty or infrequent menstruation — *including hypomenorrhea; oligomenorrhea*
626.2	Excessive or frequent menstruation — *including menometrorrhagia; menorrhagia; polymenorrhea*
626.3	Puberty bleeding — *including pubertal menorrhagia*
626.4	Irregular menstrual cycle — *including irregular periods*
626.5	Ovulation bleeding — *including regular intermenstrual bleeding*
626.6	Metrorrhagia — *including irregular intermenstrual bleeding*
626.7	Postcoital bleeding — *vaginal bleeding after sexual intercourse*
626.8	Other disorder of menstruation and other abnormal bleeding from female genital tract — *including delayed menstruation*
626.9	Unspecified disorder of menstruation and other abnormal bleeding from female genital tract — *including paramenia*

Amenorrhea: absence of menstruation.

Dysmenorrhea: painful menstruation.

Hypermenorrhea: excessive menstruation.

Polymenorrhea: frequent menstruation.

627 MENOPAUSAL AND POSTMENOPAUSAL DISORDERS

To report post-menopausal status without symptoms or disorder, see V49.81 Postmenopausal status (age-related) (natural).

627.0   Premenopausal menorrhagia — *including climacteric menorrhagia; preclimacteric menorrhagia*

627.1   Postmenopausal bleeding — *bleeding after onset of menopause*

Use this subclassification to report bleeding from the female reproductive tract (vulva, vagina, cervix, or endometrium) occurring one year or more after menopause.

Signs and symptoms of postmenopausal bleeding include vaginal bleeding, excess cervical mucus, and atrophy of vaginal mucosa. Lab work such as analysis of cytologic smears from cervix and endocervical canal, blood work to assess hormone levels, and dilation and curettage (D&C) may show pathological findings in the endometrium.

Therapies include estrogen creams to correct estrogen deficiency, D&C, and hysterectomy for endometrial carcinoma.

Associated conditions include hormonal imbalances, cancer, atrophic changes of vagina or endometrium, and adverse effects of estrogen therapy.

627.2   Menopausal or female climacteric states — *including climacteric syndrome*

627.3   Postmenopausal atrophic vaginitis — *including senile (atrophic) vaginitis*

627.4   States associated with artificial menopause — *including postartificial menopause syndromes*

627.8   Other specified menopausal and postmenopausal disorder — *including atrophic menopausal cervix; postmenopausal endometrium (atrophic)*

627.9   Unspecified menopausal and postmenopausal disorder — *menopausal disorder NOS*

628 INFERTILITY, FEMALE

This rubric classifies the inability to conceive for at least a one-year period after regular intercourse in the absence of contraceptive measure. There are three basic types of infertility: functional, anatomic, and psychogenic.

Functional infertility is due to impairment of the complex hormonal interactions involved in female reproduction. Anatomic infertility can be the result of congenital malformation, scarring or adhesions due to previous infection, atrophy due to hormone deficiency, or any other condition that mechanically impairs or prevents conception. An example of psychogenic infertility is the failure to ovulate due to the stress of marital discords (codes 628.0 and 306.59).

As appropriate, code first the underlying cause, as in adiposogenital dystrophy (253.8) or anterior pituitary disorder (253.0-253.4).

628.0   Female infertility associated with anovulation — (Use additional code for any associated (condition) 256.4) — *including anovulatory cycle*

628.1   Female infertility of pituitary-hypothalamic origin — (Code first underlying disease, as: 253.0–253.4, 253.8) — *code adiposogenital dystrophy first*

ABBREVIATIONS

BBT: basal body temperature

DHEA: dehydroepiandrosterone

FSH: follicle-stimulating hormone

HCG: human chorionic gonadotropin

HMG: human menopausal gonadotropin

LH: luteinizing hormone

LHRH: luteinizing hormone-releasing hormone

LPD: luteal phase deficiency

ZIFT: zygote intrafallopian tube transfer

✔5th   Needs fifth-digit   **OK**   Valid three-digit code

628.2   Female infertility of tubal origin — (Use additional code for any associated (condition) 614.6) — *including tubal occlusion; tubal stenosis*

628.3   Female infertility of uterine origin — (Use additional code for any associated (condition) 016.70–016.76) — *including infertility associated with congenital anomaly of uterus; nonimplantation*

628.4   Female infertility of cervical or vaginal origin — *including infertility associated with anomaly of cervical mucus, or congenital structural anomaly*

628.8   Female infertility of other specified origin — *other specified cause*

628.9   Female infertility of unspecified origin — *unknown cause*

629.0   Hematocele, female, not elsewhere classified

629.1   Hydrocele, canal of Nuck — *including cyst of canal of Nuck (acquired)*

629.8   Other specified disorder of female genital organs — *including hydrocele of round ligament; ulcer of genital organ*

629.9   Unspecified disorder of female genital organs — *including habitual aborter without current pregnancy*

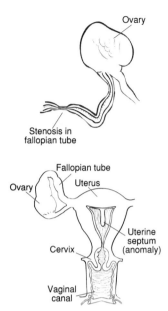

Chapter 11

630-677
Complications of Pregnancy, Childbirth, and the Puerperium

This chapter classifies diseases and disorders that occur during pregnancy, childbirth, and the six weeks immediately following childbirth.

630-633 Ectopic and Molar Pregnancy

Ectopic and molar pregnancy is abnormal products of conception or implantation of normal products of conception in an anatomic location other than the uterus. Use an additional code from rubric 639 to identify any complications.

630 HYDATIDIFORM MOLE OK

Hydatidiform mole is an abnormal product of conception in which the epithelial covering of the chorionic villi proliferates with dissolution and cystic cavitation of the avascular stroma of the villi. The result is a mass of cells that resembles a bunch of grapes. This condition also is called cystic or vesicular mole.

Signs and symptoms of hydatidiform mole include bleeding, usually in the first trimester, larger than expected uterus for gestational age, nausea and vomiting, preeclampsia, and passage of vesicular tissue.

Lab work positive for hydatidiform mole reveals HCG greater than 100,000 mIU/ml. Amniography reveals honeycomb appearance of mole; exam of flat plate of abdomen fails to show fetal skeleton after 15 weeks; ultrasound reveals abnormalities of fetus and gestational sac. Therapies include suction curettage to evacuate mole before completion of 20 weeks of gestation, primary hysterectomy in patients not desiring further pregnancies, and prophylactic chemotherapy in patients whose HCG titer rises or plateaus following pregnancy.

Associated conditions include malignancy in 20 percent of all patients with hydatidiform mole pregnancies. However, these malignancies are excluded from this rubric and are reported with 236.1.

631 OTHER ABNORMAL PRODUCT OF CONCEPTION OK

Included in this rubric are carneous mole, Breus' mole, and blighted ovum.

632 MISSED ABORTION OK

ICD-9 defines a missed abortion as the retention of a fetus for at least four weeks after fetal demise but before completion of 22 weeks of gestation. In the United States, this period of time varies according to state law and may be as few as 19 weeks.

Signs and symptoms of missed abortion include disappearance of normal signs of pregnancy and failure of uterus to grow.

Diagnostic tests include pelvic exam that may reveal brownish vaginal discharge, no fresh bleeding, and closed cervix, though no adnexal abnormalities. Lab work may reveal negative beta HCG and significantly low plasma fibrinogen level in midtrimester missed abortion. An ultrasound will show there is no fetal cardiac activity. Therapies include dilation and curettage or dilation and evacuation if pregnancy has not reached second trimester. If pregnancy is into second trimester, laminaria, suppositories, or amniotic injections of prostaglandin are used to induce delivery of the products of conception.

A missed abortion may occur at any time during the pregnancy before completion of 22 weeks of gestation but usually occurs during the second trimester. Retention of abnormal products of conception is excluded from this rubric and reported with 630 or 631. Also excluded from this rubric are failed induced abortion, classified to rubric 638, and fetal death (656.4).

633 ECTOPIC PREGNANCY

Ectopic pregnancy is implantation of fertilized ovum in anatomic location other than the uterus. The fallopian tube is the most common site of ectopic pregnancy, but it may occur in other locations of the body such as the abdomen, ovary, or cervix.

633.0   Abdominal pregnancy — *including intraperitoneal pregnancy*

633.1   Tubal pregnancy — *including fallopian pregnancy; rupture of (fallopian) tube due to pregnancy*

Tubal pregnancy is implantation of fertilized ovum in the fallopian tube, more often on the right than the left. This condition is more common in women who have had previous tubal disease, such as endometriosis of the fallopian tube, tubal surgeries, or infertility due to tubal disease. Tubal pregnancy may occur in any patient, though approximately 40 percent of these pregnancies occur in women between the ages of 20 years and 29 years old.

Signs and symptoms of tubal pregnancy include mild to severe abdominal pain and occasionally nausea and vomiting before rupture. Abnormal uterine bleeding after a rupture occurs in approximately 75 percent of cases. In tubal pregnancy, the pelvic exam shows adnexal tenderness and possible severe pain on palpation or movement of cervix and uterus. Pregnancy tests positive in 82.5 percent of cases. Lab work shows elevated urine urobilinogen and ultrasound may reveal empty uterine cavity with products of conception outside the uterus. Laparoscopy may allow direct visualization of ectopic pregnancy as will laparotomy (performed more often when profound hemorrhage is suspected).

Therapies include laparoscopy or laparotomy to remove the ectopic pregnancy. If patient is concerned about fertility, fimbrioplasty and salpingostomy are performed to leave the fallopian tube in place. If fertility is not an issue, the tube is removed, the tubal disease corrected, and there is lysis of adhesions in the opposite adnexa. In cases with minimal or no bleeding and without rupture, there is milking of the pregnancy from the fimbriated end of the tube.

633.2   Ovarian pregnancy — *fertilized ovum implants on ovary*

Ovarian pregnancy is implantation of fertilized ovum within the ovary.

633.8   Other ectopic pregnancy — *including intraligamentous pregnancy; mesometric pregnancy*

This subclassification reports implantation of fertilized ovum in other specified sites such as the cervix, the uterine musculature (mesometric), or uterine cornu (horn). Signs and symptoms of other ectopic pregnancy include mild to severe abdominal pain, occasionally nausea and vomiting before rupture. Frequently after rupture, there is abnormal uterine bleeding in approximately 75 percent of cases. Therapies, depending on implantation site, include termination using such procedures as wedge resection of the uterus, fimbrioplasty, supracervical hysterectomy, unilateral salpingo-oophorectomy, and total abdominal hysterectomy.

633.9   Unspecified ectopic pregnancy — *unknown*

634-639 Other Pregnancy with Abortive Outcome

634 SPONTANEOUS ABORTION

The definition of spontaneous abortion is complete or incomplete expulsion of the products of conception before completion of 22 weeks of gestation. Spontaneous abortions may be complete with the expulsion of the entire products of conception, or incomplete with the retention of part of the products of conception, usually the placenta.

In an incomplete abortion, the amniotic sac and fetus may be expelled without the chorion and decidua and only the embryo may be expelled, or the amniotic sac may rupture with passage of the fetus alone. Incomplete abortion requires evacuation of remaining tissue by curettage.

Most spontaneous abortions are associated with abnormal products of conception such as abnormal karyotype. Overall, about 10 percent are thought to have chromosomal abnormalities. The amniotic sac and fetus may be expelled without the chorion and decidua, and only the embryo may be expelled or the amniotic sac may rupture with passage of the fetus alone. Fever and abdominal pain may indicate infection.

In pregnancies of about 14 weeks or less, although as soon as possible, therapies include suction, sharp curettage, or both to remove remaining conceptus. If bleeding is brisk, a five-percent dextrose solution is administered in lactated ringers with 10 units of oxytocin per 500 ml; antibiotics are used to control infection. In pregnancies greater than 14 weeks of gestation, oxytocin intravenously is administered or prostaglandin E2 is inserted by vaginal suppository to expedite the abortion.

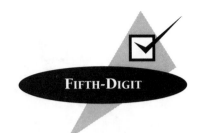

FIFTH-DIGIT

The following fourth-digit subclassification is for use with categories 634-638:

.0 complicated by genital tract and pelvic infection

.1 complicated by delayed or excessive hemorrhage

.2 complicated by damage to pelvic organs and tissues

.3 complicated by renal failure

.4 complicated by metabolic disorder

.5 complicated by shock

.6 complicated by embolism

.7 with other specified complications

.8 with unspecified complication

.9 without mention of complication

The following fifth-digit suclassification is used to identify stage of abortion with categories 634-637:

0 unspecified

1 incomplete

2 complete

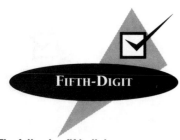

First-digit graphic with checkmark

FIFTH-DIGIT

The following fifth-digit suclassification is used to identify stage of abortion with categories 634-637:

0 unspecified

1 incomplete

2 complete

634.0 ☑5th Spontaneous abortion complicated by genital tract and pelvic infection — *miscarriage complicated by salpingitis*

634.1 ☑5th Spontaneous abortion complicated by delayed or excessive hemorrhage — *miscarriage complicated by excessive bleeding*

Severe hemorrhage must be present for this code to be assigned correctly.

634.2 ☑5th Spontaneous abortion complicated by damage to pelvic organs or tissues — *miscarriage complicated by uterine rupture*

634.3 ☑5th Spontaneous abortion complicated by renal failure — *miscarriage complicated by renal failure*

Spontaneous abortion complicated by renal failure is expulsion of the products of conception before completion of 22 weeks of gestation, complicated by renal failure in the mother.

634.4 ☑5th Spontaneous abortion complicated by metabolic disorder — *miscarriage complicated by diabetes mellitus*

Spontaneous abortion complicated by metabolic disorder is expulsion of the products of conception before completion of 22 weeks of gestation, complicated by metabolic disorders such as diabetes mellitus.

634.5 ☑5th Spontaneous abortion complicated by shock — *miscarriage complicated by shock*

Spontaneous abortion complicated by shock is expulsion of the products of conception before completion of 22 weeks of gestation, complicated by maternal shock, which is an acute peripheral circulatory failure due to an aberration of circulatory control or loss of circulating fluid. Signs and symptoms of spontaneous abortion complicated by shock include hypotension, coldness of skin, tachycardia, anxiety, or sudden disturbance of mental equilibrium.

634.6 ☑5th Spontaneous abortion complicated by embolism — *miscarriage complicated by embolism*

Spontaneous abortion complicated by embolism is expulsion of the products of conception before completion of 22 weeks of gestation, complicated by sudden blocking of an artery by a clot or foreign material in the mother.

634.7 ☑5th Spontaneous abortion with other specified complications — *miscarriage complicated by other specified complication*

634.8 ☑5th Spontaneous abortion with unspecified complication — *miscarriage with unspecified complication*

634.9 ☑5th Spontaneous abortion without mention of complication — *miscarriage without mention of complication*

☑5th   Needs fifth-digit   **OK**   Valid three-digit code

635 LEGALLY INDUCED ABORTION

A legally induced abortion is the intentional expulsion of the products of conception from the uterus by medical professionals working within the boundaries of law.

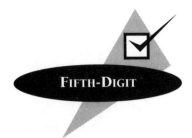

The following fifth-digit suclassification is used to identify stage of abortion with categories 634-637:

0 unspecified

1 incomplete

2 complete

635.0 ✓5th Legally induced abortion complicated by genital tract and pelvic infection — *therapeutic, complicated by salpingitis*

635.1 ✓5th Legally induced abortion complicated by delayed or excessive hemorrhage — *therapeutic, complicated by excessive bleeding*

635.2 ✓5th Legally induced abortion complicated by damage to pelvic organs or tissues — *therapeutic, complicated by uterine rupture*

635.3 ✓5th Legally induced abortion complicated by renal failure — *therapeutic, complicated by renal failure*

635.4 ✓5th Legally induced abortion complicated by metabolic disorder — *therapeutic, complicated by diabetes mellitus*

635.5 ✓5th Legally induced abortion complicated by shock — *therapeutic, complicated by shock*

635.6 ✓5th Legally induced abortion complicated by embolism — *therapeutic, complicated by embolism*

635.7 ✓5th Legally induced abortion with other specified complications — *therapeutic, with other specified complication*

635.8 ✓5th Legally induced abortion with unspecified complication — *therapeutic, with unknown complication*

635.9 ✓5th Legally induced abortion without mention of complication — *therapeutic abortion*

636 ILLEGALLY INDUCED ABORTION

An illegally induced abortion is the intentional expulsion of the products of conception from the uterus by individuals working outside the boundaries of law.

636.0 ✓5th Illegally induced abortion complicated by genital tract and pelvic infection — *criminal, complicated by salpingitis*

636.1 ✓5th Illegally induced abortion complicated by delayed or exececssive hemorrhage — *criminal, complicated by excessive bleeding*

636.2 ✓5th Illegally induced abortion complicated by damage to pelvic organs or tissue — *criminal, complicated by uterine rupture*

636.3 ✓5th Illegally induced abortion complicated by renal failure — *criminal, complicated by renal failure*

636.4 ✓5th Illegally induced abortion complicated by metabolic disorder — *criminal, complicated by diabetes mellitus*

636.5 ✓5th Illegally induced abortion complicated by shock — *criminal, complicated by shock*

636.6 ✓5th Illegally induced abortion complicated by embolism — *criminal, complicated by embolism*

636.7 ✓5th Illegally induced abortion with other specified complications — *criminal, with other specified complication*

636.8 ✓5th Illegally induced abortion with unspecified complication — *criminal, with unknown complication*

636.9 ✓5th Illegally induced abortion without mention of complication — *criminal abortion*

637 UNSPECIFIED ABORTION

Use this rubric when documentation does not support a choice of a legally or an illegally induced abortion.

637.0 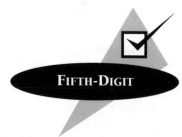5th Legally unspecified abortion complicated by genital tract and pelvic infection — *complicated by salpingitis*

637.1 5th Legally unspecified abortion complicated by delayed or excessive hemorrhage — *complicated by excessive bleeding*

637.2 5th Legally unspecified abortion complicated by damage to pelvic organs or tissues — *complicated by uterine rupture*

637.3 5th Legally unspecified abortion complicated by renal failure — *complicated by renal failure*

637.4 5th Legally unspecified abortion complicated by metabolic disorder — *complicated by diabetes mellitus*

637.5 5th Legally unspecified abortion complicated by shock — *complicated by shock*

637.6 5th Legally unspecified abortion complicated by embolism — *complicated by embolism*

637.7 5th Legally unspecified abortion with other specified complications — *with other specified complication*

637.8 5th Legally unspecified abortion with unspecified complication — *with unknown complication*

637.9 5th Legally unspecified abortion without mention of complication — *without mention of complication*

638 FAILED ATTEMPTED ABORTION

A failed attempted abortion is the attempt although failed intentional expulsion of the products of conception from the uterus.

638.0 Failed attempted abortion complicated by genital tract and pelvic infection — *failed therapeutic, complicated by salpingitis*

638.1 Failed attempted abortion complicated by delayed or excessive hemorrhage — *failed therapeutic, complicated by excessive bleeding*

638.2 Failed attempted abortion complicated by damage to pelvic organs or tissues — *failed therapeutic, complicated by ruptured fallopian tube*

638.3 Failed attempted abortion complicated by renal failure — *failed therapeutic, complicated by renal failure*

638.4 Failed attempted abortion complicated by metabolic disorder — *failed therapeutic, complicated by diabetes mellitus*

638.5 Failed attempted abortion complicated by shock — *failed therapeutic, complicated by shock*

638.6 Failed attempted abortion complicated by embolism — *failed therapeutic, complicated by embolism*

638.7 Failed attempted abortion with other specified complication — *failed therapeutic, with other specified complication*

638.8 Failed attempted abortion with unspecified complication — *failed therapeutic, with unspecified complication*

638.9 Failed attempted abortion without mention of complication — *failed therapeutic, without mention of complication*

FIFTH-DIGIT

The following fifth-digit suclassification is used to identify stage of abortion with categories 634-637:

0 unspecified

1 incomplete

2 complete

5th Needs fifth-digit   **OK** Valid three-digit code

639 COMPLICATIONS FOLLOWING ABORTION AND ECTOPIC AND MOLAR PREGNANCIES

This rubric reports complications that follow an abortion or an ectopic or molar pregnancy. It is used when the complication (not the abortion or the ectopic or molar pregnancy) is the reason for the current episode of care. For example, a patient is readmitted one week after treatment for tubal pregnancy, presenting with generalized sepsis. Codes 639.0 *General tract and pelvic infection* and 038.9 *Unspecified septicemia* would be used for the second admission. Code 633.1 *Tubal pregnancy* would not be used since it pertains only to the previous episode of care.

This rubric also is used when the complication cannot be identified at the fourth-digit level in code categories 634-638. For example, a patient admitted for missed abortion also develops generalized sepsis during the same episode of care. Codes 632 *Missed abortion*, 639.0, and 038.9 would be used for this admission, as the infection cannot be identified at the fourth-digit level for missed abortions.

639.0	Genital tract and pelvic infection following abortion or ectopic and molar pregnancies — *including endometritis, salpingitis, septicemia molar pregnancies*

Genital tract and pelvic infection following an abortion, especially one performed illegally, is commonly caused by both aerobic and anaerobic organisms. The infection may be localized to the products of conception or it may result in endometritis, salpingo-oophoritis, peritonitis, or septicemia.

Signs and symptoms of genital tract and pelvic infection include pain, bleeding, fever, vaginal discharge, and recent illegal abortion. Lab work shows elevated white blood count and cultures identify organisms causing infection, generally gram-negative bacilli (most commonly *Escherichia coli* and *Bacteroides fragilis*) and gram-positive cocci (particularly *enterococci* and *beta-hemolytic streptococci*). The infective agent may be reported secondarily.

639.1	Delayed or excessive hemorrhage following abortion or ectopic and molar pregnancies — *secondary*
639.2	Damage to pelvic organs and tissues following abortion or ectopic and molar pregnancies — *including laceration or perforation of bladder, broad ligament, periurethral tissue or uterus molar pregnancies*
639.3	Renal failure following abortion or ectopic and molar pregnancies — *secondary*
639.4	Metabolic disorders following abortion or ectopic and molar pregnancies — *secondary*
639.5	Shock following abortion or ectopic and molar pregnancies — *secondary*
639.6	Embolism following abortion or ectopic and molar pregnancies — *secondary*
639.8	Other specified complication following abortion or ectopic and molar pregnancies — *secondary*
639.9	Unspecified complication following abortion or ectopic and molar pregnancies — *secondary*

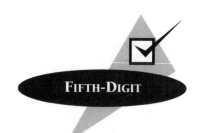

FIFTH-DIGIT

The following fifth-digit subclassification is for use with categories 640-648 to denote the current episode of care:

0 unspecified as to episode of care or not applicable

1 delivered, with or without mention of antepartum condition

2 delivered, with mention of postpartum complication

3 antepartum condition or complication

4 postpartum condition or complication

640-648 Complications Mainly Related to Pregnancy

Codes in this section describe conditions that affect the management of labor, pregnancy or delivery, and the puerperium, even if the condition was present before pregnancy.

640 HEMORRHAGE IN EARLY PREGNANCY

Early pregnancy is defined as before the completion of 22 weeks gestation.

640.0 ✔5th Threatened abortion — *potential abortion marked by bloody uterine discharge*

Signs and symptoms of threatened abortion include bleeding and uterine cramping without cervical dilation.

Therapies include bed rest and observation. Use the fifth-digit 0 if the episode of care is unspecified or not applicable; fifth-digit 1 when the threatened abortion is treated successfully and the patient goes on to deliver at term; and fifth-digit 3 if the threatened abortion is treated successfully without delivery.

640.8 ✔5th Other specified hemorrhage in early pregnancy — *including menstruation during pregnancy*

This subclassification reports bleeding during pregnancy that does not pose a threat of aborting the fetus. Bleeding may occur at any time during the pregnancy, although it is most prevalent during the first trimester when the risk of aborting the fetus is greater than during either the second or third trimester. The patient's pelvic exam reveals no evidence of spontaneous abortion, either complete or incomplete; CBC may indicate anemia if heavy bleeding is present; and an ultrasound is negative for placental abnormalities. Associated conditions that would be reported instead of 640.8 include placenta previa (641.1), premature separation of placenta (641.2), and coagulation defects in mother (641.3).

Medical record documentation must indicate that the patient did not deliver during the current episode of care. If medical record documentation indicates that the physician was concerned about the likelihood of abortion, although there was no abortion, see 640.0 *Threatened abortion*. If medical record documentation such as ultrasound reports indicates a hemorrhagic condition affecting the placenta or antepartum, see category 641 *Antepartum hemorrhage*, abruptio placentae, and placenta previa for alternative code selections.

640.9 ✔5th Unspecified hemorrhage in early pregnancy — *early pregnancy hemorrhage NOS*

641 ANTEPARTUM HEMORRHAGE, ABRUPTIO PLACENTAE, AND PLACENTA PREVIA

Antepartum hemorrhage, abruptio placentae, and placenta previa present with bleeding before the onset of labor (antepartum hemorrhage), premature separation of a normal placenta (abruptio placentae), and implantation of the placenta over or near the internal cervical os (placenta previa).

✔5th Needs fifth-digit   **OK** Valid three-digit code

641.0 ✔5th Placenta previa without hemorrhage — *low implantation of placenta without hemorrhage*

The definition of placenta previa without hemorrhage is implantation of the placenta over or near the internal os of the cervix. With total previa, the placenta completely covers the internal cervical os. Vaginal exam is contraindicated if placenta previa suspected; ultrasound locates exact position of placenta. Therapies include bed rest if patient is not near term; if patient is at term, delivery of the fetus is usually by cesarean section.

If the fetus is not delivered during this episode of care, use the fifth digit 3 to indicate an antepartum condition.

641.1 ✔5th Hemorrhage from placenta previa — *marginal placenta previa with hemorrhage; low lying placenta with hemorrhage*

The definition of hemorrhage from placenta previa is implantation of the placenta over or near the internal os of the cervix with bleeding. With total previa, the placenta completely covers the internal cervical os. With partial previa, the placenta covers a portion of the internal cervical os.

Signs and symptoms of hemorrhage from placenta previa include sudden painless vaginal bleeding beginning late in pregnancy, followed by painless massive bright red bleeding. Vaginal exam is contraindicated if placenta previa is suspected; ultrasound locates exact position of placenta. Therapies include bed rest if bleeding is minor and patient is not near term, if bleeding is substantial, blood transfusion and tocolytic agents are administered. If the fetus is not delivered during this episode of care, use the fifth digit 3 to indicate an antepartum condition.

Excluded from this subclassification is hemorrhage from vasa previa, reported with 663.5.

641.2 ✔5th Premature separation of placenta — *including ablatio placentae; Couvelaire uterus; premature separation of normally implanted placenta; abruptio placentae*

Premature separation of placenta is separation of the placenta from the site of uterine implantation before delivery of the fetus. There are two forms of placental separation: concealed, in which the hemorrhage is confined to the uterine cavity; and external, in which blood drains through the cervix. The placenta may detach either entirely or partially. Etiologies are numerous and difficult to ascertain but include advanced maternal age, multiparity, uterine distention, vascular deficiency and/or deterioration, uterine anomalies, cigarette smoking, and alcohol abuse.

Signs and symptoms of premature separation of placenta include abdominal or back pain and visible hemorrhage, depending on degree of separation and blood loss; irritable abdomen; and tender and often hypertonic uterus.

To avoid precipitating greater hemorrhage, pelvic exam is contraindicated until diagnosis of abruptio placentae established. CBC may show reduced platelets and anemia, depending on degree of hemorrhage; ultrasound determines degree of separation and viability of the fetus. Therapies include fetal monitoring to determine if fetus is in any distress, blood transfusion if severe hemorrhage is present, delivery of fetus if either bleeding persists or separation is total.

641.3 ✔5th Antepartum hemorrhage associated with coagulation defects — *antepartum or intrapartum hemorrhage associated with afibrinogenemia, hyperfibrinolysis; hypofibrinogenemia*

641.8 ✔5th Other antepartum hemorrhage — *antepartum or intrapartum hemorrhage associated with trauma or uterine leiomyoma*

641.9 ✔5th Unspecified antepartum hemorrhage — *antepartum hemorrhage NOS; spots of pregnancy*

642 HYPERTENSION COMPLICATING PREGNANCY, CHILDBIRTH, AND THE PUERPERIUM

Hypertension complicating pregnancy, childbirth and the puerperium may be benign, preexisting, chronic, or secondary to renal disease.

642.0 ✔5th Benign essential hypertension complicating pregnancy, childbirth, and the puerperium — *elevated arterial blood pressure; essential or chronic hypertension specified as complicating, or as a reason for obstetric care during pregnancy, childbirth, or the puerperium*

Benign essential hypertension complicating pregnancy, childbirth, and the puerperium, is blood pressure of 140/90 or greater before the onset of pregnancy or in the first trimester of pregnancy. Signs and symptoms of benign essential hypertension complicating pregnancy, childbirth, and the puerperium include a history of chronic benign hypertension. Examination reveals hypertension without other signs of preeclampsia such as proteinuria or nondependent edema. EKG may reveal left ventricular hypertrophy and lab work often shows elevated serum creatinine. A chest x-ray may reveal cardiomegaly. Therapies include antihypertensive drugs of established long-term safety for mother and fetus such as methyldopa, clonidine, and labetalol.

642.1 ✔5th Hypertension secondary to renal disease, complicating pregnancy, childbirth, and the puerperium — *elevated arterial blood pressure due to kidney disease; hypertension secondary to renal disease*

Hypertension secondary to renal disease, complicating pregnancy, childbirth, and the puerperium is preexisting renal disease that results in hypertension. Blood pressure is 140/90 or greater before the onset of pregnancy or in the first trimester of pregnancy. Signs and symptoms of hypertension secondary to renal disease, complicating pregnancy, childbirth, and the puerperium, include history of chronic renal disease with resultant hypertension. Examination reveals hypertension, edema. EKG may reveal left ventricular hypertrophy and lab work often shows elevated BUN and serum creatinine levels. Chest x-ray may reveal cardiomegaly. Fetal monitoring, fetal nonstress tests, and oxytocin challenge tests determine if pregnancy should be continued. Often, delivery, usually by cesarean section, is prescribed if blood pressure can no longer be controlled and fetus has completed over 22 weeks of gestation.

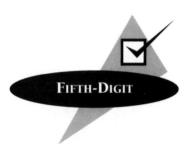

FIFTH-DIGIT

The following fifth-digit subclassification is for use with categories 640-648 to denote the current episode of care:

0 unspecified as to episode of care or not applicable

1 delivered, with or without mention of antepartum condition

2 delivered, with mention of postpartum complication

3 antepartum condition or complication

4 postpartum condition or complication

✔5th   Needs fifth-digit   **OK**   Valid three-digit code

Therapies include antihypertensive drugs of established long-term safety for mother and fetus such as methyldopa, clonidine, and labetalol.

642.2 ✔5th Other pre-existing hypertension complicating pregnancy, childbirth, and the puerperium — *hypertensive heart and renal disease or malignant hypertension specified as complicating, or as a reason for obstetric care during pregnancy, childbirth, or the puerperium*

642.3 ✔5th Transient hypertension of pregnancy — *gestational hypertension; transient hypertension, so described, in pregnancy, childbirth, or the puerperium*

642.4 ✔5th Mild or unspecified pre-eclampsia — *pre-eclampsia NOS or toxemia (pre-eclamptic) NOS*

Mild or unspecified pre-eclampsia is the development of borderline hypertension, albuminuria, and unresponsive edema between the 20th week of pregnancy and the end of the first week postpartum. Signs and symptoms of mild or unspecified pre-eclampsia include weight gain of more than two pounds in one week and nondependent edema of hands and feet. Examination shows hypertension of 140/90 or slightly higher or rise in systolic pressure of 20 mm Hg or diastolic of 15 mm Hg, and nondependent edema of face or hands. Lab work reveals albuminuria of 1+ or greater and rising serum creatinine. Therapies include bed rest and delivery once fetus has reached a suitable age of gestation to be viable and antihypertensive drugs of established long-term safety for mother and fetus such as methyldopa, clonidine, and labetalol.

Excluded from 642.4 are albuminuria in pregnancy without hypertension (646.2) and edema in pregnancy without mention of hypertension (646.1).

642.5 ✔5th Severe pre-eclampsia — *including HELLP syndrome; toxemia (pre-eclamptic), severe*

642.6 ✔5th Eclampsia complicating pregnancy, childbirth or the puerperium — *including toxemia with convulsions; eclamptic toxemia*

642.7 ✔5th Pre-eclampsia or eclampsia superimposed on pre-existing hypertension — *secondary*

642.9 ✔5th Unspecified hypertension complicating pregnancy, childbirth, or the puerperium — *childbirth, or the puerperium; hypertension NOS without mention of albuminuria or edema, complicating pregnancy, childbirth, or the puerperium*

643 EXCESSIVE VOMITING IN PREGNANCY

This category is used to describe vomiting that affects management of the pregnancy.

643.0 ✔5th Mild hyperemesis gravidarum — *hyperemesis gravidarum, mild or unspecified, starting before the end of the 22nd week of gestation*

643.1 ✔5th Hyperemesis gravidarum with metabolic disturbance — *hyperemesis gravidarum starting before the end of the 22nd week of gestation, with metabolic disturbance, such as carbohydrate depletion, dehydration or electrolyte imbalance*

643.2 ✔5th Late vomiting of pregnancy — *excessive vomiting starting after 22 completed weeks of gestation*

643.8 ✔5th Other vomiting complicating pregnancy — *vomiting due to organic disease or other cause, specified as complicating pregnancy, or as a reason for obstetric care during pregnancy*

643.9 ✔5th Unspecified vomiting of pregnancy — *vomiting as a reason for care during pregnancy, length of gestation unknown*

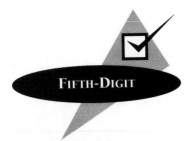

FIFTH-DIGIT

The following fifth-digit subclassification is for use with categories 640-648 to denote the current episode of care:

0 unspecified as to episode of care or not applicable

1 delivered, with or without mention of antepartum condition

2 delivered, with mention of postpartum complication

3 antepartum condition or complication

4 postpartum condition or complication

644 EARLY OR THREATENED LABOR

644.0 ✔5th Threatened premature labor — *premature labor after 22 weeks, but before 37 completed weeks of gestation*

Threatened labor is regular, painful uterine contractions at least twice every 10 minutes for a 30-minute period of time with effacement or dilation of the cervix occurring after completion of 22 weeks of gestation but before completion of 37 weeks. There is neither rupture of membranes nor delivery of the fetus. The contractions cease and the cervix stops dilating.

644.1 ✔5th Other threatened labor — *false labor after 37 completed weeks of gestation; including Braxton Hicks contractions*

644.2 ✔5th Early onset of delivery — *onset (spontaneous) of delivery before 37 completed weeks of gestation*

Early onset of delivery is delivery of an infant after completion of 22 weeks of gestation but before completion of 37 weeks. Signs and symptoms of early onset of delivery include uterine contractions lasting at least 30 seconds and occurring at 10-minute intervals (at least) during a 30-minute period of time and continued dilation and effacement of cervix over period of time despite medications to stop. Therapies include hydration and sedation once the patient is admitted in premature labor, tocolysis to try to prevent progression, and when this fails, delivery of the infant.

Only the fifth-digits 0 or 1 are valid for this subcategory code. The fifth-digit 0, unspecified as to episode of care or not applicable, will rarely, if ever, be assigned as the subcategory implies delivery.

645 LATE PREGNANCY

Post-term pregnancy is a normal pregnancy of more than 40 weeks, up to 42 weeks. A prolonged pregnancy is normal pregnancy that has advanced beyond 42 weeks of gestation. Postdatism may be treated by careful fetal monitoring with no intervention until there are indications the fetus is at risk. Postmaturity syndrome is a term that may be applied to both mothers and infants. In mothers, the syndrome is characterized by prolonged gestation, sometimes excessive fetal size, failing placental function, and impending fetal demise. When the term is used to describe infant pathology, it is classified to 766.2 *Post-term infant,* not "heavy for dates."

645.1 ✔5th Post term pregnancy — *pregnancy over 40 weeks to 42 weeks gestation*
645.2 ✔5th Prolonged pregnancy — *pregnancy which has advanced beyond 42 weeks gestation*

646 OTHER COMPLICATIONS OF PREGNANCY, NOT ELSEWHERE CLASSIFIED

Additional codes should be reported to further specify the complication. Do not report 646.3 Habitual aborter in the case of a current abortion (rubric 634) or if the patient is not currently pregnant (629.9). Report 646.9 *Unspecified complication of pregnancy* for herpes gestationis, insufficient weight gain in pregnancy, retinitis gravidarum, ptyalism pregnancy, pruritic gravidarum, or uterine size-date discrepancy.

✔5th Needs fifth-digit   **OK** Valid three-digit code

646.0 ✔5th Papyraceous fetus — *skin of fetus resembles paper*
646.1 ✔5th Edema or excessive weight gain in pregnancy, without mention of hypertension — *including gestational edema; maternal obesity syndrome*
646.2 ✔5th Unspecified renal disease in pregnancy, without mention of hypertension — *including gestational proteinuria; albuminuria or nephropathy NOS in pregnancy or the puerperium*
646.3 ✔5th Pregnancy complication, habitual aborter — *miscarried at least three times*
646.4 ✔5th Peripheral neuritis in pregnancy
646.5 ✔5th Asymptomatic bacteriuria in pregnancy
646.6 ✔5th Infections of genitourinary tract in pregnancy — *secondary*
646.7 ✔5th Liver disorders in pregnancy — *including icterus gravis, or necrosis of liver, or acute yellow atrophy of liver (obstetric) (true)*
646.8 ✔5th Other specified complications of pregnancy — *including fatigue during pregnancy; herpes gestationis; pruritic gravidarum; ptyalism in pregnancy*
646.9 ✔5th Unspecified complication of pregnancy — *pregnancy complication NOS*

647 INFECTIOUS AND PARASITIC CONDITIONS IN THE MOTHER CLASSIFIABLE ELSEWHERE, BUT COMPLICATING PREGNANCY, CHILDBIRTH, OR THE PUERPERIUM

Use additional codes to further specify the complications.

647.0 ✔5th Maternal syphilis complicating pregnancy, childbirth, or the puerperium — *secondary*

This subclassification reports a pregnancy complicated by an infection of microorganism *Treponema pallidum*, which causes venereal disease that leads to many structural and cutaneous lesions and may be transmitted to the fetus in utero.

647.1 ✔5th Maternal gonorrhea complicating pregnancy, childbirth, or the puerperium — *secondary*
647.2 ✔5th Other maternal venereal diseases complicating pregnancy, childbirth, or the puerperium — *secondary*
647.3 ✔5th Maternal tuberculosis complicating pregnancy, childbirth, or the puerperium — *secondary*

This subclassification reports a pregnancy complicated by infection by *Mycobacterium* and characterized by the formation of tubercles and caseous necrosis in the tissues.

647.4 ✔5th Maternal malaria complicating pregnancy, childbirth, or the puerperium — *secondary*

This subclassification reports a pregnancy complicated by a febrile disease caused by protozoa that are parasitic in the red blood cells. Symptoms, including fever, chills, and sweating, occur at intervals corresponding with a new generation of the parasites.

647.5 ✔5th Maternal rubella complicating pregnancy, childbirth, or the puerperium — *secondary*

This subclassification reports a pregnancy complicated by infection with a mild viral disease (German measles) known to cause birth defects.

647.6 ✔5th Other maternal viral disease complicating pregnancy, childbirth, or the puerperium — *secondary*

647.8 ✔5th Other specified maternal infectious and parasitic disease complicating pregnancy, childbirth, or the puerperium — *secondary*

647.9 ✔5th Unspecified maternal infection or infestation complicating pregnancy, childbirth, or the puerperium — *secondary*

648 OTHER CURRENT CONDITIONS IN THE MOTHER CLASSIFIABLE ELSEWHERE, BUT COMPLICATING PREGNANCY, CHILDBIRTH, OR THE PUERPERIUM

This rubric includes the listed conditions when complicating the pregnant state, aggravated by the pregnancy, or when it is the main reason for the obstetric care. Use an additional code to describe the condition. Excluded from this rubric are conditions both known or suspected of having affected the fetus, which are reported with codes from rubric 655 *Known or suspected fetal abnormality affecting management of mother.*

648.0 ✔5th Maternal diabetes mellitus complicating pregnancy, childbirth, or the puerperium — *secondary*

This subclassification reports pregnancy complicated by insulin- or non-insulin-dependent diabetes mellitus affecting the management and health of the mother and fetus during pregnancy. Signs and symptoms of diabetes mellitus include history of diabetes, insulin- or non-insulin-dependent, with associated conditions such as ketoacidosis. Blood glucose may reveal hyper- or hypoglycemia during pregnancy. Urine culture and sensitivity may reveal asymptomatic urinary tract infection and markedly elevated glycosylated hemoglobin. Other lab work includes tests for electrolyte levels, BUN, and creatinine to evaluate any renal involvement. Ultrasound, fetal biophysical profiles, and other fetal tests may be performed to monitor fetal growth and detect any major congenital anomalies.

Patients with diabetes mellitus are more apt to develop pre-eclampsia or eclampsia. If medical record documentation indicates that either condition is present, assign an additional code.

This category excludes gestational diabetes (648.8).

648.1 ✔5th Thyroid dysfunction complicating pregnancy, childbirth, or the puerperium — *secondary*

648.2 ✔5th Maternal anemia complicating pregnancy, childbirth, or the puerperium — *secondary*

Signs and symptoms of anemia include fatigue, palpitations, tachycardia, dyspnea, and pallor. In anemia, the CBC hemoglobin is 10g/100 ml. Red cells may be microcytic and hypochromic; reticulocytes and platelets may be normal or increased in number. For patients with iron deficiency anemia, lab work reveals serum iron below 30mcg/100 ml and elevated total iron binding capacity. For patients with folic acid anemia, lab work reveals low vitamin B_{12} levels. Therapies include iron therapy (oral, IV, or parenteral). Associated conditions include sickle cell anemia, sickle cell trait, and major and minor thalassemia. Anemia may be found in as many as 80 percent of pregnancies and is due mostly to dietary iron deficiency. Although rare, anemia also may be due to folic acid deficiency.

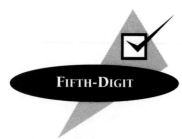

FIFTH-DIGIT

The following fifth-digit subclassification is for use with categories 640-648 to denote the current episode of care:

0 unspecified as to episode of care or not applicable

1 delivered, with or without mention of antepartum condition

2 delivered, with mention of postpartum complication

3 antepartum condition or complication

4 postpartum condition or complication

✔5th   Needs fifth-digit   **OK**   Valid three-digit code

648.3 ✓5th Maternal drug dependence complicating pregnancy, childbirth, or the puerperium — *secondary*

648.4 ✓5th Maternal mental disorders complicating pregnancy, childbirth, or the puerperium — *secondary*

648.5 ✓5th Maternal congenital cardiovascular disorders complicating pregnancy, childbirth, or the puerperium — *secondary*

648.6 ✓5th Other maternal cardiovascular diseases complicating pregnancy, childbirth, or the puerperium — *secondary*

648.7 ✓5th Bone and joint disorders of maternal back, pelvis, and lower limbs, complicating pregnancy, childbirth, or the puerperium — *secondary*

648.8 ✓5th Abnormal maternal glucose tolerance, complicating pregnancy, childbirth, or the puerperium — *secondary*

This subclassification is reported when the patient has had an abnormal glucose tolerance or gestational diabetes although a definitive diagnosis of diabetes mellitus has not been made.

648.9 ✓5th Other current maternal conditions complicating pregnancy, childbirth, or the puerperium — *secondary*

This rubric reports conditions affecting the management of the pregnancy and delivery in the absence of combination codes. This code and the appropriate code from another chapter of ICD-9-CM indicate the treatment of the condition that is affecting management of the pregnancy.

650-659 Normal Delivery, and Other Indications for Care in Pregnancy, Labor, and Delivery

650 NORMAL DELIVERY OK

The definition of delivery in a completely normal case is spontaneous vaginal delivery of a single live infant after completion of 38 to 42 weeks of gestation, with cephalic presentation, without instrumentation, and with no antepartum or postpartum conditions or complications.

Examine the medical record documentation to determine if there were any conditions, early in the pregnancy, that affected management of the patient. This category is appropriate to use if an episiotomy was performed, membranes were ruptured artificially, or the placenta was extracted manually. If forceps or vacuum extraction were used to assist delivery, see category 669 Other complications of labor and delivery, not elsewhere classified. Rubric 650 is for use as a single diagnosis code and is not to be used with any other code in the range 630-676. Use additional code to indicate outcome of delivery (V27).

651 MULTIPLE GESTATION

Use an additional code from rubric V27 to indicate the outcome of delivery in multiple births, identifying livebirths and stillborn births in cases of multiple births. If one or more fetus is malpositioned, also report a code from subclassification 652.6.

651.0 ✓5th Twin pregnancy — *two fetuses*
651.1 ✓5th Triplet pregnancy — *three fetuses*
651.2 ✓5th Quadruplet pregnancy — *four fetuses*

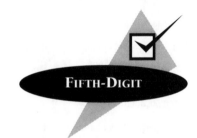

FIFTH-DIGIT

The following fifth-digit subclassification is for use with categories 651-659 to denote the current episode of care:

0 unspecified as to episode of care or not applicable

1 delivered, with or without mention of antepartum condition

2 delivered, with mention of postpartum complication

3 antepartum condition or complication

4 postpartum condition or complication

651.3 ✔5th Twin pregnancy with fetal loss and retention of one fetus — *including vanishing twin syndrome (651.33)*

651.4 ✔5th Triplet pregnancy with fetal loss and retention of one or more

651.5 ✔5th Quadruplet pregnancy with fetal loss and retention of one or more

651.6 ✔5th Other multiple pregnancy with fetal loss and retention of one or more fetus(es)

651.8 ✔5th Other specified multiple gestation

651.9 ✔5th Unspecified multiple gestation — *including superfecundation; superfetation*

652 MALPOSITION AND MALPRESENTATION OF FETUS

Any obstructed labor (660.0) would be sequenced first, followed by a code from this rubric to identify malposition of fetus.

652.0 ✔5th Unstable lie of fetus — *changing fetal position*

652.1 ✔5th Breech or other malpresentation successfully converted to cephalic presentation — *including cephalic version NOS*

652.2 ✔5th Breech presentation without mention of version — *including breech delivery (assisted) (spontaneous) NOS*

Breech presentation without mention of version is presentation of buttocks first without successful version. There are three forms of breech presentation: frank, in which the legs of the fetus extend over the abdomen and thorax so that the feet lie beside the face; complete, in which the fetal position is maintained so that the legs are flexed and crossed; and incomplete, in which one or both lower legs and feet are prolapsed into the vagina. Foot or knee presentations are subdivisions of incomplete breech presentation and are coded to 652.8.

In breech presentation, the abdominal exam (four maneuvers of Leopold) identifies fetal back on one side and the small parts on opposite side. Lower fetal pole is less distinct, especially if engagement has occurred. Fetal heart tones are heard near the midline, slightly above and to one side of the umbilicus. If cervix is slightly dilated and membranes are ruptured, vaginal exam may allow palpation and identification of presenting part; ultrasound reveals breech presentation. Delivery may be by cesarean section, breech extraction, manual assist, or spontaneous, depending on various obstetrical factors, including age and weight of fetus and type of breech.

652.3 ✔5th Transverse or oblique presentation of fetus — *oblique lie; transverse lie*

652.4 ✔5th Fetal face or brow presentation of fetus — *mentum presentation*

652.5 ✔5th High fetal head at term — *failure of head to enter pelvic brim*

652.6 ✔5th Multiple gestation with malpresentation of one fetus or more

652.7 ✔5th Prolapsed arm of fetus — *arm protrudes through birth canal*

652.8 ✔5th Other specified malposition or malpresentation of fetus — *including compound presentation; nuchal hitch (arm)*

652.9 ✔5th Unspecified malposition or malpresentation of fetus — *malpresentation NOS*

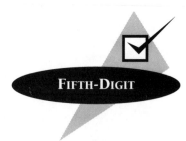

FIFTH-DIGIT

The following fifth-digit subclassification is for use with categories 651-659 to denote the current episode of care:

0 unspecified as to episode of care or not applicable

1 delivered, with or without mention of antepartum condition

2 delivered, with mention of postpartum complication

3 antepartum condition or complication

4 postpartum condition or complication

✔5th   Needs fifth-digit   **OK**   Valid three-digit code

653 DISPROPORTION

If labor is obstructed, sequence the obstruction (660.1) first, followed by a code from this rubric to report the disproportion.

653.0 ✓5th Major abnormality of bony pelvis, not further specified, in pregnancy — *pelvic deformity NOS*

653.1 ✓5th Generally contracted pelvis in pregnancy — *contracted pelvis NOS*

653.2 ✓5th Inlet contraction of pelvis in pregnancy — *inlet contraction (pelvis)*

653.3 ✓5th Outlet contraction of pelvis in pregnancy — *outlet contraction (pelvis)*

653.4 ✓5th Fetopelvic disproportion — *including cephalopelvic disproportion NOS; disproportion of mixed maternal and fetal origin, with normally formed fetus*

Fetopelvic disproportion is condition in which the presenting part of a normally formed fetus is too large to pass through the pelvic canal. Upon palpation of the abdomen, a large presenting part of the fetus in proportion to mother's pelvic canal is revealed. Ultrasound determines fetal size. Therapies include cesarean delivery.

653.5 ✓5th Unusually large fetus causing disproportion — *disproportion of fetal origin with normally formed fetus*

Use this subclassification to report an unusually large fetus too large to pass through the pelvic canal. Upon palpation of the abdomen, a large fetus in proportion to mother's pelvic canal is revealed. Ultrasound determines fetal size. Therapies include cesarean delivery.

653.6 ✓5th Hydrocephalic fetus causing disproportion — *large head of fetus disproportionate to maternal pelvis*

653.7 ✓5th Other fetal abnormality causing disproportion — *including conjoined twins; fetal ascites; fetal myelomeningocele; fetal sacral teratoma*

653.8 ✓5th Fetal disproportion of other origin

653.9 ✓5th Unspecified fetal disproportion — *disproportion NOS*

654 ABNORMALITY OF ORGANS AND SOFT TISSUES OF PELVIS

If labor is obstructed, sequence the obstruction (660.2) first, followed by a code from this rubric to report the abnormality of organs and soft tissues of pelvis.

654.0 ✓5th Congenital abnormalities of pregnant uterus complicating pregnancy, childbirth, or the puerperium — *including double uterus; uterus bicornis*

654.1 ✓5th Tumors of body of pregnant uterus — *fibroids*

654.2 ✓5th Previous cesarean section complicating pregnancy, childbirth, or the puerperium — *scar from previous cesarean delivery*

Use this subclassification to report delivery of a fetus complicated by a uterine scar caused by a previous cesarean section. Therapies include vaginal or repeat cesarean delivery.

654.3 ✓5th Retroverted and incarcerated gravid uterus — *uterus is tilted so that it cannot rise above the sacral promontory*

654.4 ✓5th Other abnormalities in shape or position of gravid uterus and of neighboring structures — *including cystocele; pendulous abdomen; rectocele*

654.5 ✓5th Cervical incompetence complicating pregnancy, childbirth, or the puerperium — *presence of Shirodkar suture with or without cervical incompetence*

Use this subclassification to report dilation of the cervix, usually leading to second-trimester abortion. The etiology may be congenital or due to

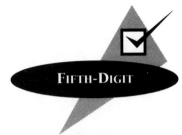

FIFTH-DIGIT

The following fifth-digit subclassification is for use with categories 651-659 to denote the current episode of care:

0 unspecified as to episode of care or not applicable

1 delivered, with or without mention of antepartum condition

2 delivered, with mention of postpartum complication

3 antepartum condition or complication

4 postpartum condition or complication

acquired causes such as previous surgical dilation, conization, breech extraction, or other trauma of delivery. Signs and symptoms of cervical incompetence include history of previous late spontaneous abortions. A cervical exam allows passage of No. 8 Hegar dilator past the internal cervical os. Hysterosalpingostomy demonstrates widened cervical os. Therapies include McDonald, Shirodkar, or other cerclage procedure (placement of encircling suture about the cervical os using heavy nonabsorbable suture or mercilene tape) to prevent protrusion and consequent rupture of the amniotic sac, followed by removal of suture at 38 weeks or when labor begins.

654.6 ✓5th Other congenital or acquired abnormality of cervix complicating pregnancy, childbirth, or the puerperium — *including cicatricial cervix; cervical polyp; stenosis or stricture of cervix*

654.7 ✓5th Congenital or acquired abnormality of vagina complicating pregnancy, childbirth, or the puerperium — *septate vagina; vaginal stenosis or stricture*

654.8 ✓5th Congenital or acquired abnormality of vulva complicating pregnancy, childbirth, or the puerperium — *including fibrosis of perineum; persistent hymen; rigid perineum*

654.9 ✓5th Other and unspecified abnormality of organs and soft tissues of pelvis complicating pregnancy, childbirth, and the puerperium — *including uterine scar NEC; dystocia syndrome*

655 KNOWN OR SUSPECTED FETAL ABNORMALITY AFFECTING MANAGEMENT OF MOTHER

Report codes in this rubric when the listed conditions in the fetus are reasons for observation or obstetrical care of the mother or for termination of the pregnancy.

655.0 ✓5th Central nervous system malformation in fetus affecting management of mother — *including fetal or suspected fetal; anencephaly, hydrocephalus or spina bifida (with myelomeningocele)*

655.1 ✓5th Chromosomal abnormality in fetus affecting management of mother — *known to have damaged or mutated chromosome resulting in abnormality*

655.2 ✓5th Hereditary disease in family possibly affecting fetus, affecting management of mother

655.3 ✓5th Suspected damage to fetus from viral disease in mother, affecting management of mother — *including maternal rubella*

655.4 ✓5th Suspected damage to fetus from other disease in mother, affecting management of mother — *including maternal alcohol addiction or maternal listerosis or maternal toxoplasmosis*

655.5 ✓5th Suspected damage to fetus from drugs, affecting management of mother — *including drug damage*

655.6 ✓5th Suspected damage to fetus from radiation, affecting management of mother — *including radiation damage*

655.7 ✓5th Decreased fetal movements — *reduction in fetal movements*

655.8 ✓5th Other known or suspected fetal abnormality, not elsewhere classified, affecting management of mother — *including suspected damage to fetus from environmental toxins or intrauterine contraceptive device*

655.9 ✓5th Unspecified fetal abnormality affecting management of mother

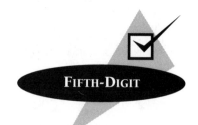

FIFTH-DIGIT

The following fifth-digit subclassification is for use with categories 651-659 to denote the current episode of care:

0 unspecified as to episode of care or not applicable

1 delivered, with or without mention of antepartum condition

2 delivered, with mention of postpartum complication

3 antepartum condition or complication

4 postpartum condition or complication

✓5th   Needs fifth-digit   **OK**   Valid three-digit code

656 OTHER FETAL AND PLACENTAL PROBLEMS AFFECTING MANAGEMENT OF MOTHER

Report codes in this rubric when the listed conditions in the fetus are a reason for observation or obstetrical care of the mother or for termination of the pregnancy.

656.0 ✓5th Fetal-maternal hemorrhage affecting management of mother — *leakage (microscopic) of fetal blood into maternal circulation*

656.1 ✓5th Rhesus isoimmunization affecting management of mother — *including anti-D [Rh] antibodies; Rh incompatibility*

656.2 ✓5th Isoimmunization from other and unspecified blood-group incompatibility affecting management of mother — *including ABO isoimmunization*

656.3 ✓5th Fetal distress affecting management of mother — *including metabolic acidemia*

The definition of fetal distress is metabolic abnormalities, notably hypoxia and acidosis, which affect the functions of vital organs of the fetus. Fetal distress can occur at any time during pregnancy and during or because of the stress of uterine contractions and medications. In fetal distress, the fetal heart monitor reveals acceleration or deceleration of fetal heart rate, flattened heart rate baseline, and extreme and variable deceleration of uterine tachysystole and tetanic contractions. Fetal scalp blood sampling (blood pH) reveals fetal distress. Therapies include administration of oxygen to mother.

Excluded from this subclassification are abnormal fetal acid-base balance (656.8); abnormality in fetal heart rate or rhythm (659.7); or meconium in liquor (656.8).

656.4 ✓5th Intrauterine death affecting management of mother — *including fetal death NOS; fetal death after completion of 22 weeks' gestation; missed delivery*

656.5 ✓5th Poor fetal growth affecting management of mother — *"light for dates"; "placental insufficiency"; "small for dates"*

656.6 ✓5th Excessive fetal growth affecting management of mother — *"large for dates"*

656.7 ✓5th Other placental conditions affecting management of mother — *including abnormal placenta; placental infarct*

656.8 ✓5th Other specified fetal and placental problems affecting management of mother — *including abnormal acid-base balance; intrauterine abscess; lithopedion*

656.9 ✓5th Unspecified fetal and placental problem affecting management of mother — *unknown*

657 POLYHYDRAMNIOS

This code requires a fifth-digit. Assign a 0 for fourth-digit placement with this code, and then assign the appropriate fifth-digit.

657.0 ✓5th Polyhydramnios — *excessive amniotic fluid*

658 OTHER PROBLEMS ASSOCIATED WITH AMNIOTIC CAVITY AND MEMBRANES

Amniotic fluid embolism (673.1) is excluded from this rubric.

658.0 ✓5th Oligohydramnios — *presence of abnormally low amount of amniotic fluid*

658.1 ✓5th Premature rupture of membranes in pregnancy — *rupture of amniotic sac less than 24 hours prior to onset of labor*

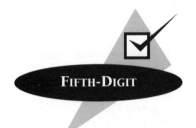

FIFTH-DIGIT

The following fifth-digit subclassification is for use with categories 651-659 to denote the current episode of care:

0 unspecified as to episode of care or not applicable

1 delivered, with or without mention of antepartum condition

2 delivered, with mention of postpartum complication

3 antepartum condition or complication

4 postpartum condition or complication

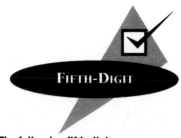

FIFTH-DIGIT

The following fifth-digit subclassification is for use with categories 651-659 to denote the current episode of care:

0 unspecified as to episode of care or not applicable

1 delivered, with or without mention of antepartum condition

2 delivered, with mention of postpartum complication

3 antepartum condition or complication

4 postpartum condition or complication

658.2 ✓5th Delayed delivery after spontaneous or unspecified rupture of membranes — *prolonged rupture of membranes NOS; rupture of amniotic sac 24 hours or more prior to the onset of labor*
658.3 ✓5th Delayed delivery after artificial rupture of membranes
658.4 ✓5th Infection of amniotic cavity — *including amnionitis; membranitis; chorioamnionitis*
658.8 ✓5th Other problems associated with amniotic cavity and membranes — *including amnion nodosum; amniotic cyst; infarct of amnion; cyst of chorion*
658.9 ✓5th Unspecified problem associated with amniotic cavity and membranes — *unknown*

659 OTHER INDICATIONS FOR CARE OR INTERVENTION RELATED TO LABOR AND DELIVERY, NOT ELSEWHERE CLASSIFIED

An "elderly" pregnant woman is one who is 35 years of age or older. A primigravida is delivery of a first child, while a multigravida is delivery of a second or greater pregnancy. Supervision only of the pregnancy of an elderly primigravida is reported with V23.81; of an elderly multigravida with V23.82.

659.0 ✓5th Failed mechanical induction of labor — *failure of induction of labor by surgical or other instrumental methods*
659.1 ✓5th Failed medical or unspecified induction of labor — *including failed induction NOS; failure of induction of labor by medical methods, such as oxytocic drugs*
659.2 ✓5th Maternal pyrexia during labor, unspecified — *fever while the patient is in labor*
659.3 ✓5th Generalized infection during labor — *including septicemia during labor*
659.4 ✓5th Grand multiparity, with current pregnancy — *birth to six or more children previously*
659.5 ✓5th Elderly primigravida — *beyond the age norm for a first pregnancy*
659.6 ✓5th Elderly multigravida — *age at delivery at least 35, and has experienced at least one pregnancy previously*
659.7 ✓5th Abnormality in fetal heart rate or rhythm — *depressed fetal heart tones, including brachycardia, tachycardia*
659.8 ✓5th Other specified indications for care or intervention related to labor and delivery — *including age less than 16 years at expected date of delivery*
659.9 ✓5th Unspecified indication for care or intervention related to labor and delivery — *unknown*

660-669 Complications Occurring Mainly in the Course of Labor and Delivery

660 OBSTRUCTED LABOR
Additional codes may be required to report the cause of the obstruction, and should be sequenced secondarily to the code from this rubric.

660.0 ✓5th Obstruction caused by malposition of fetus at onset of labor — *secondary*
660.1 ✓5th Obstruction by bony pelvis during labor and delivery — *secondary*
660.2 ✓5th Obstruction by abnormal pelvic soft tissues during labor and delivery — *secondary*
660.3 ✓5th Deep transverse arrest and persistent occipitoposterior position during labor and delivery
660.4 ✓5th Shoulder (girdle) dystocia during labor and delivery — *impacted shoulders*
660.5 ✓5th Locked twins — *one twin is in breech position, the other high in head position, rendering vaginal delivery impossible*
660.6 ✓5th Unspecified failed trial of labor — *failed trial of labor*

✓5th   Needs fifth-digit   **OK**   Valid three-digit code

660.7 ✔5th Unspecified failed forceps or vacuum extractor — *application of ventouse or forceps*

660.8 ✔5th Other causes of obstructed labor — *other specified causes of obstructed labor NEC*

660.9 ✔5th Unspecified obstructed labor — *dystocia NOS or fetal dystocia NOS or maternal dystocia NOS*

661 ABNORMALITY OF FORCES OF LABOR

661.0 ✔5th Primary uterine inertia — *weakness of uterus during first stage of labor; including failure of cervical dilation; hypotonic uterine dysfunction, primary*

661.1 ✔5th Secondary uterine inertia — *weakness of uterus in second stage of labor; including arrested active phase of labor; hypotonic uterine dysfunction, secondary*

661.2 ✔5th Other and unspecified uterine inertia — *including desultory labor; irregular labor; slow slope active phase of labor*

661.3 ✔5th Precipitate labor — *rapid labor and delivery*

Precipitate labor is cervical dilation of five centimeters or more per hour for primigravidas and 10 centimeters or more per hour for multigravidas. Usually, precipitate labor is the result of extraordinary forceful uterine contractions or low birth canal resistance.

661.4 ✔5th Hypertonic, incoordinate, or prolonged uterine contractions — *including cervical spasm; dyscoordinate labor; hourglass contraction of uterus; retraction ring (Band's) (pathological); uterine spasm*

661.9 ✔5th Unspecified abnormality of labor — *unknown*

662.0 ✔5th Prolonged first stage of labor

662.1 ✔5th Unspecified prolonged labor — *unknown*

662.2 ✔5th Prolonged second stage of labor

662.3 ✔5th Delayed delivery of second twin, triplet, etc.

663.0 ✔5th Prolapse of cord, complicating labor and delivery — *including presentation of cord; an emergent situation*

663.1 ✔5th Cord around neck, with compression, complicating labor and delivery — *cord tightly around neck*

663.2 ✔5th Other and unspecified cord entanglement, with compression, complicating labor and delivery — *including entanglement of cords of twins in mono-amniotic sac; knot in cord (with compression)*

663.3 ✔5th Other and unspecified cord entanglement, without mention of compression, complicating labor and delivery — *unknown*

663.4 ✔5th Short cord complicating labor and delivery — *lacks appropriate amount of slack, increasing risk of placental abruption*

663.5 ✔5th Vasa previa complicating labor and delivery — *umbilical cord is presenting part*

663.6 ✔5th Vascular lesions of cord complicating labor and delivery — *including bruising; hematoma; thrombosis of vessels*

663.8 ✔5th Other umbilical cord complications during labor and delivery — *including velamentous insertion of umbilical cord; ruptured umbilical cord*

663.9 ✔5th Unspecified umbilical cord complication during labor and delivery — *unknown*

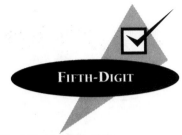

FIFTH-DIGIT

The following fifth-digit subclassification is for use with categories 660-669 to denote the current episode of care.

0 unspecified as to episode of care or not applicable

1 delivered, with or without mention of antepartum condition

2 delivered, with mention of postpartum complication

3 antepartum condition or complication

4 postpartum condition or complication

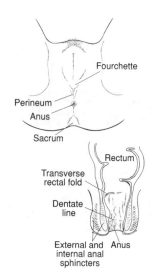

664 TRAUMA TO PERINEUM AND VULVA DURING DELIVERY

This category includes a laceration, rupture, or a tear to perineum and vulva during delivery due to damage from instruments such as forceps and from an extension of an episiotomy.

664.0 ✔5th First-degree perineal laceration during delivery — *perineal laceration, rupture or tear involving fourchette, hymen, labia, skin, vagina or vulva*

664.1 ✔5th Second-degree perineal laceration during delivery — *perineal laceration, rupture or tear (following episiotomy) involving pelvic floor, perineal muscles, or vaginal muscles*

664.2 ✔5th Third-degree perineal laceration during delivery — *perineal laceration, rupture or tear (following episiotomy) involving anal sphincter, rectovaginal septum or sphincter, NOS*

664.3 ✔5th Fourth-degree perineal laceration during delivery — *secondary*

664.4 ✔5th Unspecified perineal laceration during delivery — *including central laceration*

664.5 ✔5th Vulvar and perineal hematoma during delivery

664.8 ✔5th Other specified trauma to perineum and vulva during delivery — *unknown*

664.9 ✔5th Unspecified trauma to perineum and vulva during delivery — *unknown*

665 OTHER OBSTETRICAL TRAUMA

665.0 ✔5th Rupture of uterus before onset of labor

665.1 ✔5th Rupture of uterus during and after labor — *rupture of uterus NOS*

665.2 ✔5th Obstetrical inversion of uterus — *failure of placenta to separate from uterus, facilitating the turning of the uterus inside out*

665.3 ✔5th Obstetrical laceration of cervix

665.4 ✔5th High vaginal laceration during and after labor — *laceration of vaginal wall or sulcus without mention of perineal laceration*

665.5 ✔5th Other obstetrical injury to pelvic organs — *injury to bladder or urethra*

665.6 ✔5th Obstetrical damage to pelvic joints and ligaments — *including avulsion of inner symphyseal cartilage; damage to coccyx; separation of symphysis pubis*

665.7 ✔5th Obstetrical pelvic hematoma — *hematoma of vagina*

665.8 ✔5th Other specified obstetrical trauma — *unknown*

665.9 ✔5th Unspecified obstetrical trauma — *obstetrical trauma NOS*

666 POSTPARTUM HEMORRHAGE

Postpartum hemorrhage is vaginal bleeding in excess of 500 ml during third stage of labor, in the immediate postpartum period or after first 24 hours following delivery. Therapies include manual exploration of uterine cavity for retained placenta and curettage of the uterine cavity.

Postpartum hemorrhage may be associated with a retained, trapped, or adherent placenta (666.0). It also may occur within the first 24 hours following delivery of the fetus but not be associated with a retained portion of the placenta and/or membranes (code 666.1). Delayed or secondary postpartum hemorrhage refers to hemorrhage occurring after the first 24 hours after delivery of the fetus and usually is associated with a retained portion of the placenta and/or membranes (666.2). Code 666.3 includes postpartum coagulation defects, as seen in hypofibrinogenemia or thrombocytonia.

Postpartum hemorrhage due to etiologies other than a retained placenta or membranes is classified elsewhere. Other etiologies for postpartum hemorrhage include lacerations of the cervix, vagina or perineum; rupture of the uterus; a hypotonic myometrium due to general anesthesia; and overdistension of the uterus due to abnormally large fetus or multiple gestation.

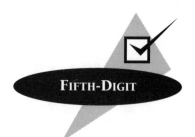

FIFTH-DIGIT

The following fifth-digit subclassification is for use with categories 660-669 to denote the current episode of care:

0 unspecified as to episode of care or not applicable

1 delivered, with or without mention of antepartum condition

2 delivered, with mention of postpartum complication

3 antepartum condition or complication

4 postpartum condition or complication

✔5th Needs fifth-digit   **OK** Valid three-digit code

666.0 ✓5th Third-stage postpartum hemorrhage — *including hemorrhage associated with retained, trapped, or adherent placenta; retained placenta NOS*

666.1 ✓5th Other immediate postpartum hemorrhage — *including atony of uterus; hemorrhage within the first 24 hours following delivery of placenta; postpartum hemorrhage (atonic) NOS*

666.2 ✓5th Delayed and secondary postpartum hemorrhage — *including hemorrhage after the first 24 hours following delivery; hemorrhage associated with retained portions of placenta or membranes; postpartum hemorrhage specified as delayed or secondary; retained products of conception NOS*

666.3 ✓5th Postpartum coagulation defects — *including postpartum afibrinogenemia or fibrinolysis*

667 RETAINED PLACENTA OR MEMBRANES, WITHOUT HEMORRHAGE

667.0 ✓5th Retained placenta without hemorrhage — *including placenta accreta, retained placenta NOS, or retained placenta, total, no hemorrhage*

667.1 ✓5th Retained portions of placenta or membranes, without hemorrhage — *retained products of conception, following delivery, without hemorrhage*

668 COMPLICATIONS OF THE ADMINISTRATION OF ANESTHETIC OR OTHER SEDATION IN LABOR AND DELIVERY

This rubric includes complications arising from the administration of a general or local anesthetic, analgesic, or other sedation in labor or delivery. Additional codes may be required to further identify the specific complications. This rubric excludes a reaction to a spinal or lumbar puncture or a spinal headache (349.0).

668.0 ✓5th Pulmonary complications of the administration of anesthesia or other sedation in labor and delivery — *pressure collapse of lung or inhalation or aspiration of stomach contents or secretions following anesthesia or other sedation; use additional code to further specify complication*

668.1 ✓5th Cardiac complications of the administration of anesthesia or other sedation in labor and delivery — *use additional code to further specify complication*

668.2 ✓5th Central nervous system complications of the administration of anesthesia or other sedation in labor and delivery — *cerebral anoxia following anesthesia or other sedation; use additional code to further specify complication*

668.8 ✓5th Other complications of the administration of anesthesia or other sedation in labor and delivery — *other specified complications of anesthesia or other sedation*

668.9 ✓5th Unspecified complication of the administration of anesthesia or other sedation in labor and delivery — *anesthesia complication NOS, obstetric*

669 OTHER COMPLICATIONS OF LABOR AND DELIVERY, NOT ELSEWHERE CLASSIFIED

669.0 ✓5th Maternal distress — *metabolic disturbance*

669.1 ✓5th Shock during or following labor and delivery — *obstetric shock*

669.2 ✓5th Maternal hypotension syndrome — *low arterial blood pressure in the mother*

669.3 ✓5th Acute renal failure following labor and delivery

669.4 ✓5th Other complications of obstetrical surgery and procedures — *cardiac arrest or failure following cesarean or other obstetrical surgery or procedure, including delivery NOS*

669.5 ✓5th Forceps or vacuum extractor delivery without mention of indication — *delivery by ventouse*

669.6 ✓5th Breech extraction, without mention of indication

669.7 ✓5th Cesarean delivery, without mention of indication

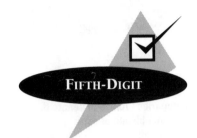

FIFTH-DIGIT

The following fifth-digit subclassification is for use with categories 660-669 to denote the current episode of care:

0 unspecified as to episode of care or not applicable

1 delivered, with or without mention of antepartum condition

2 delivered, with mention of postpartum complication

3 antepartum condition or complication

4 postpartum condition or complication

669.8 ✔5th Other complications of labor and delivery

669.9 ✔5th Unspecified complication of labor and delivery — *including sudden death during childbirth*

670-677 Complications of the Puerperium

Categories 671 and 673-676 include the listed conditions even if they occur during pregnancy or childbirth.

670 MAJOR PUERPERAL INFECTION

Select the appropriate fifth-digit subclassification for this code and use a 0 as the fourth-digit.

This rubric excludes infection following abortion (639.0); minor genital tract infection following delivery (646.6); puerperal pyrexia (672); and urinary tract infection following delivery (646.6).

670.0 ✔5th Major puerperal infection — *including infection and inflammation in the days following childbirth; puerperal endometritis, fever, pelvic cellulitis or sepsis*

671 VENOUS COMPLICATIONS IN PREGNANCY AND THE PUERPERIUM

671.0 ✔5th Varicose veins of legs in pregnancy and the puerperium — *distended tortuous veins of the lower extremities associated with pregnancy*

671.1 ✔5th Varicose veins of vulva and perineum in pregnancy and the puerperium — *distended tortuous veins on the external female genitalia and perineum associated with pregnancy*

671.2 ✔5th Superficial thrombophlebitis in pregnancy and the puerperium — *inflammation and blood clot of superficial vein following childbirth; thrombophlebitis (superficial)*

671.3 ✔5th Deep phlebothrombosis, antepartum — *inflammation and blood clot of deep vein in pregnant patient; deep-vein thrombosis, antepartum*

671.4 ✔5th Deep phlebothrombosis, postpartum — *inflammation and blood clot of deep vein in pregnant patient; deep-vein thrombosis, postpartum*

671.5 ✔5th Other phlebitis and thrombosis in pregnancy and the puerperium — *including cerebral venous thrombosis; thrombosis of intracranial venous sinus*

671.8 ✔5th Other venous complications in pregnancy and the puerperium — *including hemorrhoids*

671.9 ✔5th Unspecified venous complication in pregnancy and the puerperium — *including phlebitis NOS; thrombosis NOS*

672 PYREXIA OF UNKNOWN ORIGIN DURING THE PUERPERIUM

Select the appropriate fifth-digit subclassification for this code, and use a 0 as the fourth-digit.

672.0 ✔5th Pyrexia of unknown origin during the puerperium — *including postpartum fever NOS; puerperal fever NOS; puerperal pyrexia NOS*

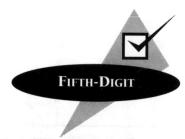

FIFTH-DIGIT

The following fifth-digit subclassification is for use with categories 670-676 to denote the current episode of care:

0 unspecified as to episode of care or not applicable

1 delivered, with or without mention of antepartum condition

2 delivered, with mention of postpartum complication

3 antepartum condition or complication

4 postpartum condition or complication

✔5th   Needs fifth-digit   **OK**   Valid three-digit code

673 OBSTETRICAL PULMONARY EMBOLISM

This rubric reports pulmonary emboli in pregnancy, childbirth, or the puerperium, or specified as puerperal. Excluded are emboli following abortion (639.6).

673.0 ✓5th Obstetrical air embolism — *bubble of air blocking artery in the lung, associated with pregnancy*

673.1 ✓5th Amniotic fluid embolism — *bubble of amniotic fluid blocking artery in mother's lung*

673.2 ✓5th Obstetrical blood-clot embolism — *puerperal pulmonary embolism NOS*

673.3 ✓5th Obstetrical pyemic and septic embolism — *blockage of the artery in the lung, associated with infection in pregnancy*

673.8 ✓5th Other obstetrical pulmonary embolism — *including fat embolism*

674 OTHER AND UNSPECIFIED COMPLICATIONS OF THE PUERPERIUM, NOT ELSEWHERE CLASSIFIED

674.0 ✓5th Cerebrovascular disorders in the puerperium — *secondary*

674.1 ✓5th Disruption of cesarean wound — *dehiscence or disruption of uterine wound*

674.2 ✓5th Disruption of obstetrical perineal wound — *including breakdown of perineum; secondary perineal tear; disruption of episiotomy wound*

674.3 ✓5th Other complications of obstetrical surgical wounds — *including hematoma, hemorrhage or infection of cesarean or perineal wound*

674.4 ✓5th Placental polyp

674.8 ✓5th Other complications of the puerperium — *including hepatorenal syndrome, following delivery; postpartum cardiomyopathy or subinvolution of the uterus; puerperal cardiac thrombosis*

674.9 ✓5th Unspecified complications of the puerperium — *including sudden death of unknown cause during the puerperium*

675 INFECTIONS OF THE BREAST AND NIPPLE ASSOCIATED WITH CHILDBIRTH

Included in this rubric are the listed conditions as they occur during childbirth, pregnancy, or in the puerperium.

675.0 ✓5th Infection of nipple associated with childbirth — *abscess of the nipple*

675.1 ✓5th Abscess of breast associated with childbirth — *including mammary abscess; purulent abscess*

675.2 ✓5th Nonpurulent mastitis associated with childbirth — *including lymphangitis of breast; interstitial mastitis*

675.8 ✓5th Other specified infection of the breast and nipple associated with childbirth

675.9 ✓5th Unspecified infection of the breast and nipple associated with childbirth — *unknown*

676 OTHER DISORDERS OF THE BREAST ASSOCIATED WITH CHILDBIRTH AND DISORDERS OF LACTATION

Included in this rubric are the listed conditions as they occur during childbirth, pregnancy, or in the puerperium.

676.0 ✓5th Retracted nipple associated with childbirth — *drawing back of the projected surface of the mammary gland*

676.1 ✓5th Cracked nipple associated with childbirth — *fissure of nipple*

676.2 ✓5th Engorgement of breasts associated with childbirth — *abnormally high accumulation of milk in the breast ducts*

676.3 ✓5th Other and unspecified disorder of breast associated with childbirth — *including absence of milk secretion by the breast*

676.4 ✓5th Failure of lactation — *agalactia*

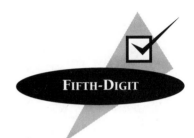

FIFTH-DIGIT

The following fifth-digit subclassifications are for use with categories 670-676 to denote the current episode of care.

0 unspecified as to episode of care or not applicable

1 delivered, with or without mention of antepartum condition

2 delivered, with mention of postpartum complication

3 antepartum condition or complication

4 postpartum condition or complication

676.5 ✔5th Suppressed lactation
676.6 ✔5th Galactorrhea — *including Chiari-Frommel syndrome*
676.8 ✔5th Other disorders of lactation — *including galactocele*
676.9 ✔5th Unspecified disorder of lactation — *unknown*

677 LATE EFFECT OF COMPLICATION OF PREGNANCY, CHILDBIRTH, AND THE PUERPERIUM OK

Code first any sequelae. This category is to be used to indicate conditions in 632-648.9 and 651-676.9 as the cause of the late effect classifiable elsewhere. The "late effects" include conditions specified as such, or as sequelae, which may occur at any time after the puerperium.

✔5th   Needs fifth-digit   OK   Valid three-digit code

Chapter 12

680-709
Diseases of the Skin and Subcutaneous Tissue

This chapter classifies diseases and disorders of the epidermis, dermis, and subcutaneous tissue, nails, scar tissue, sebaceous glands, sweat glands, and hair and hair follicles.

680-686 Infections of Skin and Subcutaneous Tissue

This range of codes classifies infections of skin and subcutaneous tissue is diseases and disorders such as boils, carbuncles, furuncles, cellulitis, abscess, lymphadenitis, local infections, and pilonidal cysts. When assigning a code from categories 680-686, also assign a code (as a secondary code) to identify the infective organism, such as *staphylococcus* (code 041.1). Excluded from this range are certain infections of the skin classified to Chapter 1 Parasitic and Infectious Diseases of ICD-9, including erysipelas (035); erysipeloid of Rosenbach (027.1); herpes (rubrics 053 and 054); molluscum contagiosum (078.0); and viral warts (078.1).

680 CARBUNCLE AND FURUNCLE

Carbuncles and furuncles are infections caused by either aerobic or anaerobic bacterial organisms. A carbuncle is a collection of pus contained in a cavity or sac. A furuncle is a painful nodule formed by circumscribed inflammation of the skin and subcutaneous tissue that encloses a central core.

Signs and symptoms of carbuncle and furuncle include pain, fluctuating or fixed mass, fever, chills, and malaise with furuncle in active stage. A gram stain and culture (if open wound or pus is present) may be performed to identify infective organism. Therapies include antimicrobials (penicillin).

Use an additional code to identify the infective organism, typically *streptococcus* or *staphylococcus*. Use the appropriate fourth digit to indicate the anatomic location of the furuncle or carbuncle. Excluded from this rubric are carbuncles of the eye, lacrimal apparatus, and orbit, classified to rubrics in the nervous system chapter of ICD-9, and those of the genital system, classified to the chapter on diseases of the genitourinary system.

680.0	Carbuncle and furuncle of face — *single boil or cluster of boils on sites including ear, nose, temple*	
680.1	Carbuncle and furuncle of neck — *single boil or cluster of boils, neck*	
680.2	Carbuncle and furuncle of trunk — *including back, breast, chest, flank, groin, perineum, umbilicus, abdominal wall*	
680.3	Carbuncle and furuncle of upper arm and forearm — *including arm, axilla, shoulder*	
680.4	Carbuncle and furuncle of hand — *including finger, thumb, wrist*	
680.5	Carbuncle and furuncle of buttock — *including anus, gluteal region*	

680.6	Carbuncle and furuncle of leg, except foot — *including ankle, knee, thigh, hip*
680.7	Carbuncle and furuncle of foot — *including heel, toe*
680.8	Carbuncle and furuncle of other specified sites — *including head except face; scalp*
680.9	Carbuncle and furuncle of unspecified site — *unknown site*

681 CELLULITIS AND ABSCESS OF FINGER AND TOE

Cellulitis and abscess of finger and toe are infections often caused by group A *streptococci* or *Staphylococcus aureus* but may be caused by other organisms. Cellulitis is an infection of the dermis and subcutaneous tissues. An abscess is a collection of pus resulting from an acute or chronic localized infection associated with tissue destruction.

Signs and symptoms of cellulitis and abscess of finger and toe include erythema, warmth, edema, and pain.

Lab work reveals elevated sedimentation rate and mild leukocytosis with left shift. Gram stain and culture of lesion identify infective organism. Therapies include antimicrobials (penicillin or cephalosporin). Associated conditions include surgical wounds, cutaneous ulcers of the skin, and diabetes mellitus.

Use an additional code to identify the infective organism, typically streptococcus or staphylococcus. When cellulitis occurs with chronic skin ulcer (category 707), code both conditions.

681.00	Unspecified cellulitis and abscess of finger — *sudden, severe inflammation of finger not otherwise specified*
681.01	Felon — *cellulitis in fleshy tip of finger; Whitlow*
681.02	Onychia and paronychia of finger — *in or around fingernail; panaritium, perionychia*
681.10	Unspecified cellulitis and abscess of toe — *sudden, severe inflammation of toe not otherwise specified*
681.11	Onychia and paronychia of toe — *in or around toenail; panaritium, perionychia*
681.9	Cellulitis and abscess of unspecified digit — *unknown*

682 OTHER CELLULITIS AND ABSCESS

Cellulitis and abscess are infections caused by *streptococci*, *staphylococci*, or other organisms. Cellulitis is an infection of the dermis and subcutaneous tissues, more severe in patients with resistance to infection (e.g., diabetics). An abscess is a collection of pus resulting from an acute or chronic localized infection associated with tissue destruction.

Signs and symptoms of other cellulitis and abscess include edema, warmth, redness, pain, and interference with function. Gram stain and culture of lesion identify infective organism. Blood work usually reveals negative cultures, while serological testing, specifically measurement of anti-DNAse B, confirms streptococcal etiology. Therapies include antimicrobials (penicillin).

Use an additional code to identify the infective organism, typically streptococcus. Abscess and lymphangitis are included in this code category. Sequencing should follow the guidelines for selection of the principal diagnosis. When cellulitis or abscess occurs with chronic skin ulcer (category 707), code both conditions.

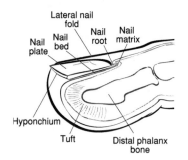

Lateral nail fold
Nail root
Nail matrix
Nail plate
Nail bed
Hyponchium
Tuft
Distal phalanx bone

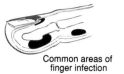

Common areas of finger infection

✔5th   Needs fifth-digit   **OK**   Valid three-digit code

682.0   Cellulitis and abscess of face — *including cheek, chin, forehead, nose, temple, submandibular region*

682.1   Cellulitis and abscess of neck — *sudden severe suppurative inflammation and edema in muscle or subcutaneous tissue*

682.2   Cellulitis and abscess of trunk — *including back, chest, flank, groin, perineum, umbilicus, abdominal wall*

682.3   Cellulitis and abscess of upper arm and forearm — *including axilla, shoulder*

682.4   Cellulitis and abscess of hand, except fingers and thumb — *including wrist*

682.5   Cellulitis and abscess of buttock — *including gluteal region*

682.6   Cellulitis and abscess of leg, except foot — *including ankle, knee, thigh, hip*

682.7   Cellulitis and abscess of foot, except toes — *including heel*

682.8   Cellulitis and abscess of other specified site — *including scalp, pterygopalatine fossa, head, except face*

682.9   Cellulitis and abscess of unspecified site — *unknown site*

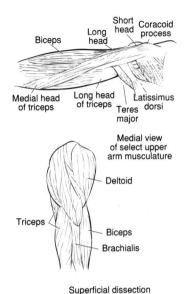

Medial view
of select upper
arm musculature

Superficial dissection
of right arm and shoulder

683 ACUTE LYMPHADENITIS OK

The definition of acute lymphadenitis is sudden, severe inflammation of the lymph nodes. The infection may be due to streptococci, staphylococci or other organisms. Therapies include antimicrobials (penicillin).

Use an additional code to identify the infective organism, typically streptococcus. Abscess and acute lymphangitis are included in this code category. Chronic or subacute, mesenteric and unspecified lymphadenitis are excluded. Sequencing should follow the guidelines for selection of principal diagnosis. When cellulitis or abscess associated with acute lymphadenitis occurs with chronic skin ulcer (category 707), code both conditions.

684 IMPETIGO OK

Impetigo is a superficial skin infection. There are two types of impetigo: bullous and vesicular. With bullous impetigo, fragile bullae form rapidly, break early and heal centrally, leaving crusted erosions. Vesicular impetigo originates as small vesicles or pustules that break, exposing a red, moist base, and secrete a honey-yellow to white-brown crust. Usually caused by *streptococci, staphylococci* or both, impetigo occurs most frequently after a minor skin injury such as a cut, scrape, or insect bite but infrequently may also develop on healthy skin.

Signs and symptoms of impetigo include skin lesions, itching, and mild pain. Blood work reveals elevated sedimentation rate. Gram stain and culture of lesion identify infective organism, and antistreptolysin-O (ASO) titers detect streptococcal infection. Therapies include triple antibiotic ointment (bacitracin, Polysporin, and neomycin applied three times daily).

Excluded from this rubric is impetigo herpetiformis, reported with 694.3.

685 PILONIDAL CYST

Pilonidal cyst is a hair-containing cyst or sinus located at the sacrococcygeal area, which often has a sinus that opens at a postanal dimple.

Signs and symptoms of pilonidal cyst include edema, warmth, redness, pain, and interference with function. A gram stain and culture of lesion identify infective organism. Blood work usually identifies negative culture. Therapies include incision and drainage or circumferential excision. Use the appropriate fourth digit to indicate the presence or absence of an abscess.

685.0 Pilonidal cyst with abscess — *cyst and abscess in sacrococcygeal tissue, including sinus or fistula*

685.1 Pilonidal cyst without mention of abscess — *cyst in sacrococcygeal tissue, including sinus or fistula*

686 OTHER LOCAL INFECTIONS OF SKIN AND SUBCUTANEOUS TISSUE

This rubric classifies other local infections of skin and subcutaneous tissue is infection of skin and subcutaneous tissue including pyoderma, pyogenic granuloma, granuloma, or dermatitis due to a pus-forming organism such as those classified to rubric 041. Therapies include antibiotics, and incision and drainage of larger lesions.

686.00 Unspecified pyoderma — *dermatitis unknown*

686.01 Pyoderma gangrenosum — *persistent, debilitating dermatitis with boggy blue-red ulcers*

686.09 Other pyoderma — *not elsewhere classified*

686.1 Pyogenic granuloma of skin and subcutaneous tissue — *septic, suppurative, telangiectaticum*

686.8 Other specified local infections of skin and subcutaneous tissue — *including dermatitis vegetans; Andrew's pustular bacteride; Brandt's syndrome; Danbold-Closs syndrome; Spiegler-Fendt sarcoid*

686.9 Unspecified local infection of skin and subcutaneous tissue — *skin infection or fistula, unknown*

690-698 Other Inflammatory Conditions of Skin and Subcutaneous Tissue

Excluded from this range of codes is panniculitis, classified to 739.30-739.39.

690 ERYTHEMATOSQUAMOUS DERMATOSIS

Erythematosquamous dermatosis is an inflammatory, scaly condition of the skin predominantly affecting the scalp and face.

Signs and symptoms of erythematosquamous dermatosis include dandruff, itching, dry skin, and crusted scalp lesion ("cradle cap") in infants. Therapies include hydrocortisone cream for facial lesions, and dandruff shampoo for scalp and other hairy areas.

Excluded from this rubric are eczematous dermatitis of eyelid (373.31); parakeratosis variegata (696.2); psoriasis (rubric 696); and seborrheic keratosis (702).

690.10 Unspecified seborrheic dermatitis — *not otherwise specified*

690.11 Seborrhea capitis — *exclusive to scalp; cradle cap*

690.12 Seborrheic infantile dermatitis — *itchy and scaly inflammation of skin in infants*

690.18 Other seborrheic dermatitis — *not otherwise specified, including Unna's disease*

690.8 Other erythematosquamous dermatosis — *including parakeratosis*

691 ATOPIC DERMATITIS AND RELATED CONDITIONS

691.0 Diaper or napkin rash — *psoriasiform napkin eruption; ammonia dermatitis*

691.8 Other atopic dermatitis and related conditions — *including atopic dermatitis; Besnier's prurigo; atopic neurodermatitis; prurigo-asthma syndrome; intrinsic eczema*

✔5th Needs fifth-digit   **OK** Valid three-digit code

692 CONTACT DERMATITIS AND OTHER ECZEMA

This rubric classifies rash as a result of a substance that comes in contact with skin. Initially, the rash is limited to the site of contact but may spread.

Signs and symptoms of contact dermatitis and other eczema include transient redness to severe swelling, itching, and vesiculation. Therapies include identification and elimination of offending agent, topical corticosteroid gel in less acute situations, emollient, and other protective ointment for dry dermatitis.

Use the appropriate fourth digit to indicate the causative agent. An E code from the table of drugs and chemicals should be reported secondarily to report an adverse effect from a drug or chemical.

Excluded from this rubric are allergy NOS (995.3); contact dermatitis of eyelids (373.32); dermatitis due to substance taken internally (rubric 693); eczema of external ear (380.22); perioral dermatitis (695.3); and urticarial reactions (708.0-708.9, 995.1).

692.0	Contact dermatitis and other eczema due to detergents — *allergic reaction*
692.1	Contact dermatitis and other eczema due to oils and greases — *allergic reaction*
692.2	Contact dermatitis and other eczema due to solvents — *including chlorocompound, cyclohexane, ester, glycol, hydrocarbon, ketone groups*
692.3	Contact dermatitis and other eczema due to drugs and medicines in contact with skin — *including arnica, fungicides, iodine, keratolytics, mercurials, neomycin, pediculocides, phenols, scabicides; dermatitis medicamentosa*
692.4	Contact dermatitis and other eczema due to other chemical products — *including acids, adhesive plaster, alkalis, caustics, dichromate, insecticide, nylon, plastic, rubber*
692.5	Contact dermatitis and other eczema due to food in contact with skin — *including cereals, fish, flour, fruit, meat, milk*
692.6	Contact dermatitis and other eczema due to plants (except food) — *including lacquer tree; poison ivy, oak, sumac; primrose; ragweed*

692.7 Contact dermatitis and other eczema due to solar radiation

This subclassification reports photodamage to skin. Photodamage is a serious medical condition that has been identified with an increased risk of premalignant skin lesions, such as actinic keratosis, and skin malignancies such as basal cell carcinoma and melanoma.

692.70	Unspecified dermatitis due to sun — *unknown*
692.71	Contact dermatitis and other eczema due to sunburn — *first, second, or third degree*

Interestingly, no differentiation is made between first, second, and third degree sunburn in ICD-9, but this differentiation is made in ICD-10-CM.

Do not use a sunburn code to report a burn received in a tanning booth. Instead, report that burn with 692.82.

692.72	Acute dermatitis due to solar radiation — *Berlogue dermatitis, photoallergic response, phototoxic response, polymorphus light eruption*

Use this subclassification to report acute contact photosensitive reaction due to solar radiation. Contact photosensitive reaction is categorized as photoallergic or phototoxic. Sunburn is excluded from this code, see 692.71.

Photoallergic contact dermatitis is an allergic dermatitis caused by a photosensitizing substance plus sunlight in a sensitized person. The clinical presentation is similar to allergic contact dermatitis except that sunlight must be present to induce the reaction. If the photosensitizer acts internally, it is photodrug dermatitis; if it acts externally, it is a photocontact dermatitis. Some examples of oral photodrug dermatitis photosensitizes are diuretics such as Diuril, hypoglycemics such as Orinase, and phenothiazine such as Thorazine. Examples of topical photocontact dermatitis photosensitizes are antimicrobials such as bithionol and antihistamines such as Benadryl. Report an E code secondarily to identify drug if the dermatitis is drug induced.

Phototoxic contact dermatitis is a nonimmunologic reaction that occurs two hours to six hours after the skin has been exposed to a photosensitizing agent and solar radiation. The clinical presentation is similar to sunburn. Some examples of phototoxic dermatitis are phototoxic tar dermatitis (dermatitis associated with coal tar, creosote, or pitch), phytophotodermatitis, dermatitis bullosa striata pratensis (grass or meadow dermatitis), and berloque (perfume) dermatitis.

692.73   Actinic reticuloid and actinic granuloma — *skin growths the result of persistent inflammation of the skin as a reaction to solar rays*

Use this subclassification to report severe and chronic form of photosensitivity (actinic reticuloid) and skin lesion (actinic granuloma). Usually affecting males between the ages of 45 years and 70 years of age, actinic reticuloid requires complete avoidance of sunlight and other forms of ultraviolet radiation since it is resistant to treatment with sunscreens and steroids.

Actinic granuloma begins as papules and nodules. These lesions grow very slowly and eventually become annular. Persistent for years, actinic granuloma is believed to be due to defective repair of connective tissue damaged by sun and heat.

692.74   Other chronic dermatitis due to solar radiation — *including solar elastosis, chronic solar skin damage*

Use this subclassification to report other specified and unspecified forms of chronic dermatitis due to solar radiation. Included are conditions such as actinic cheilitis, actinic solar elastosis, Favre-Racouchot syndrome, "sailor's skin" and "farmer's skin."

692.75   Disseminated superficial actinic porokeratosis (DSAP)
692.79   Other dermatitis due to solar radiation — *including hydroa aestivale; photodermatitis, photosensitiveness*
692.81   Dermatitis due to cosmetics
692.82   Dermatitis due to other radiation — *infrared lights, ultraviolet lights, tanning beds, x-rays*

Use this subclassification to report dermatitis due to forms of radiation other than solar radiation, such as x-rays, radiation from tanning beds, infrared rays, ionizing radiation, ultraviolet light (excluding sunlight), and gamma rays.

692.83   Dermatitis due to metals — *including jewelry*

Use this subclassification to report dermatitis due to exposure to or contact with metals or metallic salts. Nickel, the chromates, and mercury are the most common causes of metal dermatitis in the United States. Other metals associated with dermatitis are rhodium, platinum, cobalt, tungsten, cadmium, beryllium, vanadium, zinc, and tungsten. Metals and metal salts can occur in soap and detergents, cosmetics, hair dyes, and tattoos.

692.89   Contact dermatitis and other eczema due to other specified agent — *not elsewhere specified, including dermatitis due to weather, dyes, furs, preservatives, blister beetle dermatitis, enema rash, caterpillar dermatitis*

692.9   Contact dermatitis and other eczema, due to unspecified cause

693 DERMATITIS DUE TO SUBSTANCES TAKEN INTERNALLY

Use this rubric to report dermatitis due to the ingestion of drugs, chemicals, foodstuffs, or other substances. The condition usually manifests with an abrupt onset of diffuse, symmetric erythematous eruptions. The cause may be an allergic reaction, adverse effect, drug interaction, idiosyncratic reaction, or some other cause.

Excluded from this rubric is adverse effect NOS of drugs and medicines (995.2); allergy NOS (995.3); contact dermatitis (rubric 692); and urticarial reactions (708.0-708.9, 995.1).

693.0   Dermatitis due to drugs and medicines taken internally — *dermatitis medicamentosa not otherwise specified*

The definition of dermatitis due to drugs and medicines taken internally is systemic erythematous inflammation of skin, also known as dermatitis medicamentosa or drug eruption. The condition may mimic inflammatory skin conditions such as eczema, toxic erythema, and erythroderma. Onset may be sudden (e.g., urticaria or angioedema after penicillin) or delayed.

Signs and symptoms of dermatitis due to drugs and medicines taken internally include mild rash to toxic epidermal microlysis, malaise, fever, arthralgia, and headache. Therapies include cessation of offending drug; lubricant for dry, itching, maculopapular eruption; and corticosteroid for existing rash.

ICD-9-CM coding rules regarding poisonings and adverse effects must be followed using the table of drugs and chemicals.

693.1   Dermatitis due to food taken internally — *infested food*

693.8   Dermatitis due to other specified substances taken internally — *not specified elsewhere*

693.9   Dermatitis due to unspecified substance taken internally — *unknown*

694 BULLOUS DERMATOSES

Use this rubric to report cutaneous lesions of bullous dermatoses. The primary lesion in many diseases, bullae are large blisters that form at some level of the skin.

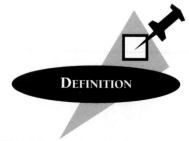

DEFINITION

Nikolsky's sign: sloughing of the outer layer of epidermis from the basal layer upon minor trauma, as in the rubbing of skin, and seen in pemphigus and other blistering skin disease.

694.0	Dermatitis herpetiformis — *including dermatosis herpetiformis; Duhring's disease, Brocq-Duhring disease; hydroa herpetiformis*
694.1	Subcorneal pustular dermatosis — *including Sneddon-Wilkinson disease*
694.2	Juvenile dermatitis herpetiformis — *juvenile pemphigoid*
694.3	Impetigo herpetiformis — *rare dermatosis of third trimester with multiply symptoms*
694.4	Pemphigus — *including erythematosus, foliaceus, vegetans, vulgaris; Senear-Usher syndrome*
694.5	Pemphigoid — *including bullous, herpes circinatus bullosus, senile dermatitis herpetiformis*

The definition of pemphigoid is chronic, benign eruption, including benign pemphigus and bullous pemphigoid. Pemphigoid is seen chiefly in the elderly and in individuals with autoimmune disease. Signs and symptoms of pemphigoid include tense bullae on normal or reddened skin. Immunofluorescence studies confirm diagnosis. Therapies include prednisone.

694.60	Benign mucous membrane pemphigoid without mention of ocular involvement — *cicatricial pemphigoid, mucosynechial atrophic bullous dermatitis*
694.61	Benign mucous membrane pemphigoid with ocular involvement — - *cicatricial pemphigoid, mucosynechial atrophic bullous dermatitis*
694.8	Other specified bullous dermatosis — *not specified elsewhere*
694.9	Unspecified bullous dermatosis — *unknown*

695 ERYTHEMATOUS CONDITIONS

Use this subclassification to report red skin lesions, which can be caused by a number of conditions.

695.0	Toxic erythema — *erythema venenatum*

Use this rubric to report erythematous eruption of a wide anatomic area caused by bacterial or other toxins or administration of medications in toxic dosages.

695.1	Erythema multiforme — *including toxic epidermal necrolysis, erythema iris; herpes iris; syndromes: Lyell's; Stevens-Johnson, Baader', Flessinger-Rendu, Klauder's*
695.2	Erythema nodosum — *painful inflammation of tissue of lower extremities usually caused by a hypersensitivity reaction, and sometimes seen as a manifestation of disease, as in sarcoidosis*
695.3	Rosacea — *erythematosa acne; rhinophyma; perioral dermatitis; rosacea acne*
695.4	Lupus erythematosus — *including discoid lupus erythematosus, not disseminated*

Use this subclassification to report lupus erythematosus, a chronic disease that causes inflammation of the connective tissue of the skin only. Occurring worldwide, this disease affects nine times as many women as men, usually those of childbearing age, and can lead to scarring and permanent disfigurement.

▶5th Needs fifth-digit   **OK** Valid three-digit code

Signs and symptoms of lupus erythematosus include erythematous, round scaling papules usually on malar prominences, bridge of nose, scalp, and external auditory canals. Thickened areas of skin may later scar.

Lab work reveals leukopenia, positive LE cells test in only 10 percent of patients. Skin biopsy shows immunoglobulins or complement components. Therapies include reduced exposure to sunlight, topical corticosteroid for lesions, and antimalarials (Plaquenil).

This subcategory includes discoid lupus erythematosus but excludes systemic lupus erythematosus, and excludes lupus vulgaris NOS (017.0) and systemic lupus erythematosus (710.0).

695.81   Ritter's disease — *generalized staph syndrome causing exfoliation and raw skin in infants*

695.89   Other specified erythematous condition — *including erythema intertrigo; pityriasis rubra; dermatitis epidemica; syndromes: Savill's; Sweet's, Wilson-Brocq, Bury's, Leiner's*

695.9   Unspecified erythematous condition — *unknown*

696 PSORIASIS AND SIMILAR DISORDERS

Use this subclassification to report a common skin disease characterized by patches of inflamed, red skin, covered by silvery scales and sometimes accompanied by painful swelling and stiffness of the joints (arthritis). With psoriasis, new cells are produced 10 times faster than normal, but the rate at which old cells are shed is unchanged. Consequently, the stratum corneum becomes thickened with flaky, immature skin cells. Occurring predominantly over the elbows, knees, scalp, and trunk, psoriasis tends to run in families, affects men and women equally and usually appears between the ages of 10 years and 30 years.

Therapies include moderate exposure to sunlight or phototherapy and use of emollient for mild cases; ointment containing coal tar or anthralin for moderate cases; and topical corticosteroids and oral methotrexate for severe cases.

696.0   Psoriatic arthropathy — *psoriasis associated with joint disease*

696.1   Other psoriasis and similar disorders — *including acrodermatitis continua, dermatitis repens, Willan-Plumbe syndrome*

696.2   Parapsoriasis — *including parakeratosis variegata; parapsoriasis lichenoides chronica; pityriasis lichenoides et varioliformis; Brocq's parapsoriasis; Mucah-Haberman syndrome; Wise's disease*

696.3   Pityriasis rosea — *pityriasis circinata (et maculata)*

696.4   Pityriasis rubra pilaris — *including Devergie's disease, lichen ruber acuminatus*

696.5   Other and unspecified pityriasis — *not otherwise specified*

696.8   Other psoriasis and similar disorders — *not otherwise specified*

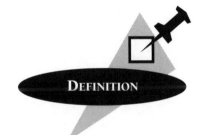

DEFINITION

Koebner's phenomenon: appearance of skin disease lesions at the site of trauma, on scars, or at points rubbed by clothing, in diseases like psoriasis, lichen planus, and certain dermatoses; also called the isomorphic effect.

697 LICHEN

Excluded from this rubric are obtusus corneus (698.3); congenital pilaris (757.39); ruber acuminatus (696.4); sclerosus of atrophicus (701.9); scrofulosus (017.0); simplex chronicus (698.3); congenital spinulosus (757.39); and urticatus (698.2).

697.0   Lichen planus — *planopilaris, ruber planus*

Use this subclassification to report inflammatory cutaneous and mucous membrane condition characterized by pruritic, violaceous, and flattop papules with fine white streaks and symmetric distribution. Signs and symptoms of lichen planus include chronic papules, acute lesions of skin and mucous membranes, and severe itching. Histopathology of skin lesion confirms diagnosis. Therapies include topical, intralesional, systemic steroids; antihistamines; psoralens plus long-wave ultraviolet light; and oral griseofulvin.

697.1   Lichen nitidus — *Pinkus' disease*

697.8   Other lichen, not elsewhere classified — *including ruber moniliforme, striata*

697.9   Unspecified lichen — *unknown*

698 PRURITUS AND RELATED CONDITIONS

Use this rubric to report conditions characterized by intense itching and/or burning sensation of the skin. Most cases of generalized pruritus are due to dry skin but may be due to a variety of dermatologic or systemic conditions. Therapies include elimination of soaps or detergents, cessation of all but necessary medications, application of moisturizers while skin is wet, tranquilizers in severe cases, and topical or systemic corticosteroids as well as antihistamines and antiserotonin drugs.

Pruritus (itching) may be related to a wide variety of conditions classifiable elsewhere, such as scabies, atopic dermatitis, sunburn, uremia, and contact dermatitis. In most cases, the pruritus is an integral part of the disease and is not reported separately. Excluded from this rubric is pruritus that is psychogenic in nature (306.3).

698.0   Pruritus ani — *intense anal itch*

698.1   Pruritus of genital organs — *intense genital itch*

698.2   Prurigo — *including lichen urticatus; Hebra's prurigo; urticaria papulosa; mitis prurigo; prurigo simplex*

698.3   Lichenification and lichen simplex chronicus — *including neurodermatitis; prurigo nodularis; Brocq's lichen simplex chronicus; Hyde's or Vidal's disease*

698.4   Dermatitis factitia (artefacta) — *including dermatitis ficta, neurotic excoriation*

698.8   Other specified pruritic conditions — *not classified elsewhere, including hiemalis, senilis, winter itch*

698.9   Unspecified pruritic disorder — *unknown type*

700-709 Other Diseases of Skin and Subcutaneous Tissue

Excluded from this range of codes are conditions confined to eyelids (373.0-374.9) and congenital conditions of the hair, skin, and nails (759.0-759.9).

700 CORNS AND CALLOSITIES OK

Calluses and corns are knobs of hyperkeratotic tissue caused by pressure or friction, most commonly seen in the bony prominences of the feet or hands. Benign conditions, they can cause pain that requires the treatment of a podiatrist or physician.

701 OTHER HYPERTROPHIC AND ATROPHIC CONDITIONS OF SKIN

Excluded form this rubric are dermatomyositis (710.0); hereditary edema of legs (757.0); and scleroderma (generalized) (710.3).

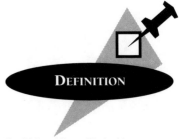

DEFINITION

701.0   Circumscribed scleroderma — *including Addison's keloid, morphea, localized dermatosclerosis, von Zambusch's disease, lichen sclerosus et atrophicus*

701.1   Acquired keratoderma — *including elastosis perforans serpiginosa; acquired ichthyosis, acquired keratoderma palmaris et plantaris; keratosis blennorrhagica*

701.2   Acquired acanthosis nigricans — *keratosis nigricans*

701.3   Striae atrophicae — *including atrophic skin spots; striae disease; senile degenerative atrophy; atrophy blanche of Milian*

701.4.   Keloid scar — *hypertrophic scar, cheloid*

Use this subclassification to report tumors consisting of actively growing hypertrophic cutaneous scar tissue. They occur as a result of trauma or irritation such as burns, incisions, vaccinations, insect bites, and other stimuli. Ulcerated keloids are prone to carcinomatous transformation, but the majority behaves as benign neoplasms. Dark-skinned races are particularly susceptible to keloid formation. Hypertrophic scars are similar to keloids except that they lack the characteristic tumor formation of keloids and do not grow beyond the margins of the original injury.

Signs and symptoms of keloid scar include history of surgery or skin trauma, overreactive visible scar formation, itching, and burning. Skin biopsy may be performed to determine histopathology. Therapies include surgical or laser excision, z-plasty when scar crosses flexion surface, cryotherapy (freezing with liquid nitrogen), radiation therapy, and injection of corticosteroid such as Kenalog-10.

In many cases, keloids and hypertrophic scars are residuals of previous trauma or surgery. If the etiology of the keloid or hypertrophic scar is known and described as a late effect, assign a secondary code describing the late effect. For example, if the diagnosis were residual keloid due a previously treated burn of the hand, codes 701.4 and 906.6 would be assigned.

701.5   Other abnormal granulation tissue — *excessive granulation*

701.8   Other specified hypertrophic and atrophic condition of skin — *including atrophia cutis senilis; cutis laxa senilis; acantholysis; pachydermatitis; Pick-Herxheimer or Gougerot-Carteaud syndrome; elastosis senilis; folliculitis ulerythematosa reticulata; confluent and reticulate papillomatosis*

701.9   Unspecified hypertrophic and atrophic condition of skin — *including skin tag, atrophoderma, pendulous abdomen, redundant skin, or unknown*

702 OTHER DERMATOSES

Excluded from this rubric is carcinoma in situ (232.0-232.9).

702.0   Actinic keratosis — *sharply outlined warty growth usually caused by sun damage to skin*

Use this subclassification to report precancerous warty lesions due to the cumulative effect of overexposure to sunlight. These lesions also are known as solar or senile keratosis, keratoderma, keratoma, acanthosis

Bulla: bleb or blister filled with serous or seropurulent fluid.

Macule: flat, discolored spot on the skin, as seen in a flat mole, freckle, or some rashes.

Papule: solid, superficial, elevated lesion of the skin.

Plaque: patch or flat area on the skin, similar to macule.

Pompholyx: itchy vesicle on the palms, fingers, and soles; a chronic condition.

Nodule: solid skin lesion that may be elevated or palpable.

Annularity: formation of rash in a ring.

Crusting: scab of serum, blood or pus; sign of inflammation or infection.

Linearity: formation of rash in a line.

Pustule: superficial, elevated, pus-filled lesion.

Excoriation: abrasion of the skin caused by scratching or rubbing; typically a sign of itching.

Wheal: hive; transient, localized and itchy edema.

verrucosa, verruca senilis, and plana senilis. Therapies include cryotherapy (freezing with liquid nitrogen) and 5-Fluorouracil.

702.1 Seborrheic keratosis
Use this subclassification to report superficial noninvasive tumor (usually multiple) originating in the epidermis. Characterized by numerous yellow or brown, sharply marginated, oval, and raised lesions, these tumors also are known as seborrheic warts or verrucae. They occur commonly in middle-aged or older patients. Therapies include shaving of the excision.

702.11	Inflamed seborrheic keratosis — *warty growth of basaloid sells not otherwise specified*
702.19	Other seborrheic keratosis
702.8	Other specified dermatoses — *including acanthotic nevus, cutaneous horn, sebaceous nevus, or not otherwise specified*

703 DISEASES OF NAIL
Excluded from this rubric are congenital anomalies of the nail (757.5) and onychia and paronychia (681.02, 681.11).

703.0   Ingrowing nail — *unguis incarnatus; with infection*

The definition of ingrowing nail is a painful condition, usually of the big toe, in which one or both edges of the nail press into the adjacent skin, leading to infection and inflammation. Common causes include poor personal hygiene, tight-fitting shoes, and incorrect nail cutting. Therapies include soaking, antibiotics to control infection, and removal of nail edge. Excluded from this subclassification is nail infection, reported with 681.9.

703.8   Other specified disease of nail — *including dystrophia unguium, hypertrophy, leukonychia, onychauxis, onycholysis, acquired polyunguia; subungual hemorrhage; horn of nail; Beau's lines; acquired anonychia; koilonychia, acquired pachyonychia, or not otherwise specified*

703.9   Unspecified disease of nail — *unknown*

704 DISEASES OF HAIR AND HAIR FOLLICLES
Excluded form this rubric are congenital anomalies (757.4).

704.00	Unspecified alopecia — *loss of hair, type unknown*
704.01	Alopecia areata — *patchy loss of hair; usually temporary*
704.02	Telogen effluvium — *temporary excessive hair loss due to stressor like childbirth, surgery, weight loss*
704.09	Other alopecia — *including folliculitis decalvans; oligotrichia, Quinquaud's disease, tinea decalvans, pseudopelade*
704.1	Hirsutism — *excessive hair growth; acquired lanuginosa, polytrichia*
704.2	Abnormalities of the hair — *atrophic hair, clastothrix, fragilitas crinium, trichorrhexis nodosa*
704.3	Variations in hair color — *canities, premature gray, heterochromia, acquired poliosis circumscripta*
704.8	Other specified disease of hair and hair follicles — *including ingrown hair, folliculitis, perifolliculitis, sycosis, Bockhart's impetigo, mentagra*
704.9	Unspecified disease of hair and hair follicles — *unknown*

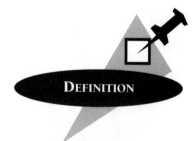

DEFINITION

Male-pattern baldness: common hair loss begins in lateral frontal area of scalp (widow's peak), and hairline retreats to subsequent baldness.

Female-pattern baldness: Thinning of the hair in the frontal, parietal, and crown regions; complete baldness is rare.

✔5th   Needs fifth-digit   **OK**   Valid three-digit code

705 DISORDERS OF SWEAT GLANDS

705.0   Anhidrosis — *diminished sweating; hypohidrosis, oligohidrosis*

705.1   Prickly heat — *heat rash, sudamina, miliaria rubra, sweat retention syndrome*

705.81 Dyshidrosis — *usually affecting hands and feet; cheiropompholyx, pompholyx*

705.82 Fox-Fordyce disease — *rare eruption of follicular papules of axillae, nipples, pubic region*

705.83 Hidradenitis — *inflammation of sweat gland; Pollitzer's disease, hidradenitis suppurativa*

Use this subclassification to report inflammation of the apocrine sweat glands occurring in the axillae, anogenital regions, nipples, and under the female breast. The condition may produce chronic abscesses or sinus tract formation. In most cases, hidradenitis is caused by the obstruction of the apocrine sweat pores due to the application of underarm deodorants, irritant depilatories, or other topical ointments or creams. Signs and symptoms of hidradenitis include large painful abscesses resulting from double comedones and extensive deep dermal inflammation, weight loss, fever, malaise, local pain, and tenderness. Gram stain and culture of lesion identify infective organism. Therapies include antimicrobials (penicillin), surgical excision, and plastic repair of affected area in chronic conditions.

Sequence an additional code secondarily to identify the infective organism, typically streptococcus or staphylococcus.

705.89 Other specified disorder of sweat glands — *not otherwise specified, including bromhidrosis, chromhidrosis, abscess, cyst, granulosis rubra nasi, urhidrosis, osmidrosis, hematidrosis*

705.9   Unspecified disorder of sweat glands — *unknown*

706 DISEASES OF SEBACEOUS GLANDS

706.0   Acne varioliformis — *frontalis, necrotica*

706.1   Other acne — *conglobata, cystic, pustular, vulgaris, comedo, blackhead*

706.2   Sebaceous cyst — *atheroma, keratin cyst, infected steatoma, wen*

Use this subclassification to report slowly developing benign cystic tumor of the skin containing follicular, keratinous, and sebaceous material. Frequently found on the scalp, ears, face, back or scrotum, and sebaceous cysts may grow very large and become infected by bacteria. Exam reveals firm, globular, movable, and nontender tumor. Therapies include for small lesions (milium), incision and expression of contents; for larger lesions, surgical excision of cyst walls.

706.3   Seborrhea — *excessive production of sebum*

706.8   Other specified disease of sebaceous glands — *including asteatosis cutis, xerosis cutis*

706.9   Unspecified disease of sebaceous glands — *unknown*

707 CHRONIC ULCER OF SKIN

Use this rubric to report chronic defect of the skin, deeper than erosion or excoriation, extending at least into the dermal layer. Chronic ulcers usually are due to chronic inflammation, ischemia, or both.

707.0   Decubitus ulcer — *bed sore, plaster ulcer, pressure ulcer; any site*

Use this subclassification to report a condition, also known as a bedsore or pressure sore that affects superficial tissues and may also deepen to affect muscle and bone. Usually occurring over a bony prominence at the sacrum, hip, heel, shoulder, or elbow, decubitus ulcers develop in patients who are bedridden, unconscious or immobile, for example, stroke or spinal cord injury victims. Intrinsic loss of pain and pressure sensations, disuse atrophy, malnutrition, anemia and infection play roles in the formation of decubitus ulcers. Herpes simplex virus is suspected in immunocompromised patients. In early stages, the condition is reversible, but left untended, a decubitus ulcer can become extensively infected, necrotic, and, ultimately, irreversible.

Signs and symptoms of decubitus ulcer include: in first stage, deep pink, red, or mottled skin that is warm, firm, or stretched tightly across area; in second stage, blistering, cracking, or abrasion of skin; in third stage, crater-like sore with involvement of underlying structures, exposure of fat; in fourth stage, necrosis extended through skin and fat to muscle; in fifth stage, advanced fat and muscle necrosis; and in sixth stage, bone destruction and osteomyelitis.

Therapies include high protein, well-balanced diet, application of absorbable gelatin sponges (Gelfoam), change in patient's position every two hours, and the use of egg-crate mattresses and protective padding (sheepskin). Other therapies include stimulation of affected area by gentle massage to facilitate circulation (thus healing), debridement (excisional, chemical, and whirlpool), or deeper surgery with closure or skin grafting for advanced stages.

707.1 Ulcer of lower limbs, except decubitus

Code first any underlying condition, as in atherosclerosis with ulceration (440.23) and diabetes (250.80-250.83). Codes in this subclassification are chosen according to ulcer site. In some cases, multiple codes may be required.

707.10	Ulcer of lower limb, unspecified — *unknown site, not calf*
707.11	Ulcer of thigh — *between hip and knee*
707.12	Ulcer of calf
707.13	Ulcer of ankle
707.14	Ulcer of heel and midfoot — *plantar surface of midfoot*
707.15	Ulcer of other part of foot — *including toes*
707.19	Ulcer of other part of lower limb — *not otherwise specified*
707.8	Chronic ulcer of other specified site — *including groin, hand, neck, perineum, sacrum, scalp, submental*
707.9	Chronic ulcer of unspecified site — *unknown skin site*

✔5th   Needs fifth-digit   **OK**   Valid three-digit code

708 URTICARIA

Use this rubric to report eruption of itching edema of the skin (hives). Often due to hypersensitivity to a drug, food, or insect stings or bites, urticaria also may be due to such stimuli as physical exercise, heat, cold, sunlight, anxiety and tension. Most episodes are acute and self-limiting over a period of one week to two weeks.

Signs and symptoms of urticaria include pruritus, wheals that may remain small or may enlarge, rings of erythema, and edema. Therapies include cessation of nonessential medication or other causative factors, oral antihistamine (Benadryl, Atarax, and Periactin), and prednisone in more severe cases (associated with angioedema).

Excluded from this rubric are angioneurotic edema (995.1); Quincke's edema (995.1); hereditary angioedema (277.6); giant urticaria (995.1); papulosa urticaria (698.2); and urticaria pigmentosa (757.33).

708.0	Allergic urticaria — *allergic hives*
708.1	Idiopathic urticaria — *hives of unknown cause*
708.2	Urticaria due to cold and heat — *hives due to heat or cold*
708.3	Dermatographic urticaria — *hives raised as a result of scratching*
708.4	Vibratory urticaria — *hives as a response to vibration*
708.5	Cholinergic urticaria — *non-allergic form of hives caused by heat or excitement*
708.8	Other specified urticaria — *including nettle rash, recurrent periodic rash, chronic hives*
708.9	Unspecified urticaria — *hives of unknown cause*

709 OTHER DISORDERS OF SKIN AND SUBCUTANEOUS TISSUE

709.00	Dyschromia, unspecified — *variation of skin pigmentation of unknown cause*
709.01	Vitiligo — *nonpigmented patches as a persistent, progressive disorder*
709.09	Other dyschromia — *including Civatte's poikiloderma, classic piebaldism, café au lait spots, xanthosis, Sutton's or Schamberg's disease, liver spots*
709.1	Vascular disorder of skin — *angioma serpiginosum, purpura annularis telangiectodes, Gougerot-Blum syndrome, Majocchi's disease*
709.2	Scar condition and fibrosis of skin — *adherent scar, cicatrix, disfigurement*
709.3	Degenerative skin disorder — *calcinosis circumscripta or cutis, colloid milium, Miescher-Leder syndrome, Wagner's disease, skin deposits*
709.4	Foreign body granuloma of skin and subcutaneous tissue
709.8	Other specified disorder of skin — *including epithelial hyperplasia, menstrual dermatosis, vesicular eruption, dermatosis papulosa nigra, macules, papules, sclerosing lipogranuloma*
709.9	Unspecified disorder of skin and subcutaneous tissue — *unknown*

710-739

Diseases of the Musculoskeletal System and Connective Tissue

This chapter classifies diseases and disorders of the bones, muscles, cartilage, fascia, ligaments, synovia, tendons, and bursa.

Connective tissue disorders classified to chapter 13 are those primarily affecting the musculoskeletal system. Injuries and certain congenital disorders of the musculoskeletal system are classified elsewhere.

Many codes for the manifestation of musculoskeletal diseases due to specified infections and other diseases and disorders classified elsewhere are included in this chapter. Also included are many codes describing the residuals of previous diseases, disorders, and injuries classified as late effects. These codes often can be identified by the term "acquired" in the description.

710-719 Arthropathies and Related Disorders

Excluded from this section are disorders of the spine (720.0-724.9).

710 DIFFUSE DISEASES OF CONNECTIVE TISSUE

This rubric reports a group of diseases in which the primary lesion appears to be damage to collagen, a protein that is the major component of connective tissue. Collagen (rheumatoid) diseases, attributed largely to disorders of the immune complex mechanisms, include myositis, sclerosis, dermal atrophy, arthritis, vasculitis, nephritis, carditis, subcutaneous nodules, polyserositis, and lupus erythematosus. Many of these conditions, such as polyarteritis nodosa (a connective tissue disease that is a form of vasculitis), are classified to other chapters.

Category 710 includes diffuse diseases of connective tissues; most are collagen diseases whose effects are not mainly confined to a single body system. For proper code assignment, follow the ICD-9-CM index carefully and read the includes and excludes notes pertaining to this category. Also excluded are those diffuse diseases affecting mainly the cardiovascular system, as in polyarteritis and other allied conditions (446.0-446.7).

Use an additional code to identify the manifestation of diffuse disease of the connective tissue, as in lung involvement (517.8) or myopathy (359.6).

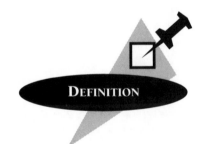

DEFINITION

Diffuse: not limited or localized; to pass through a tissue and spread.

Syndrome: set of symptoms that occur together.

Systemic: affecting the body as a whole.

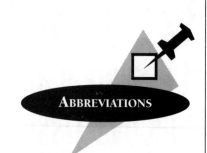

ABBREVIATIONS

CREST (syndrome): also CRST, Calcinosis, Raynaud's phenomenon, Esophageal disorder, Sclerodactyly, Telangiectasia, an induration and thickening of the skin with circulatory and organ changes in the face and hands

PSS: progressive systemic sclerosis, thickening of the skin, disseminated fibrosis and vascular irregularities in the internal organs and joints

SLE: systemic lupus erythematosus

710.0 Systemic lupus erythematosus — (Use additional code to identify manifestation, as: 359.6, 424.91, 517.8, 581.81, 582.81, 583.81) — *disseminated, including Libman-Sacks disease, L.E. cell phenomenon*

Use this code to report an inflammatory autoimmune disorder that may affect multiple organ systems. The disease is usually chronic, and the clinical course is mild to fulminating. Clinical exacerbations and remissions of manifestations involving the skin, serosal surfaces, central nervous system, kidneys, and blood cells are characteristic. Arthralgia, symmetrical arthritis, and inflammatory muscle involvement are common musculoskeletal features of acute systemic lupus erythematosus. The disease is most prevalent in women, particularly black women, of childbearing age.

No single etiology for the disease has been discovered, but initiation and expression of the disease has been associated with hormonal influences, genetic factors, loss of tolerance to autoantigens, and certain viruses and drugs. The hands and wrist are two sites commonly affected by lupus arthritis.

Signs and symptoms of systemic lupus erythematosus include fever, anorexia, malaise, weight loss, and skin lesions identical to chronic discoid lupus erythematosus, redness and edema affecting nose and cheeks revealing classic butterfly rash, photosensitivity and other ocular manifestations, joint symptoms with or without acute synovitis. Lab work reveals antinuclear antibodies in more than 95 percent of cases and may show mild normochromic, normocytic anemia, or occasionally autoimmune hemolytic anemia. Lab work also may reveal leukopenia, lymphopenia, and thrombocytopenia. Therapies include limited, symptomatic intervention, such as topical sunscreens for photosensitivity, for mild, benign forms of the disease, in addition to nonsteroidal antiinflammatory medications to control fever, joint complaints, serositis; antimalarial drugs (chloroquine, hydroxychloroquine) and topical corticosteroids for skin manifestations. Systemic corticosteroids are prescribed for more severe manifestations involving the heart and kidneys. Immunosuppressive agents (such as cyclophosphamide, chlorambucil, and azathioprine) may be prescribed in cases resistant to corticosteroids.

Associated conditions include endocarditis, renal failure due to proliferative glomerulonephritis, nephritis or nephritis syndrome, Raynaud's phenomenon, anemia, pleurisy and pleural effusion, bronchopneumonia, restrictive lung diseases, vasculitis (with resulting ileus and peritonitis), and Hashimoto's thyroiditis.

Use an additional code to identify any manifestations, as in endocarditis (424.91) or nephritis (583.81). Excluded from this code is lupus erythematosus (discoid) not otherwise specified (695.4).

710.1 Systemic sclerosis — (Use additional code to identify manifestation, as: 359.6, 517.8) — *acrosclerosis, including CRST or Weissenbach-Thibierge syndrome, scleroderma, progressive systemic sclerosis*

↙5th Needs fifth-digit   **OK** Valid three-digit code

Use this code to report widespread small vessel obliteration and fibrotic thickening of the skin and multiple organs, including the alimentary tract, kidneys, lungs, muscles, joints, nerves and heart. When localized to the face and extremities (with Raynaud's phenomena), it is called acrosclerosis. A distinct form of systemic sclerosis is CREST syndrome, which stands for subcutaneous Calcinosis, Raynaud's phenomenon, Esophageal motility dysfunction, Sclerodactyly, and Telangiectasia.

Associated conditions include Raynaud's phenomena, subcutaneous calcinosis (nodular deposition of calcium salts in the subcutaneous tissues or muscles), ulcers and infection of the finger tips, telangiectasia, malabsorption syndrome, and carpal tunnel syndrome.

Excluded from this code is circumscribed scleroderma (701.0).

710.2   Sicca syndrome — (Use additional code to identify manifestation, as: 359.6, 517.8) — *keratoconjunctivitis sicca, including Sjögren's disease*

Use this code to report Sjögren's syndrome resulting from lymphocytic infiltration of lacrimal and salivary glands. An idiopathic, autoimmune disorder, Sjögren's syndrome is characterized by xerostomia (dry mouth), keratoconjunctivitis sicca (dry eyes), and parotid gland enlargement. Primary Sjögren's syndrome presents a wide variety of clinical manifestations due to a wider involvement of the exocrine glands. The organs involved may include the skin, lung, GI tract, kidney, muscles, nerves, spleen, and thyroid. Secondary Sjögren's syndrome is limited to symptoms of the lacrimal and salivary glands.

Lab work may reveal higher frequency of human lymphocytic antigen HLA-DR3 in primary Sjögren's syndrome and of HLA-DR4 in secondary Sjögren's syndrome.

Associated conditions include rheumatoid arthritis and other collagen diseases.

710.3   Dermatomyositis — (Use additional code to identify manifestation, as: 359.6, 517.8) — *poikilodermatomyositis, polymyositis with skin involvement, including Petges-Cléjat or Unverricht-Wagner syndromes*

Use this code to report nonsuppurative inflammation of the skin, subcutaneous tissues, and muscles with necrosis of muscle fibers. The disease complex is differentiated from polymyositis by the presence of a characteristic rash of edema and erythema and a heliotrope discoloration particularly around the eyes.

Physical exam reveals prominent proximal muscle weakness. Lab work shows elevated muscle enzymes. Electromyograph (EMG) reveals myopathic patterns and muscle biopsy reveals inflammatory infiltrates.

Associated conditions include malignancy of visceral organs in adults.

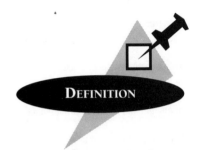

DEFINITION

Mikulicz's syndrome: complex of lacrimal and salivary gland swelling, which may include enlargement associated with other syndromes, such as Sjögren's.

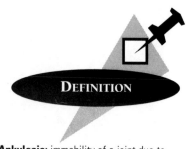

DEFINITION

Ankylosis: immobility of a joint due to disease, injury, or surgical process.

Arthropathy: any joint disease.

Arthritis: rheumatism in which inflammation is confined to the joints.

Malacia: softening of a tissue.

Myalgia: pain in a muscle or muscles.

Myositis: inflammation of a voluntary muscle.

Urethritis: inflammation of the urethra.

Dysenteric: disorder marked by inflammation of the intestines.

Helminthiasis: infection with worms.

Mycoses: disease caused by fungus.

Pyogenic: producing puss.

710.4   Polymyositis — (Use additional code to identify manifestation, as: 359.6, 517.8) — *chronic, progressive, inflammatory symmetrical weakness of limb girdles, with pain*

Use this code to report a condition identical to dermatomyositis without the characteristic skin lesions.

710.5   Eosinophilia myalgia syndrome — (Use additional code to identify manifestation, as: 359.6, 517.8) — *toxic oil syndrome*

Use this code to report a multisystem inflammatory and fibrosing illness associated with ingestion of L-tryptophan, an oral nutritional substance of amino acids. It includes toxic oil syndrome and eosinophilic fasciitis.

Signs and symptoms of eosinophilia myalgia syndrome includes history of over-the-counter use of nutritional supplements containing L-tryptophan, muscle and joint pain, weakness, swelling of arms and legs, fever, and rash. Blood work shows increased circulating eosinophils.

Associated conditions include pneumonia, cardiac and arrhythmia, pulmonary hypertension (cor pulmonale), and polyneuropathy.

710.8   Other specified diffuse disease of connective tissue — (Use additional code to identify manifestation, as: 359.6, 517.8) — *not elsewhere classified*

This subcategory includes carpal tunnel osteolysis syndrome.

710.9   Unspecified diffuse connective tissue disease — (Use additional code to identify manifestation, as: 359.6, 517.8) — *unknown collagen disease*

711 ARTHROPATHY ASSOCIATED WITH INFECTIONS

This rubric includes infections of the articular joints of bones, and must be distinguished from infections of the bones classifiable to category 730.

Direct microbial contamination may cause a primary infection of the articular joints. The routes of infection include open fractures, surgical procedures, diagnostic needle aspirations, and therapeutic drug injections.

Most of the arthropathies classified here are due to indirect (secondary) infections, and require a second code to identify the infectious organism or the underlying disease. Direct microbial infections resulting from surgical, diagnostic and therapeutic procedures are classified to categories 996-999.

Excluded from this rubric is rheumatic fever (390).

711.0 ⌐5th   Pyogenic arthritis — *due to infectious organism, including staph, strep, H. influenzae, E. coli, pneumococcus*

Use this subclassification to report acute, destructive bacterial process in a joint following infection, usually occurring as acute monoarticular (single joint) arthritis. The knee and large joints are most often involved.

Signs and symptoms of pyogenic arthritis include fever, joint pain, decreased range of motion, and swelling and redness over affected joint. Gross examination of aspirated synovial (joint) fluid confirms presence of

⌐5th   Needs fifth-digit   **OK**   Valid three-digit code

pus (pyarthrosis); gram stain and culture may detect microorganisms and crystals; examination with polarizing microscope reveals crystals. Therapies include removal of inflammatory material by aspiration or incision and drainage, antibiotic therapy that may be prolonged, and resting the joint in a stable position.

Associated conditions include systemic or localized infections, intravenous drug abuse, recent trauma or surgery, pyogenic arthropathy, septicemia, and osteomyelitis.

Not all pyogenic joint infections are classifiable to subcategory 711.0. Before assigning code 711.0, carefully review the entries in the ICD-9-CM index under the terms "Arthritis, arthritic," due to or associated "with," and the includes note under subcategory 711.4 for any bacterial organism not specifically referenced under category 041. List a code from category 041 as a secondary code to identify the specific organism responsible for the arthritis or arthropathy.

711.1 ✔5th Arthropathy associated with Reiter's disease and nonspecific urethritis — *arthritis, arthropathy, polyarthritis, polyarthropathy*

Use this subclassification to report seronegative reactive arthritis. Occurring predominantly in the lower extremities, it is triggered by urethritis, cervicitis, or dysenteric infections. The syndrome consists of a triad of nonspecific (nongonococcal or simple) urethritis, conjunctivitis (or sometimes uveitis) and arthritis, and sometimes appears with mucocutaneous lesions. There is a close correlation between this disease and the presence of the histocompatibility antigen HLA-B27.

This manifestation code includes arthropathy with Reiter's disease and nonspecific urethritis. ICD-9-CM classifies etiology first, then manifestation, to remain compatible with the dual classification concept used in the international version of ICD-9.

711.2 ✔5th Arthropathy in Behcet's syndrome — *arthritis, arthropathy, polyarthritis, polyarthropathy*

Use this subclassification to report a multisystem disorder of unknown etiology named after the Turkish dermatologist who first described it. Recurrent oral and genital ulcers, uveitis, and seronegative arthritis and central nervous system abnormalities characterize the syndrome. The arthritic component involves large and small joints with a nonspecific, self-limiting synovitis and, in more than two-thirds of the patients, commonly affects the knees and ankles. The arthritic changes resemble those of rheumatoid arthritis but are milder and lead only to shallow erosions of the articular cartilage in the more severe cases. Therapies include immunomodulating drugs and corticosteroids.

Associated conditions include cranial nerve palsies, encephalitis, mental disturbances, spinal cord lesions, convulsions and, although rarely, death.

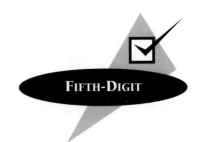

FIFTH-DIGIT

The following fifth-digit subclassification is for use with categories 711-712, 715-716, 718-719, and 730:

0 site unspecified

1 shoulder region (acromioclavicular joint, clavicle, glenohumeral joint, scapula, sternoclavicular joint)

2 upper arm (elbow joint, humerus)

3 forearm (radius, ulna, wrist joint)

4 hand (carpus, metacarpus, phalanges)

5 pelvic regions and thigh (buttock, femur, hip joint)

6 lower leg (fibula, knee joint, patella, tibia)

7 ankle and foot (ankle joint, metatarsus, phalanges, tarsus, other joints in foot)

8 other specified sites (head, neck, ribs, skull, trunk, vertebral column)

9 multiple sites

This manifestation code includes arthropathy associated with Behcet's syndrome (136.1). ICD-9-CM classifies etiology first, then manifestation, to remain compatible with the dual classification concept used in the international version of ICD-9.

711.3 ✓5th Postdysenteric arthropathy — *secondary to gastrointestinal infection*

Use this subclassification to report rare enteropathic arthropathies due to a wide range of specific dysentery-causing organisms, Shigella, and typhoid fever.

This manifestation code includes postdysenteric arthropathy, and is distinguished from subcategory 713.1 by an infectious or parasitic etiology for the enteropathic arthritis. ICD-9-CM classifies etiology first, then manifestation, to remain compatible with the dual classification concept used in the international version of ICD-9.

Excluded from this subclassification is salmonella arthritis (003.23).

711.4 ✓5th Arthropathy associated with other bacterial diseases — *secondary*

Use this subclassification to report arthropathy due to a wide variety of bacteria, excluding the pyogenic organisms identified under subcategory 711.0 and bacterial arthropathies classified elsewhere.

This manifestation code includes arthropathy associated with other bacterial diseases. ICD-9-CM classifies etiology first, then manifestation, to remain compatible with the dual classification concept used in the international version of ICD-9.

Excluded from this rubric are gonococcal arthritis (098.50) and meningococcal arthritis (036.82).

711.5 ✓5th Arthropathy associated with other viral diseases — *secondary*

Use this subclassification to report arthropathy associated with a wide variety of other viral diseases including rubella, mumps, infectious mononucleosis, lymphogranuloma venereum, variola, and many others.

This manifestation code includes arthropathy associated with other viral diseases. Arthropathy associated with viral hepatitis should also be classified here. ICD-9-CM classifies etiology first, then manifestation, to remain compatible with the dual classification concept used in the international version of ICD-9.

Excluded from this subclassification is arthropathy due to rubella (056.7).

711.6 ✓5th Arthropathy associated with mycoses — *secondary*

Use this subclassification to report arthropathy due to mycoses. Mycoses are diseases caused by fungi. A variety of fungal organisms may lodge in the synovium and create suppurative or granulomatous lesions. The synovium usually is the primary site of the joint involvement, but

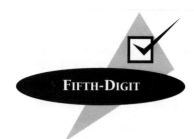

FIFTH-DIGIT

The following fifth-digit subclassification is for use with categories 711-712, 715-716, 718-719, and 730:

0 site unspecified

1 shoulder region (acromioclavicular joint, clavicle, glenohumeral joint, scapula, sternoclavicular joint)

2 upper arm (elbow joint, humerus)

3 forearm (radius, ulna, wrist joint)

4 hand (carpus, metacarpus, phalanges)

5 pelvic regions and thigh (buttock, femur, hip joint)

6 lower leg (fibula, knee joint, patella, tibia)

7 ankle and foot (ankle joint, metatarsus, phalanges, tarsus, other joints in foot)

8 other specified sites (head, neck, ribs, skull, trunk, vertebral column)

9 multiple sites

✓5th   Needs fifth-digit   **OK**   Valid three-digit code

secondary infection can spread from the marrow cavity to the subchondral bone and then into the articular tissues.

This manifestation code includes arthropathy associated with mycoses. ICD-9-CM classifies etiology first, then manifestation, to remain compatible with the dual classification concept used in the international version of ICD-9.

711.7 ✓5th Arthropathy associated with helminthiasis — *secondary*

Use this subclassification to report arthropathy due to parasitic infection of helminths (worms), hydatid cysts, or helminth larvae.

This manifestation code includes arthropathies associated with helminthiases. ICD-9-CM classifies etiology first, then manifestation, to remain compatible with the dual classification concept used in the international version of ICD-9.

711.8 ✓5th Arthropathy associated with other infectious and parasitic diseases — *secondary*

This manifestation code includes arthropathy associated with other infectious and parasitic diseases. ICD-9-CM classifies etiology first, then manifestation, to remain compatible with the dual classification concept used in the international version of ICD-9.

Excluded from this subclassification is arthropathy associated with sarcoidosis (713.7).

711.9 ✓5th Unspecified infective arthritis — *infective agent unknown*

712 CRYSTAL ARTHROPATHIES

Use this rubric to report chondrocalcinosis, arthritis and synovitis, as well as pseudogout and calcium pyrophosphate dehydrate deposition (CPDD) disease. The presence, and not the chemical composition, of crystals (apatite and hydroxyapatite, calcium pyrophosphate, calcium and dicalcium phosphate, calcium oxalate, and lipid crystals) acts as irritants. The mechanisms of initial precipitation are unknown, but predisposing conditions such as degradation of the cartilage matrix may be involved. Once the crystals have accumulated, they are taken up by phagocytic cells, initiating the inflammatory sequence. This in turn causes additional damage to the affected tissues.

The term chondrocalcinosis refers to calcification of articular cartilage. Articular chondrocalcinosis also is known as pseudogout since the disease is characterized by calcified deposits in the cartilage, but is free of the urate crystals found in gout. Aspiration and examination of synovial fluid allows precise diagnosis. Therapies include aspiration of the acutely inflamed joint, drugs such as corticosteroid injections, nonsteroidal, antiinflammatory drugs, and intravenous colchicine.

This category includes crystal (mineral) deposition arthropathies with the exception of gouty arthropathy, which is classified to code 274.0. Crystal deposition disease type I refers to gouty arthropathy due to uric acid crystals and should be classified to subcategory 274.0; type II crystal deposition disease includes the disorders classified to subcategory 712.2.

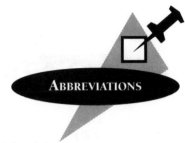

ABBREVIATIONS

Arth: arthritis

AV: acromioclavicular joint

CMC: carpometacarpal joint

E. coli: *Escherichia coli*

DJD: degenerative joint disease

H. influenzae: hemophilus influenzae

JRA: juvenile rheumatoid arthritis

MC: metacarpal joint

MT: metatarsal joint

OA: osteoarthritis

RA: rheumatoid arthritis

Staph: staphylococcus

Strep: streptococcus

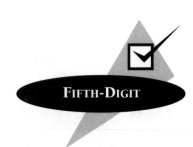

FIFTH-DIGIT

The following fifth-digit subclassification is for use with categories 711-712, 715-716, 718-719, and 730:

0 site unspecified

1 shoulder region (acromioclavicular joint, clavicle, glenohumeral joint, scapula, sternoclavicular joint)

2 upper arm (elbow joint, humerus)

3 forearm (radius, ulna, wrist joint)

4 hand (carpus, metacarpus, phalanges)

5 pelvic regions and thigh (buttock, femur, hip joint)

6 lower leg (fibula, knee joint, patella, tibia)

7 ankle and foot (ankle joint, metatarsus, phalanges, tarsus, other joints in foot)

8 other specified sites (head, neck, ribs, skull, trunk, vertebral column)

9 multiple sites

712.1 ✔5th Chondrocalcinosis due to dicalcium phosphate crystals — *crystal-induced arthritis*

This manifestation code includes chondrocalcinosis due to dicalcium phosphate crystals. ICD-9-CM classifies etiology first, then manifestation, to remain compatible with the dual classification concept used in the international version of ICD-9.

712.2 ✔5th Chondrocalcinosis due to pyrophosphate crystals — *crystal-induced arthritis*

Use this code to report chondrocalcinosis due to pyrophosphate crystals, which is a calcium pyrophosphate dehydrate deposition (CPPD) disease and type II crystal deposition disease.

This manifestation code includes chondrocalcinosis due to pyrophosphate crystals. ICD-9-CM classifies etiology first, then manifestation, to remain compatible with the dual classification concept used in the international version of ICD-9.

712.3 ✔5th Chondrocalcinosis, cause unspecified — *crystal-induced arthritis*

This manifestation code includes chondrocalcinosis due to unspecified cause. ICD-9-CM classifies etiology first, then manifestation, to remain compatible with the dual classification concept used in the international version of ICD-9.

712.8 ✔5th Other specified crystal arthropathies — *crystal-induced arthritis*

Use this code to report other specified crystal arthropathies due to lipid crystals, apatite and hydroxyapatite, calcium oxalate, calcium phosphate, and other identifiable crystals not elsewhere classifiable.

712.9 ✔5th Unspecified crystal arthropathy — *crystal-induced arthritis, type unknown*

713 ARTHROPATHY ASSOCIATED WITH OTHER DISORDERS CLASSIFIED ELSEWHERE

This rubric includes manifestation codes used to classify arthropathy associated with other disorders classified elsewhere. ICD-9-CM classifies etiology first, then manifestation, to remain compatible with the dual classification concept used in the international version of ICD-9.

Whenever the physician's diagnostic statement specifies etiology for the patient's arthropathy, a code from category 713 should be used as a secondary code. For example, the diagnosis "arthropathy due to hemochromatosis" is assigned codes 275.0 and 713.0, and the diagnosis "arthropathic multiple myeloma of the hip" is assigned codes 203.0X and 713.2. In the first case, the cause and effect relationship is stated; in the second, the relationship is implied. The term "associated with" in the code title indicates that both parts of the title may be in the physician's diagnostic statement. The word "as" in the notation "code first underlying disease as" under each subcategory indicates an incomplete list of etiologies.

713.0 Arthropathy associated with other endocrine and metabolic disorders — (Code first underlying disease, as: 243–244.9, 252.0, 253.0, 270.2, 272.0–272.9, 275.0, 279.00–279.09) — *secondary*

✔5th Needs fifth-digit   **OK** Valid three-digit code

713.1 Arthropathy associated with gastrointestinal conditions other than infections — (Code first underlying disease, as: 555.0–555.9, 556.0–556.9) — *secondary*

713.2 Arthropathy associated with hematological disorders — (Code first underlying disease, as: 202.30–202.38, 203.00, 203.01, 204.00–208.91, 282.4–282.7, 286.0–286.2) — *secondary*

713.3 Arthropathy associated with dermatological disorders — (Code first underlying disease, as: 695.1, 695.2) — *secondary*

713.4 Arthropathy associated with respiratory disorders — (Code first underlying disease, as: (diseases)) — *secondary*

713.5 Arthropathy associated with neurological disorders — (Code first underlying disease, as: 094.0, 250.60–250.63, 336.0) — *secondary*

713.6 Arthropathy associated with hypersensitivity reaction — (Code first underlying disease, as: 287.0, 999.50–999.59) — *secondary*

713.7 Other general diseases with articular involvement — (Code first underlying disease, as: 135, 277.3) — *secondary*

713.8 Arthropathy associated with other conditions classifiable elsewhere — (Code first underlying disease, as: (diseases)) — *secondary*

714 RHEUMATOID ARTHRITIS AND OTHER INFLAMMATORY POLYARTHROPATHIES

714.0 Rheumatoid arthritis — (Use additional code to identify manifestation, as: 357.1, 359.6) — *chronic rheumatic polyarthritis*

Rheumatoid arthritis is a chronic, systemic inflammatory disease of unknown etiology, characterized by a variable but prolonged course with exacerbations and remissions of joint pains and swelling. In early stages, the disease attacks the joints of the hands and feet. As the disease progresses, more joints become involved. Also known as primary progressive arthritis and proliferative arthritis, the disease often leads to progressive deformities, which may develop rapidly and cause permanent disability.

Clinical manifestations of rheumatoid arthritis are highly variable, particularly in the mode of onset, distribution, degree of severity ,and rate of progression. Joint disease is the major manifestation; systemic involvement (spleen, liver, eyes, etc.) is rare.

Signs and symptoms of rheumatoid arthritis include articular inflammation, malaise, weight loss, paresthesia, Raynaud's phenomenon, periarticular pain and stiffness, symmetrical joint swelling and stiffness, warmth, and pain and tenderness (most severe in the morning, subsiding somewhat during the day).

Lab work includes a complete blood count (CBC) to reveal anemia, elevated white blood cell count (WBC) and elevated erythrocyte sedimentation rate (ESR). Various serological tests may be used to detect rheumatoid factor, but false positive and false negative results are not unusual; typically, tests show elevated gamma globulins IgM and IgC during both acute and chronic phases. X-rays of affected joints early in the disease reveal evidence of periarticular soft tissue swelling and joint effusion; as the disease progresses, x-rays show regional osteoporosis,

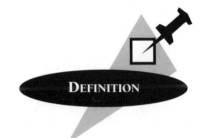

DEFINITION

Sjögren's: also Gougerot-Houser and Sicca, complex of symptoms of unknown source in middle aged women in which the following triad exists: keratoconjunctivitis sicca, xerostomia, and connective tissue disease (usually rheumatoid arthritis but sometimes systemic lupus erythematosus). Cause may be an abnormal immune response.

osteolysis of subchondral bone, and narrowing of cartilage spaces and, in the late stages, subluxation, dislocation, and ankylosis.

Therapies include medical treatment basically directed toward pain relief and reduction of inflammation with a wide variety of drugs including gold salts, corticosteroids and nonsteroidal antiinflammatory drugs for preservation of function and prevention of deformities. Physical and occupational therapy and splinting of joints are other therapies, as well as surgery such as arthrodesis, synovectomy, tendon grafts and transplantations, arthroplasty, capsulectomy, and capsulotomy.

Associated conditions include nonspecific pericarditis and pleuritis, pulmonary fibrosis, secondary amyloidosis, leukopenia, arteritis, and adverse effect of medications used to treat rheumatoid arthritis.

714.1   Felty's syndrome — *rheumatoid arthritis with splenoadenomegaly and leukopenia*

The definition of Felty's syndrome is association of rheumatoid arthritis with splenomegaly and leukopenia. Mild anemia and thrombocytopenia may accompany the variable severe neutropenia, and skin and pulmonary infections are frequent complications.

714.2   Other rheumatoid arthritis with visceral or systemic involvement — *rheumatoid carditis*

Other rheumatoid arthritis with visceral or systemic involvement occurs in the connective tissue components of the cardiovascular, reticuloendothelial, digestive, and respiratory system.

714.3 Juvenile chronic polyarthritis

Juvenile chronic polyarthritis is a rheumatoid-like disorder occurring in children (onset prior to age 17), involving one or more joints. Juvenile rheumatoid arthritis has a much more favorable prognosis than adult-onset disease.

The disease process for juvenile rheumatoid arthritis and polyarthritis is different genetically and immunologically from rheumatoid arthritis in adults," but the condition is still classified to subcategory 714.3 with the appropriate fifth digit, depending on the clinical presentation.

714.30   Polyarticular juvenile rheumatoid arthritis, chronic or unspecified — *number of joints affected unspecified, Still's disease*

Polyarticular juvenile rheumatoid arthritis, chronic or unspecified, is systemic juvenile arthritis or polyarthritis, also known as Still's disease, that interferes with growth and development.

714.31   Polyarticular juvenile rheumatoid arthritis, acute — *affecting many joints*

Polyarticular juvenile rheumatoid arthritis, acute, is systemic juvenile arthritis or polyarthritis, also known as Still's disease, described as acute. Typically, the acute phase includes high fever, erythematous rash, anemia, generalized lymphadenopathy and, in some cases, hepatosplenomegaly, iridocyclitis, and pericarditis.

✓5th   Needs fifth-digit   **OK**   Valid three-digit code

714.32   Pauciarticular juvenile rheumatoid arthritis — *affecting only a few joints*

Pauciarticular juvenile rheumatoid arthritis is a disease, also known as oligoarticular juvenile arthritis, affecting a small number of joints, usually two to five. It is associated with chronic iridocyclitis in 25 percent to 30 percent of patients and can lead to blindness.

714.33   Monoarticular juvenile rheumatoid arthritis — *affecting one joint*

Monoarticular juvenile rheumatoid arthritis is juvenile arthritis limited to one joint.

Pauciarticular juvenile arthritis may be used to describe monoarticular juvenile arthritis. In such cases, verify the diagnosis with the physician to ensure proper code assignment.

714.4   Chronic postrheumatic arthropathy — *chronic rheumatoid nodular fibrositis, Jaccoud's syndrome*

The definition of chronic postrheumatic arthropathy is a form of arthropathy of the hands and feet caused by repeated attacks of rheumatic arthritis. Also called Jaccoud's syndrome, this disease is characterized by flexion deformities, particularly of the metacarpophalangeal joints, and is associated with pronounced ulnar deviation of the fingers. Chronic rheumatoid nodular fibrositis is a variation of this disease characterized by the presence of subcutaneous nodules in the region of the previously involved joints.

714.81   Rheumatoid lung — *Caplan's syndrome, diffuse interstitial rheumatoid lung disease, fibrosing alveolitis*

Rheumatoid lung is diseases of the lung associated with rheumatoid arthritis, including Hamman-Rich syndrome (when associated with rheumatoid arthritis) and Caplan's syndrome, a syndrome of rheumatoid pneumoconiosis seen in patients with concomitant coal worker's pneumoconiosis.

714.89   Other specified inflammatory polyarthropathies — *not otherwise specified*
714.9   Unspecified inflammatory polyarthropathy — *unknown*

715 OSTEOARTHROSIS AND ALLIED DISORDERS

Osteoarthrosis and allied disorders are degenerative, rather than inflammatory, diseases of one or more joints. Also known as osteoarthritis and degenerative joint disease, osteoarthrosis is most conspicuous in the large joints and initiated by local deterioration of the articular cartilage. It progressively destroys the cartilage, remodels the subchondral bone, and causes a secondary inflammation of the synovial membrane.

Signs and symptoms of osteoarthrosis and allied disorders include pain in affected joints, muscle spasm, crepitation, and atrophy of surrounding muscles without evidence of inflammation.

Lab work is usually of little value, although examination of synovial fluid may demonstrate increased mucin content. X-rays of affected joints readily show narrowing of articular space, subchondral sclerosis and cysts, osteophyte formation, and joint remodeling.

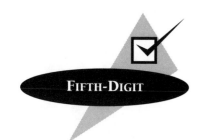

FIFTH-DIGIT

The following fifth-digit subclassification is for use with categories 711-712, 715-716, 718-719, and 730:

0 site unspecified

1 shoulder region (acromioclavicular joint, clavicle, glenohumeral joint, scapula, sternoclavicular joint)

2 upper arm (elbow joint, humerus)

3 forearm (radius, ulna, wrist joint)

4 hand (carpus, metacarpus, phalanges)

5 pelvic regions and thigh (buttock, femur, hip joint)

6 lower leg (fibula, knee joint, patella, tibia)

7 ankle and foot (ankle joint, metatarsus, phalanges, tarsus, other joints in foot)

8 other specified sites (head, neck, ribs, skull, trunk, vertebral column)

9 multiple sites

Therapies include pain and weight management, reduction of secondary inflammation of the synovial membrane, and physical and occupational therapy to help the patient maintain joint function and prevent or correct joint deformities. Surgery such as osteotomy near the joint improves biomechanics and soft tissue operations such as release of muscle contractions and neurectomy may help relieve intractable pain. For osteoarthritis of the hip, therapy includes hip preserving surgery (excision of osteophytes, curettage and bone grafting of acetabular cysts, proximal femoral osteotomy and muscle release) or hip reconstruction (cup arthroplasty, total hip replacement, femoral head replacement, and arthrodesis).

Assignment of the fourth digit to codes in this category is based on whether the disease is generalized or localized and whether it is primary or secondary.

715.0 ✔5th Osteoarthrosis, generalized — *degenerative joint disease, multiple joints; primary generalized hypertrophic osteoarthrosis*

Generalized disease is osteoarthrosis involving many joints without any known preexisting abnormality. Localized osteoarthrosis is disease confined to a limited number of sites, generally one or two of the larger weight-bearing joints, such as the hip or knee.

715.1 ✔5th Osteoarthrosis, localized, primary — *idiopathic localized osteoarthropathy*

Primary osteoarthrosis is idiopathic or due to some constitutional or genetic factor.

715.2 ✔5th Osteoarthrosis, localized, secondary — *coxae malum senilis*

Secondary osteoarthrosis is due to some identifiable initiating factor. These factors include obesity, trauma, congenital malformations, superimposition of fibrosis and scarring from previous inflammatory disease or infection, foreign bodies, malalignment of joints, metabolic or circulatory bone diseases and iatrogenic factors such as osteoarthrosis caused by continuous pressure on the joint surfaces during orthopaedic treatment of congenital deformities. Secondary osteoarthroses should be paired with a second code describing the causative injury, disorder, or disease.

715.3 ✔5th Osteoarthrosis, localized, not specified whether primary or secondary — *Otto's pelvis*

715.8 ✔5th Osteoarthrosis involving or with mention of more than one site, but not specified as generalized

715.9 ✔5th Osteoarthrosis, unspecified whether generalized or localized

716 OTHER AND UNSPECIFIED ARTHROPATHIES

716.0 ✔5th Kaschin-Beck disease — *endemic polyarthritis*

716.1 ✔5th Traumatic arthropathy — *following injury*

716.2 ✔5th Allergic arthritis — *immunological reaction following exposure to antigen*

Allergic arthritis is associated with a hypersensitive state acquired through exposure to an allergen.

Loosening of orthopaedic implants (including prostheses and other devices) due to an allergic or inflammatory reaction to chromium, cobalt, or nickel in the implant is classified as a postoperative complication. In

✔5th   Needs fifth-digit   **OK**   Valid three-digit code

such cases, use code 996.66 or 996.67 to classify the postoperative complication, followed by 716.2 to further describe the nature of the complication.

Excluded from this subclassification is arthritis associated with Henoch-Schonlein purpura or serum sickness (713.6).

716.3 ✓5th Climacteric arthritis — *menopausal*
716.4 ✓5th Transient arthropathy
716.5 ✓5th Unspecified polyarthropathy or polyarthritis — *unknown type*
716.6 ✓5th Unspecified monoarthritis — *unknown type*
716.8 ✓5th Other specified arthropathy — *not otherwise specified, including due to old epiphyseal slip, villous arthritis*
716.9 ✓5th Unspecified arthropathy — *unknown*

717 INTERNAL DERANGEMENT OF KNEE

This rubric includes degenerative disorders of the articular cartilage or meniscus of the knee, as well as the late effects of acute trauma to the knee classifiable to category 836. It excludes acute derangement of knee and current injury (836.0-836.6), ankylosis (718.5), contracture (718.4), deformity (736.4-736.6), and recurrent dislocation (718.3).

717.0 Old bucket handle tear of medial meniscus — *old bucket handle tear of unspecified cartilage*

717.1 Derangement of anterior horn of medial meniscus

717.2 Derangement of posterior horn of medial meniscus

717.3 Other and unspecified derangement of medial meniscus — *degeneration of internal semilunar cartilage*

This code includes tears of medial cartilage or the meniscus of the knee that may be described as radial, peripheral, horizontal cleavage type, flap, and complex tears.

717.40 Unspecified derangement of lateral meniscus — *unknown*

717.41 Bucket handle tear of lateral meniscus

717.42 Derangement of anterior horn of lateral meniscus

717.43 Derangement of posterior horn of lateral meniscus

717.49 Other derangement of lateral meniscus — *not otherwise specified*

This code includes tears of the lateral meniscus of the knee that may be described as radial, peripheral, horizontal cleavage type, flap, and complex tears.

717.5 Derangement of meniscus, not elsewhere classified — *including congenital discoid meniscus, cyst of semilunar cartilage*

This code includes other forms of meniscal derangements, such as cysts of any meniscus and congenital discoid lateral or medial meniscus.

717.6 Loose body in knee — *joint mice, rice bodies*

Loose body in knee is joint mice, rice bodies, and debris described as cartilaginous (cartilage only, radiolucent on x-rays), osseous (bony), osteocartilaginous, and fibrous. Osteochondritis dissecans is commonly the cause; other causes include synovial chondromatosis, osteophytes, fractured articular surfaces, and damaged menisci.

717.7	Chondromalacia of patella — *degeneration or softening of articular cartilage of patella*
717.81	Old disruption of lateral collateral ligament
717.82	Old disruption of medial collateral ligament
717.83	Old disruption of anterior cruciate ligament
717.84	Old disruption of posterior cruciate ligament
717.85	Old disruption of other ligament of knee — *capsular ligament*
717.89	Other internal derangement of knee — *not otherwise specified, including calcification, derangement of ligament, slipped patella, intraligamentous cyst, Haglund-Läwen-Fründ syndrome, Büdinger-Ludloff-Läwen disease*

This code includes old disruptions of the arcuate complex, medial capsule, lateral capsule, and popliteus.

| 717.9 | Unspecified internal derangement of knee — *unknown* |

718 OTHER DERANGEMENT OF JOINT

718.0	✔5th Articular cartilage disorder — *meniscus old rupture, old tear*
718.1	✔5th Loose body in joint — *joint mice*

Loose body in joint is joint mice, rice bodies, and debris described as cartilaginous, osseous (bony), osteocartilaginous, or fibrous in joints other than the knee.

| 718.2 | ✔5th Pathological dislocation — *spontaneous; not recurrent and not from injury* |

Pathological dislocation is dislocation of an articular joint due to a disease process (e.g., poliomyelitis), rather than trauma.

This code should be accompanied by a second ICD-9-CM code identifying the specific pathology (etiology of the pathological dislocation).

| 718.3 | ✔5th Recurrent dislocation of joint — *occurring again and again* |

Recurrent dislocation of joint is chronic, subsequent, additional, and repeated dislocations or subluxations of a joint due to trauma.

| 718.4 | ✔5th Contracture of joint — *strong resistance to stretch* |

Contracture of joint is a disorder characterized by restriction of joint motion due to contraction of the muscles that articulate the joint. The condition may be due to tonic spasm, fibrosis, loss of musculature equilibrium, or disuse atrophy.

718.5	✔5th Ankylosis of joint — *immobility*
718.6	✔5th Unspecified intrapelvic protrusion of acetabulum — *protrusio acetabuli, cause unknown*
718.8	✔5th Other joint derangement, not elsewhere classified — *flail joint, instability of joint*

This subclassification may be used as an additional code to classify instability of a joint secondary to removal of prosthesis. Use code 909.3 when the instability is described as a late effect of the prosthesis removal.

| 718.9 | ✔5th Unspecified derangement of joint — *unknown cause* |

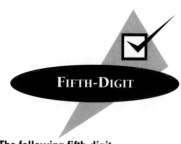

FIFTH-DIGIT

The following fifth-digit subclassification is for use with categories 711-712, 715-716, 718-719, and 730:

0 site unspecified

1 shoulder region (acromioclavicular joint, clavicle, glenohumeral joint, scapula, sternoclavicular joint)

2 upper arm (elbow joint, humerus)

3 forearm (radius, ulna, wrist joint)

4 hand (carpus, metacarpus, phalanges)

5 pelvic regions and thigh (buttock, femur, hip joint)

6 lower leg (fibula, knee joint, patella, tibia)

7 ankle and foot (ankle joint, metatarsus, phalanges, tarsus, other joints in foot)

8 other specified sites (head, neck, ribs, skull, trunk, vertebral column)

9 multiple sites

✔5th Needs fifth-digit   **OK** Valid three-digit code

719 OTHER AND UNSPECIFIED DISORDERS OF JOINT

719.0 ✔5th Effusion of joint — *hydrarthrosis, swelling of joint*

Effusion of joint is the escape of fluid from blood vessels or lymphatics into joint spaces. Hemorrhagic effusion is from blood. Hydrarthrosis is the accumulation of watery fluid in a joint. Effusion indicates synovial irritation due to disease or trauma (excluding current injury).

Therapies include aspiration of a tense effusion.

719.1 ✔5th Hemarthrosis — *blood in the joint*

Hemarthrosis is presence of gross blood in the joint spaces, excluding that due to current injury or hemophilia.

719.2 ✔5th Villonodular synovitis

Villonodular synovitis is a form of inflammation involving the synovial membranes of joints. There are two types of villonodular synovitis: pigmented and nonpigmented.

Therapies include steroidal and nonsteroidal medication to reduce inflammation and synovectomy when nonoperative therapy fails.

Villonodular synovitis may be a form of benign neoplasm of the connective tissue of the synovium, or be representative of granulomatous disease. The term "villonodular synovitis" is sometimes used to describe conditions such as xanthofibroma, giant cell tumor of tendon sheath and benign synovioma, which are classified elsewhere.

719.3 ✔5th Palindromic rheumatism — *Hench-Rosenberg syndrome, intermittent hydrarthrosis*

Palindromic rheumatism is sudden and recurring attacks of moderate to severe joint pain and swelling. The etiology is unknown but the condition has been associated with irritants and allergic reactions.

719.4 ✔5th Pain in joint — *arthralgia*
719.5 ✔5th Stiffness of joint, not elsewhere classified
719.6 ✔5th Other symptoms referable to joint — *including joint crepitus, snapping hip*
719.7 ✔5th Difficulty in walking
719.8 ✔5th Other specified disorders of joint — *not otherwise specified, including calcification, fistula*
719.9 ✔5th Unspecified disorder of joint — *unknown*

720-724 Dorsopathies

720 ANKYLOSING SPONDYLITIS AND OTHER INFLAMMATORY SPONDYLOPATHIES

720.0 Ankylosing spondylitis — *arthritis primarily of the sacroiliac joints and to varying degree, the rest of the spine and peripheral joints, with no new bone formation; Marie-Strümpell spondylitis*

Ankylosing spondylitis is a chronic, progressive inflammatory disease of unknown etiology involving primarily the small apophyseal and

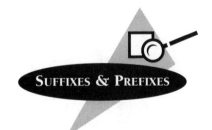

SUFFIXES & PREFIXES

Dors(o): relating to a dorsum or the back part of the body

Ossific: forming or becoming a bone

Panniculus: layer of membrane

Sacr(o): relating to the sacrum

Spondylitis: inflammation of the vertebra

Stenosis: narrowing of duct or canal

costovertebral joints of the spine and sacroiliac. This disease also is known as Marie-Strumpell or Bekhterev disease.

720.1   Spinal enthesopathy — *Romanus lesion; disorder of peripheral ligamentous or muscular attachments of spine*

720.2   Sacroiliitis, not elsewhere classified — *pain and inflammation within the joint or the junction of sacrum and hip*

720.81   Inflammatory spondylopathies in diseases classified elsewhere — (Code first underlying disease, as: 015.00–015.06) — *secondary to underlying disease*

720.89   Other inflammatory spondylopathies — *not otherwise specified*

720.9   Unspecified inflammatory spondylopathy — *unknown type*

721 SPONDYLOSIS AND ALLIED DISORDERS

Spondylosis and allied disorders are degenerative, rather than inflammatory, arthritis, osteoarthritis, and spondylarthritis of the spine. Myelopathy is a qualifying term describing diseases and disturbances of the spinal cord. Paresthesia, loss of sensation and loss of sphincter control, are among the most common forms of myelopathy.

Assignment of a fourth digit to codes in this category is based on the presence or absence of myelopathy. For coding purposes, myelopathy includes any symptomatic impingement, compression, disruption, or disturbance of the spinal cord or blood supply of the spinal cord due to spondylosis.

721.0   Cervical spondylosis without myelopathy — *cervical or cervicodorsal; in the neck*

721.1   Cervical spondylosis with myelopathy — *spondylogenic compression of cervical spinal cord; vertebral artery compression or anterior spinal artery compression syndromes*

721.2   Thoracic spondylosis without myelopathy — *upper back, T1-T12*

721.3   Lumbosacral spondylosis without myelopathy — *lower back, L1-L5*

721.41   Spondylosis with myelopathy, thoracic region — *upper back, T1-T12*

721.42   Spondylosis with myelopathy, lumbar region — *lower back, L1-L5*

721.5   Kissing spine — *including Baastrup's, Michotte's syndromes*

721.6   Ankylosing vertebral hyperostosis — *hypertrophy or exostosis causing immobility*

721.7   Traumatic spondylopathy — *including Kummell's disease*

721.8   Other allied disorders of spine — *not otherwise specified, including arthritis of coccyx*

721.90   Spondylosis of unspecified site without mention of myelopathy — *unknown cause, but without compression of spinal cord*

721.91   Spondylosis of unspecified site with myelopathy — *unknown cause, but with compression of spinal cord*

722 INTERVERTEBRAL DISK DISORDERS

722.0   Displacement of cervical intervertebral disc without myelopathy — *neuritis or radiculitis due to displacement or rupture of cervical intervertebral disc; neck, C1-C7; without compression of spinal cord*

722.10   Displacement of lumbar intervertebral disc without myelopathy — *lumbago, neuritis, radiculitis, or sciatica due to displacement of intervertebral disc; lower back, L1-L5; without compression of spinal cord*

722.11   Displacement of thoracic intervertebral disc without myelopathy — *lumbago, neuritis, radiculitis, or sciatica due to displacement of intervertebral disc; upper back, T1-T12; without compression of spinal cord*

↵5th   Needs fifth-digit   **OK**   Valid three-digit code

722.2   Displacement of intervertebral disc, site unspecified, without myelopathy — *lumbago, neuritis, radiculitis, or sciatica due to displacement of intervertebral disc; unknown site in spine; without compression of spinal cord*

722.3 Schmorl's nodes

Schmorl's nodes describe the prolapse of the nucleus pulposus into an adjoining vertebra, as seen on x-rays of the spine.

722.30   Schmorl's nodes, unspecified region — *nodule caused by prolapse of disk pulp into adjacent vertebra, unknown site in spine*

722.31   Schmorl's nodes, thoracic region — *nodule caused by prolapse of disk pulp into adjacent vertebra, upper back, T1-T12*

722.32   Schmorl's nodes, lumbar region — *nodule caused by prolapse of disk pulp into adjacent vertebra, lower back, L1-L5*

722.39   Schmorl's nodes, other spinal region — *nodule caused by prolapse of disk pulp into adjacent vertebra, cervical, C1-C7, or not otherwise specified*

722.4   Degeneration of cervical intervertebral disc — *including cervicothoracic intervertebral disc*

722.51   Degeneration of thoracic or thoracolumbar intervertebral disc

722.52   Degeneration of lumbar or lumbosacral intervertebral disc

722.6   Degeneration of intervertebral disc, site unspecified — *unknown site*

722.70   Intervertebral disc disorder with myelopathy, unspecified region — *with compression on spine, unknown site in spine*

722.71   Intervertebral cervical disc disorder with myelopathy, cervical region — *with compression on spine, in neck, C1-C7*

722.72   Intervertebral thoracic disc disorder with myelopathy, thoracic region — *with compression on spine, upper back, T1-T12*

722.73   Intervertebral lumbar disc disorder with myelopathy, lumbar region — *with compression on spine, lower back, L1-L5*

722.8 Postlaminectomy syndrome

Postlaminectomy syndrome is a complex of symptoms following laminectomy surgery. It includes conditions and syndromes described as postfusion, postmicrosurgery, and postchemonucleolysis.

722.80   Postlaminectomy syndrome, unspecified region — *unknown site on spine*

722.81   Postlaminectomy syndrome, cervical region — *neck, C1-C7*

722.82   Postlaminectomy syndrome, thoracic region — *upper back, T1-T12*

722.83   Postlaminectomy syndrome, lumbar region — *lower back, L1-L5*

722.90   Other and unspecified disc disorder of unspecified region — *including calcification, discitis, unknown site on spine*

722.91   Other and unspecified disc disorder of cervical region — *including calcification, discitis, neck, C1-C7*

722.92   Other and unspecified disc disorder of thoracic region — *including calcification, discitis, upper back, T1-T12*

722.93   Other and unspecified disc disorder of lumbar region — *including calcification, discitis, lower back, L1-L5*

723 OTHER DISORDERS OF CERVICAL REGION

723.0   Spinal stenosis in cervical region — *stricture in neck region, C1-C7*

723.1   Cervicalgia — *pain in neck region, C1-C7*

723.2   Cervicocranial syndrome — *Barre-Lieou, craniovertebral, or posterior cervical sympathetic syndromes*

723.3   Cervicobrachial syndrome (diffuse)

723.4   Brachial neuritis or radiculitis nos — *including radicular syndrome of upper limbs*

723.5	Torticollis, unspecified — *contracture of neck, cause undetermined*
723.6	Panniculitis specified as affecting neck — *cutaneous nodules caused by subcutaneous inflammatory reaction*
723.7	Ossification of posterior longitudinal ligament in cervical region
723.8	Other syndromes affecting cervical region — *not otherwise specified, including, video display tube syndrome, occipital neuralgia, Klippel's disease*

This code includes cervical instability syndromes, including C1-2 rotary instability syndrome.

723.9	Unspecified musculoskeletal disorders and symptoms referable to neck — *unknown*

724 OTHER AND UNSPECIFIED DISORDERS OF BACK

724.00	Spinal stenosis, unspecified region other than cervical — *stricture, unknown site in spine*
724.01	Spinal stenosis of thoracic region — *stricture, upper back, T1-T12*
724.02	Spinal stenosis of lumbar region — *stricture, lower back, L1-L5*
724.09	Spinal stenosis, other region other than cervical — *stricture, other site, cervical site excluded*
724.1	Pain in thoracic spine — *upper back, T1-T12*
724.2	Lumbago — *lower back, L1-L5*
724.3	Sciatica — *neuralgia of sciatic nerve*
724.4	Thoracic or lumbosacral neuritis or radiculitis, unspecified — *including vertebral bodies impingement syndrome, radicular syndrome of lower limbs*
724.5	Unspecified backache — *specifics unknown*
724.6	Disorders of sacrum — *including ankylosis, instability, or Thiele syndrome*
724.70	Unspecified disorder of coccyx — *unknown*
724.71	Hypermobility of coccyx
724.79	Other disorder of coccyx — *including pain, coccygodynia*
724.8	Other symptoms referable to back — *including ossification of posterior longitudinal ligament, sacral panniculitis, muscle spasm, stiffness in back*
724.9	Other unspecified back disorder — *specific unknown*

725-729 Rheumatism, Excluding the Back

725 POLYMYALGIA RHEUMATICA `OK`

Polymyalgia rheumatica is self-limiting disease of the elderly which often develops abruptly with joint and muscle pain and stiffness of the pelvis and shoulder girdle in association with fever, malaise, fatigue, weight loss, and anemia. The disease bears a close relationship with giant cell arteritis, and the two conditions often occur concomitantly.

726 PERIPHERAL ENTHESOPATHIES AND ALLIED SYNDROMES

Peripheral enthesopathies and allied syndromes are disorders of peripheral ligamentous or muscular attachments. The term "enthesopathy" is an obscure medical term meaning disease of the ligamentous or muscular attachments of a joint.

726.0	Adhesive capsulitis of shoulder

Adhesive capsulitis of shoulder is frozen shoulder syndrome, characterized by development of diffuse capsulitis of the glenohumeral joint with subsequent adherence of the inflamed capsule to the humeral head. Contracture due to the shrunken, adherent capsule prevents motion in the glenohumeral joint; that is, the joint is "frozen" in one position. The

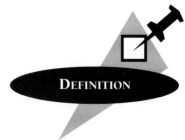

DEFINITION

Bursa: sac filled with fluid and situated in tissues.

Bursitis: inflammation of a bursa.

Capsule: cartilaginous, fatty, fibrous, or membranous structure enclosing an organ.

Capsulitis: inflammation of a capsule.

Ten(o): relating to a tendon.

Tenosynovitis: inflammation of a tendon sheath.

Fibr(o): relating to fibers.

Fibromatosis: formation of a fibrous nodule from the deep fascia.

Myo: relating to muscle.

Myositis: inflammation of a voluntary muscle.

✔5th Needs fifth-digit   `OK` Valid three-digit code

capsulitis may be caused by a variety of intrinsic and extrinsic disorders such as bicipital tendinitis, calcific supraspinatus tendinitis, basal pleurisy, and subphrenic inflammation.

Therapies include arthroscopic lavage, distension, and instillation of cortisone.

726.1 Rotator cuff syndrome of shoulder and allied disorders

Rotator cuff syndrome of shoulder and allied disorders are disorders of the ligamentous or muscular attachments of the shoulder joint and allied syndromes of the rotator cuff. The rotator cuff is a musculotendinous structure that blends with the joint capsule and is attached to the humerus. The supraspinatus is the major muscle that contributes to the formation of the rotator cuff.

726.10	Unspecified disorders of bursae and tendons in shoulder region — *rotator cuff or supraspinatus syndromes*
726.11	Calcifying tendinitis of shoulder — *hardening and inflammation of tendons due to calcium deposits*
726.12	Bicipital tenosynovitis — *inflammation of the tendon and tendon sheath surrounding the long head of the biceps*
726.19	Other specified disorders of rotator cuff syndrome of shoulder and allied disorders — *not otherwise specified, including painful arc syndrome*
726.2	Other affections of shoulder region, not elsewhere classified — *including periarthritis, scapulohumeral fibrositis, Duplay's or shoulder impingement syndromes*
726.30	Unspecified enthesopathy of elbow — *disorder of the attachment of muscle or tendon to bone, site unknown*
726.31	Medial epicondylitis of elbow — *disorder of the attachment of muscle or tendon to bone*
726.32	Lateral epicondylitis of elbow — *disorder of the attachment of muscle or tendon to bone, tennis/golfer's elbow*
726.33	Olecranon bursitis — *inflammation of bursa; elbow*

Olecranon bursitis is inflammation of the olecranon bursa. There are two olecranon bursae: one lies deep to the triceps tendon and the other between the skin and olecranon process. The latter is more commonly inflamed.

726.39	Other enthesopathy of elbow region — *not otherwise specified*
726.4	Enthesopathy of wrist and carpus — *disorder of the attachment of muscle or tendon to bone, bursitis, periarthritis*
726.5	Enthesopathy of hip region — *disorder of the attachment of muscle or tendon to bone, bursitis, periarthritis; gluteal, trochanteric, or psoas tendinitis, iliac crest spur*

Enthesopathy of hip region is a complex of conditions such as iliotibial band syndrome of hip, trochanteric bursitis, subgluteal bursitis, iliopectineal bursitis, trochanteric tendinitis (with calcification), psoas and tibiopsoas tendinitis, iliac crest spur. and snapping hip syndrome.

726.60	Unspecified enthesopathy of knee — *disorder of the attachment of muscle or tendon to bone, bursitis, periarthritis, site unknown*
726.61	Pes anserinus tendinitis or bursitis — *inflammation of the combined insertion of tendinous expansions of satirise, gracilis, and semitendinosus muscles*

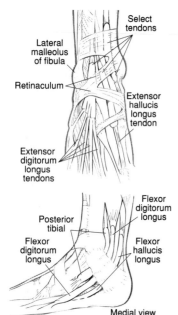

Select tendons

Lateral malleolus of fibula

Retinaculum

Extensor hallucis longus tendon

Extensor digitorum longus tendons

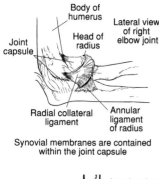

Posterior tibial

Flexor digitorum longus

Flexor digitorum longus

Flexor hallucis longus

Medial view

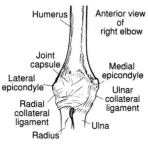

Body of humerus

Head of radius

Lateral view of right elbow joint

Joint capsule

Radial collateral ligament

Annular ligament of radius

Synovial membranes are contained within the joint capsule

Humerus

Anterior view of right elbow

Joint capsule

Lateral epicondyle

Medial epicondyle

Radial collateral ligament

Ulnar collateral ligament

Radius

Ulna

726.62 Tibial collateral ligament bursitis — *Pellegrini-Stieda syndrome*
726.63 Fibular collateral ligament bursitis — *inflammation of bursa*
726.64 Patellar tendinitis — *inflammation of patellar tendon*
726.65 Prepatellar bursitis — *inflammation of bursa*
726.69 Other enthesopathy of knee — *including infrapatellar, subpatellar*

This code includes iliotibial band syndrome of knee, infrapatellar bursitis, subpatellar bursitis, medial gastrocnemius bursitis, and semimembranosus bursitis.

726.70 Unspecified enthesopathy of ankle and tarsus — *disorder of the attachment of muscle or tendon to bone, site unknown*
726.71 Achilles bursitis or tendinitis — *including Albert's disease*
726.72 Tibialis tendinitis — *anterior or posterior*
726.73 Calcaneal spur
726.79 Other enthesopathy of ankle and tarsus — *not otherwise specified, including peroneal tendinitis*

This subclassification includes peroneal tendinitis, "pump bump" and tendinitis of the flexor hallucis longus, flexor digitorum longus, extensor hallucis longus, and extensor digitorum longus.

726.8 Other peripheral enthesopathies — *not otherwise specified*
726.90 Enthesopathy of unspecified site — *unknown site*
726.91 Exostosis of unspecified site — *bone spur NOS*

727 OTHER DISORDERS OF SYNOVIUM, TENDON, AND BURSA

727.0 Synovitis and tenosynovitis

Synovitis is inflammation of a synovial membrane, especially the synovium that lines articular joints. In a normal synovial joint, the smooth and reciprocally shaped cartilaginous opposing surfaces permit a fluid, frictionless, and painless articulation. Irregularities, disease, and damage to the articular surfaces lead to progressive degenerative changes resulting in pain and limitation of movement. The joint capsule is particularly sensitive to stretching and increased fluid pressure.

Tenosynovitis is the inflammation of a tendon and its synovial sheath. It is also known as tendosynovitis, tendovaginitis, tenontothecitis, tenontolemmitis, and vaginal or tendinous synovitis. At site of friction, the tendon is enveloped by a sheath consisting of a visceral and parietal layer of synovial membrane and is lubricated by a synovial-like fluid containing hyaluronate. The synovial sheath is in turn covered by a dense, fibrous tissue sheath. Irregularities, disease, and damage to the tendon's attachment to the articular joints may lead to progressive degenerative changes with resultant limitation of movement and pain. The synovial membranes of tendon sheaths and bursae are capable of the same inflammatory reactions to abnormal conditions as the synovial membranes of joints.

727.00 Unspecified synovitis and tenosynovitis — *synovitis NOS, tenosynovitis NOS*
727.01 Synovitis and tenosynovitis in diseases classified elsewhere — (Code first underlying disease, as: 015.00–015.96) — *secondary to an underlying disease*
727.02 Giant cell tumor of tendon sheath
727.03 Trigger finger (acquired)
727.04 Radial styloid tenosynovitis — *de Quervain's disease*
727.05 Other tenosynovitis of hand and wrist — *not otherwise specified*
727.06 Tenosynovitis of foot and ankle
727.09 Other synovitis and tenosynovitis — *including buttock, elbow, hip, knee*

5th Needs fifth-digit   **OK** Valid three-digit code

727.1   Bunion — *enlargement of the first metatarsal head caused by inflammation of bursa, frequently resulting in lateral displacement of the great toe*

A bunion is a localized friction-type bursitis located at either the medial or dorsal aspect of the first metatarsophalangeal joint. Bunions of the medial aspect are usually associated with hallux valgus.

727.2   Specific bursitides often of occupational origin — *including chronic crepitant synovitis of wrist, miner's elbow or knee*

Specific bursitises often of occupational origin is friction-type bursitis of various sites excluding bunions. Examples of these bursitises are "housemaid's knee," "student's elbow," and "weaver's bottom."

727.3   Other bursitis disorders — *not otherwise specified*

727.4 Ganglion and cyst of synovium, tendon, and bursa

Ganglion and cyst of synovium, tendon, and bursa are thin-walled cystic lesions of unknown etiology containing thick, clear, mucinous fluid, possibly due to mucoid degeneration. Arising in relation to periarticular tissues, joint capsules and tendon sheaths, ganglia are limited to the hands and feet and are most common in the dorsum of the wrist.

727.40   Unspecified synovial cyst — *round, cystic swelling of unspecified synovial site*
727.41   Ganglion of joint — *round, cystic swelling*
727.42   Ganglion of tendon sheath — *round, cystic swelling*
727.43   Unspecified ganglion — *round, cystic swelling of unspecified site*
727.49   Other ganglion and cyst of synovium, tendon, and bursa — *round cystic swelling of bursa*
727.50   Unspecified rupture of synovium — *nontraumatic, unknown site*
727.51   Synovial cyst of popliteal space — *including Baker's cyst of knee*

Synovial cyst of popliteal space is Baker's cysts, sometimes called popliteal cysts. In children, Baker's cysts are common but usually are asymptomatic and regress spontaneously. In adults, Baker's cysts, in conjunction with synovial effusion due to rheumatoid arthritis or degenerative joint disease, may produce significant impairment. When a Baker's cyst interferes with normal knee function, surgical exploration, and excision of the cyst is indicated.

Baker's cysts are classified to subcategory 727.5 for rupture of synovium because the cysts usually communicate with the knee joint through a long and tortuous duct, allowing the cyst to become distended by any synovial effusion and possibly extend down as far as the mid calf.

727.59   Other rupture of synovium — *other*

727.6 Rupture of tendon, nontraumatic

Rupture of tendon, nontraumatic, is a rupture due to pathology rather than trauma or injury. A normal tendon seldom ruptures even with strenuous activity, but if it has become damaged by disease (e.g., secondary to tenosynovitis) or degenerated due to the fraying caused by friction (e.g., due to bony erosion), it may rupture even with normal activity. Degeneration occurs in rheumatic arthritis, lupus erythematosus, hyperparathyroidism and systemic steroid use, or when steroids are injected directly into a tendon.

Therapies include reconstructive surgery to repair or replace abnormal part of ruptured tendon.

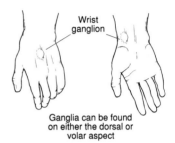

Ganglia can be found on either the dorsal or volar aspect

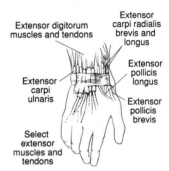

727.60 Nontraumatic rupture of unspecified tendon — *unknown tendon*
727.61 Complete rupture of rotator cuff
727.62 Nontraumatic rupture of tendons of biceps (long head)
727.63 Nontraumatic rupture of extensor tendons of hand and wrist

This subclassification includes the extensor pollicis longus, extensor pollicis brevis, extensor digitorum communis, extensor indicis, and the abductor pollicis longus tendons.

727.64 Nontraumatic rupture of flexor tendons of hand and wrist

This subclassification includes the flexor digitorum superficialis, flexor digitorum profundus, and the flexor pollicis longus tendons.

727.65 Nontraumatic rupture of quadriceps tendon
727.66 Nontraumatic rupture of patellar tendon
727.67 Nontraumatic rupture of Achilles tendon
727.68 Nontraumatic rupture of other tendons of foot and ankle — *not otherwise specified*
727.69 Nontraumatic rupture of other tendon — *not otherwise specified*
727.81 Contracture of tendon (sheath) — *acquired short Achilles tendon*
727.82 Calcium deposits in tendon and bursa — *calcification or calcific tendonitis, not otherwise specified*
727.83 Plica syndrome — *plica knee*
727.89 Other disorders of synovium, tendon, and bursa — *including abscess, hemorrhage, union of bursa or tendon, pseudobursa*
727.9 Unspecified disorder of synovium, tendon, and bursa — *specifics unknown, including sloughing tendon, slipped tendon, degeneration of synovial membrane, tenophyte*

728 DISORDERS OF MUSCLE, LIGAMENT, AND FASCIA

728.0 Infective myositis — *purulent, suppurative*

Infective myositis is inflammation of the voluntary muscles due to infection. It is usually secondary to osteomyelitis or a penetrating wound, but hematogenous infection can occur in debilitated patients or patients with suppressed immunity.

Signs and symptoms of infective myositis include marked swelling and pain, usually confined to shoulder girdle and arms, but may affect any part of the body.

728.10 Unspecified calcification and ossification — *massive calcification*
728.11 Progressive myositis ossificans — *Münchmeyer's syndrome*
728.12 Traumatic myositis ossificans — *myositis ossificans (circumscripta)*
728.13 Postoperative heterotopic calcification — *occurring at the site of surgery*
728.19 Other muscular calcification and ossification — *not otherwise specified, including polymyositis ossificans*
728.2 Muscular wasting and disuse atrophy, not elsewhere classified — *including hemiatrophy of leg, myofibrosis*
728.3 Other specific muscle disorders — *including arthrogryposis, immobility syndrome*
728.4 Laxity of ligament — *looseness or relaxation*
728.5 Hypermobility syndrome
728.6 Contracture of palmar fascia — *Dupuytren's contracture*

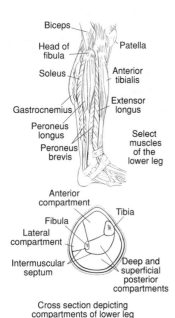

Biceps
Head of fibula
Patella
Soleus
Anterior tibialis
Gastrocnemius
Extensor longus
Peroneus longus
Peroneus brevis
Select muscles of the lower leg

Anterior compartment
Fibula
Tibia
Lateral compartment
Intermuscular septum
Deep and superficial posterior compartments

Cross section depicting compartments of lower leg

↙5th Needs fifth-digit   **OK** Valid three-digit code

728.71   Plantar fascial fibromatosis — *plantar fascia syndrome, contracture, traumatic fasciitis*

728.79   Other fibromatoses of muscle, ligament, and fascia — *not otherwise specified, including Garrod's or knuckle pads, nodular fasciitis, subcutaneous or proliferative pseudosarcomatous fibromatosis*

728.81   Interstitial myositis

728.82   Foreign body granuloma of muscle — *including talc granuloma of muscle*

728.83   Rupture of muscle, nontraumatic

728.84   Diastasis of muscle — *diastasis recti*

728.85   Spasm of muscle

728.86   Necrotizing fasciitis — (Use additional code to identify associated (condition) 041.00–041.89, 785.4)

728.89   Other disorder of muscle, ligament, and fascia — *not otherwise specified, including thecal abscess; cicatrix of muscle; calcification, contraction or cyst of ligament; contraction, eosinophilic, hernia of fascia*

728.9   Unspecified disorder of muscle, ligament, and fascia — *unknown*

729 OTHER DISORDERS OF SOFT TISSUES

729.0   Rheumatism, unspecified and fibrositis — *-- specifics unknown*

729.1   Unspecified myalgia and myositis — *unspecified generalized musculoskeletal pain, stiffness and easy fatigability*

729.2   Unspecified neuralgia, neuritis, and radiculitis — *pain along an inflamed nerve, with inflammation of the root of the associated spinal nerve, site unspecified*

729.3 Panniculitis, unspecified

Panniculitis, unspecified, is inflammation of subcutaneous fat. The term often is used solely to refer to an inflammation of the panniculus adiposa of the abdominal wall. Miscellaneous forms of panniculitis include those resulting from trauma, insulin injections, pancreatitis, allergic reactions, insect toxins, angiitis, idiopathic cold agglutinins, and sclerosing lipogranulomas.

Many variations of panniculitis, such as erythema nodosum (tuberculous and nontuberculous) and erythema pernio, are classified elsewhere. When coding panniculitis, obtain as much specific information as possible and follow the ICD-9-CM index carefully.

729.30   Panniculitis, unspecified site — *Weber-Christian disease*

729.31   Hypertrophy of fat pad, knee — *infrapatellar fat pad*

729.39   Panniculitis of other sites — *not otherwise specified*

729.4   Unspecified fasciitis — *inflammation of the fibrous tissue that acts to compartmentalize muscle*

729.5   Pain in soft tissues of limb — *not otherwise specified*

729.6   Residual foreign body in soft tissue

729.81   Swelling of limb

729.82   Cramp of limb

729.89   Other musculoskeletal symptoms referable to limbs

729.9   Other and unspecified disorders of soft tissue — *not otherwise specified, including polyalgia, nontraumatic compartment or Profichet's syndrome*

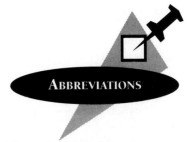

ABBREVIATIONS

MPD: myofascial pain-dysfunction syndrome, a disorder of the temporomandibular joint that results from clenching the jaw or grinding the teeth together. The muscles in the jaw then become tired and spasm causing intense pain

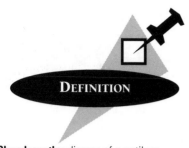

DEFINITION

Chondropathy: disease of a cartilage.

Osteochondropathy: condition affected both bone and cartilage.

Osteoarthropathy: any disease of the joints and bones.

Osteopathy: any disease of bone.

730-739 Osteopathies, Chondropathies, and Acquired Musculoskeletal Deformities

730 OSTEOMYELITIS, PERIOSTITIS, AND OTHER INFECTIONS INVOLVING BONE

Osteomyelitis, periostitis and other infections involving bone is a broad spectrum of bone infections. Osteomyelitis is an inflammation of bone and bone marrow. The condition is commonly due to a pathogen such as bacteria, virus, protozoa, or fungus. Periostitis is an inflammation of the periosteum, the thick fibrous membrane covering all the surfaces of bones except at the articular cartilage. The combination of osteomyelitis and periostitis is periosteomyelitis.

The pathogenesis of osteomyelitis, periostitis, and periosteomyelitis follows three general routes of infection. Hematogenous osteomyelitis (acute) is a form of osteomyelitis common to children where blood-borne organisms settle in the metaphyseal vascular bed of the rapidly developing long bones. Osteomyelitis may develop as an extension of a contiguous infection, particularly infections involving ischemic, diabetic, or neurotrophic ulcers. The third route of infection is by direct inoculation of pathogens through an open wound created by injury or a surgical procedure.

Signs and symptoms of osteomyelitis, periostitis, and other infections involving bone, include pain and unwillingness to move affected area, site closest to surface sometimes detectable by gentle palpation, and, occasionally, malaise, fever, chills, and anorexia.

Lab work includes aspiration with a large bore needle for gram stain and culture to confirm diagnosis and reveal pathogenic agent. Blood cultures may be positive in patients with acute hematogenous osteomyelitis. Bone scans such as scintigraphy are useful, although other factors may cause false positive results and false negative results are possible with acute hematogenous osteomyelitis.

Therapies include long-term antibiotic therapy and surgery to incise and drain involved area, decompress intraosseous, and remove necrotic debris in severe acute cases. Other surgery includes sequestrectomy, excision of multiple sinus tracts, craterization, saucerization, partial excision of bone, and bone grafting for chronic osteomyelitis.

Associated conditions include skin ulcers of various types, septicemia, diabetes, tuberculosis, poliomyelitis, neuropathy, septic arthritis, and trauma (such as compound fractures).

Osteomyelitis may result from direct inoculation from a traumatic or surgical wound. In these cases, follow the Department of Health and Human Services (DHHS) definitions regarding principal and other diagnoses and code sequencing and ICD-9-CM coding rules regarding late effects and complications of surgical and medical care where applicable.

730.0 ✔5th Acute osteomyelitis — *abscess of any bone except accessory sinus, jaw, or mastoid*

Acute osteomyelitis are diseases including periostitis and periosteomyelitis in acute and subacute forms. Clinically, patients fall into two groups: those who respond to intravenous antibiotics and those who require surgical intervention.

✔5th   Needs fifth-digit   **OK**   Valid three-digit code

730.1 ✔5th Chronic osteomyelitis — *Brodie's abscess, Busquet's disease, necrosis, sequestrum, sclerosing osteomyelitis of Garré*

Chronic osteomyelitis is persistent, recurring infection of bone and/or draining sinuses, often regarded as controllable but incurable.

730.2 ✔5th Unspecified osteomyelitis — *osteitis or osteomyelitis of unknown origin, with or without periostitis*

730.3 ✔5th Periostitis without mention of osteomyelitis — *abscess without mention of osteomyelitis*

730.7 ✔5th Osteopathy resulting from poliomyelitis — *secondary to polio*

730.8 ✔5th Other infections involving bone in diseases classified elsewhere — *secondary to underlying disease*

730.9 ✔5th Unspecified infection of bone — *unknown*

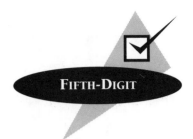

The following fifth-digit subclassification is for use with category 730:

0 site unspecified

1 shoulder region (acromioclavicular joint, clavicle, glenohumeral joint, scapula, sternoclavicular joint)

2 upper arm (elbow joint, humerus)

3 forearm (radius, ulna, wrist joint)

4 hand (carpus, metacarpus, phalanges)

5 pelvic regions and thigh (buttock, femur, hip joint)

6 lower leg (fibula, knee joint, patella, and tibia)

7 ankle and foot (ankle joint, metatarsus, phalanges, tarsus, other joints in foot)

8 other specified sites (head, neck, ribs, skull, trunk, vertebral column)

9 multiple sites

731 OSTEITIS DEFORMANS AND OSTEOPATHIES ASSOCIATED WITH OTHER DISORDERS CLASSIFIED ELSEWHERE

Osteitis deformans and osteopathies associated with other disorders classified elsewhere include the disseminated bone disorder known as Paget's disease. Characterized by slow and progressive enlargement and deformity of multiple bones, Paget's disease is associated with unexplained acceleration of both deposition and resorption of bone. During the early (osteolytic) phase of the disease, resorption exceeds deposition, and the bone, although enlarged, becomes sponge-like, weakened, and deformed. The second (osteosclerotic) phase is marked by deposition exceeding resorption resulting in the bones becoming thick and dense. The disease sometimes is associated with an invariably fatal form of malignant osteogenic sarcoma as a result of hyperactive osteoblast activity. Etiology is unknown, but there is some evidence that it may be triggered by a "slow virus" that affects primarily the osteoclasts.

731.0 Osteitis deformans without mention of bone tumor — *Paget's disease of bone*

731.1 Osteitis deformans in diseases classified elsewhere — (Code first underlying disease, as: 170.0–170.9) — *secondary to underlying disease*

731.2 Hypertrophic pulmonary osteoarthropathy — *Bamberger-Marie disease, Minkowski's, Pierre Marie-Bamberger, or thoracogenous rheumatic syndromes*

731.8 Other bone involvement in diseases classified elsewhere — (Code first underlying disease, as: 250.80–250.83) (Use additional code to specify bone condition, such as acute osteomyelitis (730.00–730.09) — *secondary to underlying disease*

732 OSTEOCHONDROPATHIES

Osteochondropathies are self-limiting disorders of unknown etiology that mostly affect children (juvenile osteochondrosis) three years to 10 years old. Four phases in the pathogenesis of the disease have been identified: necrosis; revascularization, bone deposition and resorption; bone healing; and bone deformity.

The fourth phase often is associated with degenerative arthropathy and is subject to ICD-9-CM coding rules regarding late effects where applicable. Also, many osteochondroses are identified by their eponyms (e.g., Kienbock's disease of the carpal lunate) and can be found under the main terms "Disease," "Osteochondrosis," and "Syndrome" in the ICD-9-CM index.

732.0 Juvenile osteochondrosis of spine — *marginal or vertebral epiphysis of Scheuermann or spine; vertebral epiphysitis*

732.1 Juvenile osteochondrosis of hip and pelvis — *including acetabulum, head of femur, iliac crest, symphysis pubis; coxa plana, ischiopubic synchondrosis of van Neck, Wadenström's disease, pseudocoxalgia*

732.2 Nontraumatic slipped upper femoral epiphysis — *slipped upper femoral epiphysis, not otherwise specified*

732.3 Juvenile osteochondrosis of upper extremity — *including capitulum of humerus if Panner, carpal lunate of Kienbock, head of humerus of Haas, heads of metacarpals of Mauclaire, lower ulna of Burns, radial head of Brailsford*

732.4 Juvenile osteochondrosis of lower extremity, excluding foot — *including primary patellar center of Köhler, proximal tibia of Blount, secondary patellar center of Sinding-Larsen, tibial tubercle of Osgood-Schlatter; tibia vara, Blount-Barber or Erlacher-Blount syndromes*

732.5 Juvenile osteochondrosis of foot — *astragalus of Diaz, calcaneum of Sever, second metatarsal of Freiberg, fifth metatarsal of Iselin, os tibiale externum of Haglund, tarsal navicular of Köhler, calcaneal apophysitis, epiphysitis os calcis, Mouchet's disease*

732.6 Other juvenile osteochondrosis — *apophysitis, epiphysitis, osteochondritis, osteochondrosis of site not otherwise specified*

732.7 Osteochondritis dissecans

Osteochondritis dissecans is a form of osteochondropathy in which the convex surfaces of certain pressure epiphyses are susceptible to avascular necrosis. When a small tangential segment of subchondral bone becomes separated or "dissected" from the remaining portion of the epiphysis by reactive fibrous and granulation tissue, it is designated an osteochondritis or osteochondrosis dissecans.

732.8 Other specified forms of osteochondropathy — *adult osteochondrosis of spine*

732.9 Unspecified osteochondropathy — *apophysitis, epiphysitis, osteochondritis, osteochondrosis, not specified as adult or juvenile, of site not otherwise specified*

733 OTHER DISORDERS OF BONE AND CARTILAGE

733.0 Osteoporosis

Osteoporosis is generalized bone disease characterized by decreased osteoblastic formation of matrix combined with increased osteoclastic resorption of bone, resulting in a marked decrease in bone mass. Osteoporosis often presents with osteopenia, which is a decrease in bone mineralization. Osteoporosis is classified into two major groups: primary and secondary. Primary osteoporosis implies that the condition is a fundamental disease entity and may be further broken down into involutional disease (e.g., juvenile). Secondary osteoporosis attributes the condition to an underlying clinical disease, medical condition, or medication.

Signs and symptoms of osteoporosis include chronic and intermittent back pain (due to vertebral microfractures), skeletal remodeling such as dorsal kyphosis, or loss of height.

Lab work usually shows normal results although metabolic studies may reveal a negative calcium balance. Radiographs and bone scans determine extent and severity of osteoporosis and osteopenia and may reveal fresh or old evidence of pathological fractures. Quantitative computed tomography (CT) and single and dual energy x-ray absorptiometry (DEXA) measure bone density, and bone biopsy occasionally is done for histological studies.

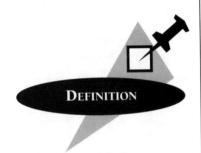

DEFINITION

Idiopathic osteoporosis: bone mass reduction, usually without abnormality of mineral or organic content, without known cause.

Osteoporosis: bone mass reduction, usually without abnormality of mineral or organic content.

Senile osteoporosis: bone mass reduction, usually without abnormality of mineral or organic content, in postmenopausal women.

5th   Needs fifth-digit   **OK**   Valid three-digit code

Therapies include medical management such as dietary manipulation, calcitonin, diphosphonate's, vitamin D, calcium and sodium fluoride, and estrogen therapy following menopause.

Associated conditions include pathological fractures; in the case of secondary osteoporosis, wide range of underlying factors such as anemia, hormone-related disorders, hepatic disease, starvation and anorexia, small intestine disease, mastocytosis, hemochromatosis, acromegaly, and conditions resulting from gastrectomy and treatment with anticonvulsants.

733.00 Unspecified osteoporosis — *wedging of vertebra not otherwise specified*

733.01 Senile osteoporosis — *bone mass reduction, usually without abnormality of mineral or organic content, in postmenopausal women*

733.02 Idiopathic osteoporosis — *bone mass reduction, usually without abnormality of mineral or organic content, not the result of disease or trauma*

733.03 Disuse osteoporosis

733.09 Other osteoporosis — *not otherwise specified, including drug-induced osteoporosis, Preiser's disease*

733.1 Pathologic fracture

A pathological fracture occurs at a site weakened by preexisting disease. These fractures are often differentiated from traumatic fractures by clinically assessing the magnitude of the trauma or stress causing the fracture. A relatively minor trauma or stress can cause a pathological fracture in bones diseased by osteoporosis and other metabolic bone disease, disseminated bone disorders, inflammatory bone diseases, Paget's disease, neoplasms, or any other condition that can compromise bone strength and integrity.

733.10 Pathologic fracture, unspecified site — *spontaneous fracture, site unknown*

733.11 Pathologic fracture of humerus — *spontaneous fracture*

733.12 Pathologic fracture of distal radius and ulna — *spontaneous fracture*

733.13 Pathologic fracture of vertebrae — *spontaneous fracture*

733.14 Pathologic fracture of neck of femur — *spontaneous fracture*

733.15 Pathologic fracture of other specified part of femur — *spontaneous fracture*

733.16 Pathologic fracture of tibia and fibula — *spontaneous fracture*

733.19 Pathologic fracture of other specified site — *spontaneous fracture, site not otherwise specified*

733.20 Unspecified cyst of bone (localized) — *unknown site*

733.21 Solitary bone cyst — *unicameral bone cyst*

733.22 Aneurysmal bone cyst

733.29 Other cyst of bone — *not otherwise specified, including fibrous dysplasia*

733.3 Hyperostosis of skull — *formation of new, abnormal bone on the inner aspect of cranial bones; leontiasis ossium, Buchem's, Morel-Moore, and Morgagni-Stewart-Morel syndromes*

733.4 Aseptic necrosis of bone

Aseptic necrosis of bone is infarction of bone tissue due to noninfectious etiologies such as fractures (avascular necrosis due to fracture), ischemic disorders, and immunosuppressive agents such as corticosteroids following renal transplants. It leads to degenerative joint disease or nonunion of fracture.

Osteonecrosis can be used to describe a wide variety of disorders, both infectious and noninfectious, resulting in bone infarction.

Some conditions falling under the general category of osteonecrosis are due to infectious etiologies and should be classified elsewhere. For example, osteonecrosis associated with acute staphylococcal osteomyelitis is classified to subcategories 730.0X and 041.1. Also,

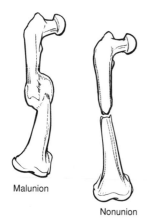

Malunion

Nonunion

Examples of malunion and nonunion
of femoral fractures

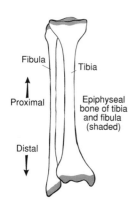

Fibula   Tibia

Proximal   Epiphyseal
bone of tibia
and fibula
(shaded)

Distal

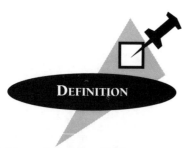

DEFINITION

Cubitus valgus deformity: forearm
angles away from the body.

Cubitus varus deformity: forearm angles
toward the body.

Valgus deformity of wrist: wrist angles
away from the body.

Varus deformity of wrist: wrist angles
toward the body.

osteonecrosis unspecified as to infectious or noninfectious etiology is classified to
subcategory 730.1X.

733.40	Aseptic necrosis of bone, site unspecified — *death of bone tissue not due to infection, unknown site*	

733.40 Aseptic necrosis of bone, site unspecified — *death of bone tissue not due to infection, unknown site*

733.41 Aseptic necrosis of head of humerus — *death of bone tissue not due to infection*

733.42 Aseptic necrosis of head and neck of femur — *death of bone tissue not due to infection*

733.43 Aseptic necrosis of medial femoral condyle — *death of bone tissue not due to infection*

733.44 Aseptic necrosis of talus — *death of bone tissue not due to infection*

733.49 Aseptic necrosis of other bone site — *death of bone tissue not due to infection, site not otherwise specified*

733.5 Osteitis condensans — *piriform sclerosis of ilium*

733.6 Tietze's disease — *painful swell and inflammation of unknown origin of rib cartilage; costochondral junction syndrome, costochondritis*

733.7 Algoneurodystrophy — *disuse atrophy of bone, Sudeck's atrophy*

733.81 Malunion of fracture — *broken bone heals in misalignment*

733.82 Nonunion of fracture — *broken bone fails to heal*

733.90 Disorder of bone and cartilage, unspecified — *specifics unknown*

733.91 Arrest of bone development or growth — *Harris lines, epiphyseal arrest*

733.92 Chondromalacia — *localized, except patella, systemic, tibial plateau*

733.99 Other disorders of bone and cartilage — *not otherwise specified, including diaphysitis, hypertrophy of bone, relapsing polychondritis, Bruck's disease, slipped rib, xiphoiditis, ossification of cartilage*

734 FLAT FOOT OK

735 ACQUIRED DEFORMITIES OF TOE

735.0 Hallux valgus (acquired) — *deformity in which the great toe angles toward other toes of that foot*

735.1 Hallux varus (acquired) — *deformity in which the great toe angles away from other toes of that foot*

735.2 Hallux rigidus — *limited motion of great toe due to painful flexion; also called hallux rigidus*

735.3 Hallux malleus — *hammer toe of big toe*

735.4 Other hammer toe (acquired) — *hammer toe, other than big toe*

735.5 Claw toe (acquired) — *contracture of toe*

735.8 Other acquired deformity of toe — *including hypertrophic, overriding, overlapping, or pigeon toe*

735.9 Unspecified acquired deformity of toe — *unknown*

736 OTHER ACQUIRED DEFORMITIES OF LIMBS

736.00 Unspecified deformity of forearm, excluding fingers — *unknown*

736.01 Cubitus valgus (acquired) — *deformity in which the forearm angles away from the body*

736.02 Cubitus varus (acquired) — *deformity in which the forearm angles toward the body*

736.03 Valgus deformity of wrist (acquired) — *deformity in which the wrist angles away from the body*

736.04 Varus deformity of wrist (acquired) — *deformity in which the wrist angles toward the body*

⤶5th   Needs fifth-digit   OK   Valid three-digit code

736.05 Wrist drop (acquired) — *paralysis or injury of extensor muscles of hand and fingers causing flexion of wrist*

Wrist drop is a condition in which the wrist remains flexed downward and is unable to be extended. It is often caused by injury to the radial nerve of the forearm or paralysis of the muscles in the hand and wrist.

736.06 Claw hand (acquired) — *contracture of hand*

A claw hand is characterized by curved or bent fingers, making the hand appear claw-like. Claw hand can be something that a child is born with (congenital) or can develop as a consequence of disorders (acquired).

736.07 Club hand, acquired

736.09 Other acquired deformities of forearm, excluding fingers — *not otherwise specified, including intrinsic swan neck hand*

736.1 Mallet finger — *constant flexion of distal joint*

736.20 Unspecified deformity of finger — *unknown*

736.21 Boutonniere deformity — *fixed flexion of proximal interphalangeal joint and hyperextension of distal interphalangeal joint*

736.22 Swan-neck deformity — *flexion of the distal interphalangeal joint and hyperextension of the proximal interphalangeal joint*

736.29 Other acquired deformity of finger — *not otherwise specified, including shallow acetabulum, acquired short ip, wandering acetabulum*

736.30 Unspecified acquired deformity of hip — *unknown*

736.31 Coxa valga (acquired) — *angle formed by the head and neck of the femur and axis of the shaft is increased*

736.32 Coxa vara (acquired) — *angle formed by the head and neck of the femur and axis of the shaft is decreased*

736.39 Other acquired deformities of hip — *not otherwise specified*

736.41 Genu valgum (acquired) — *"knock-knee;" knees close together, ankles far apart*

736.42 Genu varum (acquired) — *"bowleg," knees far apart, ankles close together*

736.5 Genu recurvatum (acquired) — *"back-knee," hyperextension of knee*

736.6 Other acquired deformities of knee — *not otherwise specified*

736.70 Unspecified deformity of ankle and foot, acquired — *unknown*

736.71 Acquired equinovarus deformity — *clubfoot*

736.72 Equinus deformity of foot, acquired — *tip-toe walking deformity*

736.73 Cavus deformity of foot, acquired — *abnormally high arch*

736.74 Claw foot, acquired — *contracture deformity*

736.75 Cavovarus deformity of foot, acquired

736.76 Other acquired calcaneus deformity — *not otherwise specified*

736.79 Other acquired deformity of ankle and foot — *not otherwise specified, including pronation of ankle or foot, varus talipes, valgus talipes*

736.81 Unequal leg length (acquired)

736.89 Other acquired deformity of other parts of limb — *not otherwise specified, including angulation or torsion of tibia; bowing of femur, fibula, tibia, winged scapula*

736.9 Acquired deformity of limb, site unspecified — *unknown*

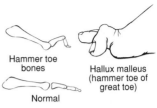

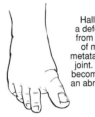

Hammer toe bones

Hallux malleus (hammer toe of great toe)

Normal

Hammertoe may affect any number of toes

Hallux rigidus is a deformity arising from limited range of motion in the metatarsophalangeal joint. The great toe becomes locked into an abnormal position

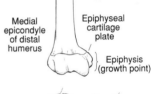

Medial epicondyle of distal humerus

Epiphyseal cartilage plate

Epiphysis (growth point)

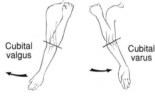

Cubital valgus

Cubital varus

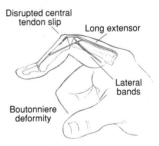

Disrupted central tendon slip

Long extensor

Lateral bands

Boutonniere deformity

Disruption of the central tendon slip causes the finger to drop. Tension from the lateral bands causes the finger tip to be fully extended

Normal distal joint

Mallet finger showing disrupted insertion of extensor tendon

737 CURVATURE OF SPINE

Curvature of spine is deformity of the spine. Kyphosis is an abnormal increase in the thoracic convexity as viewed from the side. Lordosis is the anterior convexity of the cervical and lumbar spine as viewed from the side.

737.0	Adolescent postural kyphosis — *acquired abnormal convex curve of spine*
737.10	Kyphosis (acquired) (postural)
737.11	Kyphosis due to radiation
737.12	Kyphosis, postlaminectomy
737.19	Other kyphosis (acquired) — *not otherwise specified*
737.20	Lordosis (acquired) (postural) — *not due to disease or injury*
737.21	Lordosis, postlaminectomy
737.22	Other postsurgical lordosis
737.29	Other lordosis (acquired) — *not specified elsewhere*

737.3 Kyphoscoliosis and scoliosis

Scoliosis is lateral curvature of the spine and kyphoscoliosis is a lateral curvature of the spine with extensive flexion. Scoliosis may be described as structural or nonstructural depending on whether the condition is reversible. Etiologies for nonstructural scoliosis include poor posture, pain, muscle spasms and uneven limb lengths. Structural scoliosis etiologies include idiopathic (infantile, juvenile, adolescent), osteopathic, neuropathic, and myopathic.

Specific etiologies for osteopathic scoliosis include fractures and dislocations of the spine, rickets, osteomalacia and thoracogenic conditions such as unilateral pulmonary disease, or deformities caused by unilateral surgical procedures. Neuropathic scoliosis etiologies include acquired conditions such as poliomyelitis, paraplegia, syringomyelia, and Friedreich's ataxia.

ICD-9-CM coding rules for late effects are applicable for osteopathic and neuropathic etiologies when scoliosis represents the residual of the etiology. Etiologies for myopathic scoliosis are all congenital scolioses classified in ICD-9-CM chapter 14, Congenital Anomalies (740-759).

737.30	Scoliosis (and kyphoscoliosis), idiopathic — *not due to disease or injury*
737.31	Resolving infantile idiopathic scoliosis
737.32	Progressive infantile idiopathic scoliosis
737.33	Scoliosis due to radiation
737.34	Thoracogenic scoliosis
737.39	Other kyphoscoliosis and scoliosis — *not otherwise specified*
737.40	Unspecified curvature of spine associated with other condition — (Code first associated condition as: 015.00–015.06, 138, 237.70–237.72, 252.0, 277.5, 356.1, 731.0, 733.00–733.09) — *unknown type, secondary to underlying disease*
737.41	Kyphosis associated with other condition — (Code first associated condition as: 015.00–015.06, 138, 237.70–237.72, 252.0, 277.5, 356.1, 731.0, 733.00–733.09) — *abnormal convex curve of the spine as seen in profile, secondary to underlying disease*
737.42	Lordosis associated with other condition — (Code first associated condition as: 015.00–015.06, 138, 237.70–237.72, 252.0, 277.5, 356.1, 731.0, 733.00–733.09) — *abnormal concave curve of the spine as seen in profile, secondary to underlying disease*

✔5th Needs fifth-digit   **OK** Valid three-digit code

737.43	Scoliosis associated with other condition — (Code first associated condition as: 015.00–015.06, 138, 237.70–237.72, 252.0, 277.5, 356.1, 731.0, 733.00–733.09) — *abnormal lateral curve of the spine, secondary to underlying disease*
737.8	Other curvatures of spine associated with other conditions — *not otherwise specified*
737.9	Unspecified curvature of spine associated with other condition — *unknown curvature of spine*

738 OTHER ACQUIRED MUSCULOSKELETAL DEFORMITY

Other acquired musculoskeletal deformity is a noncongenital deformity due to a variety of conditions such as degenerative disease; a late effect of fracture, dislocation or other soft tissue injury or infection; or pathological weakness of a musculoligamentous structure.

Deformities due to acute injury or illness are classified only to the acute injury or illness to which they pertain; an "acquired deformity" of the nasal septum due to acute fracture of the septum requires one code only (802.0).

738.0	Acquired deformity of nose — *overdevelopment of nasal bones*

738.1 Other acquired deformity of head

Other acquired deformity of head includes deformities of the zygoma and zygomatic arch. The zygoma is the long slender process of the temporal and malar bones on each side of the skull. The bridge formed by the articulation of the temporal and malar processes is the zygomatic arch to which the masseter muscle, which moves the lower jaw (mandible), is attached.

738.10	Unspecified acquired deformity of head — *unknown*
738.11	Zygomatic hyperplasia — *overgrowth*
738.12	Zygomatic hypoplasia — *undergrowth*
738.19	Other specified acquired deformity of head — *not otherwise specified*
738.2	Acquired deformity of neck
738.3	Acquired deformity of chest and rib — *thorax, chest, rib, xiphoid process, pectus carinatum, pectus excavatum*
738.4	Acquired spondylolisthesis

Acquired spondylolisthesis is forward slipping of one vertebral body (with the remainder of the spinal column above it) in relation to the vertebral segment immediately below, not due to congenital deformity or fracture. Acquired spondylolisthesis may be secondary to degenerative disk disease, a late effect of fracture or due to spondylolysis (not qualified as congenital) or pathological weakness of bone.

The subterm "traumatic" listed in the ICD-9-CM index under the main term "Spondylolisthesis" refers to spondylolisthesis due to birth or intrauterine trauma, rather than as a late effect of trauma occurring any time after birth. Traumatic spondylolisthesis is considered a congenital anomaly and is classified to code 756.12. Spondylolisthesis due to acute trauma is classified as a current injury and coded as an acute fracture of the vertebra. Spondylolisthesis as a late effect of trauma, such as a prior fracture of the vertebra, is classified as acquired using the appropriate ICD-9-CM code for late effect (e.g., 905.1).

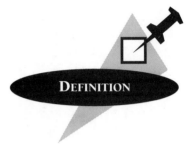

DEFINITION

Acquired: not genetic, but produced by influences outside the organism.

Genetic: determined by the genes.

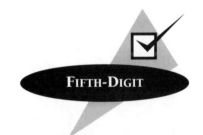

FIFTH-DIGIT

A fifth digit to further defines other acquired deformities of the head as follows:

0 unspecified deformity

1 zygomatic hyperplasia - abnormal increase in the number of cells in the zygomatic tissue

2 zygomatic hypoplasia - deficiency in the size of the zygoma or zygomatic arch

9 other specified deformity

738.5	Other acquired deformity of back or spine	
738.6	Acquired deformity of pelvis — *pelvic obliquity*	
738.7	Cauliflower ear	
738.8	Acquired musculoskeletal deformity of other specified site — *not otherwise specified, including clavicle*	
738.9	Acquired musculoskeletal deformity of unspecified site — *unknown*	

739 NONALLOPATHIC LESIONS, NOT ELSEWHERE CLASSIFIED

739.0	Nonallopathic lesion of head region, not elsewhere classified — *occipitocervical*
739.1	Nonallopathic lesion of cervical region, not elsewhere classified — *cervicothoracic*
739.2	Nonallopathic lesion of thoracic region, not elsewhere classified — *thoracolumbar*
739.3	Nonallopathic lesion of lumbar region, not elsewhere classified — *lumbosacral*
739.4	Nonallopathic lesion of sacral region, not elsewhere classified — *sacrococcygeal, sacroiliac*
739.5	Nonallopathic lesion of pelvic region, not elsewhere classified — *hip, pubic*
739.6	Nonallopathic lesion of lower extremities, not elsewhere classified — *thigh, knee, calf, foot*
739.7	Nonallopathic lesion of upper extremities, not elsewhere classified — *forearm, wrist, hand, upper arm*
739.8	Nonallopathic lesion of rib cage, not elsewhere classified
739.9	Nonallopathic lesion of abdomen and other sites, not elsewhere classified

5th Needs fifth-digit   **OK** Valid three-digit code

740-759
Congenital Anomalies

Congenital anomalies may be the result of genetic factors (chromosomes), teratogens (agents causing physical defects in the embryo), or both. The anomalies may be apparent at birth or hidden and identified sometime after birth. Whatever the cause, congenital anomalies can be attributed to nearly 50 percent of deaths to full-term newborn infants.

Codes in Chapter 14 are classified according to a principal or defining defect rather than to the cause (chromosome abnormalities are the exception). Regardless of the origin, dysmorphology — clinical structural abnormality — is generally the primary indication of a congenital anomaly and, in many cases, a syndrome may be classified according to a single anatomic anomaly rather than a complex of symptoms. For example, Apert's syndrome is classified to 755.55 *Acrocephalosyndactyly*. Rubric 755 classifies reduction deformities of the lower limb, and abnormal bony fusion in the feet is a single anatomic anomaly of the multi-complex syndrome that can include fusion in the hands and facial anomalies.

ICD-9 does not differentiate between abnormalities that are intrinsic — related to the fetus — or extrinsic — as a result of intrauterine problems, although a note in ICD-9 prior to rubric 754 *Certain congenital musculoskeletal deformities* identifies codes as specific to extrinsic factors. However, ICD-9 does make a distinction in the classification of an anomaly as compared to a deformity. An anomaly is a malformation caused by abnormal fetal development, as in transposition of great vessels or spina bifida. A deformity is an alteration in structure caused by an extrinsic force, as in intrauterine compression. The force may cause a disruption in a normal fetal structure, including congenital amputations from amniotic bands.

In some cases, two codes are necessary to describe the condition. For example, the condition thalidomide phocomelia (thalidomide influence on the developing fetus during the perinatal period) requires two codes – 755.23 *Longitudinal deficiency, combined, involving humerus, radius, and ulna (complete or incomplete)* and 760.79 *Noxious influences affecting fetus via placenta or milk*.

There is no clear distinction between what is classified to Chapter 14 and a congenital anomaly classified to another chapter in ICD-9. For example, oligohydramnios, a condition caused by a complication of pregnancy, is classified to Chapter 15, Certain Conditions Originating in the Perinatal Period (760-779). Retinoblastoma, a tumor arising in the fetal retina and diagnosed after birth, is reported with 190.5 *Malignant neoplasm of the retina* from Chapter 2, Neoplasms. The congenital absence of clotting factors is reported with codes in the rubric 286 *Coagulation defects*. Some diseases are reclassified into congenital anomalies in ICD-10, among them, fetal alcohol syndrome, while errors in metabolism are excluded.

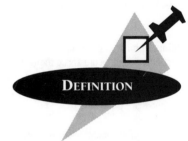

DEFINITION

Congenital anomalies: physical traits that are present at birth, though they may not be detected until some years later. They include diseases, malformations, atresias, agenesis, hypoplastic, or hyperplastic conditions. Congenital anomalies may be due to genetic factors, such as in Down syndrome, to teratogenic factors, such as radiation, infection, and metabolic disorders, or complications of pregnancy, such as placental hemorrhage or compression of the umbilical cord.

Deformation: a congenital defect resulting from intrauterine compression.

Disruption: a congenital defect resulting from interruption of blood supply or by constriction.

Malformation: a congenital defect resulting from a flawed fetal growth process.

Postnatal onset disorder: a congenital disorder not apparent at birth, but discovered sometime thereafter.

Prenatal onset disorder: a congenital disorder apparent at birth.

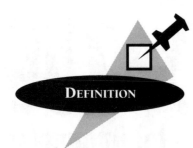

DEFINITION

Craniorachischisis (also known as Antley-Bixler syndrome): condition resulting from the failure of the neural tube fails to close in the brain and spinal cord.

Iniencephaly: in this condition, brain protrudes into the cord space through a defect in the occiput and the infant's head is tilted back at an extreme angle touching the thoracic vertebrae.

Exposure of the neural tissue or meninges is an open defect, while closed defects are covered by skin. This distinction is important, as the occult spina bifida codes are excluded from Category 741. Neural tube defects have an incidence rate of one percent to four percent of all births, and have been associated with low folic acid intake by the mother. Spina bifida is the most common of the neural tube defects.

Cerebellum (means little brain): dorsal and occipital portion of the brain, helps maintain balance, track movement, and coordinates fine voluntary movement such as piano playing.

Medulla oblongata (also known as the brain stem): continuous with the cord and regulates vital functions such as breathing, the heart beat, and serves as the reflex center for coughing, sneezing, swallowing, and vomiting.

Meningomyelocele: describes a herniated membrane (meningeo) and cord (myle) that protrudes though the vertebral column.

Polymicrogyria: describes a malformation of the brain consisting of many (poly), small (micro) folds (gyri).

740 ANENCEPHALUS AND SIMILAR ANOMALIES

Anencephalus is a usually fatal brain defect of newborn caused by a closure of the neural groove early in the first trimester of pregnancy. It can present in several forms:

- The cranial vault may be absent
- The cerebral hemispheres are missing or exist as masses attached to the base of the skull
- The brain is abnormally shaped

Anencephalus is identified in the patient record as acrania, partial or total absence of the skull, amyelencephalus, the absence of the brain and spinal cord, hemianencephaly, absence of half the brain, and hemicephaly, absence of one of the brain hemispheres. Medical management in rubric 740 is attuned to a fatal outcome, whereas the conditions falling into rubric 741 are not necessarily terminal.

740.0	Anencephalus — *Anencephalus; acrania; amyelencephalus; hemicephaly; hemiencephaly*
740.1	Craniorachischisis — *Craniorachischisis; Antley- Bixler syndrome*
740.2	Iniencephaly — *Iniencephaly; protrusion of brain into cord space*

741 SPINA BIFIDA

Citing the location of the lesion is mandatory when coding spina bifida; the "unspecified" fifth digit should be avoided. The presence of absence of hydrocephalus is a second axis in the rubric, while spina bifida occulta is excluded from this rubric and reported with 756.17.

Spina bifida, a defect in the vertebral column, presents in conjunction with several anomalies or it may occur as a solitary anomaly. Prognosis depends both on the number and severity of anomalies and on the size and location of the vertebral defect. Paralysis at the level below the defect is always present when the cord or spinal nerve roots are involved. Defects at the lumbosacral level can cause bladder and rectal problems. The child will often have orthopedic problems such as kyphosis or clubfoot. Death is usually ascribed to shunt complications, including infection and renal failure.

The circulation of the cerebrospinal fluid (CSF) is impeded, causing additional fluid pressure on the brain, in hydrocephalus, a condition that may be categorized as either communicating or non-communicating. In communicating hydrocephalus, there is no obstruction.

Type II is the most serious of the four types of malformations found in Arnold-Chiari or Chiari disease and the only type assigned to this subcategory. In this variation, the inferior poles of the cerebellum and the medulla protrude through the foramen magnum into the spinal canal. It is typically associated with other anomalies such as polymicrogyria, meningomyelocele, and hydrocephalus.

Subclassification 741.9 includes:

- Spinal hydromeningocele: fluid-filled sac composed of meninges protruding through the vertebral column defect
- Hydromyelocele: sac filled with CSF protruding through the wall of the spinal cord
- Meningocele: sac of meninges protruding through the skull or vertebral column
- Meningomyelocele: sac of meninges and cord protruding through the spinal column

✔5th   Needs fifth-digit   **OK**   Valid three-digit code

- Myelocele: protrusion of the cord through the vertebral column

- Myelocystocele: protrusion of cord substance through the spinal canal

- Rachischisis: complete fissure in the vertebral column

- Syringomyelocele: saclike protrusion of the cord which remains in communication with the central canal of the cord

Condition	Antomy Displaced	Nature of Defect	Structural Defect Location
Craniorhachischisis	C + B	Fissure	Skull and Vertebral column
Encephalocystocele	B	Hernia of brain, filled with CSF	Skull
Holoprosencephaly	B	Forebrain defect	Brain
Hydroencephalocele	B	Brain protrudes in a sac	Skull
Hydromeningocele	M	Meninges protrude, filled with CSF	Vertebral column
Iniencephaly	B	brain protrudes into cord space	Skull
Meningoencephalocele	B + M	Brain and meninges protrude	Skull
Micrencephaly	B	abnormally small brain	Brain
Microgyria	B	abnormally small convolutions of brain	Brain
Myelomeningocele	C +M	Meninges and cord protrude	Vertebral column
Hydrocephalus	B	CSF volume too great	Brain (CSF circulation)
Syringomyelocele	C	Hernia cavity communicates with cord	Cord
Myelocystocele	C	Cord substance protrudes	Cord
Myelocele	C	Cord protrudes	Vertebral column

B= Brain   **C= Skull**   **M= Meninges**

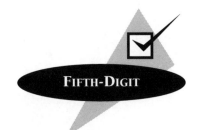

FIFTH-DIGIT

The following fifth-digit subclassification is for use with category 741:

0 unspecified region

1 cervical region

2 dorsal (thoracic) region

3 lumbar region

741.0 ✔5th Spina bifida with hydrocephalus — *Spina bifida with hydrocephalus; Arnold-Chiari syndrome, type II; Dandy-Walker syndrome with spina bifida*

741.9 ✔5th Spina bifida without mention of hydrocephalus — *Spina bifida without mention of hydrocephalus; myelocystocele; spina bifida aperta; myelocele; meningomyelocele*

742 OTHER CONGENITAL ANOMALIES OF NERVOUS SYSTEM

742.0 Encephalocele — *Encephalocele; cerebral meningocele; Arnold-Chiari syndrome Type III; encephalocystocele*

An encephalocele is a neural herniation of brain parenchyma and meninges that protrudes through a cranial defect. Encephalocele is also known as cranium bifidum with encephalocele, hydrencephalocele, and hydrencephalomeningocele. Lesions occur in the occipital region or anywhere in the cranial vault.

742.1 Microcephalus — *Microcephalus; hydromicrocephaly; micrencephaly*

In microcephalus, the head circumference is more than two standard deviations below the mean for age, sex, race and gestation. Anomalous development, such as such as a chromosomal disorder or maternal phenylketonuria, during the first seven months of gestation causes

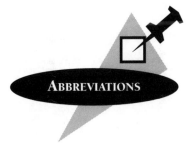

ABBREVIATIONS

Aperta: open

Hydro: water

primary microcephaly. Secondary microcephaly results from an insult, such as infection, trauma, anoxia, or metabolic disorders, during the last two months of gestation or during the perinatal period.

742.2 Congenital reduction deformities of brain — *Reduction deformities of brain; agyria; arhinencephaly; Arnold-Chiari syndrome, type IV*

742.3 Congenital hydrocephalus — *Congenital hydrocephalus; anomaly, congenital obstruction and stenosis of aqueduct of Sylvius; Dandy-Walker syndrome; atresia of foramina of Magendie and Luschka*

Ventricular enlargement, abundant cerebral spinal fluid, and, in most cases, increasing pressure are present in congenital hydrocephalus. In addition, the foramen of Magendie and the foreman of Luschka may be undeveloped, resulting in the obstruction of fluid through the aqueduct of Sylvius, which carries the cerebrospinal fluid between the midbrain and the fourth ventricle. An obstruction of the fourth ventricle outlet, as seen in Dandy-Walker syndrome (741.0 with spina bifida) describes noncommunicating hydrocephalus. Other conditions that may present include arachnoiditis, lesions such as neoplasms, cysts, and hematomas. In addition, the obstruction may be secondary to exudate, hemorrhage, or parasites.

Communicating hydrocephalus may be due to adhesions of the basilar cisterns or surface subarachnoid space following infection or hemorrhage, post developmental adhesions, vitamin A deficiency, developmental failure or erythrocyte obstruction of the arachnoid villi, or Arnold Chiari malformation (741.0).

Acquired hydrocephalus (331.3-331.4) is excluded from this rubric, as is hydrocephalus due to congenital toxoplasmosis (771.2).

Cerebral cysts, macroencephaly, (synonym for megalencephaly) an abnormally large head, large convolutions of the cerebrum, ulegyria, - abnormal convolutions of the cerebrum due to scarring — and porencephaly — a cerebral cyst with an opening into a ventricle — are abnormalities that may progress to hydrocephalus. These conditions are reported with 742.4.

742.4 Other specified congenital anomalies of brain — *Other specified anomalies of brain; macroencephaly; macrogyria; megalencephaly; proencephaly; ulegyria*

742.51 Diastematomyelia — *Diastematomyelia; longitudinal fissure in spinal cord*

Diastematomyelia reports a longitudinal fissure in the spinal cord that results in gait disturbance, muscular atrophy, and lack of sphincter control.

742.53 Hydromyelia — *Hydromyelia; hydrorhachis*

Hydromyelia reports a dilated spinal canal. It is a synonym for hydrorhachis.

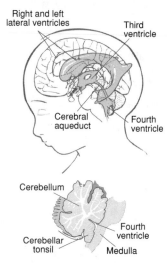

Right and left lateral ventricles
Third ventricle
Cerebral aqueduct
Fourth ventricle

Cerebellum
Fourth ventricle
Cerebellar tonsil
Medulla

Detail of section through brain stem showing part of cerebellum herniating into the brain stem (Chiari malformation)

5th Needs fifth-digit   **OK** Valid three-digit code

Amyelia is the absence of a spinal cord, whereas atelomyelia is an incompletely developed cord. Myelodysplasia and myelatelia are synonymous terms describing a defective spinal cord.

742.59   Other specified congenital anomaly of spinal cord — *Other specified anomalies of spinal cord; amyelia; atelomyelia; myelatelia; myelodysplasia*

742.8   Other specified congenital anomalies of nervous system — *Other specified anomalies of nervous system; jaw-winking syndrome; Marcus-Gunn syndrome; Riley-Day syndrome*

Marcus Gunn syndrome, also known as jaw-winking syndrome, is characterized by the onset of rapid eyelid movement, producing a winking effect, when the jaw moves. The cause is unknown.

Riley-Day syndrome, or familial dysautonomia, is primarily found in families of European-Jewish extraction. Poor sucking ability, sweating while eating, hypotonia, and insensitivity to pain characterize the condition.

742.9   Unspecified congenital anomaly of brain, spinal cord, and nervous system — *Unspecified anomaly of brain, spinal cord, and nervous system; congenital lesion of brain, nervous system or spinal cord*

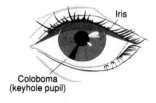

Coloboma
(keyhole pupil)

743 CONGENITAL ANOMALIES OF EYE

Any structure or organ of the body is subject to a failure or deviation in development. Congenital anomalies of the eye are classified according to the specific site affected, and the type of defect. They include:

- Anophthalmos: absence of an eye
- Cryptophthalmos: uninterrupted extension of an eyelid across the eyeball
- Microphthalmos: abnormally small eye

Physicians assess this condition according to levels of debility. Pure microphthalmos, a condition of a small eye with a tendency to angle-closing glaucoma, is reported with 743.12 if the condition causes vision complications. Simple microphthalmos (743.11) is a small eye, which is essentially normal in functionality.

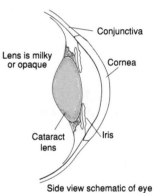

Side view schematic of eye

743.00   Unspecified clinical anophthalmos — *Clinical anophthalmos, unspecified; agenesis of entire eye or part of the eye*

743.03   Cystic eyeball, congenital — *Cystic eyeball, congenital; space occupied by eyeball is a cyst*

743.06   Cryptophthalmos — *Cryptophthalmos; adhesion of eyelid to eyeball*

743.10   Unspecified microphthalmos — *Microphthalmos, unspecified; abnormally small eye*

743.11   Simple microphthalmos — *Simple microphthalmos; a small eye which is essentially normal in function*

743.12   Microphthalmos associated with other anomalies of eye and adnexa — *Microphthalmos associated with other anomalies of eye and adnexa; abnormally small eye appearing with other eye and ocular adnexa anomalies*

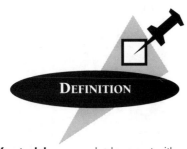

DEFINITION

Keratoglobus: corneal enlargement with a globe-shaped protrusion of the cornea, associated with congenital glaucoma (buphthalmos).

Megalocornea: enlarged cornea associated with buphthalmos.

Cataract positional terminology:

Capsular: cataract is found within the lens capsule.

Cortical: cataract that begins at the outside edges of the lens and extends inward and found at the center of the lens.

Subcapsular: cataract beginning at the back of the lens.

Total: cataract covering the entire surface of the lens.

Axenfeld's anomaly is a white line on the posterior aspect of the iris.

Rieger's anomaly is bilateral and increases the risk of glaucoma. It is associated with a family history of the disease, with other anomalies such as growth hormone deficiency, and a flat nose.

The manifestations of Peter's anomaly vary among individuals. There may be anterior displacement of Schwalbe's line, central corneal opacity, and unilateral or bilateral loss of Descemet's corneal membrane.

Descemet's corneal membrane: membrane between the endothelial layer of the cornea and the substantia propria.

Schwalbe's line: circular bundle of connective tissue forming a thickened part of Descemet's membrane.

Substantia propria: third layer from the exterior of the eye inward toward the cornea.

743.2 Buphthalmos

Buphthalmos is congenital glaucoma. In affected infants, a defect in the iridocorneal angle, an outlet in the anterior chamber of the eye, impedes aqueous circulation. Excluded from this rubric are glaucoma of childhood (365.14) and traumatic glaucoma due to birth injury (767.8).

Glaucoma is an elevated pressure in the aqueous humor. Undetected, glaucoma can lead to nerve damage and blindness. Surgery, directed toward restoring the natural circulation of the aqueous, can prevent loss of sight. A genetic abnormality or an inflammation of the eye prior to birth can cause congenital glaucoma.

743.20 Unspecified buphthalmos — *Buphthalmos, unspecified; congenital glaucoma*
743.21 Simple buphthalmos — *Simple buphthalmos; congenital glaucoma*
743.22 Buphthalmos associated with other ocular anomaly — *Buphthalmos associated with other ocular anomalies; keratoglobus or megalocornea associated with buphthalmos*

743.3 Congenital cataract and lens anomalies

Cataracts are milky or opaque areas on the lens of the eye that translate into milky or opaque disturbances in the field of vision. Infection during development, genetic error, or metabolites residing within the lens may be the cause. Excluded from this rubric are cataracts that are associated with syndromes congenital in nature although not present at birth, as in craniofacial dyostosis (756.0). These cataracts are reported with 366.44.

Other anomalies of the lens include aphakia, or congenital absence of the lens, and anomalies of shape including spherophakia (sphere shaped) or microphakia (small lens). An ectopic lens is a displaced lens.

A coloboma describes a part absent from an ophthalmological structure, due usually to a chromosomal defect, which presents as a fissure of the iris, the ciliary body, or the choroid (thus the common name "keyhole pupil"). It is typically associated with CHARGE syndrome (C/coloboma; H/heart; A/atresia of choanae; R/retarded growth and development; G/genital hypoplasia; E/ear anomalies). Coloboma may increase the risk of iridial tearing and often includes iris and choroid flaws.

743.30 Unspecified congenital cataract — *Congenital cataract, unspecified; congenital cataract NOS*
743.31 Congenital capsular and subcapsular cataract — *Capsular and subcapsular cataract; cataract within lens capsule*
743.32 Congenital cortical and zonular cataract — *Cortical and zonular cataract; cataract begins at periphery of lens and extends inward*
743.33 Congenital nuclear cataract — *Nuclear cataract; cataract located in center of lens*
743.34 Congenital total and subtotal cataract — *Total and subtotal cataract, congenital; all or part of lens covered by cataract*
743.35 Congenital aphakia — *Congenital aphakia; absence of lens*
743.36 Congenital anomalies of lens shape — *Anomalies of lens shape; microphakia; spherophakia*
743.37 Congenital ectopic lens — *Congenital ectopic lens; lens displaced*
743.39 Other congenital cataract and lens anomalies — *Other congenital cataract and lens anomalies*
743.41 Congenital anomaly of corneal size and shape — *Anomalies of corneal size and shape; microcornea*

✓5th Needs fifth-digit   **OK** Valid three-digit code

743.42 Congenital corneal opacity, interfering with vision — *Corneal opacities, interfering with vision, congenital*

743.43 Other congenital corneal opacity

743.44 Specified congenital anomaly of anterior chamber, chamber angle, and related structures — *Specified anomalies of anterior chamber, chamber angle, and related structures; Axenfeld's; Peters'*

743.45 Aniridia — *Aniridia; incomplete formation of iris*

Aniridia, the incomplete formation of the iris, results in vision loss. Typically, aniridia is bilateral and gives the appearance of black irises though it is the pupil - and not the iris - which is dark. An autosomal-dominant or autosomal-recessive gene can be a cause and, if so determined, the child may have other health or developmental problems.

743.46 Other specified congenital anomaly of iris and ciliary body — *Other specified anomalies of iris and ciliary body; anisocoria, congenital; atresia of pupil*

Anisocoria, or unequal pupils, is a common condition. In corectopia, the pupil is asymmetrically placed in the iris. Children with iris colobomata should be checked for fissure of the optic nerve and of the fundus.

743.47 Specified congenital anomaly of sclera — *Specified anomalies of sclera;*

743.48 Multiple and combined congenital anomalies of anterior segment of eye — *Multiple and combined anomalies of anterior segment; anisocoria combined with Peters' anomaly*

743.49 Other congenital anomaly of anterior segment of eye — *Other anomalies of anterior segment*

743.51 Vitreous anomaly, congenital — *Vitreous anomalies; congenital vitreous opacity*

743.52 Fundus coloboma — *Fundus coloboma; fissure in fundus*

743.53 Congenital chorioretinal degeneration — *Chorioretinal degeneration, congenital*

743.54 Congenital folds and cysts of posterior segment of eye — *Congenital folds and cysts of posterior segment*

743.55 Congenital macular change — *Congenital macular changes*

743.56 Other congenital retinal changes — *Other retinal changes, congenital*

743.57 Specified congenital anomalies of optic disc — *Specified anomalies of optic disk; coloboma of optic disk*

743.58 Congenital vascular anomalies of posterior segment of eye — *Vascular anomalies; congenital retinal aneurysm; tortuous retina vessel*

743.59 Other congenital anomalies of posterior segment of eye — *Other congenital anomalies of posterior segment*

743.61 Congenital ptosis of eyelid — *Congenital ptosis; congenital drooping of eyelid*

A severe case of ptosis is treated immediately after birth since it can disrupt visual development. In less than severe cases, treatment is delayed until the child reaches three to five years of age.

743.62 Congenital deformity of eyelid — *Congenital deformities of eyelids; ablepharon; congenital ectropion and entropion*

Ablepharon, the congenital absence of an eyelid, seldom appears as a solitary variant, which is typical of agenesis anomalies.

An accessory eyelid is an additional eyelid.

Entropion is inversion of the lower eyelid, whereas ectropion is the eversion of the lower eyelid. Both conditions require surgical correction since rubbing caused by the displacement often scars the cornea.

743.63 Other specified congenital anomaly of eyelid — *Other specified congenital anomalies of eyelid*

743.64 Specified congenital anomaly of lacrimal gland — *Specified congenital anomalies of lacrimal gland*

743.65 Specified congenital anomaly of lacrimal passages — *Specified congenital anomalies of lacrimal passages; lacrimal apparatus atresia*

The lacrimal glands produce the tears that moisten the eyes to keep them healthy. Tears are produced at each blink and pumped down and across the eye. Any excess tears drain through the tear duct and into the nose, which explains why our noses run when we cry. Excess tears can also be dangerous. Surgery may be required to open ducts obstructed by puss in an infection resulting from stagnant tears.

743.66 Specified congenital anomaly of orbit — *Specified congenital anomalies of orbit; specified anomalies of orbit NEC*

743.69 Other congenital anomalies of eyelids, lacrimal system, and orbit — *Other congenital anomalies of eyelids, lacrimal system, and orbit*

743.8 Other specified congenital anomalies of eye — *Other specified anomalies of eye; megalophthalmos; Norrie's disease*

743.9 Unspecified congenital anomaly of eye — *Unspecified anomaly of eye; congenital anomaly NOS*

744 CONGENITAL ANOMALIES OF EAR, FACE, AND NECK

Codes in this rubric are classified according to site and the impairment associated with the anomaly. The most significant codes in this rubric are those reporting hearing impairments, classified to 744.0. Congenital deafness, without mention of cause, is excluded from this rubric and is reported with codes from the series 389.0-389.9.

744.00 Unspecified congenital anomaly of ear causing impairment of hearing — *Unspecified anomaly of ear with impairment of hearing*

744.01 Congenital absence of external ear causing impairment of hearing — *Absence of external ear; agenesis of auditory canal*

744.02 Other congenital anomaly of external ear causing impairment of hearing — *Other anomalies of external ear with impairment of hearing; atresia or stricture of auditory canal (external)*

744.03 Congenital anomaly of middle ear, except ossicles, causing impairment of hearing — *Anomaly of middle ear, except ossicles; atresia or stricture of osseous meatus*

744.04 Congenital anomalies of ear ossicles — *Anomalies of ear ossicles; fusion of ear ossicles*

744.05 Congenital anomalies of inner ear — *Anomalies of inner ear; congenital anomaly of membranous labyrinth; Mondini dysplasia*

744.09 Other congenital anomalies of ear causing impairment of hearing — *Other anomalies of ear causing impairment of hearing; agenesis of ear*

744.1 Congenital anomalies of accessory auricle — *Accessory auricle; polyotia; preauricular tag; supernumerary tag*

744.21 Congenital absence of ear lobe — *Absence of ear lobe, congenital; agenesis of ear lobe*

744.22 Macrotia — *Macrotia; abnormally large external ear*

5th Needs fifth-digit   **OK** Valid three-digit code

744.23 Microtia — *Microtia; abnormally small external ear*

Microtia, external auditory canal atresia and ossicular fusion often occur together. Auricle atresia is associated with craniofacial syndromes such as Treacher-Collins and Nager syndromes, but may occur in solitary.

744.24 Specified congenital anomaly of Eustachian tube — *Specified anomalies of Eustachian tube; agenesis of Eustachian tube*

744.29 Other congenital anomaly of ear — *Other specified anomalies of ear; bat ear; melotia; Darwin's tubercle*

Large and protruding ears, called Bat ear, is a large, can be surgically modified. Polyotia is the presence of an accessory auricle. Pointed ear, Stahl's ear, and Spoke ear describe ears pointed at the top. Darwin's tubercle, a prominence on the upper posterior of the superior ridge of the auricle; is a vestigial remnant of a folded ear.

744.3 Unspecified congenital anomaly of ear — *Unspecified anomaly of ear; congenital deformity of ear, NOS*

744.4 Branchial cleft cyst or fistula; preauricular sinus

Branchial cleft relates to embryonic development of the external auricle, the external auditory meatus, and the tympanic membrane. A sinus is a blind ending tract. A fistula is an open-ended tract.

744.41 Congenital branchial cleft sinus or fistula — *Branchial cleft sinus or fistula; branchial sinus; branchial arch syndrome*

744.42 Congenital branchial cleft cyst — *Branchial cleft cyst; fluid filled space in branchial cleft*

744.43 Congenital cervical auricle — *Cervical auricle*

744.46 Congenital preauricular sinus or fistula

744.47 Congenital preauricular cyst — *Preauricular cyst; fluid filled space or sac in front of auricle*

744.49 Other congenital branchial cleft cyst or fistula; preauricular sinus — *Other branchial cleft cyst or fistula; preauricular sinus*

744.5 Congenital webbing of neck — *Webbing of neck; pterygium colli*

Pterygium colli is a webbed effect produced by an anomalous band of fascia extending from the mastoid process to the clavicle.

744.81 Macrocheilia — *Macrocheilia; congenital hypertrophy of lip*

744.82 Microcheilia — *Microcheilia; congenital hypoplasia of lip*

Microcheilia is an abnormally small lip.

744.83 Macrostomia — *Macrostomia; abnormally large mouth*

744.84 Microstomia — *Microstomia; abnormally small mouth*

Microstomia is an abnormally small mouth.

744.89 Other specified congenital anomaly of face and neck — *Other specified anomalies of face and neck; agenesis of chin*

744.9 Unspecified congenital anomaly of face and neck — *Unspecified anomalies of face and neck; congenital anomaly of face and neck, NOS*

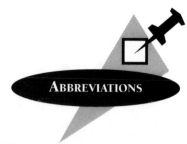

ABBREVIATIONS

ASD: atrial septal defect, a congenital defect of the heart due to incomplete closure of the atrial septum

LA, LV: left artery, left ventricle

PDA: patent ductus arteriosus

RA RV: right atrium, right ventricle

VSD: ventricular septal defect, a congenital defect of the heart due to incomplete closure of the septum between the cardiac ventricles

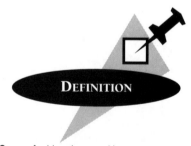

DEFINITION

Cyanosis: blue tinge to skin

Circulation, Pulmonary: superior vena cava and inferior vena cava > RA >RV> pulmonary artery > lungs > pulmonary vein > LA >LV >aorta >systemic circulation

Circulation, Systemic: LA>LV >aorta > main arteries > lesser arteries> arterioles> capillaries > venules > lesser veins > major veins > superior or inferior vena cava> RA

Great vessels: major vessels entering and leaving the heart: superior and inferior vena cava, pulmonary artery and vein, aorta

745-747 Congenital Anomalies of the Cardiovascular System

One percent of all births has a cardiac anomaly. The evaluation of an infant or child with a cardiac anomaly must determine the anomalous pattern of vascularity, cardiac enlargement, and if cyanosis present, or a combination of the possible irregularities. An anomalous vascular pattern indicates abnormal circulation. An anomalous vascularity is characterized as a transposition or transposition complex anomaly. The term "transposition" refers to the normal anterior-to-posterior relationships of the vessels. An enlarged heart requires an evaluation of the chambers to determine extent of the anomaly. Cyanosis is the most common variant, followed by volume load disorders.

745 BULBUS CORDIS ANOMALIES AND ANOMALIES OF CARDIAL SEPTAL CLOSURE

Bulbus cordis relates to embryological development of the fetal heart. Persistent truncus arteriosus is the failure of the aorticopulmonary trunk to divide at the correct developmental stage. There are four classifications and an infant born with the condition presents as cyanotic and tachypneic, and may be struggling with congestive heart failure due to the effects of the abnormally increased pulmonary artery blood flow. The infant may require the Rastelli procedure, which involves separating the pulmonary artery from the primitive truncus to create a right ventricle-to-pulmonary artery conduit.

745.0   Bulbus cordis anomalies and anomalies of cardiac septal closure, common truncus — *Common truncus; absent septum; persistent truncus arteriosus*

745.10   Complete transposition of great vessels — *Complete transposition of great vessels; classical transposition of great vessels*

745.11   Transposition of great vessels, double outlet right ventricle — *Double outlet ventricle; dextratransposition of aorta; Taussig-Bing syndrome*

Double outlet right ventricle is a cyanotic congenital heart disease, affecting more males than females, and presents within the first 24 hours after birth. The infant is often cyanotic and tachypneic, and congestive heart failure is probable. Survival depends on the existence of a ventricular septal defect, an atrial septal defect, or a patent ductus arteriosus, which allow communication between the pulmonary and systemic circulations. Many of the operative procedures work with the anomalous anatomy to achieve operational pulmonary and systemic circulations. For example, the Jantene operation creates a corrective arterial switch.

In Taussig-Bing syndrome, the aorta is in the right ventricle, the pulmonary artery is located in both ventricles, and a ventricular septal defect is present. The child is often cyanotic due to the oxygen insufficiency resulting from the anomalies.

745.12   Corrected transposition of great vessels — *Corrected transposition of great vessels; "status post transposition surgery"*

Report 745.12 to identify a newborn with a transposition syndrome subsequently corrected since this transposition often involves sequelae.

745.19   Other transposition of great vessels — *Other transposition of great vessels*

745.2   Tetralogy of Fallot — *Tetralogy of Fallot; Fallot's pentalogy*

✔5th   Needs fifth-digit   **OK**   Valid three-digit code

The tetralogy of Fallot represents eight percent of all congenital heart diseases. The anomaly, which presents by six months, is a cyanotic and transposition syndrome. A right aortic arch, abnormal origin of coronary arteries, a left superior vena cava, and an enlarged bronchial artery are characteristic. Palliative repairs are performed in the early years, with definitive repair reserved until five to seven years of age, using the Blalock-Taussig, Pohl's, or Waterston-Cooley operations. This code excludes Fallot's triad, which is reported with 746.09.

745.3 Bulbus cordis anomalies and anomalies of cardiac septal closure, common ventricle — *Common ventricle; cor triloculare biatriatum*

A single ventricle arises from the absence of a ventricular septum. Typically, there is transposition of the great vessels, cardiomegaly, cyanosis, congestive heart failure, and mixed pulmonary and system circulation.

745.4 Ventricular septal defect — *Ventricular septal defect; Eisenmenger's defect; Gerbo defect; Roger's disease*

Ventricular septal defects (VSD) may appear as solitary anomalies or present as part of a syndrome, such as Holt-Roan syndrome, trisomy 13, 18, and 21, and tetralogy of Fallot. A VSD may involve both the membranous and muscular portions of the ventricles. Approximately 80 percent involve the membranous septum. Within two months to three months of birth, the infant presents with congestive heart failure. Treatment includes patching the VSD, pulmonary artery banding, and medical therapy. Common atrioventricular canal type anomalies (745.69) and single ventricle anomalies (745.3) are excluded from this code.

Eisenmenger's syndrome is a progressive cyanotic condition characterized by a VSD, pulmonary hypertension, and combined pulmonary and systemic circulations. A small, asymptomatic VSD is a primary characteristic of Roger's disease, also reported with 745.4.

745.5 Ostium secundum type atrial septal defect — *Ostium secundum type atrial septal defect; Lutembacher's syndrome; patent or persistent foramen ovale*

Ostium secundum accounts for 90 percent of all atrial septal defects (ASD). Treatment depends on the age of the patient at evaluation and usually involves applying a patch to the ASD. An ASD left untreated can cause right heart failure, atrial fibrillation later in life, and the increased risk of blood clots leading to a stroke.

Lutembacher's syndrome, reported with 745.5, is an ASD in conjunction with mitral rheumatic stenosis. A patent foramen ovale, also reported with 745.5, is treated when other heart defects are present. The foramen ovale normally closes shortly after birth.

745.6 Endocardial cushion defects

There are three classifications of cushion defects: complete, partial, and intermediate. A complete defect presents with congestive heart failure and all types demonstrate ostium primum. A partial defect is the most common. About 40 percent of cushion anomalies are associated with trisomy-21 (Down's syndrome), which is separately reported with 758.0.

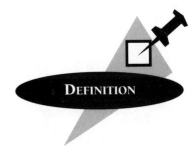

DEFINITION

Ostium primum: describes an ASD high on the septum between the two atria. The opening is normal in the fetus to compensate for the lack of an independent pulmonary circulation, which begins to function immediately after birth.

Ostium secundum: describes an ASD low on the septum between the two atria. The opening is normal in the fetus to compensate for the fetal lack of an independent pulmonary circulation, which begins to function immediately after birth.

Stenosis: refers to a narrowing of an artery in conjunction with cardiac anomalies.

745.60 Unspecified type congenital endocardial cushion defect — *Endocardial cushion defect, unspecified type*

745.61 Ostium primum defect — *Ostium primum defect; persistent ostium primum*

745.69 Other congenital endocardial cushion defect — *Other endocardial cushion defects; agenesis of atrial septum; single atrium*

745.7 Cor biloculare — *Cor biloculare; agenesis of atrial and ventricular septa*

Cor biloculare describes a heart lacking both an atrial and a ventricular septum. A two-chambered heart severely compromises the newborn and few born with the condition live to the first year.

745.8 Other bulbus cordis anomalies and anomalies of cardiac septal closure — *Other bulbus cordis anomalies and anomalies of cardiac septal closure; cor triloculare; cor unilocular; persistent bulbus cordis in left ventricle*

745.9 Unspecified congenital defect of septal closure — *Unspecified defect of septal closure; septal defect NOS*

746 OTHER CONGENITAL ANOMALIES OF HEART

Endocardial fibroelastosis is excluded from this rubric and reported with 425.3.

746.00 Unspecified congenital pulmonary valve anomaly — *Pulmonary valve anomaly, unspecified*

746.01 Congenital atresia of pulmonary valve — *Atresia, congenital; congenital absence of pulmonary valve*

Absence of the pulmonary valve is associated with hypoplastic right heart structures. An infant becomes critically ill when the foramen ovale and PDA close and result in impaired pulmonary circulation. A shunt may be placed between the aorta and the pulmonary artery or a pulmonary artery may be implanted to correct the problem.

746.02 Congenital stenosis of pulmonary valve — *Stenosis, congenital*

A ventricle may become enlarged to compensate for the slow down of blood circulation due to a narrowed valve. Severe stenosis, reported with 746.02, requires surgical repair and lifelong antibiotic prophylaxis.

746.09 Other congenital anomalies of pulmonary valve — *Other anomalies of pulmonary valve; Fallot's triad; supernumerary pulmonic cusps*

Other pulmonary insufficiencies are managed medically. The trilogy or triad of Fallot involves pulmonary stenosis, ASD, and right ventricular hypertrophy.

746.1 Congenital tricuspid atresia and stenosis — *Tricuspid atresia and stenosis, congenital; absence of tricuspid valve*

746.2 Ebstein's anomaly — *Ebstein's anomaly; malformation of tricuspid valve leaflets and atrial-septal defect*

In Ebstein's anomaly, the tricuspid valve is displaced downward, which can lead to fatigue palpitations and dyspnea. A portion of the RV is atrialized (i.e., thinned and dysplastic). Dilated tricuspid annulus and a dilated RA are present. Of the four classifications, "D" is the most severe, manifesting with nearly total atrialization of the RV and other cardiac anomalies such as ASD and Wolff-Parkinson-White syndrome.

✔5th Needs fifth-digit   **OK** Valid three-digit code

746.3   Congenital stenosis of aortic valve — *Congenital stenosis of aortic valve; congenital aortic stenosis*

746.4   Congenital insufficiency of aortic valve — *Congenital insufficiency of aortic valve; bicuspid aortic valve; congenital aortic insufficiency*

Thickened and stiffened valves may cause the stenosis or it may be due to the valve having only one or two cusps. If severe, the stenosis produces fatigue, dizziness, and fainting.

746.5   Congenital mitral stenosis — *Congenital mitral stenosis; fused commissure; parachute deformity*

Fusion of the commissures of the valve causes mitral stenosis. The valves are not calcific and the treatment is a commissurotomy.

746.6   Congenital mitral insufficiency — *Congenital mitral insufficiency; backflow from incomplete valve closure*

Mitral insufficiency is regurgitation or back flow into the RA leading to decreased systemic flow. The condition overworks the heart in its efforts to pump blood to the body's periphery.

746.7   Hypoplastic left heart syndrome — *Hypoplastic left heart syndrome; atresia of aortic valve and hypoplastic aorta and left ventricle*

Hypoplastic left heart syndrome accounts for 10 percent of all heart defects. The LV is tiny; and symptoms include stenosis or atresia of the aortic and mitral valves and coarctation of the aorta. The condition can be critical and treatments include heart transplant and palliative reconstruction. If a transplant is necessary, large amounts of donor aorta must be used in the reconstruction of the aorta. Reconstruction, if the selected treatment, is performed in stages (i.e., the Norwood procedure is performed immediately, followed by the Glenn procedure three months to six months later, and the Fontan reconstructive procedure at 18 months to 24 months of age).

746.81   Congenital subaortic stenosis — *Subaortic stenosis; Narrowing below aortic valve*

In subaortic stenosis, the LV works hard to push the blood past the coarctation of the aorta, a condition that leads to cardiomegaly and congestive heart failure. A mild condition requires no surgery unless, over time, the stenosis worsens and leads to severe tachycardia, tachypnea, and eventually into congestive heart failure. Other milder complications include fatigue, chest pain, and fainting.

746.82   Cor triatriatum — *Cor triatriatum; left atrium divided in two leading to 3 atria*

In cor triatriatum, a small extra chamber above the LA receives the blood from the pulmonary vein. This extra chamber hampers the force of the blood entering the LA and, as a result, congestive heart failure may result.

746.83   Congenital infundibular pulmonic stenosis — *Infundibular pulmonic stenosis; subvalvular stenosis*

Infundibular pulmonic stenosis is a narrowing of the outflow tract of the right ventricle below the pulmonary valve within the infundibulum. The

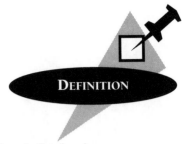

DEFINITION

Cusp: leaflet of a valve.

Wolff-Parkinson-White syndrome: condition characterized by an extra conduction pathway prior to the AV nodes, which leads to premature electrical signals to the ventricles. Symptoms include tachycardia, dizziness, palpitations, fainting, and cardiac arrest. If the patient is refractory to medication, either catheter or radiofrequency ablation is performed to restore the primacy of the AV nodes in electrical conduction.

condition is due to a fibrous diaphragm or to a long, narrow fibromuscular channel.

746.84 Congenital obstructive anomalies of heart, not elsewhere classified — *Obstructive anomalies of heart, NEC; Uhl's disease*

Uhl's disease is a RV spongiform dysplasia, characteristically with paper-thin ventricle walls.

746.85 Congenital coronary artery anomaly — *Coronary artery anomaly; arteriovenous malformation of coronary artery*

Anomalous Left Coronary Artery Originating from Pulmonary Artery (ALCAPA), is a serious condition and, if left untreated, only about 20 percent of children survive beyond adolescence. A single coronary artery is inadequate for perfusion and infarctions leave the heart dependent on collateral circulation to perfuse the left ventricle. Surgery establishes a two-coronary artery system through re-vascularization.

746.86 Congenital heart block — *Congenital heart block; complete or partial atrioventricular block*

Congenital heart block appears as both a sole congenital variant and as part of a syndrome of congenital anomalies. An isolated variant may be associated with autoimmune diseases in the mother. In these situations, the infants are born with neonatal lupus syndrome, which disappears after six months of age. The heart block does not disappear. Whatever the origin of the disorder, diminished cardiac output progresses to congestive heart failure. The infant is surgically treated with pacemaker implantation.

746.87 Congenital malposition of heart and cardiac apex — *Malposition of heart and cardiac apex; abdominal heart; dextrocardia*

There are four types of dextrocardia:

1. Dextroposition: extrinsic factor causes the heart to shift to the right, leading to hypoplastic right lung, a partial anomaly of the pulmonary venous connection to the inferior vena cava, and right-sided pulmonary collaterals.

2. Dextroversion: abnormal rotation of the cardiac loops in embryological development leads to atrioventricular or ventriculoatrial discordance, or a single ventricle, which may be part of Cantrell syndrome: omphalocele or other midline defect, lower sternal defect, anterior inferior diaphragmatic defect, parietal pericardial defect, and left ventricular diverticulum.

3. Ventriculoatrial situs inversus is associated with tetralogy of Fallot, and Kartagener's syndrome. Excluded from 746.87 is dextrocardia with complete transposition of viscera, which is reported with 759.3.

4. Levocardia: includes four variants: 1) situs solitus with normal heart, 2) levoposition (heart shifts to left in mediastinum due to dysgenesis

of left lung), 3) levoversion of situs inversus, atrioventricular and ventriculoatrial discordance, 4) situs ambiguous.

Dextrocardia and levocardia are both reported with 746.87 in ICD-9-CM, but each has its own specific code in ICD-10-CM.

Ectopic cordis is a serious anomaly in which the sternum is split and the heart protrudes (most common form), or the heart is displaced to the abdomen or neck. A newborn with the condition generally dies within a few days of birth in nearly 100 percent of cases. Ectopic cordis is reported with 746.87.

746.89   Other specified congenital anomaly of heart — *Other specified anomalies of heart; congenital cardiomegaly; bifid apex of heart; diverticula of heart*

In diverticulum of the left ventricle, the diverticulum protrudes into the epigastrium. It may or may not be an isolated anomaly.

Brugada syndrome is a combination of right bundle branch block, ST elevation, and arrhythmic right ventricular dysplasia (ARVD), which results in abnormal left ventricular electrophysiology and sudden death. The condition runs in families and is treated by implantation of an automatic cardioverter-defibrillator.

746.9   Unspecified congenital anomaly of heart — *Unspecified anomaly of heart; congenital cardiac anomaly NOS*

747 OTHER CONGENITAL ANOMALIES OF CIRCULATORY SYSTEM

747.0   Patent ductus arteriosus — *Patent ductus arteriosus; patent ductus Botalli; persistent ductus arteriosus*

Other terms for patent ductus arteriosus (PDA) are persistent ductus arteriosus, or patent ductus Botallo. The incidence is greater in females and it is one of the most common cardiovascular anomalies. The ductus arteriosus is patent during fetal life for breathing through the umbilical cord and, in most infants, closes within a few weeks of birth. A patent ductus arteriosus allows the lungs to be bypassed until birth, shunting right ventricular blood to the aorta. The condition presents two ways: if the infant is premature, the patency typically closes once the infant reaches the appropriate developmental stage. If the infant is term, with persistent patency, the infant will experience elevated left heart pressures and increased pulmonary circulation, putting undue strain on the left heart and pulmonary vasculature, leading to pulmonary vascular disease and congestive heart failure. There is an increased risk of bacterial endocarditis. PDAs are surgically corrected, no matter their size, due to probable complications.

747.10   Coarctation of aorta (preductal) (postductal) — *Coarctation of aorta (preductal) (postductal); hypoplasia of aortic arch*

Coarctation refers to a pinching in of the aortic arch, forcing the left heart to pump past the obstruction, which leads to enlargement, increased blood pressure in arteries behind the obstruction, decreased pressure in arteries

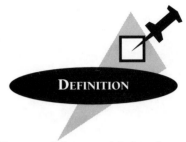

DEFINITION

Situs: normal placement of the heart in the mediastinum is intertwined with normal placement of the lungs and abdominal viscera, with cardiac apex pointing to right.

Situs Ambiguous: structures normally asymmetrical are symmetrical and the visceral locations and morphology are indeterminate. Asplenia is a situs ambiguous syndrome characterized by absence of a spleen, a hypoplastic heart, bilateral right sided bronchial trees, a horizontal liver, and stomach placement at the midline.

Situs Inversus: heart, abdominal viscera, and lungs are switched. (Dextrocardia with situs inversus allows normal cardiac function since there is ample room for proper functioning of the organs and no other associated cardiac anomaly.)

Situs Solitus: heart is out of position, while the abdominal viscera and lungs are in normal position.

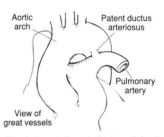

The ductus arteriosus is the natural shunt that bypasses lung circulation in the prenatal phase

Aortic ring syndrome

post obstruction, and congestive heart failure. In post obstruction, the aorta may enlarge to increase the risk of dilation, aneurysm, rupture, and stroke. Patients with coarctation are at lifelong risk for bacterial endocarditis and for myocardial infarction. The obstruction is resected as soon as possible after birth and the same procedure may need to be repeated in adulthood. The congestive failure subsides after corrective surgery, although there may be persistent pulmonary hypertension.

747.11 Congenital interruption of aortic arch — *Interruption of aortic arch; part of aortic arch is missing*

747.20 Unspecified congenital anomaly of aorta — *Anomaly of arch, unspecified*

747.21 Congenital anomaly of aortic arch — *Anomalies of aortic arch; dextroposition of aorta; aortic ring syndrome; persistent right aortic arch*

An anomalous arch in double aortic arch encircles the trachea or the esophagus, leading to tracheal compression and subsequent proclivity to repeated respiratory infections. The anomalous arch may be patent and always causes difficulty because of its position.

747.22 Congenital atresia and stenosis of aorta — *Atresia and stenosis of aorta; hypoplasia of aorta; stricture of aorta*

Aortic stenosis is a progressive condition that rarely produces symptoms in the young. Progressive elevated resistance to the pumping action of the left ventricle leads to increased LV pressure and hypertrophy. Hypertrophy weakens the heart and is prodromal to heart failure. The thicker and stiffer the ventricle walls, the weaker the pumping action. The two most common forms of aortic stenosis are valvular obstruction resulting from a defect in the valve, and subaortic obstruction, found in the Left Ventricular Outlet Tract. The condition may be an isolated phenomenon or appear in conjunction with VSD, PDA, and coarctation of the aorta.

747.29 Other congenital anomaly of aorta — *Other anomalies of aorta*

Aneurysms of the sinus of Valsalva may not be apparent until adulthood. If rupture occurs, the patient is subject to congestive heart failure and sudden death. Typically, the rupture occurs in either the right or left coronary sinus leading to an acute right-to-left shunt.

747.3 Congenital anomalies of pulmonary artery — *Anomalies of pulmonary artery; coarctation of pulmonary artery; stenosis of pulmonary artery*

Agenesis of the pulmonary artery is rare, occurring on the left more than on the right, and is usually a benign variation. When symptomatic, it results in frequent respiratory tract infections with bronchiectasis.

747.40 Congenital anomaly of great veins unspecified — *Anomaly of great veins, unspecified; anomaly NOS of pulmonary vein*

747.41 Total congenital anomalous pulmonary venous connection — *Total anomalous pulmonary venous return; TAPVR*

Total anomalous pulmonary venous return (TAPVR) allows oxygenated blood to drain into the right atrium (normally the recipient of deoxygenated blood). ASD often accompanies the condition that is treated

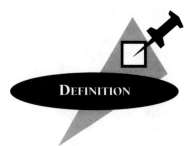

DEFINITION

Coronary sinus, left: located in left atrium.

Coronary sinus, right: located in right atrium.

↙5th Needs fifth-digit   **OK** Valid three-digit code

by severing the pulmonary return to the RA and creating a return to the LA.

747.42   Partial congenital anomalous pulmonary venous connection — *Partial anomalous pulmonary venous return PAPVR*

Partial anomalous pulmonary venous return (PAPVR) is rarely clinically significant unless associated with sinus venosus ASD, which elevates it to significant importance.

747.49   Other congenital anomalies of great veins — *Other anomalies of great veins; congenital stenosis superior or inferior vena cava*

In Scimitar syndrome, one lobe of the left lung is hypoplastic leading to a right shift by the heart. PAPVR is usually present, the thoracic aorta or the celiac axis supplies blood to the aorta, and there are diaphragmatic and thoracic defects.

Persistent left superior vena cava (LSVC), the most common thoracic venous anomaly is a remnant of a structure normally disappearing during embryological development and, if a solitary variant, is seldom symptomatic or significant.

747.5   Congenital absence or hypoplasia of umbilical artery — *Absence or hypoplasia of umbilical artery; single umbilical artery*

747.60   Congenital anomaly of the peripheral vascular system, unspecified site — *Anomaly of peripheral vascular system, unspecified site*

747.61   Congenital gastrointestinal vessel anomaly — *Gastrointestinal vessel anomaly; anomaly of blood vessel serving digestive system*

747.62   Congenital renal vessel anomaly — *Renal vessel anomaly; anomaly of blood vessel serving kidney*

747.63   Congenital upper limb vessel anomaly — *Upper limb vessel anomaly; anomaly of blood vessel serving arms or hands*

747.64   Congenital lower limb vessel anomaly — *Lower limb vessel anomaly; anomaly of blood vessel serving legs or feet*

747.69   Congenital anomaly of other specified site of peripheral vascular system — *Anomalies of other specified sites of peripheral vascular system*

747.81   Congenital anomaly of cerebrovascular system — *Anomalies of cerebrovascular system; cerebral arteriovenous malformation*

747.82   Congenital spinal vessel anomaly — *Spinal vessel anomaly; arteriovenous malformation of spinal vessel*

747.89   Other specified congenital anomaly of circulatory system — *Other specified anomalies of circulatory system; congenital aneurysm, specified site, NEC; persistent pulmonary hypertension; pseudoarteriosus*

747.9   Unspecified congenital anomaly of circulatory system — *Unspecified anomaly of circulatory system*

748 CONGENITAL ANOMALIES OF RESPIRATORY SYSTEM

Excluded from this rubric is congenital defect of the diaphragm, which is reported with 756.6.

748.0   Congenital choanal atresia — *Choanal atresia; congenital stenosis of nares (anterior or posterior)*

748.1   Other congenital anomaly of nose — *Other anomalies of nose; absent nose; cleft nose; deformity of wall of nasal sinus*

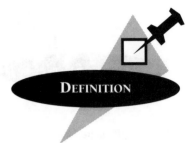

DEFINITION

Sinus venosus ASD: similar to ostium secundum (see 745.5), except that in sinus venosus ASD, the pulmonary arterial pressure is higher, the incidence of pulmonary vascular resistance is greater, and it occurs at a younger age.

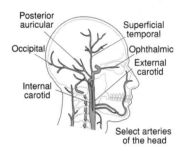

Select arteries of the head

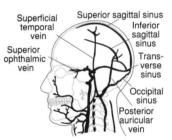

Select veins of the head

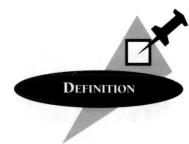

Bilateral cleft palate, lips; structure fails to join at midline.

Cheilopalatoschisis: cleft lip and cleft palate.

Cheiloschisis: cleft lip, a defect involving the lip and the nose.

Incomplete cleft palate, incomplete cleft lip: only soft palate is involved.

Incomplete cleft lip: lip is partially split.

Antimongoloid slant: downward slant of the palpebral fissures.

Clinodactyly: minor deformity of a curved, short fifth finger.

Mongoloid slant: upward slant of the palpebral fissures.

748.2	Congenital web of larynx — *Web of larynx; subglottic web of larynx*
748.3	Other congenital anomaly of larynx, trachea, and bronchus — *Other anomalies of larynx, trachea, and bronchus; agenesis of bronchus; epiglottal atresia*
748.4	Congenital cystic lung — *Congenital cystic lung; congenital polycystic lung*
748.5	Congenital agenesis, hypoplasia, and dysplasia of lung — *Agenesis, hypoplasia, and dysplasia of lung; hypoplasia of lung or lobe of lung; sequestration of lung*
748.60	Unspecified congenital anomaly of lung — *Anomaly of lung, unspecified*
748.61	Congenital bronchiectasis — *Congenital bronchiectasis; congenital dilatation of bronchus (I)*
748.69	Other congenital anomaly of lung — *Other anomalies of lung; accessory lung; azygos lobe of lung*
748.8	Other specified congenital anomaly of respiratory system — *Other specified anomalies of respiratory system; congenital cyst of mediastinum; pleural folds anomaly*
748.9	Unspecified congenital anomaly of respiratory system — *Unspecified anomaly of respiratory system; anomaly of respiratory system, NOS*

749 CLEFT PALATE AND CLEFT LIP

Cleft palate is the fourth most common birth defect and the most common facial birth defect, affecting approximately one out of every 700 infants. While it is associated with multiple defect syndromes, it is typically associated with a cleft lip, occurring in the first few weeks of fetal development, and is multi-factorial in cause. Cleft palate is repaired at six months to 12 months of age and may require follow up surgery at a later age. If the cleft involves the gum line, an alveolar bone graft is used in the restorative surgery.

749.00	Unspecified cleft palate — *Cleft palate, unspecified; unspecified anomaly of cleft palate*
749.01	Unilateral cleft palate, complete — *Unilateral cleft palate, complete; complete cleft of palate on one side only of midline*
749.02	Unilateral cleft palate, incomplete — *Unilateral cleft palate, incomplete; cleft uvula*
749.03	Bilateral cleft palate, complete — *Bilateral cleft palate, complete; complete cleft of palate on each side of midline*
749.04	Bilateral cleft palate, incomplete — *Bilateral cleft palate, incomplete; incomplete cleft of palate on both sides of midline*
749.10	Unspecified cleft lip — *Cleft lip, unspecified; notched lip, congenital*
749.11	Unilateral cleft lip, complete — *Unilateral cleft lip, complete; cleft goes totally through lip on one side of midline*
749.12	Unilateral cleft lip, incomplete — *Unilateral cleft lip, incomplete; one sided cleft not going through entire lip at midline*
749.13	Bilateral cleft lip, complete — *Bilateral cleft lip, complete; cleft goes completely through lip on both sides of midline*
749.14	Bilateral cleft lip, incomplete — *Bilateral cleft lip, incomplete; cleft does not go through entire lip at midline*
749.20	Unspecified cleft palate with cleft lip — *Cleft palate with cleft lip, unspecified*
749.21	Unilateral cleft palate with cleft lip, complete — *Unilateral cleft palate with cleft lip, complete; complete cleft through midline of palate and lip on one side of midline*
749.22	Unilateral cleft palate with cleft lip, incomplete — *Unilateral cleft palate with cleft lip, incomplete; incomplete cleft at midline of palate and lip on one side*
749.23	Bilateral cleft palate with cleft lip, complete — *Bilateral cleft palate and cleft lip, complete; complete cleft of lip and palate at both sides of midline*

✔5th   Needs fifth-digit   **OK**   Valid three-digit code

749.24   Bilateral cleft palate with cleft lip, incomplete — *Bilateral cleft palate and cleft lip, incomplete; incomplete cleft of both palate and lip at midline of both sides*

749.25   Other combinations of cleft palate with cleft lip — *Other combinations of cleft palate and cleft lip; incomplete cleft lip, unilateral with complete cleft of palate, bilateral*

750 OTHER CONGENITAL ANOMALIES OF UPPER ALIMENTARY TRACT

This rubric excludes congenital dentofacial anomalies classified to 524.0-524.9.

750.0   Tongue tie — *Tongue tie; ankyloglossia*

750.10   Congenital anomaly of tongue, unspecified — *Anomaly of tongue, unspecified; unspecified anomaly of tongue*

750.11   Aglossia — *Aglossia; agenesis of tongue*

Aglossia is absence of the tongue. It is seen in Hanhart syndrome, a condition marked by absent tongue and serious anomalies of the limbs.

750.12   Congenital adhesions of tongue — *Congenital adhesions of tongue*

750.13   Congenital fissure of tongue — *Fissure of tongue; bifid tongue; double tongue*

Bifid tongue occurs when the tongue buds fail to develop normally. It is seen most often in South America.

750.15   Macroglossia — *Macroglossia; congenital hypertrophy of tongue*

Macroglossia is an abnormally large tongue.

750.16   Microglossia — *Microglossia; congenital hypoplasia of tongue*

Microglossia is an abnormally small tongue.

750.19   Other congenital anomaly of tongue — *Other anomalies of tongue; anomalies of tongue NEC*

750.21   Congenital absence of salivary gland — *Absence of salivary gland; agenesis of salivary gland*

750.22   Congenital accessory salivary gland — *Accessory salivary gland; supernumerary salivary gland*

750.23   Congenital atresia, salivary duct — *Atresia, salivary gland; imperforate salivary duct*

750.24   Congenital fistula of salivary gland — *Congenital fistula of salivary gland*

750.25   Congenital fistula of lip — *Congenital fistula of lip; congenital (mucus) lip pits*

750.26   Other specified congenital anomalies of mouth — *Other specified anomalies of mouth; agenesis of uvula; nevus of oral mucosa*

750.27   Congenital diverticulum of pharynx — *Diverticulum of pharynx; pharyngeal pouch*

A pharyngeal pouch is an abnormal pocket in the wall of the pharynx, causing difficulty in swallowing.

750.29   Other specified congenital anomaly of pharynx

750.3   Congenital tracheoesophageal fistula, esophageal atresia and stenosis — *Tracheoesophageal fistula, esophageal atresia and stenosis; esophageal agenesis; congenital esophageal ring*

A tracheoesophageal fistula, which is an abnormal opening between the trachea and the esophagus, must be repaired immediately after birth. In esophageal atresia, the esophagus ends in a blind pouch. Even though the esophagus ends in a blind pouch, it is essential that newborns are able to suck and swallow. Surgical intervention temporarily diverts the esophagus to an opening in the neck, while the infant's nutrition is maintained by IV feedings.

Esophageal stenosis is an abnormally narrowed lumen of the esophagus associated with vomiting and dysphagia.

750.4   Other specified congenital anomaly of esophagus — *Other specified anomalies of esophagus; congenital dilatation of esophagus; giant esophagus*

750.5   Congenital hypertrophic pyloric stenosis — *Congenital hypertrophic pyloric stenosis; pyloric stricture; pyloric stenosis*

Hypertrophic pyloric stenosis is the most common cause of surgery in the young infant, excluding hernia surgery. In this condition, the outlet to the intestines becomes blocked, leading to projectile vomiting, electrolyte imbalances, and dehydration. The condition is often diagnosed between two weeks and four weeks of age. Pyloromyotomy may be delayed until an electrolyte disturbance or dehydration is corrected.

750.6   Congenital hiatus hernia — *Congenital hiatus hernia; displacement of cardia through esophageal hernia*

A hiatal hernia is an upward displacement of the stomach through the esophageal hiatus into the mediastinal cavity, leading to esophageal reflux disease. It is always corrected.

750.7   Other specified congenital anomalies of stomach — *Other specified anomalies of stomach; congenital hourglass stomach; transposition of stomach*

Cardiospasm is the failure of the cardiac sphincter to relax, leading to aperistalsis. In hourglass stomach, fibrous bands pinch in the stomach, giving it an hourglass appearance. When the stomach is transposed, it lies on the right side of the abdomen. Megalogastria is an abnormally large stomach and microgastria is an abnormally small stomach.

750.8   Other specified congenital anomalies of upper alimentary tract — *Other specified anomalies of upper alimentary tract; gastric agenesis; upper alimentary tract hypoplasia*

750.9   Unspecified congenital anomaly of upper alimentary tract — *Unspecified anomaly of upper alimentary tract; congenital anomaly of upper alimentary tract, NOS*

751 OTHER CONGENITAL ANOMALIES OF DIGESTIVE SYSTEM

751.0   Meckel's diverticulum — *Meckel's diverticulum; persistent omphalomesenteric duct; persistent vitelline duct*

Meckel's diverticulum is a sacculation of the distal ileum caused by failure of the vitelline duct to atrophy. It is the most frequently occurring digestive malformation and usually presents with massive dark red rectal bleeding which is often painless to the child. Strangulation or intussusception can occur.

751.1   Congenital atresia and stenosis of small intestine — *Atresia and stenosis of small intestine; narrowing of lumen of small intestine, congenital*

DEFINITION

Colon: large intestine, the most distal portion of the intestinal tract.

Duodenum: most proximal portion of the small intestines.

Ileum: midportion of the small intestines.

Jejunum: most distal portion of the small intestines.

Large intestine: colon.

Mediastinum: space in the chest containing the heart.

Small intestine: composed of the duodenum, ileum, jejunum.

✔5th   Needs fifth-digit   **OK**   Valid three-digit code

Atresia of the small intestine usually affects the ileum and is associated with trisomy-21 (Down syndrome) if it appears in the duodenum. It is diagnosed in utero through ultrasound or shortly after birth and treated with resection and primary anastomosis.

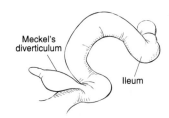

The diverticulum pouch is often found about 50 cm from the ileocecal junction

751.2 Congenital atresia and stenosis of large intestine, rectum, and anal canal — *Atresia and stenosis of large intestine, rectum and anal canal; anal genesis; colonic agenesis; anal atresia; rectal atresia*

Imperforate anus is diagnosed on birth. The infant is given a diverting colostomy and corrective surgery is performed later.

751.3 Hirschsprung's disease and other congenital functional disorders of colon — *Hirschsprung's disease and other congenital functional disorders of the colon; aganglionosis; congenital megacolon*

Hirschsprung's disease is a massive distention of the colon with associated inability to defecate due to lack of innervation of the affected portion of the colon. It has familial associations and is more commonly seen in males. The condition is often diagnosed about 48 hours after birth, as the infant is unable to pass meconium, and treatment is immediate to prevent the onset of enterocolitis.

751.4 Congenital anomalies of intestinal fixation — *Anomalies of intestinal fixation; congenital omental adhesions; congenital peritoneal adhesions; insufficient rotation of cecum or colon; universal mesentery*

Volvulus is a potential symptom of malrotation of the intestine, leading to strangulation and intestinal infarction through choking off the mesenteric artery.

751.5 Other congenital anomalies of intestine — *Other anomalies of intestine; congenital diverticulum of colon; anal duplication; megaloduodenum*

Dolichocolon is an abnormally long colon.

A persistent cloaca is the third level of a developmental anomaly involving the persistence of a urogenital sinus. In this condition, there is a single orifice behind the clitoris and agenesis of the anus and vagina. Treatment is delayed until the child is at least one year of age. A colostomy is performed after birth as a temporary measure and the infant is catheterized intermittently until corrective surgery is performed.

751.60 Unspecified congenital anomaly of gallbladder, bile ducts, and liver — *Unspecified anomaly of gallbladder, bile ducts, and liver; gallbladder anomaly NOS*

751.61 Congenital biliary atresia — *Biliary atresia; congenital hypoplastic bile duct*

Biliary atresia is the lack of patency of the extrahepatic ducts thought to be an obliterative process rather than a developmental anomaly. It is a serious condition, which may lead to cirrhosis of the liver. Approximately 10 percent of the cases are associated with multiple malformations, the most common being polysplenia (multiple right-sided spleens, a midline liver, a pre-duodenal portal vein, and cardiac malformations).

751.62 Congenital cystic disease of liver — *Congenital cystic disease of liver; congenital polycystic liver disease; fibrocystic disease of liver*

Congenital polycystic disease of the liver involves the formation of numerous cysts that block the drainage of bile.

751.69 Other congenital anomaly of gallbladder, bile ducts, and liver — *Other anomalies of gallbladder, bile ducts, and liver; gallbladder agenesis; accessory hepatic ducts; floating liver; intrahepatic gallbladder*

When the liver or gallbladder is characterized as floating, the organ is displaced and moveable.

751.7 Congenital anomalies of pancreas — *Anomalies of pancreas; pancreatic agenesis; pancreatic heterotopia*

If the pancreas either does not develop (agenesis) or is extremely underdeveloped (hypoplasia), intrauterine growth is retarded due to lack of the insulin, which would normally be secreted by the pancreas.

751.8 Other specified congenital anomalies of digestive system — *Other specified anomalies of digestive system; partial agenesis of alimentary tract; congenital malposition of digestive organs NOS*

751.9 Unspecified congenital anomaly of digestive system — *Unspecified anomaly of digestive system; congenital anomaly of digestive system NOS*

752 CONGENITAL ANOMALIES OF GENITAL ORGANS

Excluded from this rubric are syndromes associated with anomalies in the number and form of chromosomes (758.0-758.9) and testicular feminization syndrome (257.8).

752.0 Congenital anomalies of ovaries — *Anomalies of ovaries; agenesis of ovary; streak ovary; ectopic ovary*

Ovarian agenesis is associated with low set ears, a high palate, mental retardation, and edema of the extremities. The genitalia may be ambiguous. Without the estrogen produced by the ovaries, breast development and menarche do not occur.

A streak ovary contains streaks of fibrous stroma where germ cells should reside. Germ cells are absent.

752.10 Unspecified congenital anomaly of fallopian tubes and broad ligaments — *Unspecified anomaly of fallopian tubes and broad ligaments; fallopian tube anomaly NOS*

752.11 Embryonic cyst of fallopian tubes and broad ligaments — *Embryonic cyst of fallopian tubes and broad ligaments; epoophoron cyst; Gartner's duct cyst*

Gartner's duct stretches from the parovarium to the vagina. The epoophoron is a rudimentary structure composed of Gartner's duct and up to 15 transverse ducts.

752.19 Other congenital anomaly of fallopian tubes and broad ligaments — *Other anomalies of fallopian tubes and broad ligaments; agenesis of fallopian tube*

752.2 Congenital doubling of uterus — *Doubling of uterus; didelphic uterus*

A didelphic uterus is associated with a septate vagina. It has two cervices and two small uteri. An expectant mother with a didelphic uterus may have a difficult time bringing a child to term.

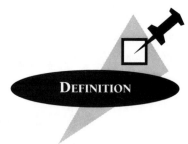

DEFINITION

Cryptorchism: both testes "hidden" in inguinal canal.

Dorsum (of penis): top of the penis.

Germ cell: cell that produces an egg (ovum) or a sperm.

Labia majora: large outer lips of the female external genitalia.

Labia minora: smaller inner lips of the female external genitalia.

Scrotum: sac containing the testes.

Ventrum (of penis): bottom of the penis.

✔5th Needs fifth-digit   **OK** Valid three-digit code

752.3 Other congenital anomaly of uterus — *Other anomalies of uterus; uterine aplasia; bicornuate uterus; uterus unicornis*

A bicornuate uterus has two uterine cavities correctable by surgery.

A unicornuate uterus has only one lateral half and usually only one fallopian tube. This condition is associated with a high rate of miscarriage.

752.40 Unspecified congenital anomaly of cervix, vagina, and external female genitalia — *Unspecified anomaly of cervix, vagina, and external female genitalia; cervical anomaly NOS*

752.41 Embryonic cyst of cervix, vagina, and external female genitalia — *Embryonic cyst of cervix, vagina, and external female genitalia; congenital cyst of canal of Nuck; embryonal vagina*

752.42 Imperforate hymen — *Imperforate hymen; hymen completely covers entrance to vagina*

752.49 Other congenital anomaly of cervix, vagina, and external female genitalia — *Other anomalies of cervix, vagina, and external female genitalia; vaginal agenesis; congenital stricture of cervical canal*

Synechia vulvae are fused labia minora. There is a tiny opening that permits the flow of urine from the urethra.

752.51 Undescended testis — *Undescended testis; cryptorchism*

In true cryptorchism, the testis is concealed within the abdominal cavity. In incomplete cryptorchism, the testis has partially descended within the inguinal canal and arrested. Both conditions are associated with low birth weight, with incidence increasing as birth weights decrease. Cryptorchism must be corrected through orchiopexy by age two or sterility will result.

752.52 Retractile testis — *Retractile testis; testis can be manually manipulated down inguinal canal and into scrotal sac*

A retractile testis can be manipulated into the scrotum without strain.

752.61 Hypospadias — *Hypospadias; urethra found on ventrum of penis*

The urethral meatus lies on the ventral portion of the penile shaft. Corrective surgery should be performed by eight months to 12 months of age.

752.62 Epispadias — *Epispadias; anaspadias*

Epispadias is rare, with the urethral meatus on the dorsal portion of the penile shaft. The penis curves upward.

752.63 Congenital chordee — *Congenital chordee; downward curve of penis*

Chordee is the downward bowing of the penis and is associated with hypospadias, although it may occur as a solitary variant.

752.64 Micropenis — *Micropenis; abnormally small penis*

Micropenis, a form of ambiguous genitalia, is caused by lack of endocrine output during fetal life, specifically lack of testosterone. Typically the penis, though small, is normal in function. Testosterone shots administered in infancy allow the penis to obtain normal size.

752.65   Hidden penis — *Hidden penis*
752.69   Other penile anomalies — *Other penile anomalies; specified penile anomaly NEC*

Penile agenesis is so rare that it occurs in one out of 30 million births. The scrotum is usually normal, though the testicles are undescended.

Penile duplication presents as a bifid penis with two corpora cavernosa and two hemialgias and may range from the glans only to duplication of the entire urogenital tract.

In torsion of the penis, the rotation is typically to the left.

752.7   Indeterminate sex and pseudohermaphroditism — *Indeterminate sex and pseudohermaphroditism; gynandrism; ovotestis; pure gonadal dysgenesis*

Indeterminate sex and pseudohermaphroditism and intersex are interchangeable terms. This category excludes all forms of this condition but gonadal dysgenesis. As in other forms of the condition, in hermaphroditism due to gonadal dysgenesis, the external genitalia do not match the genetic makeup of the individual. The fetus begins as a female and, if the chromosome pattern is XY, develop as boys. For reasons unrelated to the other causes of the condition, gonadal development is subpart, leading to the birth of an infant of ambiguous sex.

752.8   Other specified congenital anomalies of genital organs — *Other specified anomalies of genital organs; prostatic agenesis; anorchism; round ligament aplasia*
752.9   Unspecified congenital anomaly of genital organs — *Unspecified anomaly of genital organs; congenital anomaly NOS of genital organ, NEC*

753 CONGENITAL ANOMALIES OF URINARY SYSTEM

753.0   Congenital renal agenesis and dysgenesis — (Code first any associated 593.70–593.73) — *Renal agenesis and dysgenesis; renal hypoplasia*

Renal agenesis can be either bilateral or unilateral. When bilateral, the condition is terminal due to its affect on other organs. In bilateral agenesis of the kidneys, the fetus lives in an environment of oligohydramnios, which prevents normal development of the lungs. (The lungs are dependent on a moist environment for normal development.)

753.10   Unspecified congenital cystic kidney disease — *Cystic kidney disease, unspecified; unspecified cystic kidney disease*
753.11   Congenital single renal cyst — *Congenital single renal cyst*

There is evidence that a single congenital renal cyst is a marker for polycystic kidney disease.

753.12   Congenital polycystic kidney, unspecified type — *Polycystic kidney, unspecified type; unspecified polycystic kidney disease*
753.13   Congenital polycystic kidney, autosomal dominant — *Polycystic kidney, autosomal dominant*

Polycystic kidney disease, autosomal-dominant, is a progressive disease of adult onset characterized by bilateral cysts. The kidneys are enlarged and their function impaired.

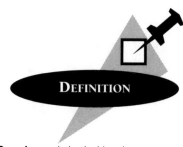

DEFINITION

Gonad: sexual gland, either the ovary or testis.

Oligohydramnios: abnormally scant amount of amniotic fluid.

Allele: different form of the same gene.

Chromosome: structure in the cell nucleus that transmits hereditary characteristics.

Genotype: genetic constitution of an organism.

✔5th   Needs fifth-digit   **OK**   Valid three-digit code

753.14 Congenital polycystic kidney, autosomal recessive — *Polycystic kidney; autosomal recessive*

Polycystic kidney disease, autosomal-recessive, has early childhood onset. There are multiple cysts in the kidneys and liver, leading to failure of both organs.

753.15 Congenital renal dysplasia — (Code first any associated 593.70–593.73) — *Renal dysplasia; abnormal development of kidney*

753.16 Congenital medullary cystic kidney — *Medullary cystic kidney; nephronophthisis*

Medullary cystic kidney is a disease of the renal tubules leading to proteinuria and renal failure.

753.17 Congenital medullary sponge kidney — *Medullary sponge kidney; congenital dilatation of collecting tubules of kidney*

A medullary sponge kidney demonstrates dilation of the tubules. It may be symptomatic if calcinosis develops in the tubules, leading to renal insufficiency.

753.19 Other specified congenital cystic kidney disease — *other specified cystic kidney disease; multicystic kidney*

753.20 Unspecified congenital obstructive defect of renal pelvis and ureter — *Unspecified obstructive defect of renal pelvis and ureter*

753.21 Congenital obstruction of ureteropelvic junction — *Congenital obstruction of uteropelvic junction; stricture of ureteropelvic junction*

Congenital obstruction of the ureteropelvic junction is the most common urinary tract anomaly. Its appearance is associated with other anomalies of the urinary tract such as horseshoe kidney, ectopic kidney, multicystic, and dysplastic kidney. The condition may be diagnosed antenatally and is corrected within the first few months of life. A pyeloplasty promotes normal growth and development of urinary tract structures.

753.22 Congenital obstruction of ureterovesical junction — *Congenital obstruction of ureterovesical junction; adynamic ureter; congenital hydroureter*

Obstruction of the ureterovesical junction often occurs with ureteropelvic obstruction.

753.23 Congenital ureterocele — *Congenital ureterocele; herniation of ureter*

753.29 Other congentital obstructive defect of renal pelvis and ureter — *Other obstructive defects of renal pelvis and ureter*

753.3 Other specified congenital anomaly of kidney — *Other specified anomalies of kidney; accessory kidney; discoid kidney; ectopic kidney; giant kidney; horseshoe kidney*

Horseshoe and discoid kidneys are the products of fusion anomalies. A discoid kidney is fused medially at both poles, while a horseshoe kidney is fused at the lower poles. Horseshoe kidney may be associated with Wilms' tumor and anomalies of a number of body systems. An ectopic kidney is on the opposite side of its ureter.

753.4 Other specified congenital anomaly of ureter — *Other specified anomalies of ureter; ureteral agenesis; displace ureteral orifice; anomalous implantation of ureter*

Duplication occurs most frequently among ureteral anomalies.

753.5 Exstrophy of urinary bladder — *Exstrophy of urinary bladder; ectopia vesicae; extroversion of bladder*

Exstrophy of the bladder is the absence if part of the lower abdominal wall and part of the anterior bladder wall, allowing the posterior bladder wall to protrude. The bladder must be closed immediately after birth, a first stage of complex reconstructive surgeries.

753.6 Congenital atresia and stenosis of urethra and bladder neck — *Atresia and stenosis of urethra and bladder neck; imperforate urinary meatus; congenital stricture of vesicourethral orifice*

Urethral atresia is successful treated antenatally by placement of a vesicoamniotic shunt.

753.7 Congenital anomalies of urachus — *Anomalies of urachus; urachal fistula; persistent umbilical sinus*

A urachal cyst presents as an extraperitoneal mass near the umbilicus. It may become infected or rupture, possibly causing peritonitis if it drains into the peritoneum rather than through the umbilicus.

753.8 Other specified congenital anomaly of bladder and urethra — *Other specified anomalies of bladder and urethra; agenesis of bladder; accessory urethra; congenital diverticulum of bladder*

Congenital diverticulum of the bladder, also known as Hutch diverticulum, occurs where the ureter enters the bladder and may cause obstruction and deviation. The diverticulum threatens the competence of the ureterovesical valve, leading to vesicoureteral reflux.

Female hypospadias presents the urinary meatus fairly near its normal position; however, it is associated with other anomalies of the urinary-genital tract.

753.9 Unspecified congenital anomaly of urinary system — *Unspecified anomaly of urinary system; congenital anomaly NOS of any part of urinary system excluding urachus*

754 CERTAIN CONGENITAL MUSCULOSKELETAL DEFORMITIES

Defects in this rubric are limited by ICD-9 notes to those defects caused by extrinsic factors (e.g., intrauterine problems including malposition and pressure).

754.0 Congenital musculoskeletal deformities of skull, face, and jaw — *Certain congenital musculoskeletal deformities of skull, face and jaw; facial asymmetry; Potter's facies; congenital deviation of nasal septum*

Dolichocephaly is a skull that is long in relation to the anterior/posterior axis. Plagiocephaly is a lopsided and twisted skull. Potter's facies is a facial appearance characterized by deep folds under the eyes. The folds are caused by oligohydramnios related to agenesis of the kidneys.

✔5th Needs fifth-digit   **OK** Valid three-digit code

754.1   Congenital musculoskeletal deformity of sternocleidomastoid muscle — *Certain congenital musculoskeletal deformities of sternocleidomastoid muscle; congenital sternomastoid torticollis; congenital wryneck*

Sternocleidomastoid torticollis is apparent after birth. Because there are other non-muscular causes of congenital torticollis, the pediatrician must ascertain the cause. If it is muscular, the child should be checked for hip dysplasia, as it is frequently associated with muscular torticollis. Treatment involves daily stretching for the first year of life. If torticollis persists, surgery is necessary to correct the asymmetrical tilt to the face.

754.2   Congenital musculoskeletal deformity of spine — *Certain congenital musculoskeletal deformities of spine; congenital postural scoliosis*

Congenital scoliosis, an anterior/posterior plane vertebral malformation, may appear in three variants. It can be an isolated deformity or be associated with other multi-system deformities. Approximately 20 percent of the cases include genitourinary malformations, while another 20 percent show coexistent cord defects.

Lordosis is an exaggerated inward curve in the low back.

754.3 Congenital dislocation of hip

Dislocation and subluxation of the hip occur in conjunction with ligamentous laxity of the hip joint capsules. Females are affected nine times out of 10 and there is a 30 percent to 50 percent incidence among breech births. Osteoarthritis, gait abnormalities, pains, and unequal leg length may result if left untreated.

754.30   Congenital dislocation of hip, unilateral — *Congenital dislocation of hip, unilateral; congenital dislocation of hip NOS*

754.31   Congenital dislocation of hip, bilateral — *Congenital dislocation of hip, bilateral; congenital dislocation of both hips*

754.32   Congenital subluxation of hip, unilateral — *Congenital subluxation of hip, unilateral; congenital flexion deformity, hip or thigh; predislocation status of hip at birth*

754.33   Congenital subluxation of hip, bilateral — *Congenital subluxation of hip, bilateral; congenital partial dislocation of both hips*

754.35   Congenital dislocation of one hip with subluxation of other hip — *Congenital dislocation of one hip with subluxation of other hip; congenital dislocation of one hip with congenital partial dislocation of other hip*

754.4 Congenital genu recurvatum and bowing of long bones of leg

Bowing of the long bones can occur alone or as part of a series of anomalies, of which osteogenesis imperfecta is the most known.

754.40   Congenital genu recurvatum — *Genu recurvatum; hyperextension of knee joint*

754.41   Congenital dislocation of knee (with genu recurvatum) — *Congenital dislocation of knee (with genu recurvatum)*

754.42   Congenital bowing of femur — *Congenital bowing of femur*

754.43   Congenital bowing of tibia and fibula — *Congenital bowing of tibia and fibula*

754.44   Congenital bowing of unspecified long bones of leg — *Congenital bowing of unspecified long bones of leg*

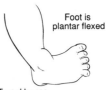

Foot is plantar flexed

Tarsal bones are inverted

The congenital deformity known as clubfoot is usually bilateral. The bones and soft tissues may be normal in shape but are locked in a tortured position.

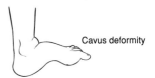

Cavus deformity

754.50 Congenital talipes varus — *Talipes varus; pes varus; unspecified congenital varus deformity of foot*

In talipes varus, the foot rotates outward, promoting walking on the outside of the sole.

754.51 Congenital talipes equinovarus — *Talipes equinovarus; equinovarus (congenital)*

Also known as clubfoot, talipes equinovarus is a condition in which the sole points straight back. As is the case with the other foot deformities, talipes equinovarus arises from improper alignment of the baby in utero.

754.52 Congenital metatarsus primus varus — *Metatarsus primus varus*

Metatarsus primus valgus is a deformity of the cuneiform bone.

754.53 Metatarsus varus

Metatarsus varus is a toeing-in deformity.

754.59 Other congenital varus deformity of feet — *Other varus deformities of feet; talipes calcaneovarus*

Talipes calcaneovarus has the foot pointing out and down.

754.60 Congenital talipes valgus — *Talipes valgus; congenital valgus deformity of foot, unspecified*

Talipes valgus is a deformity in which the foot toes in, promoting walking on the inside of the soles.

754.61 Congenital pes planus — *Congenital pes planus; congenital flat foot*

Congenital flat foot is a more severe problem than acquired flat foot.

754.62 Talipes calcaneovalgus — *Talipes calcaneovalgus; flexed foot with heel only touching ground*

Talipes calcaneovalgus, in which the foot toes out, is the most common foot deformity.

754.69 Other congenital valgus deformity of feet — *Other valgus deformities of feet*

Talipes equinovalgus is a form of clubfoot in which the heel points outward.

754.70 Unspecified talipes — *Talipes, unspecified; congenital deformity of foot, NOS*
754.71 Talipes cavus — *Talipes cavus; cavus foot (congenital)*

In talipes cavus, there is muscle imbalance and weakness due to many causes. The forefoot is adducted and the heel is valgus.

754.79 Other congenital deformity of feet — *Other deformities of feet; asymmetric talipes; talipes equinus*

754.8 Other specified nonteratogenic anomalies

Pectus excavatum produces a deep indentation in the chest at the level of the breastbone. It may be a solitary phenomenon, but has a strong association with Marfan's syndrome and cardiac anomalies. More males than females are affected by the condition. Pectus carinatum, which causes the chest to curve outward like a pigeon's breast, is associated with other anomalies and is primarily a cosmetic problem.

754.81   Pectus excavatum — *Pectus excavatum; congenital funnel chest*
754.82   Pectus carinatum — *Pectus carinatum; congenital pigeon chest*
754.89   Other specified nonteratogenic anomalies — *Other specified nonteratogenic anomalies; club hand (congenital); spade-like hand (congenital)*

755 OTHER CONGENITAL ANOMALIES OF LIMBS

Intrinsic and extrinsic factors may cause the anomalies reported by this rubric. Intrinsic factors include errors of fetal development. Extrinsic factors are the result of intrauterine problems including malposition and pressure and comprise only two percent of all congenital anomalies.

755.0 Polydactyly

Polydactyly may be genetic, solitary, or part of numerous syndromes. The supernumerary digits may be rudimentary or normally formed.

755.00   Polydactyly, unspecified digits — *Polydactyly, unspecified digits; supernumerary digits*
755.01   Polydactyly of fingers — *Polydactyly of fingers; accessory fingers*
755.02   Polydactyly of toes — *Polydactyly of toes; accessory toes*

755.1 Syndactyly

Syndactyly is genetically linked and may appear in conjunction with other syndromes. When the webbing is confined to the skin, surgery is generally performed at six months of age to enhance normal digit development. The corrective operation involves splitting the webbing and skin grafts. When all five bones are fused, the situation is more complex and surgery rarely is able to provide optimal function.

755.10   Syndactyly of multiple and unspecified sites — *Syndactyly of multiple and unspecified sites; digital webbing*
755.11   Syndactyly of fingers without fusion of bone — *Syndactyly of fingers without fusion of bone; soft tissues only are affected*
755.12   Syndactyly of fingers with fusion of bone — *Syndactyly of fingers with fusion of bone; both bony and soft tissues affected by anomalous development*
755.13   Syndactyly of toes without fusion of bone — *Syndactyly of toes without fusion of bone; soft tissue only affected*
755.14   Syndactyly of toes with fusion of bone — *Syndactyly of toes with fusion of bone; bony and soft tissue affected by anomalous development*
755.20   Congenital unspecified reduction deformity of upper limb — *Unspecified reduction deformity of upper limb; ectromelia NOS of upper limb*

Ectromelia is hypoplasia of the long bones in the upper limb. In hemimelia, a part of the bone of the upper limb is missing.

755.21   Congenital transverse deficiency of upper limb — *Transverse deficiency of upper limb; amelia of upper limb; agenesis of fingers; congenital amputation of upper limb*

Amelia is the congenital absence of the upper limb.

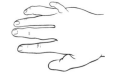

Syndactyly of digits (webbing)
Image at right depicts a case involving fusion of bone and nail

Supernumary digit

Congenital amputation of any limb may be due to constriction by fibrous amniotic bands or to teratogenic factors.

755.22 Congenital longitudinal deficiency of upper limb, not elsewhere classified — *Longitudinal deficiency of upper limb, NEC; phocomelia NOS of upper limb*

In complete phocomelia, the hands are attached to the trunk. In incomplete phocomelia, there may be a rudimentary long bone.

755.23 Congenital longitudinal deficiency, combined, involving humerus, radius, and ulna (complete or incomplete) — *Longitudinal deficiency, combined, involving humerus, radius and ulna (complete or incomplete); agenesis of arm and forearm; phocomelia, complete, of upper limb*

755.24 Congenital longitudinal deficiency, humeral, complete or partial (with or without distal deficiencies, incomplete) — *Longitudinal deficiency, radioulnar, complete or partial (with or without distal deficiencies, incomplete); agenesis of radius and ulna, with or without agenesis of some but not all distal elements*

Proximal phocomelia means the absence of a humerus.

755.25 Congenital longitudinal deficiency, radioulnar, complete or partial (with or without distal deficiencies, incomplete) — *Longitudinal deficiency, radioulnar, complete or partial (with or without distal deficiencies, incomplete); distal phocomelia of upper limb*

755.26 Congenital longitudinal deficiency, radial, complete or partial (with or without distal deficiencies, incomplete) — *Longitudinal deficiency, radial, complete or partial (with or without distal deficiencies, incomplete); radial agenesis*

755.27 Congenital longitudinal deficiency, ulnar, complete or partial (with or without distal deficiencies, incomplete) — *Longitudinal deficiency, ulnar, complete or partial (with or without distal deficiencies, incomplete); ulnar agenesis*

755.28 Congenital longitudinal deficiency, carpals or metacarpals, complete or partial (with or without incomplete phalangeal deficiency) — *Longitudinal deficiency, carpals or metacarpals, complete or partial (with or without incomplete phalangeal deficiency); aphalangia of upper limb, terminal, complete or partial*

755.29 Congenital longitudinal deficiency, phalanges, complete or partial

755.30 Congenital unspecified reduction deformity of lower limb — *Unspecified reduction deformity of lower limb; ectromelia NOS of lower limb; shortening of leg, congenital*

Ectromelia is hypoplasia of the long bones in the lower limb. In hemimelia, a part of the bone of the lower limb is missing.

755.31 Congenital transverse deficiency of lower limb — *Transverse deficiency of lower limb; amelia of lower limb; pedal agenesis*

Amelia is the congenital absence of one or more lower limbs.

755.32 Congenital longitudinal deficiency of lower limb, not elsewhere classified — *Longitudinal deficiency of lower limb, NEC; phocomelia NOS of lower limb*

755.33 Congenital longitudinal deficiency, combined, involving femur, tibia, and fibula (complete or incomplete) — *Longitudinal deficiency of lower limb, NEC; phocomelia NOS of lower limb*

Complete phocomelia of the lower limb means the direct attachment of the feet to the trunk.

5th Needs fifth-digit   **OK** Valid three-digit code

755.34 Congenital longitudinal deficiency, femoral, complete or partial (with or without distal deficiencies, incomplete) — *Longitudinal deficiency, femoral, complete or partial (with or without distal deficiencies, incomplete); femoral agenesis; proximal phocomelia of lower limb*

Proximal phocomelia of the lower limb means the absence of a femur.

755.35 Congenital longitudinal deficiency, tibiofibular, complete or partial (with or without distal deficiencies, incomplete) — *Longitudinal deficiency, tibiofibular, complete or partial (with or without distal deficiencies, incomplete; tibial agenesis; distal phocomelia of lower limb*

755.36 Congenital longitudinal deficiency, tibia, complete or partial (with or without distal deficiencies, incomplete)

755.37 Congenital longitudinal deficiency, fibular, complete or partial (with or without distal deficiencies, incomplete) — *Longitudinal deficiency, fibular, complete or partial (with or without distal deficiencies, incomplete)*

755.38 Congenital longitudinal deficiency, tarsals or metatarsals, complete or partial (with or without incomplete phalangeal deficiency) — *Longitudinal deficiency, tarsals or metatarsals, complete or partial (with or without incomplete phalangeal deficiency)*

755.39 Congenital longitudinal deficiency, phalanges, complete or partial — *Longitudinal deficiency, phalanges, complete or partial; agenesis of toe; aphalangia of lower limb, terminal, complete or partial*

755.4 Congenital reduction deformities, unspecified limb — *Reduction deformities, unspecified limb; amelia, ectromelia, hemimelia, of unspecified limb*

755.50 Unspecified congenital anomaly of upper limb — *Unspecified anomaly of upper limb*

755.51 Congenital deformity of clavicle — *Congenital deformity of clavicle; clavicular anomaly*

755.52 Congenital elevation of scapula — *Congenital elevation of scapula; Sprengel's deformity*

Sprengel's deformity connotes a hypoplastic and elevated scapula. Often, the hypoplastic trapezius, deltoid, or rhomboid is absent. The result may be torticollis, scoliosis, or limb length discrepancy.

755.53 Radioulnar synostosis — *Radioulnar synostosis; fusion of radius and ulna*

The forearm is permanently pronated. Most cases do not require surgery.

755.54 Madelung's deformity — *Madelung's deformity*

Madelung's deformity is a dysplasia of the radius involving an exaggerated radial inclination, a short forearm, dorsal dislocation of the ulnar head, and a "V" shaped proximal carpal row. The condition may arise from an abnormal fibrous band tethering the sigmoid notch of the radius proximally to the ulna.

755.55 Acrocephalosyndactyly — *Acrocephalosyndactyly; Apert's syndrome*

Apert's syndrome involves premature fusing of the cranial sutures, asymmetrical facies, webbed hands, and progressive calcification and fusion of the bones of the hands, feet, and cervical spine.

755.56 Accessory carpal bones — *Accessory carpal bones; supernumerary carpals*

755.57 Macrodactylia (fingers) — *Macrodactyly (fingers); abnormally large fingers*

755.58 Congenital cleft hand — *Cleft hand, congenital; lobster-claw hand*

Lobster-claw hand, a rare disorder, affects the phalanges of the middle finger. The corresponding metacarpal may be absent and the hand is separated into medial and lateral sections by a deep cleft.

755.59   Other congenital anomaly of upper limb, including shoulder girdle — *Other anomalies of upper limb, including shoulder girdle; cleidocranial dysostosis; cubitus valgus, congenital; cubitus varus, congenital*

Cleidocranial dysostosis, or Scheutthauer-Marie-Sainton syndrome, is genetic disease most often characterized by the absence or hypoplastic development of the collarbone.

In cubitus valgus, the forearm is adducted from the midline on extension. In cubitus varus, the forearm deviates inward when extended.

755.6 Other anomalies of lower limb, including pelvic girdle

The angle between the long axes of the neck and shaft of the femur is 120-125 degrees in the normal individual. In coxa valga this angle is increased to approximately 140 degrees, creating extreme adduction with the possibility of a superior dislocation in the immature hip. In coxa vara this angle is abnormally decreased, creating an extreme abduction. Coxa vara is much more common than coxa valga.

755.60   Unspecified congenital anomaly of lower limb — *Unspecified anomaly of lower limb*

755.61   Congenital coxa valga — *Coxa valga, congenital; angle of femoral head > 120 degrees, congenital*

755.62   Congenital coxa vara — *Coxa vara, congenital; angle femoral head < 120 degrees, congenital*

755.63   Other congenital deformity of hip (joint) — *Other congenital deformity of hip (joint); congenital anteversion of femoral neck*

755.64   Congenital deformity of knee (joint) — *Congenital deformity of knee (joint); patellar agenesis; rudimentary patella; genu varum; genu valgum*

Genu valgum (knock-knee) is a normal part of development that may require surgical intervention if it persists beyond 10 years or 12 years of age if there are more than three inches between the ankles.

755.65   Macrodactylia of toes — *Macrodactylia of toes; abnormally large toes*

755.66   Other congenital anomaly of toes — *Other anomalies of toes; congenital hallux valgus; hallux varus, congenital*

The correction of hallux valgus is postponed until skeletal maturity.

755.67   Congenital anomalies of foot, not elsewhere classified — *Anomalies of foot, NEC; astragaloscaphoid synostosis; calcaneonavicular bar*

"Coalition" and "bar" refer to an abnormal union of bones that are normally separated.

755.69   Other congenital anomaly of lower limb, including pelvic girdle — *Other anomalies of lower limb, including pelvic girdle; congenital deformity of ankle (joint), sacroiliac (joint)*

755.8   Other specified congenital anomalies of unspecified limb — *Other specified anomalies of unspecified limb*

✔5th Needs fifth-digit   **OK** Valid three-digit code

Larsen's syndrome is a genetic, multi-system disorder that presents with multiple dislocations and other bony irregularities, as well as cylindrical fingers, and unusual facies. Other symptoms include mental retardation, short stature, and cardiac abnormalities.

755.9 Unspecified congenital anomaly of unspecified limb — *Unspecified anomaly of unspecified limb; congenital anomaly NOS of unspecified limb*

756 OTHER CONGENITAL MUSCULOSKELETAL ANOMALIES
756.0 Congenital anomalies of skull and face bones — *Anomalies of skull and face bones; agenesis of skull; acrocephaly; Crouzon's disease*

Acrocephaly is a pointed vault of the skull.

Craniosynostosis is an abnormal fusing of the cranial sutures. In the newborn, the cranial sutures are open, serving two desired outcomes: normal delivery with a malleable head and the ability of the skull to grow to accommodate the growing brain. The sagittal suture is the most frequently occurring site of synostosis and is the least likely to be associated with genetics. Any bilateral craniosynostosis is a flag for a possible genetic relationship.

Corrective surgery is performed primarily for cosmetic reasons, although in some cases, the facial bones are affected or the brain does not have enough room and the surgery is justified for both cosmetic and medical reasons.

Oxycephaly describes a cone-shaped head.

Platybasia is an upward thrust of the odontoid bone through the foramen magnum, causing pressure on the midbrain.

Trigonocephaly is a triangular-shaped head.

Crouzon's disease combines craniosynostosis, exophthalmos, hypoplastic midface, flat sphenoids, and a large mandible. Genetic and spontaneous causes are split 50 percent. Asymmetrical exophthalmos and the large jaw are correctable.

Hypertelorism is an abnormal distance between the eyes.

First arch syndrome refers to the developmental stage of the first arch. And involves numerous craniofacial anomalies.

Oculo-auricle-vertebral (OAV) syndrome is synonymous with Goldenhar's syndrome and non-hereditary.

Greig's syndrome is a hereditary disease involving multiple deformities of the hands and feet, macrocephaly, hypertelorism, mild mental retardation, and a broad, flat nose.

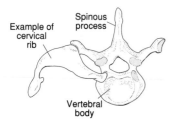

Example of cervical rib

Spinous process

Vertebral body

Superior view of C7 showing cervical rib, which usually occurs bilaterally

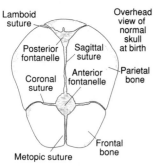

Lamboid suture

Overhead view of normal skull at birth

Posterior fontanelle

Sagittal suture

Coronal suture

Anterior fontanelle

Parietal bone

Metopic suture

Frontal bone

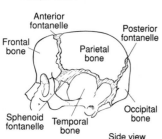

Anterior fontanelle

Posterior fontanelle

Frontal bone

Parietal bone

Sphenoid fontanelle

Temporal bone

Occipital bone

Side view

Hallman Streiff syndrome is an oculo-mandibula-facial syndrome inclusive of short stature and congenital cataracts.

Treacher-Collins, synonymous with Franceschetti's syndrome, is genetically driven and involves an eye slant, lip coloboma, micrognathia, microtia, hypoplastic zygomatic arches, and macrostomia.

756.10 Congenital anomaly of spine, unspecified — *Anomaly of spine, unspecified*

756.11 Congenital spondylolysis, lumbosacral region — *Spondylolisthesis, lumbosacral spine; downward slipping of vertebra toward sacral vertebra*

Spondylolysis is a defect in the vertebra, usually L5, filled with fibrous tissue containing nerve endings that are painful due to compression.

756.12 Congenital spondylolisthesis — *Spondylolisthesis; downward slipping of vertebra*

Spondylolisthesis is the slipping forward of one vertebra over another, often L5, and is usually associated with a spinal defect such as spina bifida occulta. Females are more often affected.

756.13 Congenital absence of vertebra — *Absence of vertebra, congenital; vertebral agenesis*

756.14 Hemivertebra — *Hemivertebra; half a vertebra*

A hemivertebra, a condition that can promote scoliosis, is treated with fusion and bone graft to render it equal in height.

756.15 Congenital fusion of spine (vertebra) — *Fusion of spine, (vertebra) congenital; congenital joining of vertebrae*

Bertolotti's syndrome involves sacralization of the L4-L5 vertebrae. An L5 transverse process forms a pseudoarthrosis with the ala of S1, increasing the tilt of the vertebra and enhancing the possibility of scoliosis.

756.16 Klippel-Feil syndrome — *Klippel-Feil syndrome; brevicollis*

A short neck caused by the fusion of existing cervical vertebrae and the absence of at least one cervical vertebra characterize Klippel-Feil syndrome, also known as brevicollis. It has a high rate of associated malformations or syndromes and affects females.

756.17 Spina bifida occulta — *Spina bifida occulta; vertebral defect covered by skin*

Spina bifida occulta is fairly benign in adults if not causing apparent problems during childhood. The disorder is vertebral, as in spina bifida aperta; however, skin covers the defect in the occulta form. In severe forms, which accounts for about 2 percent of the occulta cases, the condition is called spinal dysraphism to distinguish it from its benign presentation.

756.19 Other congenital anomaly of spine — *Other anomalies of spine; platyspondylia; supernumerary vertebra*

756.2 Cervical rib — *Cervical rib; supernumerary rib in cervical region*

A cervical rib is a supernumerary rib in the cervical region, which can lead to thoracic outlet syndrome.

✔5th   Needs fifth-digit   **OK**   Valid three-digit code

756.3 Other congenital anomaly of ribs and sternum — *Other anomalies of ribs and sternum; sternal agenesis; congenital fissure of sternum*

756.4 Chondrodystrophy — *Chondrodystrophy; achondroplasia; dyschondroplasia*

Chondrodystrophy, a defect of the cartilage growth mechanism, is primary cause of short limb dwarfism, a condition characterized by decreased length of the long bones, although the diameter is not affected. The condition is hereditary. Dyschondroplasia typically affects unilateral joints and involves knobby fingers and genu valgus.

Jeune's syndrome is an asphyxiating thoracic dystrophy.

Maffucci's syndrome, another term for Kast's syndrome, is a non-hereditary dyschondroplasia and involves soft tissue hemangiomata, cyst like bone lesions, and multiple phleboliths. The hemangiomata can enhance dysplastic.

756.50 Unspecified congenital osteodystrophy — *Osteodystrophy, unspecified*

756.51 Osteogenesis imperfecta — *Osteogenesis imperfecta; fragilitas ossium; osteopsathyrosis*

Osteogenesis imperfecta is a hereditary collagen disorder that produces very brittle bones. Type 1 is the most common and mildest form, with the affected person's stature being normal or near normal. Multiple fractures may occur prior to puberty, decreasing later in life. Type II is the most severe, causing death at or soon after birth. Types III IV are treated with intramedullary rods inserted into the long bones.

756.52 Osteopetrosis — *Osteopetrosis; abnormal density of bone*

Osteopetrosis produces an overgrowth of bone that spills into the marrow and obliterates the marrow of the bones below the head and the foramina. The loss of marrow leads to anemia and heptad-splenomegaly. Osteopetrosis can lead to sight and hearing impairments because the nerves cannot emerge through their foramina in the skull.

756.53 Osteopoikilosis — *Osteopoikilosis; multiple, scattered areas of increased bony density*

Osteopoikilosis, a rare genetic disorder, manifests in multiple areas of increased bone density, although the disorder is often asymptomatic. It is associated with other disorders such as dwarfism or scleroderma.

756.54 Polyostotic fibrous dysplasia of bone — *Polyostotic fibrous dysplasia of bone*

756.55 Chondroectodermal dysplasia — *Chondroectodermal dysplasia; Ellis-van Creveld syndrome*

Chondroectodermal dysplasia is characterized by abnormal development of hair, skin, teeth, and cartilage. Polydactyly and heart anomalies are also present.

756.56 Multiple epiphyseal dysplasia — *Multiple epiphyseal dysplasia*

756.59 Other congenital osteodystrophy — *Other osteodystrophies; Albright-(McCune)-Sternberg syndrome*

McCune-Albright syndrome, which usually affects females, involves bone disease with enhanced potential for fractures, leg deformities, endocrine disease, and skin changes. There is wide variability in degree of severity.

756.6 Congenital anomaly of diaphragm — *Anomalies of diaphragm; diaphragmatic agenesis; congenital hernia of foramen of Morgagni*

756.70 Unspecified congenital anomaly of abdominal wall — *Anomaly of abdominal wall, unspecified*

756.71 Prune belly syndrome — *Prune belly syndrome; Eagle-Barrett syndrome; prolapse of bladder mucosa*

Prune belly syndrome, also known as Eagle-Barrett disease, manifests in the absence of the lower rectus abdominus and the medial portions of the oblique muscles. There are urinary tract anomalies. About 95 percent of infants affected are males and 50 percent of all affected newborns are stillborn or die within two years of birth.

756.79 Other congenital anomalies of abdominal wall — *Other congenital anomalies of abdominal wall; exomphalos; gastroschisis; omphalocele*

An omphalocele is a defect in the abdominal wall involving the umbilicus. Large omphaloceles contain parts of the intestines that are reduced over time. The condition may be associated with a syndrome or may appear as a solitary variant.

756.81 Congenital absence of muscle and tendon — *Absence of muscle and tendon; agenesis of pectoral muscle*

756.82 Accessory muscle — *Accessory muscle; supernumerary muscle*

756.83 Ehlers-Danlos syndrome — *Ehlers-Danlos syndrome; collagen disorder, congenital*

Ehlers-Danlos syndrome, a genetic collagen disorder, causes hyperelasticity of the skin, hypermobility of the joints, and fragility of blood vessels. Wound healing is impaired.

756.89 Other specified congenital anomaly of muscle, tendon, fascia, and connective tissue — *Other specified anomalies of muscle, tendon, fascia and connective tissue; amyotrophia congenita*

Use this code for amyotrophia congenita; congenital shortening of tendon, Ayala's disease, Bakwin-Krida syndrome, elongated ligamentum patellae; Fong's syndrome; HOOD syndrome; Krabbe's syndrome; Oestreicher-Turner syndrome; popliteal web syndrome; Pyle-Cohn disease; Schwartz-(Jambul) syndrome; Touraine's syndrome, congenital trigger finger; Turner-Kieser syndrome; and Waardenburg's syndrome.

756.9 Other and unspecified congenital anomaly of musculoskeletal system — *Other and unspecified anomalies of musculoskeletal system; congenital anomaly NOS of musculoskeletal system, NEC*

✔5th Needs fifth-digit   **OK** Valid three-digit code

757 CONGENITAL ANOMALIES OF THE INTEGUMENT

757.0 Hereditary edema of legs — *Hereditary edema of legs; congenital lymphedema; Milroy's disease*

Congenital lymphedema is a disorder of lymph drainage system affecting the legs. Infection is a constant threat. Garments that avoid compression and the use of gradient pumps are the common treatments.

757.1 Ichthyosis congenita — *Ichthyosis congenita; Harlequin fetus*

Ichthyosis congenita refers to scaly skin as a result of an excessive production of skin cells.

Sjogren-Larsson syndrome manifests with dry, scaly skin, as well as mental retardation, speech abnormalities, and spasticity. Retinal degeneration is characteristic in about 50 percent of all cases.

757.2 Dermatoglyphic anomalies — *Dermatoglyphic anomalies; abnormal palmar creases*

757.31 Congenital ectodermal dysplasia — *Congenital ectodermal dysplasia; Clouston's syndrome*

Congenital ectodermal dysplasia, or hidrotic ED, is an inherited disorder primarily affecting the French. The nails are thick and there is thick skin on the palms and soles and dark skin on the elbows and knees.

757.32 Congenital vascular hamartomas — *Vascular hamartomas; birthmarks; port wine stain*

Port wine stain, or nevus flammeus, is a hemangioma that is red and flat at birth, which thickens over time.

757.33 Congenital pigmentary anomaly of skin — *Congenital pigmentary anomalies of skin; congenital poikiloderma; urticaria pigmentosa*

Urticaria pigmentosa is a self-limiting rash that tends to disappear after puberty.

757.39 Other specified congenital anomaly of skin — *Other specified anomalies of skin; accessory skin tags; keratoderma (congenital)*

Congenital pachydermatocele, or cutis pendula, causes the skin to hang in wrinkled folds.

757.4 Specified congenital anomalies of hair — *Specified anomalies of hair; congenital alopecia; persistent lanugo*

Congenital alopecia is the failure of the hair to grow or develop.

757.5 Specified congenital anomalies of nails — *Specified anomalies of nails; anonychia; congenital clubnail*

Anonychia is the absence of one or more fingernails.

757.6 Specified congenital anomalies of breast — *Specified anomalies of breast; supernumerary breast; hypoplasia of breast*

757.8 Other specified congenital anomalies of the integument — *Other specified anomalies of the integument*

757.9   Unspecified congenital anomaly of the integument — *Unspecified anomaly of the integument; congenital anomaly NOS of integument*

758 CHROMOSOMAL ANOMALIES

Chromosomes are divided into two types: autosomes and sex-linked. Of the 21 pairs, only one pair, the 23rd, is related to sex are distributed as XX in girls and as XY in boys. The other 22 pairs are called autosomes. The conditions in the 758 category involve anomalies in either the sex chromosome or autosome arrangements.

758.0   Down's syndrome — *Down's syndrome; Mongolism; Trisomy 21 or 22*

Down's syndrome is the result of an extra chromosome (trisomy) on the 21st pair of chromosomes. Characteristics include hypertrophy, hearing loss due to the angle of the ear canals, developmental delay, delay in language acquisition, and heart defects.

758.1   Patau's syndrome — *Patau's syndrome; Trisomy 13*

Patau's syndrome is also a trisomic condition involving the 13th pair of autosomes. The brain's failure to divide into lobes is a primary characteristic that can affect the senses of sight, smell, and hearing. Lip and palate (typically cleft) anomalies may be present.

758.2   Edwards' syndrome — *Edwards' syndrome; Trisomy 18*

Edwards' syndrome, a trisomic autosome 18, involves delays in growth, the respiratory system, craniofacial malformations, skeletal defects, and webbing. Mental retardation is another characteristic.

758.3   Autosomal deletion syndromes — *Autosomal deletion syndromes; antimongolism syndrome; cri-du-chat syndrome*

Autosomal deletion syndromes involve either the deletion or misplacement of genetic material. In cri-du-chat syndrome, there is deletion or misplacement of the genetic material from the fifth chromosome. The individual may be hypotonic and scoliotic.

758.4   Balanced autosomal translocation in normal individual — *Balanced autosomal translocation in normal individual*

758.5   Other conditions due to autosomal anomalies — *Other conditions due to autosomal anomalies; accessory autosomes NEC*

758.6   Gonadal dysgenesis — *Gonadal dysgenesis; ovarian dysgenesis; Turner's syndrome; XO syndrome*

Turner's syndrome, also known as XO syndrome, affects females. It is sex chromosome linked, occurring once every 2,500 births. Characteristics include short stature, ovarian dysgenesis, and associated heart, kidney and thyroid disorders. Growth hormone and estrogen are used to treat the symptoms.

758.7   Klinefelter's syndrome — *Klinefelter's syndrome; XXY syndrome*

Klinefelter's syndrome affects only males, and involves an additional X chromosome, creating a pattern of XXY instead of XY. The condition is divided in mosaic and non-mosaic patients (mosaic implies that not all cells are affected). Characteristics include delayed language development. Injections of testosterone can counter the physical anomalies of the

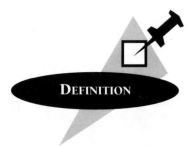

DEFINITION

Cri-du-chat: weak, mewling cry by an infant.

Hypertelorism: widely spaced eyes.

✔5th   Needs fifth-digit   **OK**   Valid three-digit code

syndrome. Associated disorders are asthma, hypostatic leg ulcers, thrombophlebitis, and osteoporosis. Male breast cancer presents a risk 20 times that of the non-Klinefelter male and there is also an increased incidence of mediastinal germ cell cancer.

A variant of Klinefelter syndrome produces two sets of abnormal sex chromosomes, for an XX YY arrangement. Another variant is XXXXY.

758.81   Other conditions due to sex chromosome anomalies — *Other conditions due to sex chromosome anomalies*

758.89   Other conditions due to chromosome anomalies — *Other conditions due to other chromosome anomalies*

MELAS syndrome is a mitochondrial myopathy that can lead to stroke-like episodes and enchephalomyopathy. Patients are increasingly fatigued in this progressive disease.

758.9   Conditions due to anomaly of unspecified chromosome — *Conditions due to anomaly of unspecified chromosome*

759 OTHER AND UNSPECIFIED CONGENITAL ANOMALIES

759.0   Congenital anomalies of spleen — *Anomalies of spleen; accessory spleen; congenital splenomegaly*

Asplenia is a serious condition associated with congenital heart anomalies.

759.1   Congenital anomalies of adrenal gland — *Anomalies of adrenal gland; aberrant adrenal gland; adrenal agenesis*

Use this code to report adrenal hypoplasia, or an absent, accessory, or aberrant adrenal gland. Excluded from this code are congenital disorders of steroid metabolism (255.2) and adrenogenital disorders (255.2).

759.2   Congenital anomalies of other endocrine glands — *Anomalies of other endocrine glands; parathyroidal agenesis; persistent thyroglossal duct*

A thyroglossal duct cyst is a fluid filled connective extending from the tongue base to the thyroid. The thyroglossal duct generally disappears during fetal development. This code reports thyroglossal duct cyst, absent parathyroid gland, accessory thyroid gland, or persistent thyroglossal or thyrolingual duct. Excluded from this code are congenital goiter (246.1) and congenital hypothyroidism (243).

759.3   Situs inversus — *Situs inversus; transposition of viscera, abdominal or thoracic or both*

Situs inversus, or Kartagener's syndrome, is a condition in which the abdominal and/or thoracic organs are in reverse position.

DEFINITION

Ectopia lentis: subluxation of the lens of the eye

Pectus carinatum: pigeon chest

Pectus excavatum: funnel chest

759.4   Conjoined twins — *Conjoined twins; craniopagus; pygopagus; thoracopagus*

Conjoined twins are born from a single ovum and a shared single placenta. They are always identical Incidence is one in every 50,000 to 80,000 births, with highest incidence in Africa and India. The twins can be joined at various sites, the most common being the thoracopagus arrangement of sharing a heart, joined at the chest, followed by omphalopagus, an anterior union at the midtrunk. Most conjoined twins miscarry or are stillborn.

759.5   Tuberous sclerosis — *Tuberous sclerosis; Bourneville's disease*

Tuberous sclerosis promotes benign tumors in the vital organs as well as in the eyes and skin, and affects both sexes. This condition can cause epileptic seizures and developmental delays and may be referred to as Bourneville's disease, Epiloia; Bourneville-Pringle syndrome; or Pringle's disease.

759.6   Other congenital hamartoses, not elsewhere classified — *Other hamartomas, NEC; Peutz-Jeghers syndrome; von Hippel-Lindau syndrome*

Von Hippel-Lindau syndrome involves abnormal growth of the blood vessels leading to hemangiomata and hemangioblastomata. They tend to grow in the retina, brain, cord, and adrenals. Predisposing the affected individuals to kidney cancer, it appears in the fourth decade.

Also use this code to report Jahnke's syndrome, Peutz-Jeghers syndrome; Sturge-Weber (-Dimitri) syndrome; Kalischer's syndrome, Krabbe's cutaneocerebral angioma syndrome; Lawford's syndrome; Milles' syndrome; Shimmer's syndrome; Sturge-Kalischer-Weber syndrome; and Weber-Dimitri syndrome.

759.7   Multiple congenital anomalies, so described — *Multiple congenital anomalies, so described; congenital anomaly NOS*

759.81   Prader-Willi syndrome — *Prader-Willi syndrome*

Prader-Willi syndrome is characterized by several conditions, including hypotonia, hypogonadism, hyperphagia, cognitive impairments, behavioral difficulties, and morbid obesity. The hypothalamus dysfunction leads to the disordered appetite (hyperphagia), which in turn causes the morbid obesity. The disorder is considered to be a deletion error in the genes.

759.82   Marfan's syndrome — *Marfan syndrome*

Marfan syndrome is a connective tissue disorder, affecting the long limbs, fingers, and toes. Arm span often exceeds height. The face is narrow and sharply featured and the chest may be excavatum or carinatum. The lens may be displaced, causing myopia. Other symptoms include loose joints, weakened aorta and cardiac valves, decreased lung elasticity, and scoliosis.

759.83   Fragile X syndrome — *Fragile X syndrome*

Fragile X syndrome occurs in males and females and involves mental retardation that is often more profound in males.

⬿5th   Needs fifth-digit   **OK**   Valid three-digit code

759.89   Other specified multiple congenital anomalies, so described — *Other specified anomalies; Laurence-Moon-Biedl syndrome*

This code can be reported to describe congenital malformation syndromes affecting multiple systems, not elsewhere classified, including Alport's syndrome; bird-headed dwarf (Seckel's syndrome); Brachmann-de Lange syndrome; Brachymorphism with ectopic lentis (Marchesani -(Weil) syndrome; Craniocarpotarsal dystrophy (Freeman-Sheldon syndrome); whistling-face syndrome; microencephaly, and dwarfism (Cockayne's syndrome). Other conditions reported with this code include Noonan's syndrome; Orodigitofacial dystosis (Bardet-Biedl) syndrome; Papillon-Lege and Psaume syndrome; Rubinstein-Taybi's syndrome; Smith-Lemli Opitz syndrome; Synophthalmus; and a congenital thoracogastroschisis, umbilical fistula, or cyst.

Laurence-Moon-Biedl syndrome, reported with this code, involves obesity, mental retardation, polydactyly or syndactyly, renal disease, retinitis pigmentosa, genital hypoplasia, and, in males, hypogonadism.

759.9   Unspecified congenital anomaly — *Congenital anomaly, unspecified*

Chapter 15

760-779

Certain Conditions Originating in the Perinatal Period

This chapter classifies conditions that begin during the perinatal period even if death or morbidity occurs later. The perinatal period is defined as the period of time occurring before, during, and up to 28 days following birth. These codes are used to classify causes or morbidity and mortality in the fetus or newborn and should never be used on the mother's coding profile. Additional codes can be used to further specify the newborn's condition.

760-763 Maternal Causes of Perinatal Morbidity and Mortality

Use these codes to report fetal or newborn conditions caused by systemic, metabolic, or infectious diseases of the mother. Maternal diseases that can affect the health or life of the fetus or newborn include hypertension, renal disease, urinary or respiratory tract infections, and circulatory diseases (pulmonary embolism, thrombophlebitis). Categories 760-763 also include fetal or newborn conditions caused by maternal nutritional disorders; maternal injury, surgery or death; maternal ingestion of drugs, chemicals or alcohol; and maternal complications of labor, delivery, or both.

These codes are reserved for use on the newborn coding profile as a secondary diagnosis to follow a code from rubrics V30 -V39 for liveborn infants. They also may be used as a principal diagnosis for a newborn that has been transferred or readmitted for a condition classifiable to codes 760-763. Assign a code from these categories only when there is evidence documented in the chart that the maternal condition has in fact affected the fetus or newborn.

760 FETUS OR NEWBORN AFFECTED BY MATERNAL CONDITIONS WHICH MAY BE UNRELATED TO PRESENT PREGNANCY

Excluded from this rubric is maternal endocrine and metabolic disorders affecting fetus or newborn (775.0-775.9).

760.0 Fetus or newborn affected by maternal hypertensive disorders — *fetus or newborn affected by maternal hypertension*

Use this code to report a fetal or newborn condition caused by maternal hypertension. The hypertension may be benign or malignant, preexisting, transient or gestational, chronic, or secondary (such as that due to renal artery stenosis). The incidence of maternal hypertension varies from 0.5 percent to 4 percent depending on the race and age of the mother, and averages 2.5 percent. The fetus or infant of a mother with hypertension has a 25 percent to 30 percent risk of prematurity and a 10 percent to 15 percent chance of being small for gestation age (SGA).

Therapies include resuscitation at birth for anoxia. Associated conditions include prematurity, alveolar conditions, respiratory distress syndrome, inadequate or erratic brain perfusion, acute tubular necrosis, necrotizing enterocolitis, hypotension, blood pressure peaks, hypovolemia, SGA, hypermagnesemia, thrombocytopenia, and neutropenia.

Use this code for the fetus or newborn when the maternal conditions have been classified to rubric 642.

760.1 Fetus or newborn affected by maternal renal and urinary tract diseases — *fetus or newborn affected by renal and urinary tract diseases*

Use this code for the fetus or newborn when the maternal conditions have been classified to rubrics 580-599.

760.2 Fetus or newborn affected by maternal infections — *fetus or newborn affected by maternal infectious disease, but fetus not manifesting that disease*

Use this code for the fetus or newborn when the maternal infectious disease has been classified to 001-136 and 487, but fetus or newborn is not manifesting the disease. Excluded from this rubric are congenital infectious diseases (771.09-771.8) and maternal genital tract and other localized infection (780.8).

760.3 Fetus or newborn affected by other chronic maternal circulatory and respiratory diseases — *fetus or newborn affected by chronic maternal circulatory and respiratory diseases*

Use this code for the fetus or newborn when the maternal conditions are classifiable to 390-459, 490-519, or 745-748.

760.4 Fetus or newborn affected by maternal nutritional disorders — *fetus or newborn affected by nutritional disorders*

Use this code for the fetus or newborn when the maternal disorders are classifiable to 260-269. Excluded from this code is fetal malnutrition (764.10-764.29).

760.5 Fetus or newborn affected by maternal injury — *fetus or newborn affected by maternal injury*

Use this code for the fetus or newborn when the maternal disorders are classifiable to 800-995.

760.6 Surgical operation on mother

Excluded from this code are cesarean section for present delivery (763.4); damage to placenta from amniocentesis, cesarean section, or surgical induction (762.1); or previous surgery to uterus or pelvic organs (763.89).

760.7 Noxious influences affecting fetus via placenta or breast milk

Use this code when the fetal or newborn condition caused by maternal ingestion of drugs or chemicals. This includes drugs taken for therapeutic purposes during pregnancy (but excludes drugs taken during labor and delivery, classified to code 763.5), drugs taken before pregnancy is known, and exposure to chemicals through the maternal work place while the fetus is in utero. Most drugs ingested during pregnancy, including their

✔5th Needs fifth-digit   **OK** Valid three-digit code

metabolites, cross the placenta and reach the fetus. Therefore, many substances have the potential for affecting the fetus. The specific effects on the fetus or newborn depend on the type of noxious substance.

Associated conditions include limb defects, skeletal and facial anomalies, mental retardation, chromosomal abnormalities, cardiac defects, and central nervous system defects.

These codes may be used regardless of the patient's age. For example, it is not uncommon for the daughters of women who ingested diethylstilbestrol (DES) during pregnancy to develop ovarian cancer from exposure of the drug through the placenta while in utero.

In addition, these codes may be used when the fetus or newborn shows signs and symptoms of acute intoxication of the noxious influence.

Excluded from this subclassification are anesthetic and analgesic drugs administered during labor and delivery (763.5) and drug withdrawal syndrome in newborn (779.5).

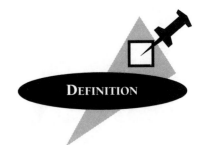

DEFINITION

Palmar grasp: flexion of the fingers upon stimulation of the palm of the hand, present at birth. This "grasp" reflex disappears in approximately six months.

760.70 Unspecified noxious substance affecting fetus or newborn via placenta or breast milk — *fetus or newborn affected by drug NEC*

760.71 Alcohol affecting fetus or newborn via placenta or breast milk — *fetal alcohol syndrome*

Use this code to report a fetal or newborn condition caused by maternal ingestion of alcohol during pregnancy. This code includes fetal alcohol syndrome (FAS), a condition diagnosed in patients born to chronic alcoholics who drank heavily during pregnancy. Lesser alcohol abuse results in a decreased severity of the manifestations of FAS. It is not known how much alcohol can be consumed safely.

Signs and symptoms of alcohol include jitteriness, diaphoresis, and convulsions; with acute intoxication, stupor or coma, confusion, lethargy, poor reflex responses; with fetal alcohol syndrome, pre- and postnatal growth retardation, short palpebral fissures, midfacial hypoplasia, low unparallel ears, flattened nasal bridge, and abnormal palmar creases. Toxicology tests of blood or urine reveal presence of alcohol. Associated conditions include cardiac defects, joint contractures, and mental retardation.

This code is used to report the effects of alcohol on the fetus or newborn, including alcohol withdrawal syndrome. Note that some newborns may suffer from both fetal alcohol syndrome and alcohol withdrawal syndrome, or fetal alcohol syndrome and acute alcohol intoxication.

760.72 Narcotics affecting fetus or newborn via placenta or breast milk

Use this code to report fetal or newborn condition caused by maternal ingestion of narcotics during pregnancy. Narcotics include opium, heroin, morphine, codeine, papaverine, and their many synthetics such as Demerol and methadone.

Signs and symptoms of narcotics include drowsiness and "nodding," small or pinpoint pupils, urinary retention, shallow irregular respirations or apnea, and, in severe cases, hypotension, hypothermia, and pulmonary edema. Toxicology tests of blood or urine reveal presence of narcotics. Therapies include drugs such as naloxone (Narcan).

This subclassification is used to report the effects of narcotics on the fetus or newborn. It excludes drug withdrawal syndrome, which is classified to code 779.5. Note that some newborns may suffer from both drug withdrawal syndrome and other physiopathological effects of narcotics in the perinatal period such as acute intoxication. Code both conditions.

760.73   Hallucinogenic agents affecting fetus or newborn via placenta or breast milk

Use this code to report the fetal or newborn condition caused by maternal ingestion of hallucinogenic agents during pregnancy. Hallucinogenic agents include lysergide (LSD), mescaline, psilocybin, sodium thiopental (STP), marijuana, phencyclidine (PCP), tetrahydrocannabinol (THC), and hashish.

Signs and symptoms of hallucinogenic agents include dilated pupils, restlessness, hyperreflexia, easy distractibility, and tachycardia. Toxicology tests of blood or urine reveal presence of hallucinogenics. Therapies include drugs such as diazepam and ammonium chloride.

This subclassification is used to report the effects of hallucinogens on the fetus or newborn. It excludes drug withdrawal syndrome, which is classified to code 779.5. Medical literature indicates that, of all hallucinogens, only chronic marijuana abuse has been associated with drug withdrawal symptoms.

760.74   Anti-infectives affecting fetus or newborn via placenta or breast milk —
fetus affected by antibiotics via placenta or breast milk

Use this code to report a fetal or newborn condition caused by maternal ingestion of anti-infectives, such as antibiotics, during pregnancy. Antibiotics that have been associated with birth defects include sulfonamides, metronidazole and tetracycline as well as antibiotics that inhibit deoxyribonucleic acid (DNA) or ribonucleic acid (RNA) synthesis such as actinomycin D, mitomycin C, adenine arabinoside, and idoxuridine.

Associated conditions include nerve damage, inhibition of bone growth, discoloration of teeth due to demineralization of enamel, and connective tissue defects.

760.75   Cocaine affecting fetus or newborn via placenta or breast milk

Use this code to report acute cocaine intoxication, caused by maternal ingestion of cocaine or coca plant derivatives during pregnancy. Cocaine addiction is associated with major problems in the newborn.

✔5th   Needs fifth-digit   **OK**   Valid three-digit code

Signs and symptoms of cocaine include hyperactivity, hyperthermia, tachycardia, dilated pupils, and, in severe cases, convulsions, coma, and circulatory collapse. Toxicology tests of blood or urine reveal presence of cocaine.

Therapies include drugs such as diazepam or chlorpromazine.

Associated conditions include infant drug withdrawal, renal system anomalies, central nervous system anomalies, and sudden infant death syndrome (SIDS).

This subclassification is used to report the effects of cocaine or coca plant derivatives on the fetus or newborn. It excludes drug withdrawal syndrome, which is classified to code 779.5. Code both conditions for newborns suffering from both drug withdrawal syndrome and other physiopathological effects of cocaine in the perinatal period.

760.76 Diethylstilbestrol (DES) affecting fetus or newborn via placenta or breast milk

760.79 Other noxious influences affecting fetus or newborn via placenta or breast milk — *including fetus or newborn affected by immune sera, medicinal agents NEC, or toxic substance NEC*

760.8 Other specified maternal conditions affecting fetus or newborn — *genital tract and other localized infection affecting fetus or newborn, but fetus or newborn manifesting that disease*

760.9 Unspecified maternal condition affecting fetus or newborn — *unknown*

761 FETUS OR NEWBORN AFFECTED BY MATERNAL COMPLICATIONS OF PREGNANCY

761.0 Fetus or newborn affected by incompetent cervix of mother

761.1 Fetus or newborn affected by premature rupture of membranes of mother

761.2 Fetus or newborn affected by oligohydramnios

Use this code to report a fetus or newborn affected by presence of less than 300 ml of amniotic fluid at term.

Associated conditions include Potter's syndrome, fetal urinary tract obstruction, intrauterine growth retardation, amniotic band syndrome, fetal compression, and fetal demise.

761.3 Fetus or newborn affected by polyhydramnios — *hydramnios (acute) (chronic)*

Use this code to report a fetus or newborn affected by presence of excessive amount of amniotic fluid during pregnancy. Polyhydramnios often is associated with maternal diabetes; however, the cause is unknown in approximately a third of all cases.

Associated conditions include esophageal atresia, anencephaly, spinal bifida, and isoimmunization.

761.4 Fetus or newborn affected by ectopic pregnancy of mother — *including abdominal, intraperitoneal, and tubal*

Use this code to report a fetus or newborn affected by implantation of a fertilized ovum in an area other than the uterus, for example, the cervix, uterine tube, ovary, or abdominal or pelvic cavity. This condition frequently occurs when the mother has some type of infertility. The most frequent site of ectopic pregnancy is within the fallopian tube. It is rare for the fetus to complete the weeks of gestation necessary to be viable.

761.5 Fetus or newborn affected by multiple pregnancy of mother — *including triplet, twin births*

761.6 Fetus or newborn affected by maternal death

761.7 Fetus or newborn affected by malpresentation before labor — *including breech presentation, external version, oblique lie, transverse lie, unstable lie*

761.8 Fetus or newborn affected by other specified maternal complications of pregnancy — *including spontaneous abortion, fetus*

761.9 Fetus or newborn affected by unspecified maternal complication of pregnancy — *unknown*

762 FETUS OR NEWBORN AFFECTED BY COMPLICATIONS OF PLACENTA, CORD, AND MEMBRANES

762.0 Fetus or newborn affected by placenta previa

Use this code to report a fetus or newborn affected by implantation of the placenta over or near the internal os of the cervix. There are two forms of placental previa: total, in which the placenta completely covers the internal cervical os, and partial, in which the placenta covers a portion of the internal cervical os. Placenta previa often results in a fetus being delivered prior to term.

Associated conditions include prematurity, alveolar conditions and respiratory distress syndrome, inadequate or erratic brain perfusion, hypotension, blood pressure peaks, infections including meningitis and sepsis, and SGA.

762.1 Fetus or newborn affected by other forms of placental separation and hemorrhage — *including abruptio placentae; antepartum hemorrhage; damage to placenta from amniocentesis; cesarean section or surgical induction; blood loss; premature separation of placenta; rupture of marginal sinus*

762.2 Fetus or newborn affected by other forms of other and unspecified morphological and functional abnormalities of placenta — *including dysfunction, infarction, insufficiency; yellow vernix syndrome*

762.3 Fetus or newborn affected by placental transfusion syndromes — (Use additional code 772.0, 776.4) — *placental and cord abnormality resulting in twin-to-twin or other transplacental transfusion*

762.4 Fetus or newborn affected by prolapsed cord — *cord -presentation*

762.5 Fetus or newborn affected by other compression of umbilical cord — *including cord around neck; entanglement; knot, torsion*

762.6 Fetus or newborn affected by other and unspecified conditions of umbilical cord — *including short cord, thrombosis, varices, velamentous insertion, vasa previa*

762.7 Fetus or newborn affected by chorioamnionitis — *including amnionitis, membranitis, placentitis*

✔5th Needs fifth-digit   **OK** Valid three-digit code

762.8 Fetus or newborn affected by other specified abnormalities of chorion and amnion — *not elsewhere classified*

762.9 Fetus or newborn affected by unspecified abnormality of chorion and amnion — *unknown*

763 FETUS OR NEWBORN AFFECTED BY OTHER COMPLICATIONS OF LABOR AND DELIVERY

763.0 Fetus or newborn affected by breech delivery and extraction

763.1 Fetus or newborn affected by other malpresentation, malposition, and disproportion during labor and delivery — *including abnormality of bony pelvis, contracted pelvis, persistent occipitoposterior position, shoulder presentation, transverse lie*

763.2 Fetus or newborn affected by forceps delivery — *fetus or newborn affected by forceps extraction*

763.3 Fetus or newborn affected by delivery by vacuum extractor

763.4 Fetus or newborn affected by cesarean delivery

763.5 Fetus or newborn affected by maternal anesthesia and analgesia — *reactions and intoxications from maternal opiates and tranquilizers during labor and delivery*

763.6 Fetus or newborn affected by precipitate delivery — *rapid second stage*

763.7 Fetus or newborn affected by abnormal uterine contractions — *including fetus or newborn affected by contraction ring, hypertonic labor, hypotonic uterine dysfunction, uterine inertia or dysfunction*

763.81 Abnormality in fetal heart rate or rhythm before the onset of labor

763.82 Abnormality in fetal heart rate or rhythm during labor

763.83 Abnormality in fetal heart rate or rhythm, unspecified as to time of onset

763.89 Other specified complications of labor and delivery affecting fetus or newborn — *including fetus or newborn affected by abnormality of maternal soft tissues, destructive operation on live fetus to facilitate delivery, induction of labor (medical), previous surgery to uterus or pelvic organs*

763.9 Unspecified complication of labor and delivery affecting fetus or newborn

764-779 Other Conditions Originating in the Perinatal Period

764 SLOW FETAL GROWTH AND FETAL MALNUTRITION

Use this code to report a condition when the fetus is considerably below the normal weight of offspring of the same gestational age. Malnutrition in a fetus may be due to defective assimilation or utilization of foods or to a maternal diet that is unbalanced or insufficient. Other factors that may cause an infant to be light for dates are genetic disorders, drugs, small maternal stature, placenta previa, multiple pregnancies, hypertension, anemia, and renal disease.

This condition may be described with such terms as "small for gestational age," "low birth weight," or "intrauterine growth retardation" (IUGR).

Associated conditions include genetic disorders such as Down syndrome, Edwards' syndrome, autosomal trisomy, and Turner syndrome.

764.0 ✓5th "Light-for-dates" without mention of fetal malnutrition — *infants underweight for gestational age; "small for dates"*

764.1 ✓5th "Light-for-dates" with signs of fetal malnutrition — *infants "light-for-dates;" infant showing signs of fetal malnutrition, such as dry peeling skin and loss of subcutaneous tissue; intrauterine malnutrition*

FIFTH-DIGIT

The following fifth-digit subclassification is for use with categories 764-765 to denote birthweight:

0 unspecified

1 less than 500 grams (less than 1.1 lbs)

2 500-749 grams (1.11 to 1.67 lbs)

3 750-999 grams (1.68 to 2.23 lbs)

4 1000-1249 grams (2.24 to 2.78 lbs)

5 1250-1499 grams (2.79 to 3.34 lbs)

6 1500-1749 grams (3.35 to 3.9 lbs)

7 1750-1999 grams (3.91 to 4.5 lbs)

8 2000-2499 grams (4.51 to 5.59 lbs)

9 2500 grams or more (5.6 lbs and over)

764.2 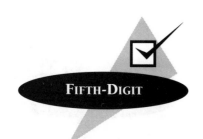5th Fetal malnutrition without mention of "light-for-dates" — *infants, not underweight for gestational age, showing signs of fetal malnutrition, such as dry peeling skin and loss of subcutaneous tissue; intrauterine malnutrition*

764.9 5th Unspecified fetal growth retardation — *including intrauterine growth retardation; undeveloped fetus or newborn*

765 DISORDERS RELATING TO SHORT GESTATION AND UNSPECIFIED LOW BIRTHWEIGHT

Use this code to report short gestation and unspecified low birthweight in disorders in a viable infant born before completing 37 weeks of gestation.

Associated conditions include alveolar conditions and respiratory distress syndrome, inadequate or erratic brain perfusion, hypotension, blood pressure peaks, infections including meningitis and sepsis, and SGA.

765.0 5th Extreme fetal immaturity — *implies birthweight of less than 1000 grams and/or a gestation of less than 28 completed weeks*

765.1 5th Other preterm infants — *implies a birthweight of 1000 to 24999 grams and/or a gestation of 28-37 completed weeks; including prematurity NOS*

766 DISORDERS RELATING TO LONG GESTATION AND HIGH BIRTHWEIGHT

Use this code to report disorders in a viable infant born after 42 weeks of gestation and/or described as "heavy," "large-for-dates," or greater than 4,500 grams birthweight.

766.0 Exceptionally large baby relating to long gestation — *implies a birthweight of 4500 grams or more*

Use this code to report an infant weighing over the 90th percentile for gestational age. Approximately 1 percent to 3 percent of neonates in the United States are considered large for gestational age. A baby may be exceptionally large when the mother has a large frame, is obese, or has diabetes. Associated conditions include hypoxia during labor and birth trauma.

766.1 Other "heavy-for-dates" infants not related to gestation period — *fetus or infant "heavy-" or "large-for-dates," regardless of period of gestation*

766.2 Post-term infant, not "heavy-for-dates" — *including postmaturity NOS, Ballantyne (-Runge) syndrome, Clifford's syndrome, Runge's syndrome*

767 BIRTH TRAUMA

The definition of birth trauma is injury to the fetus or newborn during delivery. Such injury may be due to breech presentation or forceps delivery.

767.0 Subdural and cerebral hemorrhage, birth trauma — *due to birth trauma or to intrapartum anoxia or hypoxia; including subdural hematoma (localized), tentorial tear; secondary code to identify cause*

The definition of subdural and cerebral hemorrhage is hemorrhage in or around the brain.

Signs and symptoms of subdural and cerebral hemorrhage include seizures, abnormally large head, diminished tone and/or resistance of skeletal muscles, retinal hemorrhage, positive transillumination of skull, or poor Moro's response (reaction to sudden loud noises).

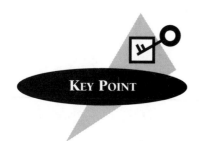

KEY POINT

In the United States, 97 percent of newborns have a birthweight of between 2500 grams (5.5 pounds) and 4500 grams (10 pounds).

FIFTH-DIGIT

The following fifth-digit subclassification is for use with categories 764-765 to denote birthweight:

0 unspecified

1 less than 500 grams (less than 1.1 lbs)

2 500-749 grams (1.11 to 1.67 lbs)

3 750-999 grams (1.68 to 2.23 lbs)

4 1000-1249 grams (2.24 to 2.78 lbs)

5 1250-1499 grams (2.79 to 3.34 lbs)

6 1500-1749 grams (3.35 to 3.9 lbs)

7 1750-1999 grams (3.91 to 4.5 lbs)

8 2000-2499 grams (4.51 to 5.59 lbs)

9 2500 grams or more (5.6 lbs and over)

5th   Needs fifth-digit   **OK**   Valid three-digit code

Lab work reveals red blood cells in cerebral spinal fluid. Computed tomography (CT) scan of head confirms diagnosis.

Therapies include fluid removal by daily subdural taps.

Associated conditions include hypoxia while in utero, anoxia while in utero, and prematurity.

767.1 Injuries to scalp, birth trauma — *including caput succedaneum, cephalhematoma, chignon (from vacuum extraction), massive epicranial subaponeurotic hemorrhage*

The definition of injuries to scalp is injuries to the scalp such as caput succedaneum, subgaleal hemorrhage, and cephalhematoma. Caput succedaneum, edema of the presenting portion of the scalp, usually is a mild trauma resulting from the pressure of the fetal scalp against the uterine cervix during labor and delivery. Subgaleal hemorrhage is a greater trauma manifested by a boggy feeling over the entire scalp, and cephalhematoma is hemorrhage of the periosteum.

767.2 Fracture of clavicle, birth trauma
767.3 Other injuries to skeleton, birth trauma — *including fracture of long bones, skull*
767.4 Injury to spine and spinal cord, birth trauma — *including dislocation, fracture, laceration, rupture*
767.5 Facial nerve injury, birth trauma — *including facial palsy, Bell's paralysis of newborn*
767.6 Injury to brachial plexus, birth trauma — *including brachial, Erb (-Duchenne), and Klumpke (-Déjérine) paralysis or palsy*

Use this code to report injury of the brachial plexus nerve during delivery. Damage of this nerve can affect the muscles of the arm and shoulder.

767.7 Other cranial and peripheral nerve injuries, birth trauma — *including phrenic nerve paralysis*
767.8 Other specified birth trauma — *including eye damage; hematoma or liver (subcapsular), testes, vulva; rupture of liver, spleen; scalpel wound; traumatic glaucoma; hematoma of sternocleidomastoid; ruptured stomach due to injury at birth; ruptured viscera; torticollis due to birth injury*
767.9 Unspecified birth trauma — *birth injury NOS*

768 INTRAUTERINE HYPOXIA AND BIRTH ASPHYXIA

Use this code to report reduction of oxygen resulting in impending or actual cessation of life. The condition may be brought on by events such as acute blood loss, aspiration of meconium, or a tight nuchal cord.

Signs and symptoms of intrauterine hypoxia and birth asphyxia include low Apgar score, pale or cyanotic color, poor or absent respirations, and poor reflexes and muscle tone. Fetal monitor shows irregular heart rhythm. Blood gases show hypercapnia and hypoxia. Therapies include endotracheal intubation and ventilation, and IV fluids with glucose.

Associated conditions include hypoglycemia, respiratory or metabolic acidosis, coma and seizures due to anoxic brain damage, fluid retention and hyponatremia due to acute tubular necrosis, sepsis, and bowel disorders such as necrotizing enterocolitis.

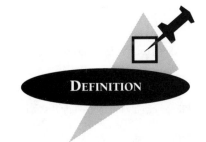

DEFINITION

Erb's palsy: usually due to forced traction at delivery, this birth injury affects one or more cervical nerve root and causes paralysis of the arm and diaphragm. In most cases, the paralysis is temporary and physical therapy improves function.

Klumpke's palsy: paralysis of wrist and hand, present at birth, involving the seventh and eighth cervical nerves and first thoracic nerve. In most cases, the paralysis is temporary and physical therapy improves function.

Bell's palsy of newborn: hemiparalysis of the face, due to birth trauma to, or intrauterine pressures upon, the facial nerve. The paralysis usually resolves within two months to three months.

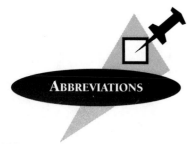

ABBREVIATIONS

ABGs: arterial blood gasses

BPD: bronchopulmonary dysplasia

CDH: congenital diaphragmatic hernia

CPAP: continuous positive airway pressure

ECMO: extracorporeal membrane oxygenation

ET: expiratory time

IMV: intermittent mandatory ventilation

IT: inspiratory time

MAS: meconium aspiration syndrome

PEEP: positive end expiratory pressure

PIE: pulmonary interstitial emphysema

PIP: peak inspiratory pressure

PM: pneumomediastinum

PPH: persistent pulmonary hypertension

RDS: respiratory distress syndrome

TTNB: transient tachypnea of the newborn

768.0   Fetal death from asphyxia or anoxia before onset of labor or at unspecified time — *secondary*

768.1   Fetal death from asphyxia or anoxia during labor — *secondary*

768.2   Fetal distress before onset of labor, in liveborn infant — *secondary; fetal metabolic acidemia first noted during labor, in liveborn infant*

Use this code to report hypoxia and acidosis affecting the functions of vital organs, such as the heart and lungs, of a fetus to the point of temporary injury or permanent injury or death.

768.3   Fetal distress first noted during labor, in liveborn infant

768.4   Fetal distress, unspecified as to time of onset, in liveborn infant — *secondary, fetal metabolic acidemia unknown as to time of onset, in liveborn infant*

768.5   Severe birth asphyxia — *secondary; birth asphyxia with neurologic involvement*

768.6   Mild or moderate birth asphyxia — *secondary;*

768.9   Unspecified birth asphyxia in liveborn infant — *including anoxia NOS, asphyxia NOS, hypoxia NOS*

769 RESPIRATORY DISTRESS SYNDROME `OK`

Use this code to report insufficient lung maturity of the fetus or newborn resulting in severe hypoxemia and multiple organ failure or death if left untreated. Also known as hyaline membrane disease and respiratory distress syndrome of the premature infant, this condition occurs primarily in premature infants (before completion of 37 weeks of gestation) or infants whose mothers are diabetic. It also may develop in infants whose mothers have toxemia or hypertension.

Signs and symptoms of respiratory distress syndrome include rapid labored respirations, substernal retractions, nasal alae flaring and "grunting" retractions, and low Apgar scores. Chest x-ray shows diffuse pulmonary atelectasis with overdistended alveolar ducts; blood gases show hypoxia. Therapies include IV fluids and electrolytes, oxygen therapy via nasal prongs, facemask, nasopharyngeal tube and endotracheal tube, and ventilation (CPAP, IPPV, and PEEP).

Associated conditions include respiratory or metabolic acidosis, hypoxemia, multiple organ failure, and atelectasis.

This category includes Type I respiratory distress syndrome or distress of the newborn. Type II respiratory distress syndrome or distress of the newborn is reported with 770.6, as is transient tachypnea of newborn.

770 OTHER RESPIRATORY CONDITIONS OF FETUS AND NEWBORN

770.0   Congenital pneumonia — *infective pneumonia acquired prenatally*

770.1   Meconium aspiration syndrome — *including aspiration of contents of birth canal NOS; meconium aspiration below vocal cords; fetal aspiration and meconium pneumonitis*

770.2   Interstitial emphysema and related conditions of newborn — *including pneumomediastinum, pneumopericardia, and pneumothorax originating in the perinatal period*

770.3   Pulmonary hemorrhage of fetus or newborn — *including hemorrhage of alveolar, intraalveolar, and massive pulmonary originating in the perinatal period*

770.4   Primary atelectasis of newborn — *including pulmonary immaturity NOS*

770.5 Other and unspecified atelectasis of newborn — *including atelectasis NOS, partial, and secondary originating in the perinatal period; pulmonary collapse*

770.6 Transitory tachypnea of newborn — *including idiopathic tachypnea, wet lung syndrome*

770.7 Chronic respiratory disease arising in the perinatal period — *including bronchopulmonary dysplasia, interstitial pulmonary fibrosis of prematurity, Wilson-Mikity syndrome, bubbly lung syndrome*

770.8 Other newborn respiratory problems after birth — *including apneic spells NOS, cyanotic attacks NOS, respiratory distress NOS, and respiratory failure NOS originating in the perinatal period; fetal acidosis, fetal anoxia, fetal asphyxia, fetal hypercapnia, and fetal hypoxia affecting newborn; respiratory depression, anaerosis, and lung paralysis of newborn*

770.9 Unspecified respiratory condition of fetus and newborn — *unknown*

771 INFECTIONS SPECIFIC TO THE PERINATAL PERIOD

Excluded from this rubric are congenital pneumonia (770.1); congenital syphilis (090.0-090.9); maternal infectious disease as a cause of mortality or morbidity in fetus or newborn, but fetus or newborn not manifesting the disease (760.2); ophthalmia neonatorum due to gonococcus (098.40); and other infections not specifically classified to this category.

771.0 Congenital rubella — *congenital rubella pneumonitis*

Use this code to report a fetal infection of the virus rubella while in utero. Maternal rubella infection that occurs within a month before conception and through the second trimester is associated with newborn disease. As many as 66 percent of newborns are free of any abnormality.

Signs and symptoms of congenital rubella include hepatosplenomegaly, "blueberry muffin" skin, and purpuric lesions. Lab work, such as immunofluorescence or enzyme immunoassays, reveals elevated antirubella IgM or IgG titers. Therapies include management of complications.

Associated conditions include hemolytic and hypoplastic anemia, pneumonia, meningoencephalitis, glaucoma and cataracts, thrombocytopenia, cardiac deformities such as patent ductus arteriosus, and other birth defects such as microcephaly and mental retardation.

771.1 Congenital cytomegalovirus infection — *congenital cytomegalic inclusion disease*

Use this code to report fetal infection of cytomegalovirus (CMV), a member of the herpes virus family, while in utero.

This category includes only congenital CMV infections; that is, those acquired up until the moment of birth, including passage through birth canal. Noncongenital CMV infections of the newborn, for example, those acquired through breast milk, in the nursery or home, or through postnatal blood transfusion, are classified elsewhere.

771.2 Other congenital infection specific to the perinatal period — *including herpes simplex, listeriosis, malaria, toxoplasmosis, tuberculosis*

771.3 Tetanus neonatorum — *tetanus omphalitis*

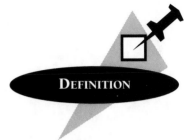

DEFINITION

Type I respiratory distress syndrome: chest x-ray shows reticulogranular pattern of the lung parenchyma with aerated areas outnumbering atelectatic areas.

Type II respiratory distress syndrome: chest x-ray shows reticulogranular pattern of the lung parenchyma with atelectatic areas outnumbering aerated areas.

Type III respiratory distress syndrome: chest x-ray shows reticulogranular pattern of the lung parenchyma with atelectatic areas outnumbering aerated areas and prominent air bronchograms.

Type IV respiratory distress syndrome: chest x-ray shows severe diffuse atelectatic areas with almost total loss of heart borders.

771.4	Omphalitis of the newborn — *including infection of naval cord and umbilical stump*
771.5	Neonatal infective mastitis
771.6	Neonatal conjunctivitis and dacryocystitis — *including ophthalmia neonatorum NOS*
771.7	Neonatal Candida infection — *including neonatal moniliasis, thrush in newborn*
771.8	Other infection specific to the perinatal period — *including intra-amniotic infection of fetus NOS, clostridial, and Escherichia coli; intrauterine sepsis of fetus; neonatal urinary tract infection; septicemia; septic umbilical cord*

772 FETAL AND NEONATAL HEMORRHAGE

Blood loss in this rubric is classified according to the site of hemorrhage. Typically, in fetal and neonatal hemorrhage, the infant will be hypotensive and pale. Hypovolemic shock should be corrected immediately.

Excluded from this rubric are hematological disorders of fetus and newborn (776.0-776.9).

772.0	Fetal blood loss — *including fetal blood loss from cut end of co-twin's cord, placenta, ruptured ord, and vasa previa; exsanguination; hemorrhage into co-twin, mother's circulation*
772.1	Fetal and neonatal intraventricular hemorrhage — *from any perinatal cause*
772.2	Fetal and neonatal subarachnoid hemorrhage of newborn — *from any perinatal cause*
772.3	Umbilical hemorrhage after birth — *slipped umbilical ligature*
772.4	Fetal and neonatal gastrointestinal hemorrhage
772.5	Fetal and neonatal adrenal hemorrhage
772.6	Fetal and neonatal cutaneous hemorrhage — *including bruising, ecchymoses, petechiae, superficial hematoma in fetus or newborn*
772.8	Other specified hemorrhage of fetus or newborn — *including hemopericardium, hemothorax of newborn*
772.9	Unspecified hemorrhage of newborn — *unknown*

773 HEMOLYTIC DISEASE OF FETUS OR NEWBORN, DUE TO ISOIMMUNIZATION

In isoimmunization, the mother develops antibodies against an antigen derived from a genetically dissimilar fetus.

773.0	Hemolytic disease due to Rh isoimmunization of fetus or newborn — *premature destruction of red blood cells due to incompatibility of Rh fetal-maternal blood grouping and positive Coombs test; including anemia, erythroblastosis, hemolytic disease, jaundice due to Rh antibodies, isoimmunization, and maternal/fetal incompatibility; Rh hemolytic disease, Rh isoimmunization*

Use this code to report incompatibility that occurs when an RH-negative mother carries and RH-positive fetus. Antibodies cross the placenta into the fetus and lead to hemolysis of the fetal blood.

Signs and symptoms of hemolytic disease due to Rh isoimmunization include scalp edema, cardiomegaly, hepatomegaly, splenomegaly, pale skin, and severe generalized edema.

Associated conditions include erythroblastosis fetalis, hydrops fetalis, ascites, polyhydramnios, pleural effusion, heart failure, anemia, and asphyxia during delivery due to enlarged liver.

✓5th   Needs fifth-digit   **OK**   Valid three-digit code

773.1 Hemolytic disease due to ABO isoimmunization of fetus or newborn — *including ABO hemolytic disease, ABO isoimmunization; anemia, erythroblastosis, hemolytic disease, jaundice due to ABO antibodies, isoimmunization, maternal/fetal incompatibility*

Use this code to report incompatibility that occurs when a mother with blood type O carries a fetus with blood type A or B. Antibodies cross the placenta into the fetus and cause hemolysis of the fetal blood.

Signs and symptoms of hemolytic disease due to ABO isoimmunization include scalp edema, cardiomegaly, hepatomegaly, splenomegaly, pale skin, and severe generalized edema.

Associated conditions include erythroblastosis fetalis, hydrops fetalis, ascites, polyhydramnios, pleural effusion, heart failure, anemia, and asphyxia during delivery due to enlarged liver.

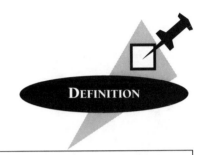

DEFINITION

773.2 Hemolytic disease due to other and unspecified isoimmunization of fetus or newborn — *including erythroblastosis NOS, hemolytic disease NOS, jaundice or anemia due to unknown blood-group incompatibility*

773.3 Hydrops fetalis due to isoimmunization — (Use additional code 773.0–773.2) — *secondary to identify type of isoimmunization*

Use this code to report gross edema of the entire body of the fetus with associated anemia due to mother-fetus blood incompatibility. The condition has a high mortality rate, especially in premature infants. Blood work reveals mother-fetus Rh and ABO incompatibility. Therapies include exchange blood transfusions, resuscitation and mechanical ventilation at birth, and thoracentesis.

Associated conditions include erythroblastosis fetalis, respiratory failure, pleural effusion, alloimmune hemolytic anemia, high output cardiac failure, and hypoproteinemia.

773.4 Kernicterus due to isoimmunization of fetus or newborn — (Use additional code 773.0–773.2) — *secondary to identify type of isoimmunization*

Use this code to report significantly large accumulation of bilirubin in the brain that may result in brain damage because of an incompatibility of fetal and maternal blood.

Signs and symptoms of kernicterus due to isoimmunization include jaundice, high fever, seizures, blunted Moro reflex, opisthotonic posturing, incomplete flexion of extremities, vomiting, and high-pitched cry. Therapies include phototherapy and exchange blood transfusions.

Associated conditions include mental retardation and hemolytic disease.

773.5 Late anemia due to isoimmunization of fetus or newborn

Apgar score: Named for American anesthesiologist Virginia Apgar, an assessment of a newborn taken at birth and again at five minutes, with possible scores of 0-10. The score is the sum of points gained in review of heart rate, respiratory effort, muscle tone, reflex irritability, and color. Each of these categories is assigned a score:

Heart rate:	0, absent;	1, slow;	2 normal
Respiration:	0 absent;	1, weak;	2 strong
Muscle tone:	0 limp;	1, some flexion;	2, well flexed
Reflex:	0, absent;	1, some motion;	2, cry, sneeze
Color:	0, total blue;	1 extremity blue;	2, completely pink

A score of 0-3 represents severe distress; 4-7 moderate distress; and 8-10 no difficulty. The score at five minutes is generally higher than the score at birth, and is a better benchmark of infant health. The two scores are generally expressed together, separated by a hash mark, as in 7/9.

774 OTHER PERINATAL JAUNDICE

Jaundice is also known as hyperbilirubinemia, which refers to the excess of bilirubin. The excess bilirubin may be caused by an overproduction of bilirubin; an impaired ability to secrete bilirubin; or a mixture of both causes.

774.0	Perinatal jaundice from hereditary hemolytic anemias — (Code first underlying disease 282.0–282.9) — *secondary to underlying disease*
774.1	Perinatal jaundice from other excessive hemolysis — *secondary to identify cause; including jaundice from bruising, drugs or toxins transmitted from mother, infection, polycythemia, swallowed maternal blood*
774.2	Neonatal jaundice associated with preterm delivery — *including hyperbilirubinemia of prematurity; jaundice due to delayed conjugation associated with preterm delivery*
774.30	Neonatal jaundice due to delayed conjugation, cause unspecified — *including Lucey-Driscoll syndrome*
774.31	Neonatal jaundice due to delayed conjugation in diseases classified elsewhere — (Code first underlying disease, as: 243, 277.4) — *secondary to underlying disease*
774.39	Other neonatal jaundice due to delayed conjugation from other causes — *including jaundice due to delayed conjugation from causes such as breast milk inhibitors and delayed development of conjugating system*
774.4	Perinatal jaundice due to hepatocellular damage — *including fetal or neonatal hepatitis, giant cell hepatitis, inspissated bile syndrome*
774.5	Perinatal jaundice from other causes — (Code first underlying disease, as: 271.1, 277.00, 277.01, 751.61) — *secondary to underlying cause*
774.6	Unspecified fetal and neonatal jaundice — *including icterus neonatorum, neonatal hyperbilirubinemia (transient), physiologic jaundice NOS*
774.7	Kernicterus of fetus or newborn not due to isoimmunization — *including bilirubin encephalopathy, kernicterus of newborn NOS*

Use this code to report significantly large accumulation of bilirubin in the brain that may result in brain damage not due to a fetal/maternal blood incompatibility (ABO incompatibility). The condition may be caused by a large influx of red blood cells through the umbilicus at the time of delivery.

Signs and symptoms of kernicterus not due to isoimmunization include jaundice, high fever, seizures, blunted Moro reflex, opisthotonic posturing, incomplete flexion of the extremities, vomiting, and high-pitched cry. Therapies include phototherapy and exchange blood transfusions.

Associated conditions include mental retardation.

5th Needs fifth-digit   **OK** Valid three-digit code

775 ENDOCRINE AND METABOLIC DISTURBANCES SPECIFIC TO THE FETUS AND NEWBORN

This rubric includes transitory endocrine and metabolic disturbances caused by the infant's response to maternal endocrine and metabolic factors, the infant's removal from them, or the infant's adjustment to extrauterine existence.

775.0   Syndrome of "infant of diabetic mother" — *maternal diabetes mellitus affecting fetus or newborn (with hypoglycemia)*

Use this code to report a syndrome with manifestations including macrosomia, birth asphyxia, hypoglycemia, cardiorespiratory disorders, and congenital malformations.

Signs and symptoms of syndrome of "infant of a diabetic mother" include large size, obesity, listlessness, limpness, poor feeding, and red florid complexion due to excessive amount of blood.

775.1   Neonatal diabetes mellitus — *diabetes mellitus syndrome in newborn*
775.2   Neonatal myasthenia gravis
775.3   Neonatal thyrotoxicosis — *hyperthyroidism (transient)*
775.4   Hypocalcemia and hypomagnesemia of newborn — *including cow's mile hypocalcemia, hypocalcemic tetany, hypoparathyroidism, phosphate-loading hypocalcemia*
775.5   Other transitory neonatal electrolyte disturbances — *including dehydration*
775.6   Neonatal hypoglycemia
775.7   Late metabolic acidosis of newborn
775.8   Other transitory neonatal endocrine and metabolic disturbances — *amino acid metabolic disorders described as transitory; including tyrosinemia*
775.9   Unspecified endocrine and metabolic disturbances specific to the fetus and newborn — *unknown*

776 HEMATOLOGICAL DISORDERS OF FETUS AND NEWBORN

776.0   Hemorrhagic disease of newborn — *including diathesis, vitamin K deficiency, Minot's disease*
776.1   Transient neonatal thrombocytopenia — *due to exchange transfusion, idiopathic maternal thrombocytopenia, isoimmunization*
776.2   Disseminated intravascular coagulation in newborn
776.3   Other transient neonatal disorders of coagulation — *including transient coagulation defect, newborn*
776.4   Polycythemia neonatorum — *including plethora; polycythemia due to donor twin transfusion, maternal-fetal transfusion*
776.5   Congenital anemia — *anemia following fetal blood loss*
776.6   Anemia of neonatal prematurity

Use this code to report a condition in viable infant born before completing 37 weeks of gestation in which the number of erythrocytes per cu mm and the quantity of hemoglobin are reduced. The hemoglobin nadir for premature infants is 6.5-9.0 g/100 ml as opposed to 9.5-11.0 g/100 ml for term infants. The extent of the anemia is directly related to the birth weight.

Signs and symptoms of anemia of prematurity include tachycardia, tachypnea, poor feeding, apnea, and dyspnea. Lab work shows abnormally low hemoglobin. Therapies include packed red blood cells, particularly when blood removed for testing exceeds 10 percent of estimated volume, and iron supplement.

Associated conditions include alveolar conditions and respiratory distress syndrome, inadequate or erratic brain perfusion, hypotension, blood pressure peaks, and infections including meningitis and sepsis.

776.7   Transient neonatal neutropenia — *including isoimmune and maternal transfer neutropenia*

776.8   Other specified transient hematological disorders of fetus or newborn — *other specified*

776.9   Unspecified hematological disorder specific to fetus or newborn — *unknown*

777 PERINATAL DISORDERS OF DIGESTIVE SYSTEM

Excluded from this rubric is intestinal obstruction classifiable to 560.0-560.9.

777.1   Fetal and newborn meconium obstruction — *including congenital fecaliths, meconium ileus NOS, meconium plug syndrome, delayed passage of meconium*

Meconium obstruction is obstruction of the digestive tract due to the fetal tar-like meconium.

Signs and symptoms of meconium obstruction include no stools for first 24 hours to 48 hours of life, abdominal distention, symptoms of distal intestinal obstruction and incomplete obstruction, and vomiting. Radiology tests, such as contrast enema, locate obstruction. Therapies include contrast enema (therapeutic) and saline enemas.

This subcategory includes meconium plug syndrome but excludes meconium ileus (277.01).

777.2   Neonatal intestinal obstruction due to inspissated milk

777.3   Neonatal hematemesis and melena due to swallowed maternal blood — *swallowed blood syndrome in newborn*

777.4   Transitory ileus of newborn

777.5   Necrotizing enterocolitis in fetus or newborn — *including pseudomembranous enterocolitis in newborn*

777.6   Perinatal intestinal perforation — *including meconium peritonitis*

777.8   Other specified perinatal disorder of digestive system — *other specified*

777.9   Unspecified perinatal disorder of digestive system — *unknown*

778 CONDITIONS INVOLVING THE INTEGUMENT AND TEMPERATURE REGULATION OF FETUS AND NEWBORN

778.0   Hydrops fetalis not due to isoimmunization — *including idiopathic hydrops*

Use this code to report gross edema of the entire body of the fetus with associated anemia. Nonimmune fetal hydrops can be caused by a wide variety of diseases and disorders involving many different body systems. The infant mortality rate is very high, particularly with premature infants. Therapies include vigorous resuscitation including mechanical ventilation at birth, thoracentesis for pleural effusion, and diuresis. Associated conditions include erythroblastosis fetalis, anemia, hypoproteinemia, respiratory failure, and pleural effusion.

DEFINITION

Farber's test: an analysis of meconium in a constipated newborn, to rule out intestinal bowel obstruction. If the meconium contains traces of squamous cells and lanugo, it can be assumed the bowel is not obstructed. The squamous cells and lanugo would have been ingested when the fetus swallowed amniotic fluid, and their presence is indicative of a patent and functional digestive system. Treatment with enemas will usually clear the meconium plug.

↳5th   Needs fifth-digit   **OK**   Valid three-digit code

Most diagnostic studies, such as fetal ultrasounds and maternal blood examination, are performed in utero and are not reported in the newborn's chart.

Excluded from this subclassification is hydrops fetalis due to isoimmunization (773.3).

778.1   Sclerema neonatorum — *including subcutaneous fat necrosis, Underwood's disease*

778.2   Cold injury syndrome of newborn

778.3   Other hypothermia of newborn

778.4   Other disturbance of temperature regulation of newborn — *including dehydration fever, environmentally-induced pyrexia, hyperthermia, transitory fever*

778.5   Other and unspecified edema of newborn — *including edema neonatorum*

778.6   Congenital hydrocele — *congenital hydrocele of tunica vaginalis*

Use this code to report a collection of fluid in the tunica vaginalis of the testicle or along the spermatic cord, or a serous dilation of a cervical duct of an infant. Almost all neonatal hydroceles are communicating and close spontaneously.

Therapies include surgery to repair persistent hydrocele (lasting more than one year) by inguinal incision and ligation of sac.

778.7   Breast engorgement in newborn — *noninfective mastitis*

778.8   Other specified condition involving the integument of fetus and newborn — *including urticaria neonatorum*

778.9   Unspecified condition involving the integument and temperature regulation of fetus and newborn — *unknown*

779 OTHER AND ILL-DEFINED CONDITIONS ORIGINATING IN THE PERINATAL PERIOD

779.0   Convulsions in newborn — *including fits and seizures in newborn*

779.1   Other and unspecified cerebral irritability in newborn — *other and unknown*

779.2   Cerebral depression, coma, and other abnormal cerebral signs in fetus or newborn — *including CNS dysfunction in newborn NOS*

779.3   Feeding problems in newborn — *including regurgitation, slow feeding, and vomiting in newborn*

779.4   Drug reactions and intoxications specific to newborn — *including Gray syndrome from chloramphenicol administration in newborn*

Use this code to report toxic conditions and adverse drug reactions in neonates, especially premature infants, caused by the body's immature detoxification and excretion mechanisms. Gray syndrome, or gray baby syndrome, is a condition caused by an infant's inability to efficiently conjugate and eliminate the antibiotic chloramphenicol.

779.5   Drug withdrawal syndrome in newborn — *drug withdrawal syndrome in infant of dependent mother*

Use this code to report complex of syndromes in newborns adversely affected by mothers who are addicted to, or frequent abusers of, drugs. Narcotics and cocaine and coca plant derivatives are the most frequently abused drugs capable of causing withdrawal symptoms in the newborn, but barbiturates, other tranquilizers, amphetamines, other stimulants, and other addictive substances can cause the syndrome.

Signs and symptoms of drug withdrawal syndrome in newborn include irritability, tremulousness, tachypnea, vomiting or diarrhea, fever, and convulsions. Toxicology tests of blood or urine identify drug. Therapies include close monitoring for seizure activity or arrhythmias, detoxification tailored for drug of dependence, drugs such as phenytoin sodium (Dilantin) or phenobarbital for seizures, exchange transfusions in emergencies.

Associated conditions include fetal alcohol syndrome, dehydration, hypocalcemia, and seizures.

779.6 Termination of pregnancy (fetus) — *including fetal death due to induced abortion and termination of pregnancy*

779.8 Other specified conditions originating in the perinatal period — *including atheromatosis of colon, toxemia, uremia, Harlequin color change syndrome, hypertonicity of infancy, papyraceous fetus, strophulus*

779.9 Unspecified condition originating in the perinatal period — *including congenital debility NOS, stillbirth NEC*

✓5th Needs fifth-digit   **OK** Valid three-digit code

Chapter 16

780-799
Symptoms, Signs, and Ill-Defined Conditions

This chapter includes symptoms, signs and abnormal results of laboratory or other investigative procedures, as well as ill-defined conditions for which there are no other, more specific diagnoses classifiable elsewhere.

In general, codes from this chapter are used to report symptoms, signs, and ill-defined conditions that point with equal suspicion to two or more diagnoses or represent important problems in medical care that may affect management of the patient. In addition, this chapter provides codes to classify abnormal findings that are reported without a corresponding definitive diagnosis. Codes for such findings can be located in the alphabetic index under such terms as "Abnormal, abnormality, abnormalities," "Decrease, decreased," "Elevation," and "Findings, abnormal, without diagnosis."

Codes from this chapter also are used to report symptoms and signs that existed on initial encounter but proved to be transient and without a specified cause. Also included are provisional diagnoses for patients who fail to return for further investigation, cases referred elsewhere for further investigation before being diagnosed, and cases in which a more definitive diagnosis was not available for other reasons.

Do not assign a code from categories 780-799 when the symptoms, signs, and abnormal findings pertain to a definitive diagnosis. For example, a patient with acute appendicitis would not need additional codes for abdominal pain (rubric 789) and abdominal rigidity (789.4). These signs and symptoms are integral to acute appendicitis and add no value to the patient's coding profile when assigned as secondary codes.

However, you may use a code from this chapter to report symptoms, signs, and abnormal findings that pertain to a particular clinical diagnosis if they represent important problems in medical care. Such problems may be useful to record because they may affect length of stay or level of nursing care and/or monitoring. Such problems also may require additional diagnostic or clinical evaluation or may affect treatment plans. In these cases, list the definitive condition as the principal diagnosis and the symptoms secondarily.

List as a secondary diagnosis any symptoms, signs, and abnormal findings that are not integral to the principal diagnosis but provide important clinical information. For example, a patient with benign prostatic hypertrophy (rubric 600) admitted in acute urinary retention might have acute urinary retention listed as a secondary diagnosis (788.2). Acute urinary retention is not integral to the disease process for benign prostatic hypertrophy, but is an indication for catheterization or surgery. Acute urinary retention can be viewed as an "important medical problem" when the medical record documentation shows the need for clinical evaluation or diagnostic procedures to rule out pathology other than benign prostatic hypertrophy as the etiology. Therapeutic treatment (e.g., catheterization prior to

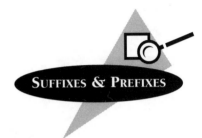

SUFFIXES & PREFIXES

Dys - difficult or painful

Neo - new

Pan - entire

Para - beyond, beside

Poly - many

Supra - above, excessive

Syn - with

Trans - across

-algia - pain

-dynia - pain

-cele - protrusion or hernia

-emesis - vomiting

-emia - blood condition

-oma - neoplasm

-phagia - eating

-pnea - breathing

-rhea - discharge

surgery) includes increased nursing care and/or monitoring such as catheter care or extended length of hospital stay.

List as the principal diagnosis any symptoms, signs, and abnormal findings that, after study, cannot be attributed to a definitive diagnosis classifiable to another ICD-9-CM chapter. Also list as the principal diagnosis any symptom, sign, or abnormal finding that points to contrasting or comparative diagnoses (e.g., it points with equal suspicion to two or more diagnoses). List the contrasting or comparative diagnoses as secondary.

780-789 Symptoms

The definition of a symptom is subjective observation reported to physician by patient but not confirmed by physician. These observations depart from the structure, function, or sensation that the patient normally experiences.

780 GENERAL SYMPTOMS

780.0 Alteration of consciousness

This subclassification reports impaired consciousness due to dysfunction of the cerebral hemispheres, the upper brainstem, or both. This subcategory includes coma, transient alteration of awareness, persistent vegetative state, and other alterations such as drowsiness, semicoma, somnolence, stupor, torpor, or suppressed or impaired awareness or unconsciousness.

Coma is a state of profound stupor or unconsciousness from which the patient cannot be aroused by external stimuli. The etiology may be trauma, intracranial neoplasm, infection and toxic reaction to infection, poisoning and adverse effects of drugs and chemicals, hypertensive and atherosclerotic cerebrovascular disease, or thrombosis.

Transient alteration of awareness refers to symptoms of staring or transient loss of awareness. This condition has been associated with migraines, epileptic seizures, transient ischemic attacks, or psychological disorders, but in many cases the etiology is unknown.

Lab work may identify cause based on blood work (hematocrit, respiratory gases, WBC, BUN), urinalysis, (sugar, acetone, albumin, sedatives) and levels of glucose, sodium, potassium, bicarbonate, chloride, alcohol, bromide. A gastric lavage reveals suspected poisoning. A lumbar puncture (if infection suspected as etiology) and culture identify presence of white blood cells and infective organism.

Therapies depend on etiology and may include, if cause unknown, temperature, pulse, respirations, blood pressure checked at frequent intervals, and glucose infusion.

Associated conditions include epidural/subdural hematoma, cerebral infarct or hemorrhage, brain tumor or abscess, brain stem infarction, tumor, hemorrhage, trauma, concussion, cerebral lacerations or contusion, cardiac arrhythmia, shock, epilepsy, infection, subarachnoid hemorrhage, catatonia, hypoglycemia, and diabetic acidosis.

780.01	Coma — *persistent unconsciousness*	
780.02	Transient alteration of awareness — *alternating states of consciousness and unconsciousness*	
780.03	Persistent vegetative state — *awake without consciousness*	

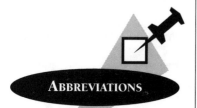

ABBREVIATIONS

ABG: arterial blood gas

BUN: blood urea nitrogen

CBC: complete blood count

FBS: fasting blood sugar

GTT: glucose tolerance test

PUO: pyrexia (fever) unknown origin

RBC: red blood cell (count)

WBC: white blood cell (count)

↙5th Needs fifth-digit   **OK** Valid three-digit code

780.09   Other alteration of consciousness — *not specified elsewhere, including drowsiness, semicoma, somnolence, stupor*

780.1   Hallucinations — *including auditory, visual, gustatory, olfactory, tactile*

Use this subclassification to report sensory perception of an object or event without corresponding external stimuli. Hallucinations generally take one of five forms, as follows:

- Auditory (perception of nonexistent voices or sounds)

- Visual (perception of nonexistent people, places, or other visual stimuli such as flashes of light)

- Olfactory (perception of nonexistent odors)

- Tactile (perception of nonexistent contact stimuli such as crawling insects on skin)

- Gustatory (perception of unpleasant tastes)

Hallucinations may be due to drugs or toxic substances or due to chronic conditions such as schizophrenia, depression, bipolar affective disorders, and organic brain syndromes.

780.2   Syncope and collapse — *blackout, fainting, Gower's syndrome*

Syncope is caused by a decrease in cerebral blood flow due to decreased cardiac output and results in sudden, brief loss of consciousness. Arrhythmia is the most common etiology (heart rates of less than 30 beats to 35 beats per minute and more than 150 beats to 180 beats per minute). If cardiovascular disease is present, alterations may be less pronounced.

Signs and symptoms of syncope and collapse include motionlessness, paleness, diaphoresis, weak pulse, and shallow breathing. Physical exam reveals hypotension and postural changes in heart rate and blood pressure. Lab work may show elevated fasting blood sugar (confirming hyperglycemia) and elevated cardiac serum isoenzyme (identifying acute myocardial infarction). Hematocrit may detect anemia. An electrocardiogram (EKG) may suggest arrhythmia, conduction abnormality, ventricular hypertrophy, or myocardial infarction and a computed tomography (CT) scan of head and brain confirms focal neurological deficit or intracranial process. Therapies depend on etiology.

Associated conditions include seizure disorder, arrhythmias, hypovolemia, myocardial infarction, drug toxicity, and transient ischemic attack.

780.3 Convulsions

Convulsions are a series of jerking movements of the face, trunk, or extremities, with involuntary contracture of voluntary muscles. Etiology is an acute focal or generalized disturbance in cerebral function. A small focus of diseased tissue in the cerebrum discharges abnormally in response to certain endogenous or exogenous stimuli. Spread of the discharge to other portions of the cerebrum results in convulsive activity and loss of consciousness. Codes in this subclassification are selected based on whether the convulsions are febrile in origin.

Associated conditions include hyperpyrexia (acute infection, heat stroke), central nervous system infections (meningitis, encephalitis, brain abscess), cerebral trauma (skull fracture, birth injury), cerebral edema (hypertensive encephalopathy, eclampsia), metabolic disturbances (hypoglycemia, hypoparathyroidism), and cerebral hypoxia (Adams-Stokes syndrome, anesthesia).

This subcategory classifies convulsive disorders and seizures that are ill-defined, as well as a sudden, acute symptomatic manifestations of other conditions. Classify to rubric 345, epilepsy, convulsive or seizure disorders described as irreversible, intractable, recurrent, repetitive, chronic, or requiring maintenance with phenobarbital or Dilantin for control. Also excluded from this subclassification is neonatal convulsion (779.0).

780.31 Febrile convulsions — *pyrexial seizure*
780.39 Other convulsions — *not originating with fever*
780.4 Dizziness and giddiness — *light-headedness, vertigo not otherwise specified*

Use this subclassification to report the illusion of movement or a feeling of unsteadiness or light-headedness.

Associated conditions include brain stem ischemia, head trauma, multiple sclerosis, posterior fossa tumor, acoustic neuroma, labyrinthitis, Menière's disease, vestibular neuritis, herpes zoster, and toxic levels of drugs.

780.5 Sleep disturbances
Excluded from this subclassification are sleep disturbances that are not organic in nature (307.40-307.49).

780.50 Unspecified sleep disturbance — *unknown*
780.51 Insomnia with sleep apnea — *cessation of breathing causes sleeplessness*

There are three types of sleep apnea: obstructive, central, and mixed; of the three, obstructive sleep apnea (OSA) is the most common. Despite the difference in the root cause of each type, people with untreated sleep apnea stop breathing repeatedly during their sleep, sometimes hundreds of times during the night and often for a minute or longer, according to the American Sleep Apnea Association.

Obstructive sleep apnea is caused by a blockage of the airway, usually when the soft tissue in the rear of the throat collapses and closes during sleep. In central sleep apnea, the airway is not blocked but the brain fails to signal the muscles to breathe. Mixed sleep apnea is a combination of the two. The condition arouses sleep apnea victims from sleep in order for them to resume breathing, resulting in fragmented sleep.

Sleep apnea affects more than 12 million Americans, according to the National Institutes of Health. Males are more prone to sleep apnea than females. Risk of sleep apnea increases for those overweight and age over 40 years, although sleep apnea can strike anyone at any age.

Untreated, sleep apnea can cause high blood pressure and other cardiovascular disease, memory problems, weight gain, impotency, and headaches. Several treatment options exist, and research into additional options continues.

780.52 Other insomnia — *sleeplessness not associated with apnea*

780.53 Hypersomnia with sleep apnea — *cessation of breathing causes sleepiness*

780.54 Other hypersomnia — *sleepiness not associated with apnea*

780.55 Disruptions of 24-hour sleep-wake cycle — *inversion of sleep rhythm, irregular sleep-wake cycle*

780.56 Dysfunctions associated with sleep stages or arousal from sleep

780.57 Other and unspecified sleep apnea — *unknown or not elsewhere classified*

Other and unspecified sleep apnea involve the abnormal cessation of breathing during sleep not classified elsewhere. Sleep apnea is due to either a failure of ventilatory drive as seen in disease of the central nervous system or obstruction of the upper airway as seen in massive obesity or tonsillar hypertrophy. Central sleep apnea is a form of obstructive apnea due to a hereditary failure of the ventilatory drive in males.

Interestingly, in ICD-10-CM sleep apnea is classified as a disease of the nervous system rather than a sign and symptom.

780.59 Other sleep disturbances

780.6 Fever — *pyrexia, PUO, FUO, chills with fever*

Use this code to report an abnormal elevation of body temperature (at least 38.3 C or 101 F) for a minimum of three weeks without the etiology being determined despite exhaustive investigation. Fever that is ill-defined or unspecified also is classified here.

Therapies depend on etiology, but include cooling blankets, cold compresses, antibiotics, and antipyretics (aspirin, acetaminophen). Associated conditions include infections, connective tissue disorders, and occult neoplasm (leukemia, lymphoma).

780.7 Malaise and fatigue

Excluded from this rubric is fatigue during combat (308.0-308.9), heat (992.6), and pregnancy (646.8), and fatigue or malaise related to neurasthenia (300.5) and senile asthenia (797).

780.71 Chronic fatigue syndrome — *severe, prolonged fatigue impairing daily function, without proven physical or psychological cause*

Chronic fatigue syndrome (CFS) also is known as myalgic encephalomyelitis, postviral fatigue syndrome, and chronic fatigue and immune dysfunction syndrome. It is marked by unrelenting exhaustion, muscle pain, cognitive disorders that patients call "brain fog," and a profound weakness that does not go away with a few good nights of sleep. There is no known cause. CFS may begin after a bout with a cold, bronchitis, hepatitis, or an intestinal bug. For some, it follows a bout of infectious mononucleosis or during a period of high stress. Unlike flu symptoms, CFS symptoms, such as a chronic headache, muscle and joint

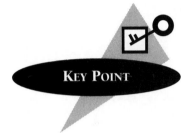

KEY POINT

Metric Conversion

Fahrenheit	to	Celsius
98.6		37.00
99.0		37.22
99.4		37.44
99.8		37.67
100.2		37.89
100.6		38.11
101.4		38.56
101.8		38.78
102.2		39.00
102.6		39.22
103.4		39.67
103.8		39.89
104.2		40.11
104.6		40.33
105.0		40.56
105.4		40.78
105.8		41.00
106.2		41.22
106.6		41.44
107.0		41.67
107.4		41.89
107.8		42.11
107.0		42.22

aches, and fatigue, either hang on or come and go frequently for more than six months. Some patients are bedridden; others can work or attend school at least part time, since any exertion typically worsens symptoms.

CFS is diagnosed two to four times more often in females than males and it is estimated that as many as 500,000 people in the United States have a CFS-like condition. There is no effective treatment for CFS. However, nonsteroidal anti-inflammatory drugs, such as ibuprofen, reduce body aches or fever, and nonsedative antihistamines relieve any prominent allergic symptoms, such as runny nose.

780.79   Other malaise and fatigue — *including asthenia, postviral syndrome, Stiller's asthenia, neurasthenia, albionarc*

780.8   Hyperhidrosis — *night sweats, diaphoresis, excessive sweating*

780.9   Other general symptoms — *including amnesia, hypokinesia, generalized pain, autopagnosia, paramnesia*

781 SYMPTOMS INVOLVING NERVOUS AND MUSCULOSKELETAL SYSTEMS

Excluded from this rubric are depression not otherwise specified (311); pain in the limb (729.5); and disorders relating to the back (724.0-724.9), hearing (388.0-389.9), joint (718.0-719.9), limb (729.0-729.9), neck (723.0-723.9), or vision (368.0-369.9).

781.0   Abnormal involuntary movements — *spasms, tremors, head movements, fasiculations; not otherwise specified*

781.1   Disturbances of sensation of smell and taste — *anosmia, parageusia, parosmia*

781.2   Abnormality of gait — *ataxic, paralytic, spastic, staggering*

781.3   Lack of coordination — *muscular incoordination, ataxia not otherwise specified*

781.4   Transient paralysis of limb — *including transient monoplegia*

781.5   Clubbing of fingers — *enlargement of soft tissues of distal fingers*

781.6   Meningismus — *irritation of lining of brain or spinal cord; Dupre's syndrome, meningism*

781.7   Tetany — *extremity muscle spasms; carpopedal spasm, magnesium deficiency syndrome*

Tetany is a type of cramp that causes the muscles of the hands and feet to cramp rhythmically, as well as spasms of the larynx with difficulty in breathing, nausea, vomiting, convulsions, and there is considerable pain. The disorder stems from a mineral imbalance, such as a lack of calcium, potassium, or magnesium, or an acid or alkaline condition of the body.

Associated conditions include poorly controlled hypoparathyroidism, hypophosphatemia, osteomalacia, renal disorders, or malabsorption syndromes. Treatment is directed at restoring metabolic balance, as by intravenous administration of calcium in cases of hypocalcemia (calcium deficiency).

781.8   Neurological neglect syndrome — *asomatognosia, hemi-akinesia, hemi-spatial neglect, sensory neglect, visuospatial neglect*

781.91   Loss of height — *not due to osteoporosis*

781.92   Abnormal posture

✔5th   Needs fifth-digit   **OK**   Valid three-digit code

781.99   Other symptoms involving nervous and musculoskeletal systems — *including acragnosis, acroagnosis, acute catatonia, floppy infant syndrome, growing pains; not otherwise specified*

782 SYMPTOMS INVOLVING SKIN AND OTHER INTEGUMENTARY TISSUE
Symptoms relating to possible breast disorders (611.71-611.79) are excluded from the rubric.

782.0   Disturbance of skin sensation — *anesthesia, burning, prickling, numbness, tingling, hperesthsia, hypoesthesia, paresthesia, Berger's paresthesia, pseudohemianesthesia*

782.1   Rash and other nonspecific skin eruption — *exanthem*

782.2   Localized superficial swelling, mass, or lump — *subcutaneous nodules*

782.3   Edema — *fluid in soft tissue; localized, anasarca, dropsy, Secretan's syndrome*

Use this code to report the accumulation of excessive amounts of fluid (water and sodium) in the intercellular tissue spaces of the body. Edema results when the balance of the lymphatic system, which normally transports excess interstitial fluid back to the intravascular space, is compromised. Pitting edema is a type of edema that retains for a time the indentation produced by pressure that forces fluid into the underlying tissues. Nonpitting edema is a type of edema that leaves no indentation when pressure is applied because fluid has coagulated in the tissues. Edema may occur at any site of the body, indicating different causes.

Excluded from this code are ascites (789.5), edema of newborn (778.5), edema of pregnancy (642.0-642.9, 646.1), fluid retention (276.6), hydrops fetalis (773.3, 778.0), hydrothorax (511.8), and nutritional edema (260, 262).

782.4   Jaundice, unspecified, not of newborn — *bilirubin causing yellow cast to skin; cholemia, icterus*

Use this code to report yellow discoloration of the skin and/or mucous membranes due to excessive levels of bilirubin in the blood. Pruritus, dark urine, and clay-colored stools commonly accompany jaundice. Etiologies for jaundice include congestive heart failure, carcinoma of the papilla of Vater or pancreas, cholecystitis and cholelithiasis, Kaye or Byler cholestasis, Laennec's or primary cirrhosis of the liver, liver abscess, hepatitis, acute or chronic pancreatitis, Dubin-Johnson syndrome, hemolytic anemia, glucose-6-phosphate dehydrogenase (G6PD) deficiency, and drug-induced hepatic insult. Lab work may include urine and fecal urobilinogen, serum bilirubin, liver enzyme tests, serum cholesterol, prothrombin, and complete blood count (CBC). Liver biopsy may rule out hepatic etiology.

Therapies depend on etiology (e.g., cholecystectomy for jaundice due to cholecystitis); dietary management, including increased carbohydrates, decreased proteins and fewer high-fat foods; frequent skin cleansing, and topical antipruritic medications for pruritus.

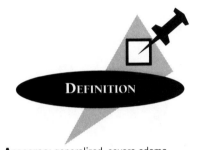

DEFINITION

Anasarca: generalized, severe edema, often observed in renal diseases when fluid retention continues for an extended period of time.

Jaundice in newborn (774.0-774.7) and jaundice due to isoimmunization (773.0-773.2, 773.4) are excluded from this code.

782.5	Cyanosis — *deficient oxygen in blood, causing blue cast to skin*
782.61	Pallor — *pale skin*
782.62	Flushing — *ruddy skin, excessive blushing*
782.7	Spontaneous ecchymoses — *hemorrhagic spots with the appearance of freckles; petechiae*

Ecchymoses is defined as a purplish, flat bruise that occurs when blood leaks out into the top layers of skin; the bruise is not raised but may be irregular in shape. Spontaneous ecchymoses is often a symptom of a coagulation disorder. Sometimes diagnostic tests are necessary to determine the diagnosis, such as serologic tests, biopsies, culture plus antimicrobial sensitivity, dermatrophy, and test media-ring worm.

782.8	Changes in skin texture — *induration, thickening, scabs, scales*
782.9	Other symptoms involving skin and integumentary tissues — *not otherwise specified*

783 SYMPTOMS CONCERNING NUTRITION, METABOLISM, AND DEVELOPMENT

783.0	Anorexia — *loss of appetite*

This code reports loss of appetite. This is a common symptom of gastrointestinal (GI) and endocrine disorders as well as psychological disturbances. Investigation of organ-specific pathology (function studies of thyroid, liver, kidney; upper GI; gallbladder series), barium enema, and blood work allow assessment of nutritional status.

Associated conditions include hypopituitarism, hypothyroidism, ketoacidosis, appendicitis, cirrhosis, Crohn's disease, gastritis, hepatitis, chronic renal failure, pernicious anemia, alcoholism, anorexia nervosa, and cancer.

This subcategory does not include anorexia nervosa. Anorexia nervosa is a psychophysiological condition classified to 307.1. Also excluded is loss of appetite with a nonorganic origin (307.59).

783.1	Abnormal weight gain
783.21	Loss of weight
783.22	Underweight
783.3	Feeding difficulties and mismanagement — *typically in elderly, infants*
783.40	Lack of normal physiological development, unspecified — *inadequate development, lack of development in childhood*
783.41	Failure to thrive — *failure to gain weight in childhood*
783.42	Delayed milestones — *including late walker, late talker*
783.43	Short stature — *growth failure, physical retardation in childhood*
783.5	Polydipsia
783.6	Polyphagia

Polyphagia refers to eating to the point of being focused only on eating (or excessive eating) before feeling full; these can be symptoms of various disorders. It can be intermittent or persistent and depending on the cause, it may or may not result in weight gain. Common causes include anxiety, premenstrual syndrome, bulimia, diabetes mellitus, gestational diabetes, Graves' disease, hyperthyroidism, hypoglycemia, and drugs such as corticosteroids, cyproheptadine, and tricyclic antidepressants.

Excluded from this subclassification are disorders of eating of nonorganic origin (307.50-307.59).

783.7   Adult failure to thrive

783.9   Other symptoms concerning nutrition, metabolism, and development

784 SYMPTOMS INVOLVING HEAD AND NECK

Excluded from this rubric are encephalopathy not otherwise specified (348.3) and specific symptoms involving neck classifiable to rubric 723.

784.0   Headache

Use this code to report pain in the cranial vaults, orbits, or nape of neck. About 90 percent of all headaches are benign. The basic etiologies of the headache are muscle contraction (tension headache), vascular (migraine or cluster headache), or a combination.

Excluded from this code are atypical face pain (350.2), migraine (346.0-346.9), and tension headache (307.81).

784.1   Throat pain

784.2   Swelling, mass, or lump in head and neck

784.3   Aphasia

Use this code to report impaired expression or comprehension of written or spoken language due to disease or injury of one or more of the brain's language centers: Broca's area, Wernicke's area, or arcuate fasciculus. Broca's area controls the muscle for speech (expressive aphasia). Wernicke's area controls the auditory and visual comprehension for speech (receptive aphasia). The arcuate fasciculus aids in control of the content of speech and enables repetition.

Associated conditions include Alzheimer's disease, brain tumor, cerebrovascular accident, encephalitis, head trauma, and heroin overdose.

784.40   Unspecified voice disturbance — *unknown*

784.41   Aphonia — *loss of voice*

784.49   Other voice disturbance — *change, hoarseness, hypernasality, dysphonia, plicae dysphonia ventricularis, rhinolalia, trachyphonia; not otherwise specified*

784.5   Other speech disturbance — *including dysarthria, dysphasia, slurred speech*

784.60   Symbolic dysfunction, unspecified — *unknown variety*

784.61   Alexia and dyslexia — *organic inability or difficulty in reading*

784.69   Other symbolic dysfunction — *including acalculia, agnosia, Bianchi's or Gerstmann's syndrome, palilalia, agraphia, apraxia*

784.7   Epistaxis — *nosebleed*

Use this code to report nosebleed. Typically occurring unilaterally, epistaxis may be spontaneous or induced from the front or back of the nose. The majority of nosebleeds occur within the anterior-inferior nasal septum (Kiesselbach's plexus), but they also can occur at the point where the inferior turbinates meet the nasopharynx. In nonsevere cases, a complete blood count may reveal acute blood loss anemia, prothrombin, and activated partial thromboplastin time measurements. Therapies include application of external pressure, insertion into nose of cotton treated with vasoconstrictor and local anesthetic, and humidified oxygen. In severe cases, therapies may include IV hydration, pinching in of nares to control bleeding in absence of nasal fracture, and anterior or posterior nasal packing if other measures prove ineffective in controlling bleeding.

Associated conditions include maxillofacial injury, nasal fracture, nasal tumors, orbital floor fracture, acute sinusitis, hypertension, cirrhosis, hepatitis, renal failure, skull fracture, aplastic and acute blood loss anemia, coagulation disorders, hereditary hemorrhagic telangiectasia (Rendu-Osler-Weber disease), leukemia, polycythemia vera, systemic lupus erythematosus, infectious mononucleosis, influenza, and anticoagulant use (adverse effect).

784.8   Hemorrhage from throat — *bleeding*

784.9   Other symptoms involving head and neck — *including choking sensation, sternutation, mouth breathing, sneezing, or halitosis; not otherwise specified*

785 SYMPTOMS INVOLVING CARDIOVASCULAR SYSTEM

Excluded from this rubric is heart failure, not otherwise specified (428.9).

785.0   Unspecified tachycardia — *rapid heart beat*

This code reports a heart rate greater than 100 beats per minute caused by the heart making an effort to deliver more oxygen to the body tissues by increasing the rate at which blood passes through the vessels. Usually, the patient will complain of palpitations or racing of the heart. Tachycardia may be the result of excitement, exercise, pain or fever as well as caffeine and tobacco. However, it may be an early sign of a life-threatening disorder such as cardiogenic or septic shock.

Associated conditions include neurogenic shock, adult respiratory distress syndrome, chronic obstructive pulmonary disease, pneumothorax, pulmonary embolism, cardiac dysrhythmia, cardiogenic shock, congestive heart failure, hypertensive crisis, myocardial infarction, thyrotoxicosis, anemia, diabetic ketoacidosis, hyponatremia, anaphylactic shock, and septic shock.

Excluded from this code is paroxysmal tachycardia (427.0-427.2).

785.1   Palpitations — *awareness of heart beat*

785.2   Undiagnosed cardiac murmurs — *mitral or systolic click syndrome, heart murmur not otherwise specified*

   ↙5th   Needs fifth-digit   **OK**   Valid three-digit code

785.3   Other abnormal heart sounds — *cardiac dullness, friction fremitus, precardial friction*

785.4   Gangrene — *phagedena, spreading cutaneous gangrene, gangrenous cellulitis*

Use this code to report the death of tissue due to loss of vascular supply. Gangrene may be wet (bacterial infection with cellulitis) or dry (affected area is dry and shriveled).

Associated conditions include diabetes with microangiopathy, ischemia due to atherosclerosis or embolism, and Raynaud's phenomenon. Code first any associated underlying disease.

This subcategory excludes gas gangrene due to tissue invasion by Clostridium perfringens or other clostridia (classified to code 040.0) and gangrene to a variety of specific sites. Refer to the ICD-9-CM index under "Gangrene, gangrenous" for specific code assignments since some specific types of gangrene are classified to other chapters.

785.5 Shock without mention of trauma

Use this subclassification to report a condition in which the blood flow to peripheral tissues and perfusion are inadequate to sustain life due to insufficient cardiac output or maladapted distribution of peripheral blood flow. The principal deficiency is a reduction in perfusion of vital tissues resulting in inadequate oxygen delivery. This facilitates aerobic metabolism, which results in anaerobic respiration. The result is increased production and accumulation of lactic acid (metabolic acidosis) with compensatory hyperventilation and respiratory alkalosis. Eventually, the homeostatic mechanisms that serve to maintain acid-base balance fail, leading to cell death and subsequent organ failure.

Cardiogenic shock is shock resulting from decreased cardiac output in heart disease. Associated conditions include disturbance of heart rate or rhythm, acute myocardial infarction, valvular heart disease, cardiomyopathy, hypoxemia secondary to pulmonary or neurologic disease, tension pneumothorax, pericardial tamponade, massive pulmonary embolism, prosthetic valve malfunction, and mixed acid-base balance disorder.

Shock due to anesthetic (995.4), anaphylactic shock (995.0), electric shock (994.8), shock following abortion (639.5), shock from lightning (994.0), shock following an obstetrical procedure (669.1), postoperative shock (998.0), or traumatic shock (958.4) are excluded from this classification.

785.50   Unspecified shock — *unknown cause*

785.51   Cardiogenic shock — *failure of peripheral circulation due to heart insufficiency*

785.59   Other shock without mention of trauma — *including endotoxic, gram-negative, hypervolemic, septic shock; not otherwise specified*

785.6   Enlargement of lymph nodes — *lymphadenopathy, swollen glands*

785.9   Other symptoms involving cardiovascular system — *including strong pulse, weak pulse, bruit; not otherwise specified*

786 SYMPTOMS INVOLVING RESPIRATORY SYSTEM AND OTHER CHEST SYMPTOMS

786.00   Unspecified respiratory abnormality — *unknown*

786.01   Hyperventilation — *rapid breathing*

786.02   Orthopnea — *difficult respiration except when patient is upright*

786.03   Apnea — *momentary cessation in breathing*

This subclassification excludes sleep apnea (780.51, 780.53, and 780.57).

786.04   Cheyne-Stokes respiration

Cheyne-Stokes respiration is defined as an abnormal breathing pattern that is first shallow and infrequent and then increases gradually to abnormally deep and rapid, before fading away completely for about 5 seconds to 30 seconds, before the next cycle of shallow breathing begins. Cheyne-Stokes respiration is often accompanied by changes in the level of consciousness; it most commonly occurs in seriously ill patients with brain or heart disorders. It may occur during sleep.

Therapies include treating the associated heart or brain disorder and prescribing the drug aminophylline.

786.05   Shortness of breath

786.06   Tachypnea — *quick, shallow breathing*

786.07   Wheezing — *whistling noises during breathing*

786.09   Other dyspnea and respiratory abnormalities — *including snoring, yawning, paroxysmal dyspnea, respiratory distress; not otherwise specified*

786.1   Stridor — *harsh sound associated with respiration in patients with airway obstruction*

786.2   Cough

786.3   Hemoptysis — *cough with hemorrhage*

Use this code to report coughing up or spitting out of blood or bloody sputum from the lungs or tracheobronchial tree. Expectoration of 200 ml of blood in a single episode suggests severe bleeding. Expectoration of 400 ml in 3 hours, or more than 600 ml in 16 hours, is life threatening. Bleeding into the respiratory tract by bronchial or pulmonary vessels causes hemoptysis, which reflects change in the vascular walls and blood-clotting mechanisms. Lab work, including complete count, sputum culture and smear, and coagulation studies, may reveal anemia or infection. Chest x-ray, pulmonary arteriography, or lung scan may rule out disease such as carcinoma, tuberculosis, and pneumonia. Bronchoscopy (with biopsy), in severe hemoptysis, locates bleeding site. Therapies include placement of patient in Trendelenburg position to promote drainage of blood from lung and cough suppressants to prevent blood from spreading throughout the lungs.

Associated conditions include chronic bronchitis, bronchogenic carcinoma, bronchiectasis, laryngeal cancer, bronchial adenoma, lung abscess, pneumonia (Klebsiella, pneumococcal), pulmonary arteriovenous fistula, pulmonary contusion, pulmonary edema, pulmonary embolism with infarction, pulmonary hypertension (primary), pulmonary tuberculosis and silicosis, tracheal trauma, ruptured aortic aneurysm,

✔5th   Needs fifth-digit   **OK**   Valid three-digit code

Wegener's granulomatosis, systemic lupus erythematosus, and coagulation disorder.

786.4   Abnormal sputum — *in color, amount, odor, quantity*

786.50   Unspecified chest pain — *unknown cause*

Use this code to report localized discomfort occurring in the chest. Among possible etiologies are acute myocardial infarction, angina, chest trauma, and peptic ulcer disease. Findings vary depending on suspected etiology (for example, electrocardiogram (EKG) for acute myocardial infarction, chest x-ray for chest trauma). Therapies include analgesics for pain control.

786.51   Precordial pain — *chest pain near heart*

786.52   Painful respiration — *pleurodynia, Prinzmetal-Massumi syndrome, pleuritic pain*

Use this code to report a form of chest pain due to painful inhalation, expiration, or both. It may be due to pain in the chest wall (rib cage and sternum), pleura, or accessory muscles of respiration.

786.59   Other chest pain — *not otherwise specified, including discomfort, pressure, tightness in chest*

786.6   Swelling, mass, or lump in chest

786.7   Abnormal chest sounds — *rales, tympany, friction sounds, abnormal percussion*

786.8   Hiccough — *singultus, spastic diaphragm*

A hiccough, or hiccups, is defined as repetitive, involuntary spasmodic contractions of the diaphragm. Hiccups are a symptom, not a disease. Hiccups involve the diaphragm (large, thin muscle which separates the chest from the abdomen) and phrenic nerve (nerve that connects the diaphragm to the brain). Almost everybody gets hiccups, even a fetus in a mother's womb.

Hiccups are caused by an irritation of nerves from the brain that control breathing muscles, especially the diaphragm. Causes are numerous for prolonged or recurrent hiccup episodes and include diseases of the pleura, pneumonia, uremia, alcoholism, use of certain prescription or non-prescription drugs, pregnancy, and disorders of the stomach, esophagus, bowel or pancreas. There is no known prevention for hiccups, though prolonged episodes may require surgery to cut the phrenic nerve.

786.9   Other symptoms involving respiratory system and chest — *breath-holding spell*

787 SYMPTOMS INVOLVING DIGESTIVE SYSTEM

787.0 Nausea and vomiting

Often, nausea and vomiting are symptoms of metabolic or microbial toxins or reactions to drugs, radiation, or motion (i.e., seasickness). Therapies depend on etiology and include antiemetics (Inapsine, Reglan, Compazine, and Norzine).

Excluded from these codes are hematemesis not otherwise specified (578.0); excessive vomiting in pregnancy (643.0-643.9); regurgitation of food in newborn (779.3); habitual vomiting (536.2); and psychogenic vomiting not otherwise specified (307.54).

787.01	Nausea with vomiting
787.02	Nausea alone
787.03	Vomiting alone
787.1	Heartburn — *pyrosis, waterbrash*
787.2	Dysphagia — *difficulty in swallowing, cricopharyngeal syndrome*

Use this code to report difficulty in swallowing. Pre-esophageal dysphagia is difficulty in emptying material from the oral pharynx into the esophagus. Esophageal dysphagia is difficulty in passing food down the esophagus. The most common symptom of esophageal disorders, dysphagia is classified as phase 1, 2, or 3. Phase 1, transfer phase, typically results from a neuromuscular disorder. Phase 2, transport phase, usually indicates spasm or carcinoma. Phase 3, entrance phase, results from lower esophageal narrowing by diverticula, esophagitis, and other disorders. Endoscopy with biopsy visualizes any gross pathology and provides specimens. Esophageal manometry measures esophageal pressure of upper and lower sphincters and detects abnormal contractions and peristalsis. Esophageal acidity test (usually performed with manometry) or acid perfusion test (Bernstein test) detect gastric acid reflux.

Associated conditions include amyotrophic lateral sclerosis, myasthenia gravis, Parkinson's disease, oral cavity tumor, carcinoma (laryngeal, esophageal, gastric), pharyngitis (chronic), airway obstruction, progressive systemic sclerosis, achalasia, and dysphagia lusoria. Associated esophageal conditions include esophageal compression (external), esophageal diverticulum, esophageal leiomyoma, esophageal obstruction by foreign body, esophagitis (corrosive, monilial, reflux), and lower esophageal ring. Other associated conditions include mediastinitis, Plummer-Vinson syndrome, systemic lupus erythematosus, hypocalcemia, syphilis, botulism, lead poisoning, and tetanus.

787.3	Flatulence, eructation, and gas pain — *bloating, tympanites, abdominal distension*
787.4	Visible peristalsis — *hyperperistalsis*
787.5	Abnormal bowel sounds — *absent or hyperactive*
787.6	Incontinence of feces — *encopresis, incontinence of sphincter ani*
787.7	Abnormal feces — *bulky stools*
787.91	Diarrhea — *loose, copious stools*
787.99	Other symptoms involving digestive system — *tenesmus, swelling, neuralgia, change in bowel habits*

788 SYMPTOMS INVOLVING URINARY SYSTEM

Excluded from this rubric are hematuria (599.7), nonspecific findings on examination of the urine (791.0-791.9), small kidney of unknown cause (589.0-589.9), and uremia not otherwise specified (586).

788.0	Renal colic — *kidney or ureter*
788.1	Dysuria — *painful urination, strangury*

⌐5th Needs fifth-digit   **OK** Valid three-digit code

788.2 Retention of urine

Signs and symptoms of retention of urine include distended abdomen, pain, and urgency. Therapies include catheterization and surgery,such as transurethral resection of prostate in males. Associated conditions include benign prostatic hypertrophy, neurogenic bladder, carcinoma of prostate, urethral stricture, and urinary tract infection.

Inability to void is a common sequela to pelvic and perineal surgery or surgery performed under spinal anesthesia. The condition is not necessarily a postoperative complication. Documentation should support the condition as a medical management problem and not solely reflect prophylactic measures such as bladder catheterization.

788.20	Unspecified retention of urine — *unknown type*
788.21	Incomplete bladder emptying
788.29	Other specified retention of urine — *not otherwise specified*

788.3 Incontinence of urine

Signs and symptoms of incontinence of urine include stress, urge, overflow or total incontinence; intermittent leakage resulting from sudden physical strain; dribble resulting from urinary retention; inability to suppress sudden urge to urinate; and continuous leakage. Cystoscopy with biopsy visualizes any gross pathology and provides specimens. Cystometry tests bladder compliance, capacity, and residual volume. Therapies include bladder retraining and surgery such as creation of urinary diversion.

Associated conditions include cerebrovascular accident, diabetic neuropathy, Guillain-Barre syndrome, multiple sclerosis, spinal cord injury, benign prostatic hypertrophy, bladder calculi, bladder cancer, prostatic cancer, chronic prostatitis, and urethral stricture.

Code first any underlying condition, as congenital ureterocele (753.23). Excluded from this subclassification is urinary incontinence of nonorganic origin (307.6). Female stress incontinence is reported with 625.6.

788.30	Unspecified urinary incontinence — *unknown type of enuresis, bladder neck syndrome*
788.31	Urge incontinence — *inability to control flow upon urge*
788.32	Stress incontinence, male — *inability to control flow upon pressure*
788.33	Mixed incontinence urge and stress (male)(female) — *urge and stress*
788.34	Incontinence without sensory awareness — *no sensory warning*
788.35	Post-void dribbling — *inability to control flow after urination*
788.36	Nocturnal enuresis — *bed-wetting*
788.37	Continuous leakage — *constant flow*
788.39	Other urinary incontinence — *not otherwise specified*
788.41	Urinary frequency — *frequent micturition*
788.42	Polyuria — *copious micturition*
788.43	Nocturia — *frequent nighttime micturition*
788.5	Oliguria and anuria — *deficient secretion or suppression of urine*
788.61	Splitting of urinary stream — *intermittent urinary stream*
788.62	Slowing of urinary stream — *weak stream*
788.69	Other abnormality of urination — *not otherwise specified*
788.7	Urethral discharge — *penile discharge, urethrorrhea*
788.8	Extravasation of urine — *escape of urine into adjacent tissues*
788.9	Other symptoms involving urinary system — *not otherwise specified, including extrarenal uremia, tenesmus*

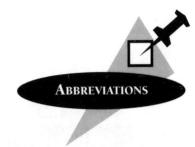

ABBREVIATIONS

BPH: benign prostatic hypertrophy

SI: stress urinary incontinence

789 OTHER SYMPTOMS INVOLVING ABDOMEN AND PELVIS

789.0 ✓5th Abdominal pain — *cramps, colic*

Use this subclassification to report localized pain or discomfort affecting the abdominal area. It may be due to drug use, the effect of toxins, or disorders of the gastrointestinal, reproductive, genitourinary, musculoskeletal, or vascular system. Blood work shows hematocrit, WBC, and differential and platelet counts. Urinalysis may identify urinary tract infection or kidney disease. Other lab work may reveal elevated liver enzymes (in hepatic disease), elevated serum bilirubin (in hepatobiliary disease), elevated serum amylase (in pancreatitis), or bacteria and parasites in stool culture (in acute diarrhea). Abdominal x-ray (supine and upright or decubitus and flat) may reveal intestinal disease or obstruction, while an ultrasound may identify aneurysms. Intravenous pyelogram (IVP) may identify renal disease or ureteral obstruction, while a sigmoidoscopy reveals condition of sigmoid colon and rectum. Associated conditions include peritonitis, perforated peptic ulcer, gallbladder disease, appendicitis, colitis, pancreatitis, lymphadenitis, pelvic inflammatory disease, intestinal obstruction, ruptured liver or spleen, ovarian cyst, ectopic pregnancy, endometriosis, pneumonia, myocardial ischemia, leukemia, nephritis, uremia, herpes zoster, and ureteral obstruction.

789.1 Hepatomegaly — *enlarged liver*
789.2 Splenomegaly — *enlarged spleen*
789.3 ✓5th Abdominal or pelvic swelling, mass, or lump — *diffuse or generalized swelling or mass*
789.4 ✓5th Abdominal rigidity — *inflexibility, turgidity*
789.5 Ascites — *fluid in peritoneal cavity*

Ascites is accumulation of serous fluid in the peritoneal cavity. Signs and symptoms of ascites include abdominal discomfort, distention, dyspnea, and a flat or an inverted umbilicus. Abdominal percussion transmits fluid wave and reveals shifting dullness. Paracentesis to remove fluid (typically 50 ml to 100 ml) may reveal the following:

- High WBC (more than 300 cells/ml to 500 cells/ml suggests infection)

- Sanguineous fluid (indicative of neoplasm or tuberculosis)

- Milky or chylous fluid (common with lymphoma)

- Concentrations of protein (less than 3 g/100 ml suggests liver disease or systemic disorder)

Therapies include bed rest, sodium restriction (20 mEq/day to 40 mEq/day), spironolactone such as Aldactone (100 mg/day to 300 mg/day, orally), monitoring of body weight and urinary sodium, and peritoneal-jugular shunting.

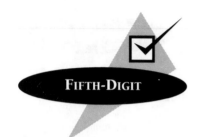

FIFTH-DIGIT

The following fifth-digit subclassification is to be used for codes 789.0, 789.3, 789.4, and 789.6:

0 unspecified site

1 right upper quadrant

2 left upper quadrant

3 right lower quadrant

4 left lower quadrant

5 periumbilic

6 epigastric

7 generalized

9 other specified site or multiple sites

✓5th   Needs fifth-digit   **OK**   Valid three-digit code

Associated conditions include chronic or subacute liver disease (most commonly cirrhosis from alcoholism), chronic active hepatitis, severe alcoholic hepatitis without cirrhosis, hepatic vein obstruction, systemic disease (heart failure, nephrotic syndrome), carcinomatosis, and tubercular peritonitis.

If the physician documents malignant ascites, assign code 197.6 instead.

789.6 ✔5th Abdominal tenderness — *rebound tenderness*
789.9 Other symptoms involving abdomen and pelvis — *including umbilical bleeding or discharge; not otherwise specified*

790-796 Nonspecific Abnormal Findings

790 NONSPECIFIC FINDINGS ON EXAMINATION OF BLOOD

Excluded from this rubric are abnormalities of platelets (287.0-287.9), thrombocytes (287.0-287.9), or white blood cells (288.0-288.9).

790.01 Precipitous drop in hematocrit — *drop in red blood cell count*
790.09 Other abnormality of red blood cells — *including morphology, volume, anisocytosis, poikilocytosis; not otherwise specified*
790.1 Elevated sedimentation rate — *sed rate*
790.2 Abnormal glucose tolerance test — *GTT*
790.3 Excessive blood level of alcohol — *indicative of alcohol consumption*
790.4 Nonspecific elevation of levels of transaminase or lactic acid dehydrogenase (LDH) — *a marker for hemolysis, pulmonary embolism, liver malignancy*
790.5 Other nonspecific abnormal serum enzyme levels — *acid phosphatase, alkaline phosphate, amylase, lipase*
790.6 Other abnormal blood chemistry — *cobalt, copper, iron, lithium, magnesium, mineral, zinc*

Use this code to report an abnormal finding on blood chemistry tests for which there is no corresponding diagnosis, such as copper, iron, lithium, and magnesium.

790.7 Bacteremia — *bacteria in the blood*

Use this code to report the presence of live bacteria circulating in the bloodstream. Bacteremia frequently results from surgical procedures (e.g., incision and drainage of an abscess or dental extractions). It also may result from colonization of indwelling urinary catheters or other invasive apparatus. Therapies include antibiotics.

Associated conditions include abscessed teeth, urinary tract infection, and infected medical device.

The term "bacteremia" is sometimes used ambiguously by clinicians to mean septicemia, which is bacteremia with clinical signs and symptoms of systemic infection and classified to rubric 038. To ensure proper classification, verify with the physician any reports of bacteremia with signs and symptoms of systemic infection such as fever, chills, prostration, nausea and vomiting, diarrhea, metastatic abscesses, and skin eruptions.

790.8	Unspecified viremia — *virus in the blood*
790.91	Abnormal arterial blood gases
790.92	Abnormal coagulation profile — *bleeding time, coagulation time, PTT, PT*
790.93	Elevated prostate specific antigen (PSA)
790.94	Euthyroid sick syndrome
790.99	Other nonspecific findings on examination of blood — *not otherwise specified, including proteinemia*

791 NONSPECIFIC FINDINGS ON EXAMINATION OF URINE

Excluded from this rubric are hematuria (599.7), specific findings indicating abnormality of amino-acid transport and metabolism (270.0-270.9), and specific findings indicating abnormality of carbohydrate transport and metabolism (271.0-271.9).

791.0   Proteinuria — *protein in urine; albuminuria, Bence-Jones proteinuria*

Proteinuria is defined as urinary protein excretion of greater than 150 mg per day. The types of proteinuria can be classified as glomerular, tubular, or overflow. Glomerular disease is the most common cause, resulting in urinary loss of albumin and immunoglobulins. Tubular proteinuria occurs when tubulointerstitial disease prevents the proximal tubule from reabsorbing low-molecular-weight proteins. Tubular diseases include hypertensive nephrosclerosis and tubulointerstitial nephropathy caused by nonsteroidal anti-inflammatory drugs. In overflow proteinuria, low-molecular-weight proteins inhibit the reabsorption of filtered proteins.

Lab tests include a quantitative measurement of protein excretion, which can be done with a 24-hour urine specimen or the urine protein-to-creatinine ratio (UPr/Cr). Dipstick analysis is used in most outpatient settings to semiquantitatively measure the urine protein concentration. The sulfosalicylic acid (SSA) turbidity test qualitatively screens for proteinuria.

Therapy depends on urine to protein concentration. Proteinuria of more than 2 g per 24 hours (moderate to heavy) requires aggressive work-up. If the creatinine clearance is normal and if there is a clear diagnosis such as diabetes or uncompensated congestive heart failure, the underlying medical condition can be treated with close follow-up of proteinuria and renal function (creatinine clearance). Benign causes include fever, intense activity or exercise, dehydration, emotional stress and acute illness. More serious causes include glomerulonephritis and multiple myeloma. Common secondary causes are diabetic nephropathy, amyloidosis, and systemic lupus erythematosus.

This subclassification excludes postural proteinuria (593.6) and proteinuria arising during pregnancy or the puerperium (642.0-642.9, 646.2).

791.1	Chyluria — *excess lymphatic fluid in urine*
791.2	Hemoglobinuria — *blood in urine seen in a lab exam*
791.3	Myoglobinuria — *myoglobin in the urine*
791.4	Biliuria — *bile pigments in the urine*
791.5	Glycosuria — *sugar in the urine*

✔5th Needs fifth-digit   **OK** Valid three-digit code

791.6   Acetonuria — *acetone in the urine; ketonuria*

791.7   Other cells and casts in urine — *not otherwise specified*

791.9   Other nonspecific finding on examination of urine — *crystalluria, melanuria, cocciurea, uricosuria, elevated 18-ketosteriods, catecholamines, indolacetic acid, or VMA*

792 NONSPECIFIC ABNORMAL FINDINGS IN OTHER BODY SUBSTANCES

A nonspecific abnormal finding in chromosomal analysis (795.2) is excluded from the rubric.

792.0   Nonspecific abnormal finding in cerebrospinal fluid

792.1   Nonspecific abnormal finding in stool contents — *mucus, pus, fat, abnormal color, occult stool*

792.2   Nonspecific abnormal finding in semen — *abnormal spermatozoa*

792.3   Nonspecific abnormal finding in amniotic fluid — *fluid surround fetus*

792.4   Nonspecific abnormal finding in saliva

792.5   Cloudy (hemodialysis) (peritoneal) dialysis affluent

792.9   Other nonspecific abnormal finding in body substances — *peritoneal, pleural, synovial, vaginal or other fluid, not elsewhere specified*

793 NONSPECIFIC ABNORMAL FINDINGS ON RADIOLOGICAL AND OTHER EXAMINATION OF BODY STRUCTURE

This rubric includes nonspecific abnormal findings in thermography, ultrasound (echogram), and x-ray. Abnormal results of function studies and radioisotope scans (794.0-794.9) are excluded from the rubric.

793.0   Nonspecific abnormal findings on radiological and other examination of skull and head — *upon x-ray, ultrasound, thermography*

793.1   Nonspecific abnormal findings on radiological and other examination of lung field — *coin lesion or shadow upon x-ray, ultrasound, thermography*

793.2   Nonspecific abnormal findings on radiological and other examination of other intrathoracic organs — *heart shadow, mediastinal shift upon x-ray, ultrasound, thermography*

793.3   Nonspecific abnormal findings on radiological and other examination of biliary tract — *nonvisualization of gallbladder upon x-ray, ultrasound, thermography*

793.4   Nonspecific abnormal findings on radiological and other examination of gastrointestinal tract — *upon x-ray, ultrasound, thermography*

793.5   Nonspecific abnormal findings on radiological and other examination of genitourinary organs — *filling defect of bladder, kidney or ureter upon x-ray, ultrasound, thermography*

793.6   Nonspecific abnormal findings on radiological and other examination of abdominal area, including retroperitoneum — *upon x-ray, ultrasound, thermography*

793.7   Nonspecific abnormal findings on radiological and other examination of musculoskeletal system — *upon x-ray, ultrasound, thermography*

793.8   Nonspecific abnormal findings on radiological and other examination of breast — *abnormal mammogram or abnormality upon x-ray, ultrasound, thermography*

793.9   Nonspecific abnormal findings on radiological and other examination of other site of body — *placenta, skin, subcutaneous tissue upon x-ray, ultrasound, thermography*

794 NONSPECIFIC ABNORMAL RESULTS OF FUNCTION STUDIES

This rubric includes nonspecific abnormal findings in radioisotope scans, uptake studies, and scintiphotography.

794.00	Unspecified abnormal function study of brain and central nervous system — *unknown*
794.01	Nonspecific abnormal echoencephalogram
794.02	Nonspecific abnormal electroencephalogram (EEG)
794.09	Other nonspecific abnormal result of function study of brain and central nervous system — *including brain scan; not otherwise specified*
794.10	Nonspecific abnormal response to unspecified nerve stimulation — *unknown*
794.11	Nonspecific abnormal retinal function studies — *ERG*
794.12	Nonspecific abnormal electro-oculogram (EOG)
794.13	Nonspecific abnormal visually evoked potential — *VEP*
794.14	Nonspecific abnormal oculomotor studies
794.15	Nonspecific abnormal auditory function studies
794.16	Nonspecific abnormal vestibular function studies
794.17	Nonspecific abnormal electromyogram (EMG)
794.19	Other nonspecific abnormal result of function study of peripheral nervous system and special senses
794.2	Nonspecific abnormal results of pulmonary system function study — *lung scan, ventilatory capacity, vital capacity*
794.30	Nonspecific abnormal unspecified cardiovascular function study — *unknown*
794.31	Nonspecific abnormal electrocardiogram (ecg) (ekg) — *Q-T interval prolongations, Romano-Ward syndrome*
794.39	Other nonspecific abnormal cardiovascular system function study — *ballistocardiogram, phonocardiogram, vectorcardiogram*
794.4	Nonspecific abnormal results of kidney function study — *renal function test*
794.5	Nonspecific abnormal results of thyroid function study — *thyroid scan, thyroid uptake*
794.6	Nonspecific abnormal results of other endocrine function study — *pituitary, thymus, adrenal, hypothalamus*
794.7	Nonspecific abnormal results of basal metabolism function study — *BMR*
794.8	Nonspecific abnormal results of liver function study — *liver scan*
794.9	Nonspecific abnormal results of other specified function study — *bladder, pancreas, placenta, spleen*

795 NONSPECIFIC ABNORMAL HISTOLOGICAL AND IMMUNOLOGICAL FINDINGS

Excluded from this rubric are nonspecific abnormalities of red blood cells (790.01-790.09).

795.0	Nonspecific abnormal Papanicolaou smear of cervix — *dyskaryotic cervical smear, Pap smear*
795.1	Nonspecific abnormal Papanicolaou smear of other site — *Pap smear other than cervical*
795.2	Nonspecific abnormal findings on chromosomal analysis — *abnormal karyotype*
795.3	Nonspecific positive culture findings — *nose, sputum, throat, wound*
795.4	Other nonspecific abnormal histological findings
795.5	Nonspecific reaction to tuberculin skin test without active tuberculosis — *Mantoux test, PPD positive, positive TB skin test*
795.6	False positive serological test for syphilis — *Wassermann reaction*

⮯5th Needs fifth-digit   **OK** Valid three-digit code

795.71   Nonspecific serologic evidence of human immunodeficiency virus (HIV) — *nonspecific findings only*

795.79   Other and unspecified nonspecific immunological findings — *raised antibody titer, raised immunoglobulin level*

796 OTHER NONSPECIFIC ABNORMAL FINDINGS

Refer to the ICD-9-CM Index before assigning a code from this rubric to ensure a more specific code cannot be found.

796.0   Nonspecific abnormal toxicological findings — *heavy metals or drugs in blood, urine or other tissue*

796.1   Abnormal reflex

796.2   Elevated blood pressure reading without diagnosis of hypertension — *no formal diagnosis of hypertension; incidental finding*

796.3   Nonspecific low blood pressure reading

796.4   Other abnormal clinical finding

796.5   Abnormal finding on antenatal screening

796.9   Other nonspecific abnormal finding — *not elsewhere specified*

797-799 Ill-Defined and Unknown Causes of Morbidity and Mortality

797 SENILITY WITHOUT MENTION OF PSYCHOSIS OK

Senile psychoses (290.0-290.9) are excluded from this code.

798 SUDDEN DEATH, CAUSE UNKNOWN

798.0   Sudden infant death syndrome — *crib death, SIDS*

Sudden infant death syndrome (SIDS) is defined as "the sudden death of an infant under one year of age which remains unexplained after a thorough case investigation, including performance of a complete autopsy, examination of the death scene, and review of the clinical history."

According to the National SIDS Resource Center, most researchers now believe that babies who die of SIDS are born with one or more conditions that make them especially vulnerable to stresses that occur in the normal life of an infant, including both internal and external influences. Maternal risk factors include cigarette smoking during pregnancy; maternal age less than 20 years; poor prenatal care; low weight gain; anemia; use of illegal drugs; and history of sexually transmitted disease or urinary tract infection.

Most deaths from SIDS occur by the end of the sixth month, with the greatest number occurring between 2 months and 4 months of age. A SIDS death occurs quickly and is often associated with sleep, with no signs of suffering, More deaths are reported in the fall and winter (in both the Northern and Southern Hemispheres) and there is a 60 percent to 40 percent male-to-female ratio. A death is diagnosed as SIDS only after all other alternatives have been eliminated: SIDS is a diagnosis of exclusion and includes investigations of the autopsy, death scene, and review of victim, and family case history.

798.1   Instantaneous death

798.2   Death occurring in less than 24 hours from onset of symptoms, not otherwise explained — *without sign of disease or trauma*

798.9   Unattended death — *found dead*

799 OTHER ILL-DEFINED AND UNKNOWN CAUSES OF MORBIDITY AND MORTALITY

799.0   Asphyxia — *lack of oxygen*

Use this code to report a lack of oxygen in respiration resulting in threatened or actual cessation of breath.

Therapies depend on etiology (e.g., removal of foreign body obstructing trachea or electrical defibrillation for cardiopulmonary arrest), and may include closed cardiac massage if heart beat and carotid pulse are absent and placement of patient in Trendelenburg position to promote drainage of water from lungs (fresh water victim). Other therapies, dependant on etiology, include mechanical ventilation, intensive respiratory therapy, IV administration of sodium bicarbonate, inhalation or injection of beta-agonists (epinephrine, Isuprel, Alupent, Brethine) to reduce bronchospasm, and administration of corticosteroids and antibiotics.

799.1   Respiratory arrest — *cardiorespiratory failure*

Use this code to report a cessation of breathing, identified as primary, secondary, or complete. Primary respiratory arrest may be due to airway obstruction, decreased respiratory drive, or respiratory muscle weakness. Secondary respiratory arrest may be a result of cardiac arrest. Therapies include cardiopulmonary resuscitation, intubation, and ventilation.

799.2   Nervousness

799.3   Unspecified debility — *specifics unknown*

799.4   Cachexia — *wasting disease; general ill health and poor nutrition*

This protein-wasting syndrome, called cachexia, most commonly occurs with lung, pancreatic, stomach, bowel, and prostate cancers, and rarely with breast cancer. It also affects people with AIDS, uncontrolled rheumatoid arthritis, severe infections, chronic lung and bowel disease, and heart failure. The cause is usually related to liver metastasis with resulting pain and loss of appetite. Sometimes the cause is mechanical, such as when a tumor grows into the stomach or blocks the intestine.

Undiagnosed and untreated cachexia is life threatening. It can decrease the effectiveness of cancer treatments such as chemotherapy and radiation therapy, and magnify their side effects.

799.8   Other ill-defined conditions — *including abiotrophy, abulia, autodigestion, autotoxemia, hemiabiotrophy, pseudoataxia, pseudotabes, stasis toxemia, toxinfection; not elsewhere classified*

799.9   Other unknown and unspecified cause of morbidity or mortality — *unknown cause of morbidity or mortality*

⌐5th   Needs fifth-digit   **OK**   Valid three-digit code

Chapter 17

800–999
Injury and Poisoning

800-829 Fractures

The coder should routinely review the radiology reports to learn the exact location of a fracture, and to express it as such with the code. If the clinician reports a proximal femur as opposed to an intertrochanteric, the radiology report will state that the fracture is intertrochanteric. This coded information is crucial to achieve an accurate evaluation of patient outcomes and utilization data. A fracture is a break in a bone resulting from two possible causes — the direct or indirect application of undue force against the bone, and pathological changes resulting in spontaneous fractures. This chapter includes only those fractures that have arisen as a result of an injury. It also excludes malunions and nonunions of fractured bones.

The clinician always determines whether a fracture is open or closed; therefore, this is one of the first determinations to be made by the coder.

Closed fractures are contained beneath the skin, while open or compound fractures connote an associated open wound.

Terms that typically describe closed fractures include:

Comminuted — a splintering of the fractured bone

Depressed — a portion of the skull broken and driven inward from a forceful blow.

Fissured — a fracture that does not split the bone

Greenstick — occurs in children; the bone is somewhat bent and partially broken

Impacted — one fractured bone end wedged into another

Linear — straight line

March — a synonym for stress fracture, a thin fracture with no evidence of soft tissue involvement that may be due to either repetitive motion or premature use of a fractured part

Simple — intact ligaments and skin

Slipped epiphysis — separation of the growing end of the bone (epiphysis) from shaft of bone that occurs in children and young adults who still have active epiphyses

Spiral — resembles a helix

Open fractures have a distinctive vocabulary. They are always compound, with a wound leading to the fracture, or the broken bone ends protruding through the skin. There is a very high risk of infection with open fractures since the tissues are exposed to

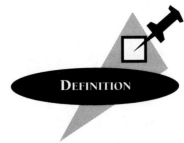

DEFINITION

Descriptive terms used for anatomical parts of bones include:

Condyle – rounded protuberance resembling a knuckle that allows articulation of the joint of the bone to occur as well as presenting surfaces for soft tissue attachments and insertions.

Process – somewhat pointed outgrowth of a bone that provides convenient surfaces for attachments and insertions of soft tissues.

Ramus – branching section of a bone that provides surfaces for attachments and insertions of soft tissues.

Symphysis – line showing where two bones have fused at a later developmental stage although the two bones originated as separate bones.

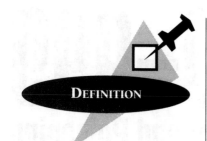

DEFINITION

Articulation describes movement of a joint. Some joints move freely (diarthrosis), while others may move only fractionally (amphiarthrosis) or do not move at all (synarthrosis).

Examples:

Amphiarthrosis - the vertebral bodies articulating against each other.

Diarthrosis - femur and tibia.

Synarthrosis - fusion of two halves of the pubis.

Extradural hemorrhage - The meninges, tough membranous protectors of the central nervous system, are arranged in three layers, the thickest and toughest being the outside membrane, the dura. Extradural hemorrhage is the most distant from the brain. Subdural hemorrhage occurs between the dura and the arachnoid membranes, while subarachnoid hemorrhage occurs beneath the arachnoid membrane and outside the innermost membrane, the pia.

Dura mater - hard membrane.

Arachnoid mater - spider web-like membrane.

Pia mater - thin or delicate membrane.

Mater means "mother" in Latin. It is likely that the mother's protective role toward her child is the reason that the meningeal layers were given this designation.

contaminants. Also, there may be missiles or foreign bodies embedded in the tissues that must be removed during surgery. Puncture wounds may be present.

Both open and closed fractures may earn the descriptive term of "complicated." A complicated fracture is one in which a bone fragment has injured an internal organ. For example, the ribs may injure the lungs, liver, and spleen, depending on the nature and direction of the force causing the fracture.

If there is no mention in the medical record as to whether the fracture is open or closed, assume that the fracture is closed.

800 FRACTURE OF VAULT OF SKULL

The vault of the skull is composed of three bones: the frontal bone and two parietal bones. Fractures of the vault may be accompanied by cerebral contusion or laceration; subarachnoid, subdural or extradural hemorrhage; or an unspecified cause of hemorrhage.

Cerebral contusions and lacerations constitute severe injury. One of the great problems associated with head trauma is that the brain sustains a double blow — the initial blow that causes the brain to travel to the opposite side of the skull, smiting the interior skull with significant force. This second blow is called contrecoup. Such force applied to the brain causes swelling and increased intracranial pressure that is very dangerous. Serious head trauma has a high mortality rate, nearly 50 percent. In addition to edema, a second complication is hemorrhage resulting from laceration of blood vessels. If the fracture is open, the brain is exposed to bacteria, compounding the danger.

Major trauma to the forebrain with no injury to the brainstem may result in survival of the patient in a chronic vegetative state for several years.

Patients who have survived severe head trauma often deal with posttraumatic epilepsy for many years.

800.0	5th	Closed fracture of vault of skull without mention of intracranial injury
800.1	5th	Closed fracture of vault of skull with cerebral laceration and contusion
800.2	5th	Closed fracture of vault of skull with subarachnoid, subdural, and extradural hemorrhage
800.3	5th	Closed fracture of vault of skull with other and unspecified intracranial hemorrhage
800.4	5th	Closed fracture of vault of skull with intercranial injury of other and unspecified nature
800.5	5th	Open fracture of vault of skull without mention of intracranial injury
800.6	5th	Open fracture of vault of skull with cerebral laceration and contusion
800.7	5th	Open fracture of vault of skull with subarachnoid, subdural, and extradural hemorrhage
800.8	5th	Open fracture of vault of skull with other and unspecified intracranial hemorrhage
800.9	5th	Open fracture of vault of skull with intracranial injury of other and unspecified nature

5th Needs fifth-digit   **OK** Valid three-digit code

801 FRACTURE OF BASE OF SKULL

Included in the description for base of skull are the following bones:

Occiput — bone at the base of the skull; contains the foramen magnum, the opening in the bone that allows the spinal cord to join the brain.

Sinuses — butterfly-shaped sphenoid sinus and the ethmoid sinus. The sinuses introduce air into the skull, lightening what would be excessive weight.

Orbital roof — the orbit has a roof and a floor. The roof is considered part of the skull base, an exception is frontal bone that forms part of the roof of the orbit as part of the skull vault.

Sphenoid bone — large bone containing the sphenoid sinus, forming part of the back of the orbit.

Temporal bones (2) — adjoin the parietal, sphenoid, and occipital bones.

Cranial fossae — anterior, middle and posterior - The three fossae form the floor of the cranial cavity (on the superior aspect of the base of the skull) and provide a surface to support the various lobes of the brain. The frontal lobes rest on the anterior fossa, the temporal lobes on the middle fossa, and the pons and medulla oblongata are contained within the posterior fossa, with the cerebellum expanding over the medulla oblongata.

801.0 ✓5th Closed fracture of base of skull without mention of intracranial injury

801.1 ✓5th Closed fracture of base of skull with cerebral laceration and contusion

801.2 ✓5th Closed fracture of base of skull with subarachnoid, subdural, and extradural hemorrhage

801.3 ✓5th Closed fracture of base of skull with other and unspecified intracranial hemorrhage

801.4 ✓5th Closed fracture of base of skull with intracranial injury of other and unspecified nature

801.5 ✓5th Open fracture of base of skull without mention of intracranial injury

801.6 ✓5th Open fracture of base of skull with cerebral laceration and contusion

801.7 ✓5th Open fracture of base of skull with subarachnoid, subdural, and extradural hemorrhage

801.8 ✓5th Open fracture of base of skull with other and unspecified intracranial hemorrhage

801.9 ✓5th Open fracture of base of skull with intracranial injury of other and unspecified nature

802 FRACTURE OF FACE BONES

The facial bones are comprised of the following bones:

Nasal bone — adjoins frontal bone to form the superior aspect of nose), the Mandible - lower jawbone

Maxilla — upper jawbone

Zygomatic bones — two bones of the cheek (2)

Lacrimal bones — two bones of the tear ducts

Vomer — inferior and interior support for nasal conchae

Orbital plate — two bones of the eye

Palate

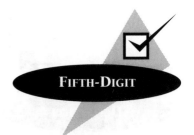

FIFTH-DIGIT

The following fifth-digit subclassification is for use with the appropriate codes in categories 800, 801, 803, and 804:

0 unspecified state of consciousness

1 with no loss of consciousness

2 with brief [less than one hour] loss of consciousness

3 with moderate [1-24 hours] loss of consciousness

4 with prolonged [more than 24 hours] loss of consciousness and return to pre-existing conscious level

5 with prolonged [more than 24 hours] loss of consciousness, without return to pre-existing conscious level

6 with loss of consciousness of unspecified duration

9 with concussion, unspecified

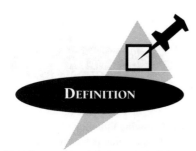

DEFINITION

Alveolar process: inferior aspect of the maxilla and the upper teeth have their origins superior to the alveolar process.

Blowout fracture: fracture of the orbital floor.

Body of a bone: main part of the bone.

Coronoid process: comes from corona, meaning crown. Always look for it on the superior aspect of the bone.

Malar: another term for zygomatic bone.

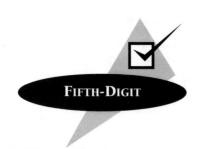

FIFTH-DIGIT

The following fifth-digit subclassification is for use with the appropriate codes in categories 800, 801, 803, and 804:

0 unspecified state of consciousness

1 with no loss of consciousness

2 with brief [less than one hour] loss of consciousness

3 with moderate [1-24 hours] loss of consciousness

4 with prolonged [more than 24 hours] loss of consciousness and return to pre-existing conscious level

5 with prolonged [more than 24 hours] loss of consciousness, without return to pre-existing conscious level

6 with loss of consciousness of unspecified duration

9 with concussion, unspecified

The orbit is one of the most complex bony structures in the skull. The frontal, mandible, lacrimal, orbital plate, zygomatic, and sphenoid bones fit together to form support and protect the eyeball.

802.0	Nasal bones, closed fracture
802.1	Nasal bones, open fracture
802.2 ✔5th	Mandible, closed fracture
802.3 ✔5th	Mandible, open fracture
802.4	Malar and maxillary bones, closed fracture
802.5	Malar and maxillary bones, open fracture
802.6	Orbital floor (blow-out), closed fracture
802.7	Orbital floor (blow-out), open fracture
802.8	Other facial bones, closed fracture
802.9	Other facial bones, open fracture

803 OTHER AND UNQUALIFIED SKULL FRACTURES

Use these codes when the record lacks specific information regarding the trauma to the head.

803.0 ✔5th Other closed skull fracture without mention of intracranial injury

803.1 ✔5th Other closed skull fracture with cerebral laceration and contusion

803.2 ✔5th Other closed skull fracture with subarachnoid, subdural, and extradural hemorrhage

803.3 ✔5th Closed skull fracture with other and unspecified intracranial hemorrhage

803.4 ✔5th Other closed skull fracture with intracranial injury of other and unspecified nature

803.5 ✔5th Other open skull fracture without mention of intracranial injury

803.6 ✔5th Other open skull fracture with cerebral laceration and contusion

803.7 ✔5th Other open skull fracture with subarachnoid, subdural, and extradural hemorrhage

803.8 ✔5th Other open skull fracture with other and unspecified intracranial hemorrhage

803.9 ✔5th Other open skull fracture with intracranial injury of other and unspecified nature

804 MULTIPLE FRACTURES INVOLVING SKULL OR FACE WITH OTHER BONES

This subcategory is used when bones of the skull or face are fractured, together with bones in other parts of the body. If there is more specific information about the nature of the various fractures, code more specifically.

804.0 ✔5th Closed fractures involving skull or face with other bones, without mention of intracranial injury

804.1 ✔5th Closed fractures involving skull or face with other bones, with cerebral laceration and contusion

804.2 ✔5th Closed fractures involving skull or face with other bones with subarachnoid, subdural, and extradural hemorrhage

804.3 ✔5th Closed fractures involving skull or face with other bones, with other and unspecified intracranial hemorrhage

804.4 ✔5th Closed fractures involving skull or face with other bones, with intracranial injury of other and unspecified nature

804.5 ✔5th Open fractures involving skull or face with other bones, without mention of intracranial injury

804.6 ✔5th Open fractures involving skull or face with other bones, with cerebral laceration and contusion

✔5th Needs fifth-digit   **OK** Valid three-digit code

804.7 ✔5th Open fractures involving skull or face with other bones with subarachnoid, subdural, and extradural hemorrhage

804.8 ✔5th Open fractures involving skull or face with other bones, with other and unspecified intracranial hemorrhage

804.9 ✔5th Open fractures involving skull or face with other bones, with intracranial injury of other and unspecified nature

805-809 Fracture of Neck and Trunk

805 FRACTURE OF VERTEBRAL COLUMN WITHOUT MENTION OF SPINAL CORD INJURY

The vertebral column forms a protective shield around the spinal column, much as the cranium protects the brain. It allows movement through articulation of the cervical, thoracic, and lumbar vertebrae (sacral vertebrae are fused). Each vertebra has a body and a neural arch, which encase the spinal cord. Each vertebra has several prominent aspects called processes for the attachment of muscles, tendons, and other soft tissues.

The two transverse processes of the cervical vertebrae have a small foramen, the foramen transversarium, through which the vertebral artery and vein and a plexus of sympathetic nerves travel. The first cervical vertebra is called the atlas and supports the globe of the head; it has no vertebral body; instead, the part of the vertebra that would have been the body is fused with the second cervical vertebra to form an osseous pivot around which the head turns. The second cervical vertebra is called the axis.

The thoracic (dorsal) vertebrae accept the heads of the ribs. The lumbar vertebrae are the largest of the moveable vertebrae, or true vertebrae.

Below the thoracic vertebrae are the five lumbar vertebrae, which are larger than the thoracic and cervical vertebrae and support a great amount of weight.

The sacrum consists of five large vertebrae that are fused in the adult. The female sacrum is shorter and wider than the male sacrum.

The composition of the coccyx varies from three to five fused segments, though the typical configuration is four.

The spinal cord, protected by the vertebral column, shares the three meningeal layers, the dura, arachnoid, and pia maters with the brain. It is described anatomically in relation to the vertebrae at each level, but the cord is not identical to the column. In addition to nerve tracts to the brain, enclosed within the column, the spinal nerves exit the column to innervate specific muscle groups bilaterally, according to their level on the vertebral column. The part of the cord that extends below the lumbar level resembled a horse's tail to early anatomists, hence its name — cauda equina.

Similar to the brain, the cord has both gray and white matter. Hemorrhage into the gray matter is known as hematomyelia; its symptoms, which are often permanent, include muscle wasting, diminished tendon reflexes, and muscle weakness. Spinal concussion, the same contrecoup action described in the brain, can result in loss of cord function after a very severe blow or jarring.

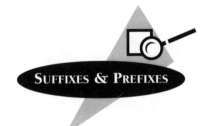

SUFFIXES & PREFIXES

Hemato - myel- ia: hemato [blood] myel [double meaning - bone marrow, spinal cord] ia [condition]

Quadri- plegia: quadri [four] plegia [stroke, blow]

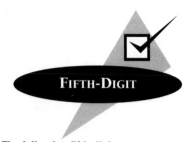

FIFTH-DIGIT

The following fifth-digit subclassification is for use with codes 805.0-805.1:

0 cervical vertebra, unspecified level

1 first cervical vertebra

2 second cervical vertebra

3 third cervical vertebra

4 fourth cervical vertebra

5 fifth cervical vertebra

6 sixth cervical vertebra

7 seventh cervical vertebra

8 multiple cervical vertebra

805.0 ✓5th Closed fracture of cervical vertebra without mention of spinal cord injury

805.1 ✓5th Open fracture of cervical vertebra without mention of spinal cord injury

805.2 Closed fracture of dorsal (thoracic) vertebra without mention of spinal cord injury

805.3 Open fracture of dorsal (thoracic) vertebra without mention of spinal cord injury

805.4 Closed fracture of lumbar vertebra without mention of spinal cord injury

805.5 Open fracture of lumbar vertebra without mention of spinal cord injury

805.6 Closed fracture of sacrum and coccyx without mention of spinal cord injury

805.7 Open fracture of sacrum and coccyx without mention of spinal cord injury

805.8 Closed fracture of unspecified part of vertebral column without mention of spinal cord injury

805.9 Open fracture of unspecified part of vertebral column without mention of spinal cord injury

806 FRACTURE OF VERTEBRAL COLUMN WITH SPINAL CORD INJURY

A transverse cord injury will cause immediate total paralysis and sensory loss below the level of the injury. It is sometimes referred to as a complete injury. An incomplete lesion will result in partial motor and sensory loss. Depending on the site of injury, outcomes vary, ranging from respiratory paralysis (injury above C-5 level), C4-C5 — quadriplegia (paralysis of 4 limbs), C-5-C6 - paralysis of the legs and partial paralysis of the arms, with abduction and flexion of the arms as movement potentials. C6-C7 allows shoulder movement and elbow flexion, though the lower limbs are paralyzed. Complete loss of bowel and bladder control is associated with injury to the third, fourth, and fifth sacral nerve roots or to the juncture at L-1. Posterior cord syndrome is an incomplete injury resulting in motor paralysis and loss of posterior spinal column sensory function.

Paralysis to both legs and the lower portion of the body is termed paraplegia.

The documentation in the medical record should be clear for coding these injuries as either complete or incomplete. Resort to "unspecified" only if the physician fails to make the distinction.

806.00 Closed fracture of C1-C4 level with unspecified spinal cord injury

806.01 Closed fracture of C1-C4 level with complete lesion of cord

806.02 Closed fracture of C1-C4 level with anterior cord syndrome

806.03 Closed fracture of C1-C4 level with central cord syndrome

806.04 Closed fracture of C1-C4 level with other specified spinal cord injury

806.05 Closed fracture of C5-C7 level with unspecified spinal cord injury

806.06 Closed fracture of C5-C7 level with complete lesion of cord

806.07 Closed fracture of C5-C7 level with anterior cord syndrome

806.08 Closed fracture of C5-C7 level with central cord syndrome

806.09 Closed fracture of C5-C7 level with other specified spinal cord injury

806.10 Open fracture of C1-C4 level with unspecified spinal cord injury

806.11 Open fracture of C1-C4 level with complete lesion of cord

806.12 Open fracture of C1-C4 level with anterior cord syndrome

806.13 Open fracture of C1-C4 level with central cord syndrome

806.14 Open fracture of C1-C4 level with other specified spinal cord injury

806.15 Open fracture of C5-C7 level with unspecified spinal cord injury

806.16 Open fracture of C5-C7 level with complete lesion of cord

806.17 Open fracture of C5-C7 level with anterior cord syndrome

806.18 Open fracture of C5-C7 level with central cord syndrome

806.19 Open fracture of C5-C7 level with other specified spinal cord injury

✓5th   Needs fifth-digit   **OK**   Valid three-digit code

806.20	Closed fracture of T1-T6 level with unspecified spinal cord injury
806.21	Closed fracture of T1-T6 level with complete lesion of cord
806.22	Closed fracture of T1-T6 level with anterior cord syndrome
806.23	Closed fracture of T1-T6 level with central cord syndrome
806.24	Closed fracture of T1-T6 level with other specified spinal cord injury
806.25	Closed fracture of T7-T12 level with unspecified spinal cord injury
806.26	Closed fracture of T7-T12 level with complete lesion of cord
806.27	Closed fracture of T7-T12 level with anterior cord syndrome
806.28	Closed fracture of T7-T12 level with central cord syndrome
806.29	Closed fracture of T7-T12 level with other specified spinal cord injury
806.30	Open fracture of T1-T6 level with unspecified spinal cord injury
806.31	Open fracture of T1-T6 level with complete lesion of cord
806.32	Open fracture of T1-T6 level with anterior cord syndrome
806.33	Open fracture of T1-T6 level with central cord syndrome
806.34	Open fracture of T1-T6 level with other specified spinal cord injury
806.35	Open fracture of T7-T12 level with unspecified spinal cord injury
806.36	Open fracture of T7-T12 level with complete lesion of cord
806.37	Open fracture of T7-T12 level with anterior cord syndrome
806.38	Open fracture of T7-T12 level with central cord syndrome
806.39	Open fracture of T7-T12 level with other specified spinal cord injury
806.4	Closed fracture of lumbar spine with spinal cord injury
806.5	Open fracture of lumbar spine with spinal cord injury
806.60	Closed fracture of sacrum and coccyx with unspecified spinal cord injury
806.61	Closed fracture of sacrum and coccyx with complete cauda equina lesion
806.62	Closed fracture of sacrum and coccyx with other cauda equina injury
806.69	Closed fracture of sacrum and coccyx with other spinal cord injury
806.70	Open fracture of sacrum and coccyx with unspecified spinal cord injury
806.71	Open fracture of sacrum and coccyx with complete cauda equina lesion
806.72	Open fracture of sacrum and coccyx with other cauda equina injury
806.79	Open fracture of sacrum and coccyx with other spinal cord injury
806.8	Closed fracture of unspecified vertebra with spinal cord injury
806.9	Open fracture of unspecified vertebra with spinal cord injury

807 FRACTURE OF RIB(S), STERNUM, LARYNX, AND TRACHEA

Twelve pairs of ribs form the thoracic cage, which protects the critical organs in the thorax and abdomen. The true ribs are the first eight ribs and the false ribs are the last four ribs. The floating ribs are the last two of the false ribs.

All of the ribs, except the floating ribs, are connected to the sternum (the breastbone) with costal cartilage.

Flail chest is one of the most dangerous thoracic injuries, resulting from an injury causing at least four fractured ribs in two locations, and pulmonary contusion, leading to hypoventilation. In flail chest, the movement of the chest is paradoxical (opposite of the natural ventilatory movement). On inhalation, the chest contracts and on expiration the chest expands. Generally, thoracic injuries carry a high mortality risk, with death attributed to hypoxemia, hypovolemia, or myocardial failure.

Fractures of the scapula, the sternum, or the first rib are indicative of applied forces.

When coding rib fractures, review the documentation to capture multiple fractures. In inpatient reimbursement, some payment algorithms are constructed according to the number of ribs fractured, making complete capture of all injuries important in all cases.

DEFINITION

Hyoid bone - a U-shaped bone that anchors the digastric muscle, primarily, allowing the mandible to open

Sternum - a sword-shaped bone ending in a point (xiphoid process)

Trachea - a cartilaginous tube forming the airway in the upper thorax, containing the larynx, or "voice box"

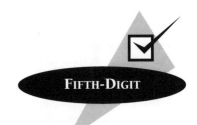

FIFTH-DIGIT

The following fifth-digit subclassification is for use with codes 807.0-807.1:

0 rib(s), unspecified

1 one rib

2 two ribs

3 three ribs

4 four ribs

5 five ribs

6 six ribs

7 seven ribs

8 eight or more ribs

9 multiple ribs, unspecified

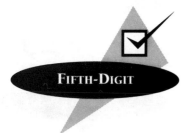

The following fifth-digit subclassification is for use with codes 807.0-807.1:

0 rib(s), unspecified
1 one rib
2 two ribs
3 three ribs
4 four ribs
5 five ribs
6 six ribs
7 seven ribs
8 eight or more ribs
9 multiple ribs, unspecified

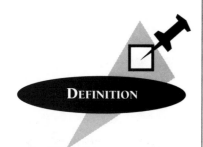

DEFINITION

Cancellous bone: describes a bone that produces bone marrow, hence is highly vascular.

The humerus in the upper arm corresponds to the femur in the thigh. The radius and ulna in the forearm correspond to the tibia and fibula in the lower leg. All are long bones, and as such, have a shaft, a head, a proximal and distal portion, and various condyles, processes, tuberosities, and trochanters. The head of a long bone always has a neck, a narrow portion that supports the head. Necks are susceptible to damage. Since the long bones contain bone marrow, a fracture presents a risk of a fatty embolic event, as well as a hemorrhagic threat. They also have epiphyseal plates that allow for growth and deactivate in adults. Fractures of the plates can be subtle and difficult to diagnose.

Caudal: - pertaining to the tail.

Cephalic: - pertaining to the head.

807.0 ✔5th	Closed fracture of rib(s)
807.1 ✔5th	Open fracture of rib(s)
807.2	Closed fracture of sternum
807.3	Open fracture of sternum
807.4	Flail chest
807.5	Closed fracture of larynx and trachea
807.6	Open fracture of larynx and trachea

808 FRACTURE OF PELVIS

The pelvis includes the ilium, the ischium, the pubis, and the sacrum, which form a bony circle to protect the pelvic contents, provide stability for the vertebral column, (sacrum) and provide an appropriate surface for femoral articulation for ambulation.

The innominate bone, or hipbone, refers to the three bones making up the hipbone - the pubis, ilium and ischium. The acetabulum is the socket for the femoral head and is found anterior to the rings of the ischium on the lateral inferior surface of the ilium. When the acetabulum is fractured, the head of the femur functions as a hammer, striking against its socket with undue force.

Note that the term, hip fracture, which is often used to describe a fracture of the acetabulum, excludes the femur. A fracture of the shaft of the femur, or of the head of the femur, is anatomically distinct from a disruption of the socket of the femoral head.

Pelvic fractures in an individual age 55 and older are associated with a 9.5 percent mortality rate within one year. In fractures of the pelvic ring (circle), the mortality risk to the patient is quite immediate, due to the hemorrhagic capability of cancellous bone. While the issue of application of external fixation may be debated, all agree that the disruption must be stabilized as soon as possible to insure a positive outcome.

808.0	Closed fracture of acetabulum
808.1	Open fracture of acetabulum
808.2	Closed fracture of pubis
808.3	Open fracture of pubis
808.41	Closed fracture of ilium
808.42	Closed fracture of ischium
808.43	Multiple closed pelvic fractures with disruption of pelvic circle
808.49	Closed fracture of other specified part of pelvis
808.51	Open fracture of ilium
808.52	Open fracture of ischium
808.53	Multiple open pelvic fractures with disruption of pelvic circle
808.59	Open fracture of other specified part of pelvis
808.8	Unspecified closed fracture of pelvis
808.9	Unspecified open fracture of pelvis

809 ILL-DEFINED FRACTURES OF BONES OF TRUNK

Although this category includes a number of excludes notes, an example is a combination of rib and pelvic fractures, poorly defined in documentation.

809.0	Fracture of bones of trunk, closed
809.1	Fracture of bones of trunk, open

✔5th Needs fifth-digit   **OK** Valid three-digit code

810-819 Fracture of Upper Limb

810 FRACTURE OF CLAVICLE

The clavicle, or collarbone, has a shaft and articulating ends — the sternal and acromial ends. The acromial end articulates with the scapula, the shoulder bone.

810.0 5th Closed fracture of clavicle
810.1 5th Open fracture of clavicle

811 FRACTURE OF SCAPULA

The scapula articulates with the clavicle and the humerus, the long bone in the upper arm. Its socket, the glenoid fossa, receives the humoral head. The coracoid process superior to the glenoid fossa provides a surface for attachments of muscles and tendons.

811.0 5th Closed fracture of scapula
811.1 5th Open fracture of scapula

812 FRACTURE OF HUMERUS

In addition to possession of an anatomical neck, the humerus includes a surgical neck, described as that portion of the anatomical neck most likely to fracture.

812.00	Closed fracture of unspecified part of upper end of humerus
812.01	Closed fracture of surgical neck of humerus
812.02	Closed fracture of anatomical neck of humerus
812.03	Closed fracture of greater tuberosity of humerus
812.09	Other closed fractures of upper end of humerus
812.10	Open fracture of unspecified part of upper end of humerus
812.11	Open fracture of surgical neck of humerus
812.12	Open fracture of anatomical neck of humerus
812.13	Open fracture of greater tuberosity of humerus
812.19	Other open fracture of upper end of humerus
812.20	Closed fracture of unspecified part of humerus
812.21	Closed fracture of shaft of humerus
812.30	Open fracture of unspecified part of humerus
812.31	Open fracture of shaft of humerus
812.40	Closed fracture of unspecified part of lower end of humerus
812.41	Closed fracture of supracondylar humerus
812.42	Closed fracture of lateral condyle of humerus
812.43	Closed fracture of medial condyle of humerus
812.44	Closed fracture of unspecified condyle(s) of humerus
812.49	Other closed fracture of lower end of humerus
812.50	Open fracture of unspecified part of lower end of humerus
812.51	Open fracture of supracondylar humerus
812.52	Open fracture of lateral condyle of humerus
812.53	Open fracture of medial condyle of humerus
812.54	Open fracture of unspecified condyle(s) of humerus
812.59	Other open fracture of lower end of humerus

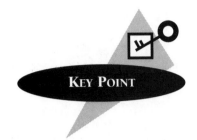

KEY POINT

All anatomical descriptions are based on the patient or skeleton visualized in the anatomical position, which is on its feet, with the palms turned to the front. This allows for mutual understanding of the words, superior, inferior, medial, lateral, proximal and distal, cephalic, and caudal. In the anatomical position, the thumbs are envisioned as lateral, and the little finger is medial. The outside of the ankle is lateral, and the inside is medial. The humoral head is proximal to the head of the body, and the end that articulates with the radius and ulna is distal or caudal to the head of the body. References to proximal or distal are always made in relation to the head of the body.

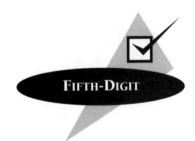

FIFTH-DIGIT

The following fifth-digit subclassification is for use with category 810:

0 unspecified part

1 sternal end of clavicle

2 shaft of clavicle

3 acromial end of clavicle

The following fifth-digit subclassification is for use with category 811:

0 unspecified part

1 acromial process

2 coracoid process

3 glenoid cavity and neck of scapula

9 other

813 FRACTURE OF RADIUS AND ULNA

The radius and ulna operate in tandem, with a hinge-like motion for bending and capabilities for pronation and supination for the hand and wrist. In the anatomical position, the hands are supinated and in the pronated position when the palms are down.

Monteggia's fracture is a common fracture at the proximal end of the ulna, combined with dislocation of the radial head. In a child, closed reduction may suffice, though adults require open reduction and internal fixation (ORIF). Reduction is the repositioning of a bone into proper alignment. Dislocations, which are the disruption of the joint, are also reduced.

Another common fracture is Colles' fracture, which is a transverse fracture of the distal radius, displacing the hand. This injury typically occurs when an individual puts out their hand to break their fall.

813.00	Unspecified fracture of radius and ulna, upper end of forearm, closed
813.01	Closed fracture of olecranon process of ulna
813.02	Closed fracture of coronoid process of ulna
813.03	Closed Monteggia's fracture
813.04	Other and unspecified closed fractures of proximal end of ulna (alone)
813.05	Closed fracture of head of radius
813.06	Closed fracture of neck of radius
813.07	Other and unspecified closed fractures of proximal end of radius (alone)
813.08	Closed fracture of radius with ulna, upper end (any part)
813.10	Unspecified open fracture of upper end of forearm
813.11	Open fracture of olecranon process of ulna
813.12	Open fracture of coronoid process of ulna
813.13	Open Monteggia's fracture
813.14	Other and unspecified open fractures of proximal end of ulna (alone)
813.15	Open fracture of head of radius
813.16	Open fracture of neck of radius
813.17	Other and unspecified open fractures of proximal end of radius (alone)
813.18	Open fracture of radius with ulna, upper end (any part)
813.20	Unspecified closed fracture of shaft of radius or ulna
813.21	Closed fracture of shaft of radius (alone)
813.22	Closed fracture of shaft of ulna (alone)
813.23	Closed fracture of shaft of radius with ulna
813.30	Unspecified open fracture of shaft of radius or ulna
813.31	Open fracture of shaft of radius (alone)
813.32	Open fracture of shaft of ulna (alone)
813.33	Open fracture of shaft of radius with ulna
813.40	Unspecified closed fracture of lower end of forearm
813.41	Closed Colles' fracture
813.42	Other closed fractures of distal end of radius (alone)
813.43	Closed fracture of distal end of ulna (alone)
813.44	Closed fracture of lower end of radius with ulna
813.50	Unspecified open fracture of lower end of forearm
813.51	Open Colles' fracture
813.52	Other open fractures of distal end of radius (alone)
813.53	Open fracture of distal end of ulna (alone)
813.54	Open fracture of lower end of radius with ulna
813.80	Closed fracture of unspecified part of forearm
813.81	Closed fracture of unspecified part of radius (alone)

✔5th   Needs fifth-digit   **OK**   Valid three-digit code

813.82	Closed fracture of unspecified part of ulna (alone)
813.83	Closed fracture of unspecified part of radius with ulna
813.90	Open fracture of unspecified part of forearm
813.91	Open fracture of unspecified part of radius (alone)
813.92	Open fracture of unspecified part of ulna (alone)
813.93	Open fracture of unspecified part of radius with ulna

814 FRACTURE OF CARPAL BONES

The eight carpal bones are functionality linked to the placement of each bone and its articulation with various partners.

Two rows of bones, with the scaphoid bone common to each row, act as a bridge to provide stability. The first row (proximal) is comprised of the scaphoid, lunate, pisiform, and triquetrum. The second row (distal) is comprised of the scaphoid, trapezium, trapezoid, capitate, and hamate.

Fractures of the distal radius and ulna are typically referred to as wrist fractures. They articulate with the proximal carpals, though, technically, they are the bones of the forearm. The carpals, which form the wrist, are considered part of the hand.

Carpal fractures usually occur as a result of extreme dorsiflexion or extension of the wrist and require significant force to happen at all.

814.00	Unspecified closed fracture of carpal bone
814.01	Closed fracture of navicular (scaphoid) bone of wrist
814.02	Closed fracture of lunate (semilunar) bone of wrist
814.03	Closed fracture of triquetral (cuneiform) bone of wrist
814.04	Closed fracture of pisiform bone of wrist
814.05	Closed fracture of trapezium bone (larger multangular) of wrist
814.06	Closed fracture of trapezoid bone (smaller multangular) of wrist
814.07	Closed fracture of capitate bone (os magnum) of wrist
814.08	Closed fracture of hamate (unciform) bone of wrist
814.09	Closed fracture of other bone of wrist
814.10	Unspecified open fracture of carpal bone
814.11	Open fracture of navicular (scaphoid) bone of wrist
814.12	Open fracture of lunate (semilunar) bone of wrist
814.13	Open fracture of triquetral (cuneiform) bone of wrist
814.14	Open fracture of pisiform bone of wrist
814.15	Open fracture of trapezium bone (larger multangular) of wrist
814.16	Open fracture of trapezoid bone (smaller multangular) of wrist
814.17	Open fracture of capitate bone (os magnum) of wrist
814.18	Open fracture of hamate (unciform) bone of wrist
814.19	Open fracture of other bone of wrist

815 FRACTURE OF METACARPAL BONE(S)

The metacarpals are the bones of the hand distal to the carpals and proximal to the phalanges (fingers). The fingers have three joints: the section next to the metacarpals is the proximal phalanx, the midsection is the middle phalanx, and the farthest section is the distal phalanx. The numbering convention selects the thumb as the first metacarpal and the medial finger (pinkie) as the fifth finger.

The anatomy of each phalanx is described in terms of base, body, and head. The base is the end portion closest to the head of the body, the body is the midsection of the bone, and the

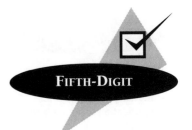

FIFTH-DIGIT

The following fifth-digit subclassification is for use with category 814:

0 carpal bone, unspecified

1 navicular [scaphoid] of wrist

2 lunate [semilunar] bone of wrist

3 triquetral [cuneiform] bone of wrist

4 pisiform

5 trapezium bone [larger multangular]

6 trapezoid bone [smaller multangular]

7 capitate bone [os magnum]

8 hamate [unciform] bone

9 other

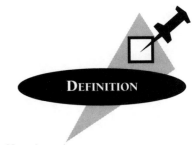

DEFINITION

Meta: beyond

Phalanx (phalanges, pl): a sharp projecting mass, hence, a finger or toe.

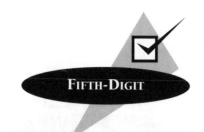

FIFTH-DIGIT

The following fifth-digit subclassification is for use with category 815:

0 metacarpal bone(s), site unspecified

1 base of thumb [first] metacarpal

2 base of other metacarpal bone(s)

3 shaft of metacarpal bone(s)

4 neck of metacarpal bone(s)

9 multiple sites of metacarpus

head is the distal end of the bone. The distal phalanx has an additional descriptor, a tuberosity. Two sesamoid bones are located closed to the distal joint of the first metacarpal (thumb).

Because they project and perform many functions, the metacarpals and phalanges account for 10 percent of all fractures, of which 50 percent are work-related.

815.0 ✔5th Closed fracture of metacarpal bones
815.1 ✔5th Open fracture of metacarpal bones

816 FRACTURE OF ONE OR MORE PHALANGES OF HAND

816.00 Closed fracture of unspecified phalanx or phalanges of hand
816.01 Closed fracture of middle or proximal phalanx or phalanges of hand
816.02 Closed fracture of distal phalanx or phalanges of hand
816.03 Closed fracture of multiple sites of phalanx or phalanges of hand
816.10 Open fracture of phalanx or phalanges of hand, unspecified
816.11 Open fracture of middle or proximal phalanx or phalanges of hand
816.12 Open fracture of distal phalanx or phalanges of hand
816.13 Open fractures of multiple sites of phalanx or phalanges of hand

817 MULTIPLE FRACTURES OF HAND BONES
Use these categories only if the documentation is extremely sketchy.

817.0 Multiple closed fractures of hand bones
817.1 Multiple open fractures of hand bones

818 ILL-DEFINED FRACTURES OF UPPER LIMB
818.0 Ill-defined closed fractures of upper limb
818.1 Ill-defined open fractures of upper limb

819 MULTIPLE FRACTURES INVOLVING BOTH UPPER LIMBS, AND UPPER LIMB WITH RIB(S) AND STERNUM
819.0 Multiple closed fractures involving both upper limbs, and upper limb with rib(s) and sternum
819.1 Multiple open fractures involving both upper limbs, and upper limb with rib(s) and sternum

820-829 Fracture of Lower Limb

820 FRACTURE OF NECK OF FEMUR
The proximal femur bears the brunt of accidents leading to fractures, compared to the other bones used for locomotion. Lower extremity fractures in children may suggest child abuse.

Fractures of the femoral shaft are relatively uncommon, while fractures of the neck are among the most frequent. Femoral neck fractures are classified in ICD-9 as transcervical, or petrochanteric, with subdivisions. Radiologists often use the terminology intracapsular and extracapsular. A subcapital or intracapsular fracture of the femoral neck has the highest risk of avascular necrosis, which occurs when a severe injury disrupts the blood supply to the bone. This fracture also is inherently more unstable after surgery than an intertrochanteric fracture since the weakest part of the bone is now supporting the point of greatest stress.

✔5th Needs fifth-digit   **OK** Valid three-digit code

Preferred treatments for the various fractures include the following:

Shaft fracture - intramedullary nailing; promotes fast weight-bearing capability

Transcervical fracture - hemiarthroplasty or total hip replacement

Intertrochanteric fracture - fixation with sliding implant

820.00	Closed fracture of unspecified intracapsular section of neck of femur
820.01	Closed fracture of epiphysis (separation) (upper) of neck of femur
820.02	Closed fracture of midcervical section of femur
820.03	Closed fracture of base of neck of femur
820.09	Other closed transcervical fracture of femur
820.10	Open fracture of unspecified intracapsular section of neck of femur
820.11	Open fracture of epiphysis (separation) (upper) of neck of femur
820.12	Open fracture of midcervical section of femur
820.13	Open fracture of base of neck of femur
820.19	Other open transcervical fracture of femur
820.20	Closed fracture of unspecified trochanteric section of femur
820.21	Closed fracture of intertrochanteric section of femur
820.22	Closed fracture of subtrochanteric section of femur
820.30	Open fracture of unspecified trochanteric section of femur
820.31	Open fracture of intertrochanteric section of femur
820.32	Open fracture of subtrochanteric section of femur
820.8	Closed fracture of unspecified part of neck of femur
820.9	Open fracture of unspecified part of neck of femur

821 FRACTURE OF OTHER AND UNSPECIFIED PARTS OF THE FEMUR

In children and adolescents, whose skeletons are still immature, distal epiphyseal fracture, presenting as valgus instability, results in a significant number of injuries. These fractures occur in normal play and sports activity, and are easy to overlook if the evaluation seems to point to a ligamentous sprain, rather than a physeal fracture.

821.00	Closed fracture of unspecified part of femur
821.01	Closed fracture of shaft of femur
821.10	Open fracture of unspecified part of femur
821.11	Open fracture of shaft of femur
821.20	Closed fracture of unspecified part of lower end of femur
821.21	Closed fracture of femoral condyle
821.22	Closed fracture of lower epiphysis of femur
821.23	Closed supracondylar fracture of femur
821.29	Other closed fracture of lower end of femur
821.30	Open fracture of unspecified part of lower end of femur
821.31	Open fracture of femoral condyle
821.32	Open fracture of lower epiphysis of femur
821.33	Open supracondylar fracture of femur
821.39	Other open fracture of lower end of femur

822 FRACTURE OF PATELLA

The anatomy of the knee joint and associated muscles, tendons, and ligaments predispose the occurrence of patellar fractures in conjunction with sprains or ruptures of the ligaments. Typically, injuries are due to direct application of force or twisting. A severely injured knee remains prone to re-injury, instability, or arthritis.

822.0	Closed fracture of patella
822.1	Open fracture of patella

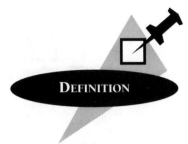

DEFINITION

Cervicotrochanteric: describes the trochanter end of the femoral neck.

Hemiarthroplasty: is the replacement of the femoral head.

Intramedullary nailing: intra [within] medulla [marrow].

Pertrochanteric: per [through, across].

Supracondylar: - supra [above] condyle

Total hip replacement: the replacement of the acetabular cup and the femoral head with prostheses.

Transcervical: trans [across] cervix [neck].

Trochanter: the two large protuberances at base of femoral neck and proximal to the shaft (femoral condyles are found at distal end).

Valgus: pointing outward, as in bowlegged.

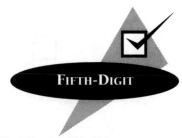

FIFTH-DIGIT

The following fifth-digit subclassification is for use with category 823:

0 tibia alone

1 fibula alone

2 fibula with tibia

823 FRACTURE OF TIBIA AND FIBULA

The malleolus is the distal end of the tibia and fibula and classified to the ankle in ICD-9 as the malleolus. The lateral malleolus is part of the fibula and the medial malleolus is part of the tibia.

823.0	✔5th	Closed fracture of upper end of tibia and fibula
823.1	✔5th	Open fracture of upper end of tibia and fibula
823.2	✔5th	Closed fracture of shaft of tibia and fibula
823.3	✔5th	Open fracture of shaft of tibia and fibula
823.8	✔5th	Closed fracture of unspecified part of tibia and fibula
823.9	✔5th	Open fracture of unspecified part of tibia and fibula

824 FRACTURE OF ANKLE

A bimalleolar fracture is a fracture of both the lateral and medial aspects of the malleolus. Pott's fracture is any fracture of the malleolus. Dupuytren's fracture is a fracture dislocation of the ankle with the talus downwardly displaced. The talus is one the major ankle (tarsal) bones. A trimalleolar fracture involves a fracture of the medial malleolus and fibula and a fracture of the posterior lip of the tibia's articulating surface.

Open reduction and internal fixation is the method of treatment for bimalleolar and trimalleolar fractures.

824.0	Closed fracture of medial malleolus
824.1	Open fracture of medial malleolus
824.2	Closed fracture of lateral malleolus
824.3	Open fracture of lateral malleolus
824.4	Closed bimalleolar fracture
824.5	Open bimalleolar fracture
824.6	Closed trimalleolar fracture
824.7	Open trimalleolar fracture
824.8	Unspecified closed fracture of ankle
824.9	Unspecified open fracture of ankle

825 FRACTURE OF ONE OR MORE TARSAL AND METATARSAL BONES

The tarsal bones are the heel bone (calcaneus, os calcis), talus (astragalus), navicular (scaphoid), cuboid, and the lateral, medial, and intermediate cuneiform bones.

825.0	Closed fracture of calcaneus
825.1	Open fracture of calcaneus
825.20	Closed fracture of unspecified bone(s) of foot (except toes)
825.21	Closed fracture of astragalus
825.22	Closed fracture of navicular (scaphoid) bone of foot
825.23	Closed fracture of cuboid bone
825.24	Closed fracture of cuneiform bone of foot
825.25	Closed fracture of metatarsal bone(s)
825.29	Other closed fracture of tarsal and metatarsal bones
825.30	Open fracture of unspecified bone(s) of foot (except toes)
825.31	Open fracture of astragalus
825.32	Open fracture of navicular (scaphoid) bone of foot
825.33	Open fracture of cuboid bone
825.34	Open fracture of cuneiform bone of foot,
825.35	Open fracture of metatarsal bone(s)
825.39	Other open fractures of tarsal and metatarsal bones

✔5th   Needs fifth-digit   **OK**   Valid three-digit code

826 FRACTURE OF ONE OR MORE PHALANGES OF FOOT

There are five metatarsals and phalanges (toes), with the heads at the distal portion of the bone.

826.0   Closed fracture of one or more phalanges of foot
826.1   Open fracture of one or more phalanges of foot

827 OTHER, MULTIPLE, AND ILL-DEFINED FRACTURES OF LOWER LIMB

Use these categories only if the documentation is extremely sketchy.

827.0   Other, multiple and ill-defined closed fractures of lower limb
827.1   Other, multiple and ill-defined open fractures of lower limb

828 MULTIPLE FRACTURES INVOLVING BOTH LOWER LIMBS, LOWER WITH UPPER LIMB, AND LOWER LIMB(S) WITH RIB(S) AND STERNUM

828.0   Multiple closed fractures involving both lower limbs, lower with upper limb, and lower limb(s) with rib(s) and sternum
828.1   Multiple fractures involving both lower limbs, lower with upper limb, and lower limb(s) with rib(s) and sternum, open

829 FRACTURE OF UNSPECIFIED BONES

829.0   Closed fracture of unspecified bone
829.1   Open fracture of unspecified bone

830-839 Dislocation

Luxation is the term used to describe a complete dislocation, one that has separated the articulating surfaces of the joint. An incomplete dislocation or subluxation is one in which the joint surfaces maintain some articulation. A simple dislocation has not penetrated to make a communicating wound. An uncomplicated dislocation is not associated with other important injuries. Open dislocations are subject to infection. They are always compound. Reduction of a dislocation is by manipulation, open or closed. They should be performed immediately, although this does not insure a good result. Avascular necrosis, traumatic arthritis, and ectopic ossification are considered threats to complete recovery.

Some dislocations are described as anterior and posterior or lateral and medial, which describe the location of the displaced bone in relation to its proper placement. For example, if the bone lies in front of its joint, the dislocation is considered to be anterior.

Dislocation of the acromioclavicular joint ranges in severity according to the degree of damage to the acromioclavicular and coracoclavicular ligaments.

Pubic symphysis and sacroiliac dislocations result from high-energy impact and are associated with other severe pelvic injuries. Regardless of the severity of injuries, a hip dislocation must be reduced first to contain blood loss and to minimize permanent damage to the pelvic structures.

The sternoclavicular joint may sustain anterior or posterior dislocations. While an anterior dislocation is simply remedied, a posterior dislocation poses a grave risk to the patient because of potential risk to critical internal thoracic organs.

Dislocation of the patella is typically lateral. The choice of open or closed reduction depends on the degree of disruption of the nearby ligaments and tendons. Intraarticular

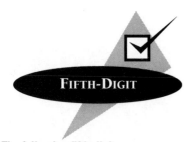

FIFTH-DIGIT

The following fifth-digit subclassification is for use with category 831:

0 shoulder, unspecified

1 anterior dislocation of humerus

2 posterior dislocation of humerus

3 inferior dislocation of humerus

4 acromioclavicular (joint)

9 other

The following fifth-digit subclassification is for use with category 832:

0 elbow, unspecified

1 anterior dislocation of elbow

2 posterior dislocation of elbow

3 medial dislocation of elbow

4 lateral dislocation of elbow

9 other

The following fifth-digit subclassification is for use with category 833:

0 wrist, unspecified part

1 radioulnar (joint), distal

2 radiocarpal (joint)

3 midcarpal (joint)

4 carpometacarpal (joint)

5 metacarpal (bone), proximal end

9 other

The following fifth-digit subclassification is for use with category 834:

0 finger, unspecified part

1 metacarpophalangeal (joint)

2 interphalangeal (joint), hand

dislocations of the patella usually require open reduction. Other dislocations of the knee are serious, requiring immediate surgery to offset the risk of vascular complications.

The ankle is seldom dislocated without an accompanying fracture and is easily reduced.

830.0	Closed dislocation of jaw
830.1	Open dislocation of jaw

831 DISLOCATION OF SHOULDER
831.0	✔5th	Closed dislocation of shoulder, unspecified
831.1	✔5th	Open dislocation of shoulder

832 DISLOCATION OF ELBOW
832.0	✔5th	Closed dislocation of elbow
832.1	✔5th	Open dislocation of elbow

833 DISLOCATION OF WRIST
833.0	✔5th	Closed dislocation of wrist
833.1	✔5th	Open dislocation of wrist

834 DISLOCATION OF FINGER
834.0	✔5th	Closed dislocation of finger
834.1	✔5th	Open dislocation of finger

835 DISLOCATION OF HIP
835.0	✔5th	Closed dislocation of hip
835.1	✔5th	Open dislocation of hip

836 DISLOCATION OF KNEE
836.0	Tear of medial cartilage or meniscus of knee, current
836.1	Tear of lateral cartilage or meniscus of knee, current
836.2	Other tear of cartilage or meniscus of knee, current
836.3	Closed dislocation of patella
836.4	Open dislocation of patella
836.50	Closed dislocation of knee, unspecified part
836.51	Closed anterior dislocation of tibia, proximal end
836.52	Closed posterior dislocation of tibia, proximal end
836.53	Closed medial dislocation of tibia, proximal end
836.54	Closed lateral dislocation of tibia, proximal end
836.59	Other closed dislocation of knee
836.60	Open dislocation of knee unspecified part
836.61	Open anterior dislocation of tibia, proximal end
836.62	Open posterior dislocation of tibia, proximal end
836.63	Open medial dislocation of tibia, proximal end
836.64	Open lateral dislocation of tibia, proximal end
836.69	Other open dislocation of knee

837 DISLOCATION OF ANKLE
837.0	Closed dislocation of ankle
837.1	Open dislocation of ankle

✔5th   Needs fifth-digit   **OK**   Valid three-digit code

838 DISLOCATION OF FOOT

838.0 ✔5th Closed dislocation of foot
838.1 ✔5th Open dislocation of foot

839 OTHER, MULTIPLE, AND ILL-DEFINED DISLOCATIONS

839.00 Closed dislocation, unspecified cervical vertebra
839.01 Closed dislocation, first cervical vertebra
839.02 Closed dislocation, second cervical vertebra
839.03 Closed dislocation, third cervical vertebra
839.04 Closed dislocation, fourth cervical vertebra
839.05 Closed dislocation, fifth cervical vertebra
839.06 Closed dislocation, sixth cervical vertebra
839.07 Closed dislocation, seventh cervical vertebra
839.08 Closed dislocation, multiple cervical vertebrae
839.10 Open dislocation, unspecified cervical vertebra
839.11 Open dislocation, first cervical vertebra
839.12 Open dislocation, second cervical vertebra
839.13 Open dislocation, third cervical vertebra
839.14 Open dislocation, fourth cervical vertebra
839.15 Open dislocation, fifth cervical vertebra
839.16 Open dislocation, sixth cervical vertebra
839.17 Open dislocation, seventh cervical vertebra
839.18 Open dislocation, multiple cervical vertebrae
839.20 Closed dislocation, lumbar vertebra
839.21 Closed dislocation, thoracic vertebra
839.30 Open dislocation, lumbar vertebra
839.31 Open dislocation, thoracic vertebra
839.40 Closed dislocation, vertebra, unspecified site
839.41 Closed dislocation, coccyx
839.42 Closed dislocation, sacrum
839.49 Closed dislocation, other vertebra
839.50 Open dislocation, vertebra, unspecified site
839.51 Open dislocation, coccyx
839.52 Open dislocation, sacrum
839.59 Open dislocation, other vertebra
839.61 Closed dislocation, sternum
839.69 Closed dislocation, other location
839.71 Open dislocation, sternum
839.79 Open dislocation, other location
839.8 Closed dislocation, multiple and ill-defined sites
839.9 Open dislocation, multiple and ill-defined sites

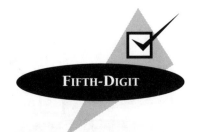

FIFTH-DIGIT

The following fifth-digit subclassification is for use with category 835:

0 dislocation of hip, unspecified

1 posterior dislocation

2 obturator dislocation

3 other anterior dislocation

The following fifth-digit subclassification is for use with category 838:

0 foot, unspecified

1 tarsal (bone), joint unspecified

2 midtarsal (joint)

3 tarsometatarsal (joint)

4 metatarsal (bone), joint unspecified

5 metatarsophalangeal (joint)

6 interphalangeal (joint), foot

9 other

840-848 Sprains and Strains of Joints and Adjacent Muscles

A sprain is not identical to a strain and should not be used as a synonym. A sprain is an injury to the ligaments, tough fibrous tissues that bind bones together at joints. A strain is an injury to the muscles or tendons that bind muscles together and does not occur at the joint.

Sprains and strains are graded. A Type I sprain connotes minor ligamentous injury; Type II, an incomplete ligamentous injury; and Type III describes a complete disruption of the ligament. The more ligaments involved in the sprain, the more serious the injury. Strains are graded from Type I - Type III. A Type III strain involves the complete tearing of muscle and separation from its tendon. Both sprains and strains manifest with swelling, pain, and

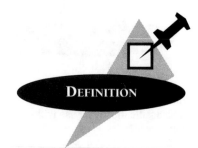

DEFINITION

Avulsion: complete separation of a soft tissue from its proper anatomical location. Hemarthrosis is the presence of blood in the joint cavity. Rupture, laceration, and tear are synonymous.

difficulty in using and are best treated according to the RICE therapy — rest of the affected part, ice, compression, and elevation.

Areas commonly sprained include the ankle, groin, knee, and neck. Ankle sprains seldom require surgery. If the patient suffers repeated injury to the weakened ankle, surgery may be performed. If two or more ligaments are involved in a knee sprain, it is serious and likely to require corrective surgery. A mild sprain may heal in two weeks to six weeks, while a severe sprain may require eight weeks to ten months to heal.

Whiplash is the sudden and forceful extension and flexion of the neck and can cause death if the movement of the neck injures the brain stem. Arms and shoulders can be affected to the point of paralysis. Whiplash accounts for 10 percent of all long-term disabilities.

840 SPRAINS AND STRAINS OF SHOULDER AND UPPER ARM

840.0	Acromioclavicular (joint) (ligament) sprain and strain
840.1	Coracoclavicular (ligament) sprain and strain
840.2	Coracohumeral (ligament) sprain and strain
840.3	Infraspinatus (muscle) (tendon) sprain and strain
840.4	Rotator cuff (capsule) sprain and strain
840.5	Subscapularis (muscle) sprain and strain
840.6	Supraspinatus (muscle) (tendon) sprain and strain
840.8	Sprain and strain of other specified sites of shoulder and upper arm
840.9	Sprain and strain of unspecified site of shoulder and upper arm

841 SPRAINS AND STRAINS OF ELBOW AND FOREARM

841.0	Radial collateral ligament sprain and strain
841.1	Ulnar collateral ligament sprain and strain
841.2	Radiohumeral (joint) sprain and strain
841.3	Ulnohumeral (joint) sprain and strain
841.8	Sprain and strain of other specified sites of elbow and forearm
841.9	Sprain and strain of unspecified site of elbow and forearm

842 SPRAINS AND STRAINS OF WRIST AND HAND

842.00	Sprain and strain of unspecified site of wrist
842.01	Sprain and strain of carpal (joint) of wrist
842.02	Sprain and strain of radiocarpal (joint) (ligament) of wrist
842.09	Other wrist sprain and strain
842.10	Sprain and strain of unspecified site of hand
842.11	Sprain and strain of carpometacarpal (joint) of hand
842.12	Sprain and strain of metacarpophalangeal (joint) of hand
842.13	Sprain and strain of interphalangeal (joint) of hand
842.19	Other hand sprain and strain

843 SPRAINS AND STRAINS OF HIP AND THIGH

843.0	Iliofemoral (ligament) sprain and strain
843.1	Ischiocapsular (ligament) sprain and strain
843.8	Sprain and strain of other specified sites of hip and thigh
843.9	Sprain and strain of unspecified site of hip and thigh

844 SPRAINS AND STRAINS OF KNEE AND LEG

844.0   Sprain and strain of lateral collateral ligament of knee

844.1   Sprain and strain of medial collateral ligament of knee

844.2   Sprain and strain of cruciate ligament of knee

844.3   Sprain and strain of tibiofibular (joint) (ligament) superior, of knee

844.8   Sprain and strain of other specified sites of knee and leg

844.9   Sprain and strain of unspecified site of knee and leg

845 SPRAINS AND STRAINS OF ANKLE AND FOOT

845.00   Unspecified site of ankle sprain and strain

845.01   Sprain and strain of deltoid (ligament) of ankle

845.02   Sprain and strain of calcaneofibular (ligament)

845.03   Sprain and strain of tibiofibular (ligament)

845.09   Other ankle sprain and strain

845.10   Sprain and strain of unspecified site of foot

845.11   Sprain and strain of tarsometatarsal (joint) (ligament)

845.12   Sprain and strain of metatarsaophalangeal (joint)

845.13   Sprain and strain of interphalangeal (joint), of toe

845.19   Other foot sprain and strain

846 SPRAINS AND STRAINS OF SACROILIAC REGION

846.0   Sprain and strain of lumbosacral (joint) (ligament)

846.1   Sprain and strain of sacroiliac (ligament)

846.2   Sprain and strain of sacrospinatus (ligament)

846.3   Sprain and strain of sacrotuberous (ligament)

846.8   Other specified sites of sacroiliac region sprain and strain

846.9   Unspecified site of sacroiliac region sprain and strain

847 SPRAINS AND STRAINS OF OTHER AND UNSPECIFIED PARTS OF BACK

847.0   Neck sprain and strain

847.1   Thoracic sprain and strain

847.2   Lumbar sprain and strain

847.3   Sprain and strain of sacrum

847.4   Sprain and strain of coccyx

847.9   Sprain and strain of unspecified site of back

848 OTHER AND ILL-DEFINED SPRAINS AND STRAINS

848.0   Sprain and strain of septal cartilage of nose

848.1   Sprain and strain of jaw

848.2   Sprain and strain of thyroid region

848.3   Sprain and strain of ribs

848.40   Sprain and strain of sternum, unspecified part

848.41   Sprain and strain of sternoclavicular (joint) (ligament)

848.42   Sprain and strain of chondrosternal (joint)

848.49   Other sprain and strains of sternum

848.5   Pelvic sprain and strains

848.8   Other specified sites of sprains and strains

848.9   Unspecified site of sprain and strain

850-854 Intracranial Injury, Excluding Those with Skull Fracture

Refer to the 800 codes.

850 CONCUSSION

850.0	Concussion with no loss of consciousness
850.1	Concussion with brief (less than one hour) loss of consciousness
850.2	Concussion with moderate (1-24 hours) loss of consciousness
850.3	Concussion with prolonged (more than 24 hours) loss of consciousness and return to pre-existing conscious level
850.4	Concussion with prolonged (more than 24 hours) loss of consciousness, without return to pre-existing conscious level
850.5	Concussion with loss of consciousness of unspecified duration
850.9	Unspecified concussion

851 CEREBRAL LACERATION AND CONTUSION

851.0	✓5th	Cortex (cerebral) contusion without mention of open intracranial wound
851.1	✓5th	Cortex (cerebral) contusion with open intracranial wound
851.2	✓5th	Cortex (cerebral) laceration without mention of open intracranial wound
851.3	✓5th	Cortex (cerebral) laceration with open intracranial wound
851.4	✓5th	Cerebellar or brain stem contusion without mention of open intracranial wound
851.5	✓5th	Cerebellar or brain stem contusion with open intracranial wound
851.6	✓5th	Cerebellar or brain stem laceration without mention of open intracranial wound
851.7	✓5th	Cerebellar or brain stem laceration with open intracranial wound
851.8	✓5th	Other and unspecified cerebral laceration and contusion, without mention of open intracranial wound
851.9	✓5th	Other and unspecified cerebral laceration and contusion, with open intracranial wound

852 SUBARACHNOID, SUBDURAL, AND EXTRADURAL HEMORRHAGE, FOLLOWING INJURY

852.0	✓5th	Subarachnoid hemorrhage following injury without mention of open intracranial wound
852.1	✓5th	Subarachnoid hemorrhage following injury, with open intracranial wound
852.2	✓5th	Subdural hemorrhage following injury without mention of open intracranial wound
852.3	✓5th	Subdural hemorrhage following injury, with open intracranial wound
852.4	✓5th	Extradural hemorrhage following injury without mention of open intracranial wound
852.5	✓5th	Extradural hemorrhage following injury with open intracranial wound

853 OTHER AND UNSPECIFIED INTRACRANIAL HEMORRHAGE FOLLOWING INJURY

853.0	✓5th	Other and unspecified intracranial hemorrhage following injury, without mention of open intracranial wound
853.1	✓5th	Other and unspecified intracranial hemorrhage following injury with open intracranial wound

---

FIFTH-DIGIT

The following fifth-digit subclassification is for use with categories 851-854:

0 unspecified state of consciousness

1 with no loss of consciousness

2 with brief [less than one hour] loss of consciousness

3 with moderate [1-24 hours] loss of consciousness

4 with prolonged [more than 24 hours] loss of consciousness and return to pre-existing conscious level

5 with prolonged [more than 24 hours] loss of consciousness, without return to pre-existing conscious level

Use fifth-digit five to designate when a patient is unconscious and dies before regaining consciousness, regardless of the duration of the loss of consciousness

6 with loss of consciousness of unspecified duration

9 with concussion, unspecified

✓5th Needs fifth-digit   **OK** Valid three-digit code

854 INTRACRANIAL INJURY OF OTHER AND UNSPECIFIED NATURE

854.0 ✓5th Intracranial injury of other and unspecified nature without mention of open intracranial wound

854.1 ✓5th Intracranial injury of other and unspecified nature with open intracranial wound

860-869 Internal Injury of Thorax, Abdomen, and Pelvis

Internal injuries can result from a blast, blunt trauma, crushing, puncture, rupture, concussion of internal organs, laceration, and hematoma.

Blast injuries result from explosive force capable of generating shock waves that damage the body. The force can emanate from a bomb, a gas leak, or any other explosion. Blast injuries are graded as primary, secondary, tertiary, and miscellaneous. A primary blast injury affects air-filled organs such as the lung, ear, and bowel. If the tympanic membrane is ruptured, the physician automatically assumes serious organ damage. Secondary injury results from injuries associated with flying objects. Tertiary injuries may result from striking objects while airborne. Morbidity and mortality are greatest if the explosion occurs within a confined space or under water.

It is important to determine the proximity of the patient to the epicenter of the blast. For example, a person 10 feet from the epicenter will sustain nine times the damage of one who is 20 feet away. The most common fatality associated with blast injury results from injury to the pulmonary system, which can result in pulmonary contusion, air embolism, free radical injury and thrombosis, lipo-oxygenation, and disseminated intravascular coagulation (DIS).

Blunt trauma has two traumatic components: compression and deceleration forces. Compression causes trauma such as rupture of the bowel, which is often a marker for more serious solid organ damage. Deceleration causes stretching and shearing injuries. A common deceleration injury is a hepatic tear along the ligamentum teres. Blunt trauma is refers to abdominal injuries. In adults, automobile accidents are to blame for 66 percent of all blunt trauma injuries.

Crush injuries involve smashing, fractures, bleeding and bruising.

A hematoma is blood free in the tissues (extravascular).

860 TRAUMATIC PNEUMOTHORAX AND HEMOTHORAX

Pneumothorax is free gas in the pleural space with lung collapse on the affected side. The medical record may state that a hemothorax is traumatic when arising from a medical procedure, but, according to ICD-9, a coder must use the 860 category for hemothorax arising from blunt or penetrating trauma unassociated with the delivery of medical care.

When hemothorax presents, the clinician suspects further damage to the lungs and heart. An evaluation must assess the integrity of the great vessels (aorta, vena cava, pulmonary artery, and pulmonary vein), as lacerations to these vessels increase mortality risks.

860.0	Traumatic pneumothorax without mention of open wound into thorax
860.1	Traumatic pneumothorax with open wound into thorax
860.2	Traumatic hemothorax without mention of open wound into thorax
860.3	Traumatic hemothorax with open wound into thorax

860.4   Traumatic pneumohemothorax without mention of open wound into thorax
860.5   Traumatic pneumohemothorax with open wound into thorax

861 INJURY TO HEART AND LUNG

861.00   Unspecified injury to heart without mention of open wound into thorax
861.01   Heart contusion without mention of open wound into thorax
861.02   Heart laceration without penetration of heart chambers or mention of open wound into thorax
861.03   Heart laceration with penetration of heart chambers, without mention of open wound into thorax
861.10   Unspecified injury to heart with open wound into thorax
861.11   Heart contusion with open wound into thorax
861.12   Heart laceration without penetration of heart chambers, with open wound into thorax
861.13   Heart laceration with penetration of heart chambers and open wound into thorax
861.20   Unspecified lung injury without mention of open wound into thorax
861.21   Lung contusion without mention of open wound into thorax
861.22   Lung laceration without mention of open wound into thorax
861.30   Unspecified lung injury with open wound into thorax
861.31   Lung contusion with open wound into thorax
861.32   Lung laceration with open wound into thorax

862 INJURY TO OTHER AND UNSPECIFIED INTRATHORACIC ORGANS

862.0   Diaphragm injury without mention of open wound into cavity
862.1   Diaphragm injury with open wound into cavity
862.21   Bronchus injury without mention of open wound into cavity
862.22   Esophagus injury without mention of open wound into cavity
862.29   Injury to other specified intrathoracic organs without mention of open wound into cavity
862.31   Bronchus injury with open wound into cavity
862.32   Esophagus injury with open wound into cavity
862.39   Injury to other specified intrathoracic organs with open wound into cavity
862.8   Injury to multiple and unspecified intrathoracic organs without mention of open wound into cavity
862.9   Injury to multiple and unspecified intrathoracic organs with open wound into cavity

863 GASTROINTESTINAL TRACT INJURY

863.0   Stomach injury without mention of open wound into cavity
863.1   Stomach injury with open wound into cavity
863.20   Small intestine injury, unspecified site, without mention of open wound into cavity
863.21   Duodenum injury without mention of open wound into cavity
863.29   Other injury to small intestine without mention of open wound into cavity
863.30   Small intestine injury, unspecified site, with open wound into cavity
863.31   Duodenum injury with open wound into cavity
863.39   Other injury to small intestine with open wound into cavity
863.40   Colon injury unspecified site, without mention of open wound into cavity
863.41   Ascending (right) colon injury without mention of open wound into cavity
863.42   Transverse colon injury without mention of open wound into cavity
863.43   Descending (left) colon injury without mention of open wound into cavity
863.44   Sigmoid colon injury without mention of open wound into cavity
863.45   Rectum injury without mention of open wound into cavity

✔5th   Needs fifth-digit   **OK**   Valid three-digit code

863.46	Injury to multiple sites in colon and rectum without mention of open wound into cavity
863.49	Other colon and rectum injury, without mention of open wound into cavity
863.50	Colon injury, unspecified site, with open wound into cavity
863.51	Ascending (right) colon injury with open wound into cavity
863.52	Transverse colon injury with open wound into cavity
863.53	Descending (left) colon injury with open wound into cavity
863.54	Sigmoid colon injury with open wound into cavity
863.55	Rectum injury with open wound into cavity
863.56	Injury to multiple sites in colon and rectum with open wound into cavity
863.59	Other injury to colon and rectum with open wound into cavity
863.80	Gastrointestinal tract injury, unspecified site, without mention of open wound into cavity
863.81	Pancreas head injury without mention of open wound into cavity
863.82	Pancreas body injury without mention of open wound into cavity
863.83	Pancreas tail injury without mention of open wound into cavity
863.84	Pancreas injury, multiple and unspecified sites, without mention of open wound into cavity
863.85	Appendix injury without mention of open wound into cavity
863.89	Injury to other and unspecified gastrointestinal sites without mention of open wound into cavity
863.90	Gastrointestinal tract injury, unspecified site, with open wound into cavity
863.91	Pancreas head injury with open wound into cavity
863.92	Pancreas body injury with open wound into cavity
863.93	Pancreas tail injury with open wound into cavity
863.94	Pancreas injury, multiple and unspecified sites, with open wound into cavity
863.95	Appendix injury with open wound into cavity
863.99	Injury to other and unspecified gastrointestinal sites with open wound into cavity

864 INJURY TO THE LIVER

The liver is protected by the fibrous membrane Glisson's capsule. If the patient is stable hemodynamically and has no other intra-abdominal injury that requires surgery, nursing and the capability of emergent surgery may allow for non-operative management of the injury.

864.0 ✔5th Liver injury without mention of open wound into cavity
864.1 ✔5th Liver injury with open wound into cavity

865 INJURY TO SPLEEN

Similar to the liver, the spleen is covered by a thick fibrous membrane, the capsule, which plays a part in grading the severity of splenic injuries.

865.0 ✔5th Spleen injury without mention of open wound into cavity
865.1 ✔5th Spleen injury with open wound into cavity

866 INJURY TO KIDNEY

The kidney's capsule protects the kidney parenchyma and is part of the injury grading system for the kidney.

866.0 ✔5th Kidney injury without mention of open wound into cavity
866.1 ✔5th Kidney injury with open wound into cavity

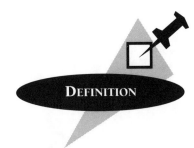

DEFINITION

Parenchymal tissue: non-structural, the essential part of an organ that does the work the organ is designed to do.

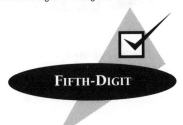

FIFTH-DIGIT

The following fifth-digit subclassification is for use with category 864:
0 unspecified injury

1 hematoma and contusion

2 laceration, minor

3 laceration, moderate

4 laceration, major

5 laceration, unspecified

9 other

The following fifth-digit subclassification is for use with category 865:
0 unspecified injury

1 hematoma with rupture of capsule

2 capsular tears, without major disruption of parenchyma

3 laceration extending into parenchyma

4 massive parenchymal disruption

9 other

The following fifth-digit subclassification is for use with category 866:
0 unspecified injury

1 hematoma without rupture of capsule

2 laceration

3 complete disruption of kidney parenchyma

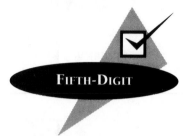

FIFTH-DIGIT

The following fifth-digit subclassification is for use with category 868:

0 unspecified intra-abdominal organ

1 adrenal gland

2 bile duct and gallbladder

3 peritoneum

4 retroperitoneum

9 other and multiple intra-abdominal organs

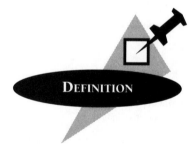

DEFINITION

Viscera: plural for viscus, organ.

867 INJURY TO PELVIC ORGANS

Pelvic organs include bladder, urethra, ureter, uterus, and other specified organ, including fallopian tube, ovary, prostate, seminal vesicle, and vas deferens.

867.0	Bladder and urethra injury without mention of open wound into cavity
867.1	Bladder and urethra injury with open wound into cavity
867.2	Ureter injury without mention of open wound into cavity
867.3	Ureter injury with open wound into cavity
867.4	Uterus injury without mention of open wound into cavity
867.5	Uterus injury with open wound into cavity
867.6	Injury to other specified pelvic organs without mention of open wound into cavity
867.7	Injury to other specified pelvic organs with open wound into cavity
867.8	Injury to unspecified pelvic organ without mention of open wound into cavity
867.9	Injury to unspecified pelvic organ with open wound into cavity

868 INJURY TO OTHER INTRA-ABDOMINAL ORGANS

The peritoneum is a serous membrane lining the abdominal cavity and reflected over the viscera. The portion covering the viscera is called the omentum (apron). The retroperitoneum lies behind the viscera and outside the cavity. The kidneys are in the retroperitoneum.

868.0	✔5th	Injury to other intra-abdominal organs without mention of open wound into cavity
868.1	✔5th	Injury to other intra-abdominal organs with open wound into cavity

869 INTERNAL INJURY TO UNSPECIFIED OR ILL-DEFINED ORGANS

Use these categories only if the documentation is extremely sketchy.

869.0	Internal injury to unspecified or ill-defined organs without mention of open wound into cavity
869.1	Internal injury to unspecified or ill-defined organs with open wound into cavity

870-879 Open Wound of Head, Neck, and Trunk

A traumatic amputation and an avulsion are essentially the same. Amputation is typically reserved to describe limb injuries and avulsion describes injuries such as the tearing or ripping of fingernails or a portion of an organ, though it can be used in reference to loss of limbs.

870 OPEN WOUND OF OCULAR ADNEXA

The ocular adnexa are the eyelid, the lacrimal apparatus, the orbit, and the periocular area.

870.0	Laceration of skin of eyelid and periocular area
870.1	Laceration of eyelid, full-thickness, not involving lacrimal passages
870.2	Laceration of eyelid involving lacrimal passages
870.3	Penetrating wound of orbit, without mention of foreign body
870.4	Penetrating wound of orbit with foreign body
870.8	Other specified open wound of ocular adnexa
870.9	Unspecified open wound of ocular adnexa

✔5th   Needs fifth-digit   **OK**   Valid three-digit code

871 OPEN WOUND OF EYEBALL

871.0	Ocular laceration without prolapse of intraocular tissue
871.1	Ocular laceration with prolapse or exposure of intraocular tissue
871.2	Rupture of eye with partial loss of intraocular tissue
871.3	Avulsion of eye
871.4	Unspecified laceration of eye
871.5	Penetration of eyeball with magnetic foreign body
871.6	Penetration of eyeball with (nonmagnetic) foreign body
871.7	Unspecified ocular penetration
871.9	Unspecified open wound of eyeball

872 OPEN WOUND OF EAR

The auricle, or pinna, is another term for the external ear. The ossicles (tiny bones) refer to the three bones facilitating hearing — the malleus, incus, and stapes.

872.00	Open wound of external ear, unspecified site, without mention of complication
872.01	Open wound of auricle, without mention of complication
872.02	Open wound of auditory canal, without mention of complication
872.10	Open wound of external ear, unspecified site, complicated
872.11	Open wound of auricle, complicated
872.12	Open wound of auditory canal, complicated
872.61	Open wound of ear drum, without mention of complication
872.62	Open wound of ossicles, without mention of complication
872.63	Open wound of Eustachian tube, without mention of complication
872.64	Open wound of cochlea, without mention of complication
872.69	Open wound of other and multiple sites, without mention of complication
872.71	Open wound of ear drum, complicated
872.72	Open wound of ossicles, complicated
872.73	Open wound of Eustachian tube, complicated
872.74	Open wound of cochlea, complicated
872.79	Open wound of other and multiple sites, complicated
872.8	Open wound of ear, part unspecified, without mention of complication
872.9	Open wound of ear, part unspecified, complicated

873 OTHER OPEN WOUND OF HEAD

873.0	Open wound of scalp, without mention of complication
873.1	Open wound of scalp, complicated
873.20	Open wound of nose, unspecified site, without mention of complication
873.21	Open wound of nasal septum, without mention of complication
873.22	Open wound of nasal cavity, without mention of complication
873.23	Open wound of nasal sinus, without mention of complication
873.29	Open wound of nose, multiple sites, without mention of complication
873.30	Open wound of nose, unspecified site, complicated
873.31	Open wound of nasal septum, complicated
873.32	Open wound of nasal cavity, complicated
873.33	Open wound of nasal sinus, complicated
873.39	Open wound of nose, multiple sites, complicated
873.40	Open wound of face, unspecified site, without mention of complication
873.41	Open wound of cheek, without mention of complication
873.42	Open wound of forehead, without mention of complication
873.43	Open wound of lip, without mention of complication
873.44	Open wound of jaw, without mention of complication

873.49   Open wound of face, other and multiple sites, without mention of complication
873.50   Open wound of face, unspecified site, complicated
873.51   Open wound of cheek, complicated
873.52   Open wound of forehead, complicated
873.53   Open wound of lip, complicated
873.54   Open wound of jaw, complicated
873.59   Open wound of face, other and multiple sites, complicated
873.60   Open wound of mouth, unspecified site, without mention of complication
873.61   Open wound of buccal mucosa, without mention of complication
873.62   Open wound of gum (alveolar process), without mention of complication
873.63   Open wound of tooth (broken), without mention of complication
873.64   Open wound of tongue and floor of mouth, without mention of complication
873.65   Open wound of palate, without mention of complication
873.69   Open wound of mouth, other and multiple sites, without mention of complication
873.70   Open wound of mouth, unspecified site, complicated
873.71   Open wound of buccal mucosa, complicated
873.72   Open wound of gum (alveolar process), complicated
873.73   Open wound of tooth (broken), complicated
873.74   Open wound of tongue and floor of mouth, complicated
873.75   Open wound of palate, complicated
873.79   Open wound of mouth, other and multiple sites, complicated
873.8   Other and unspecified open wound of head without mention of complication
873.9   Other and unspecified open wound of head, complicated

874 OPEN WOUND OF NECK

874.00   Open wound of larynx with trachea, without mention of complication
874.01   Open wound of larynx, without mention of complication
874.02   Open wound of trachea, without mention of complication
874.10   Open wound of larynx with trachea, complicated
874.11   Open wound of larynx, complicated
874.12   Open wound of trachea, complicated
874.2   Open wound of thyroid gland, without mention of complication
874.3   Open wound of thyroid gland, complicated
874.4   Open wound of pharynx, without mention of complication
874.5   Open wound of pharynx, complicated
874.8   Open wound of other and unspecified parts of neck, without mention of complication
874.9   Open wound of other and unspecified parts of neck, complicated

875 OPEN WOUND OF CHEST (WALL)

875.0   Open wound of chest (wall), without mention of complication
875.1   Open wound of chest (wall), complicated
876.0   Open wound of back, without mention of complication

876 OPEN WOUND OF BACK

876.1   Open wound of back, complicated

877 OPEN WOUND OF BUTTOCK

877.0   Open wound of buttock, without mention of complication
877.1   Open wound of buttock, complicated

⌐5th   Needs fifth-digit   **OK**   Valid three-digit code

878 OPEN WOUND OF GENITAL ORGANS (EXTERNAL), INCLUDING TRAUMATIC AMPUTATION

878.0   Open wound of penis, without mention of complication
878.1   Open wound of penis, complicated
878.2   Open wound of scrotum and testes, without mention of complication
878.3   Open wound of scrotum and testes, complicated
878.4   Open wound of vulva, without mention of complication
878.5   Open wound of vulva, complicated
878.6   Open wound of vagina, without mention of complication
878.7   Open wound of vagina, complicated
878.8   Open wound of other and unspecified parts of genital organs, without mention of complication
878.9   Open wound of other and unspecified parts of genital organs, complicated

879 OPEN WOUND OF OTHER AND UNSPECIFIED SITES, EXCEPT LIMBS

Flank (879.4) can have two meanings: (1) the part of the body found between the ribs and the uppermost crest of the ilium; or (2) the lateral side of the hip, thigh, and buttock.

879.0   Open wound of breast, without mention of complication
879.1   Open wound of breast, complicated
879.2   Open wound of abdominal wall, anterior, without mention of complication
879.3   Open wound of abdominal wall, anterior, complicated
879.4   Open wound of abdominal wall, lateral, without mention of complication
879.5   Open wound of abdominal wall, lateral, complicated
879.6   Open wound of other and unspecified parts of trunk, without mention of complication
879.7   Open wound of other and unspecified parts of trunk, complicated
879.8   Open wound(s) (multiple) of unspecified site(s), without mention of complication
879.9   Open wound(s) (multiple) of unspecified site(s), complicated

880 OPEN WOUND OF SHOULDER AND UPPER ARM

880.0 ✓5th   Open wound of shoulder and upper arm, without mention of complication
880.1 ✓5th   Open wound of shoulder and upper arm, complicated
880.2 ✓5th   Open wound of shoulder and upper arm, with tendon involvement

881 OPEN WOUND OF ELBOW, FOREARM, AND WRIST

881.0 ✓5th   Open wound of elbow, forearm, and wrist, without mention of complication
881.1 ✓5th   Open wound of elbow, forearm, and wrist, complicated
881.2 ✓5th   Open wound of elbow, forearm, and wrist, with tendon involvement

882 OPEN WOUND OF HAND EXCEPT FINGER(S) ALONE

882.0   Open wound of hand except finger(s) alone, without mention of complication
882.1   Open wound of hand except finger(s) alone, complicated
882.2   Open wound of hand except finger(s) alone, with tendon involvement

883 OPEN WOUND OF FINGER(S)

883.0   Open wound of finger(s), without mention of complication
883.1   Open wound of finger(s), complicated
883.2   Open wound of finger(s), with tendon involvement

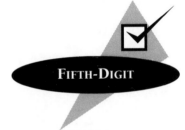

FIFTH-DIGIT

The following fifth-digit subclassification is for use with category 880:

0 shoulder region

1 scapular region

2 axillary region

3 upper arm

9 multiple sites

The following fifth-digit subclassification is for use with category 881:

0 forearm

1 elbow

2 wrist

884 MULTIPLE AND UNSPECIFIED OPEN WOUND OF UPPER LIMB

884.0   Multiple and unspecified open wound of upper limb, without mention of complication

884.1   Multiple and unspecified open wound of upper limb, complicated

884.2   Multiple and unspecified open wound of upper limb, with tendon involvement

885 TRAUMATIC AMPUTATION OF THUMB (COMPLETE) (PARTIAL)

885.0   Traumatic amputation of thumb (complete) (partial), without mention of complication

885.1   Traumatic amputation of thumb (complete) (partial), complicated

886 TRAUMATIC AMPUTATION OF OTHER FINGER(S) (COMPLETE) (PARTIAL)

886.0   Traumatic amputation of other finger(s) (complete) (partial), without mention of complication

886.1   Traumatic amputation of other finger(s) (complete) (partial), complicated

887 TRAUMATIC AMPUTATION OF ARM AND HAND (COMPLETE) (PARTIAL)

887.0   Traumatic amputation of arm and hand (complete) (partial), unilateral, below elbow, without mention of complication

887.1   Traumatic amputation of arm and hand (complete) (partial), unilateral, below elbow, complicated

887.2   Traumatic amputation of arm and hand (complete) (partial), unilateral, at or above elbow, without mention of complication

887.3   Traumatic amputation of arm and hand (complete) (partial), unilateral, at or above elbow, complicated

887.4   Traumatic amputation of arm and hand (complete) (partial), unilateral, level not specified, without mention of complication

887.5   Traumatic amputation of arm and hand (complete) (partial), unilateral, level not specified, complicated

887.6   Traumatic amputation of arm and hand (complete) (partial), bilateral (any level), without mention of complication

887.7   Traumatic amputation of arm and hand (complete) (partial), bilateral (any level), complicated

890-897 Open Wound of Lower Limb

If the patient's injury is both complicated and with tendon involvement, code both conditions to fully describe the condition and to describe the resources used to treat the injury.

Traumatic amputations: Traumatic amputation injuries are capable of amelioration due to the ability to reattach the severed part. The severed part must be kept on ice to slow the process of decay and the patient must be brought to the operating room within a six-hour to an eight-hour window. The nerves must regrow to the injured part; and grow at a rate of about an inch a month.

890 OPEN WOUND OF HIP AND THIGH

890.0   Open wound of hip and thigh, without mention of complication

890.1   Open wound of hip and thigh, complicated

890.2   Open wound of hip and thigh, with tendon involvement

↙5th   Needs fifth-digit   **OK**   Valid three-digit code

891 OPEN WOUND OF KNEE, LEG (EXCEPT THIGH), AND ANKLE

891.0   Open wound of knee, leg (except thigh), and ankle, without mention of complication

891.1   Open wound of knee, leg (except thigh), and ankle, complicated

891.2   Open wound of knee, leg (except thigh), and ankle, with tendon involvement

892 OPEN WOUND OF FOOT EXCEPT TOE(S) ALONE

892.0   Open wound of foot except toe(s) alone, without mention of complication

892.1   Open wound of foot except toe(s) alone, complicated

892.2   Open wound of foot except toe(s) alone, with tendon involvement

893 OPEN WOUND OF TOE(S)

893.0   Open wound of toe(s), without mention of complication

893.1   Open wound of toe(s), complicated

893.2   Open wound of toe(s), with tendon involvement

894 MULTIPLE AND UNSPECIFIED OPEN WOUND OF LOWER LIMB

894.0   Multiple and unspecified open wound of lower limb, without mention of complication

894.1   Multiple and unspecified open wound of lower limb, complicated

894.2   Multiple and unspecified open wound of lower limb, with tendon involvement

895 TRAUMATIC AMPUTATION OF TOE(S) (COMPLETE) (PARTIAL)

895.0   Traumatic amputation of toe(s) (complete) (partial), without mention of complication

895.1   Traumatic amputation of toe(s) (complete) (partial), complicated

896 TRAUMATIC AMPUTATION OF FOOT (COMPLETE) (PARTIAL)

896.0   Traumatic amputation of foot (complete) (partial), unilateral, without mention of complication

896.1   Traumatic amputation of foot (complete) (partial), unilateral, complicated

896.2   Traumatic amputation of foot (complete) (partial), bilateral, without mention of complication

896.3   Traumatic amputation of foot (complete) (partial), bilateral, complicated

897 TRAUMATIC AMPUTATION OF LEG(S) (COMPLETE) (PARTIAL)

897.0   Traumatic amputation of leg(s) (complete) (partial), unilateral, below knee, without mention of complication

897.1   Traumatic amputation of leg(s) (complete) (partial), unilateral, below knee, complicated

897.2   Traumatic amputation of leg(s) (complete) (partial), unilateral, at or above knee, without mention of complication

897.3   Traumatic amputation of leg(s) (complete) (partial), unilateral, at or above knee, complicated

897.4   Traumatic amputation of leg(s) (complete) (partial), unilateral, level not specified, without mention of complication

897.5   Traumatic amputation of leg(s) (complete) (partial), unilateral, level not specified, complicated

897.6   Traumatic amputation of leg(s) (complete) (partial), bilateral (any level), without mention of complication

897.7   Traumatic amputation of leg(s) (complete) (partial), bilateral (any level), complicated

900-904 Injury to Blood Vessels

Vascular trauma results from penetrating and blunt trauma. A traumatic aneurysm is a weakening in the arterial wall that bulges with the pumping of the blood, posing the threat of rupture. A traumatic fistula is an abnormal communication between an artery and a vein. (These conditions also can arise from a disease process, and are classified elsewhere in ICD 9-CM.)

Not only must the physician accurately assess the extent of trauma, but must be in control any hemorrhage as soon as possible, as mortality risk is a function of the amount of blood loss. Arterial blood loss manifests as profuse and bright red, while venous loss is steady and dark. Injury to the great vessels that enter and leave the heart is an enormous threat, as are injuries to most arteries.

900 INJURY TO BLOOD VESSELS OF HEAD AND NECK

900.00	Injury to carotid artery, unspecified
900.01	Common carotid artery injury
900.02	External carotid artery injury
900.03	Internal carotid artery injury
900.1	Internal jugular vein injury
900.81	External jugular vein injury
900.82	Injury to multiple blood vessels of head and neck
900.89	Injury to other specified blood vessels of head and neck
900.9	Injury to unspecified blood vessel of head and neck

901 INJURY TO BLOOD VESSELS OF THORAX

901.0	Thoracic aorta injury
901.1	Innominate and subclavian artery injury
901.2	Superior vena cava injury
901.3	Innominate and subclavian vein injury
901.40	Injury to unspecified pulmonary vessel(s)
901.41	Pulmonary artery injury
901.42	Pulmonary vein injury
901.81	Intercostal artery or vein injury
901.82	Internal mammary artery or vein injury
901.83	Injury to multiple blood vessels of thorax
901.89	Injury to specified blood vessels of thorax, other
901.9	Injury to unspecified blood vessel of thorax

902 INJURY TO BLOOD VESSELS OF ABDOMEN AND PELVIS

902.0	Abdominal aorta injury
902.10	Unspecified inferior vena cava injury
902.11	Hepatic vein injury
902.19	Injury to specified branches of inferior vena cava, other
902.20	Unspecified celiac and mesenteric artery injury
902.21	Gastric artery injury
902.22	Hepatic artery injury
902.23	Splenic artery injury
902.24	Injury to specified branches of celiac axis, other
902.25	Superior mesenteric artery (trunk) injury
902.26	Injury to primary branches of superior mesenteric artery
902.27	Inferior mesenteric artery injury

✔5th Needs fifth-digit   **OK** Valid three-digit code

902.29	Injury to celiac and mesenteric arteries, other
902.31	Injury to superior mesenteric vein and primary subdivisions
902.32	Inferior mesenteric vein injury
902.33	Portal vein injury
902.34	Splenic vein injury
902.39	Injury to portal and splenic veins, other
902.40	Renal vessel(s) injury, unspecified
902.41	Renal artery injury
902.42	Renal vein injury
902.49	Renal blood vessel injury, other
902.50	Unspecified iliac vessel(s) injury
902.51	Hypogastric artery injury
902.52	Hypogastric vein injury
902.53	Iliac artery injury
902.54	Iliac vein injury
902.55	Uterine artery injury
902.56	Uterine vein injury
902.59	Injury to iliac blood vessels, other
902.81	Ovarian artery injury
902.82	Ovarian vein injury
902.87	Injury to multiple blood vessels of abdomen and pelvis
902.89	Injury to specified blood vessels of abdomen and pelvis, other
902.9	Injury to blood vessel of abdomen and pelvis, unspecified

903 INJURY TO BLOOD VESSELS OF UPPER EXTREMITY

903.00	Axillary vessel(s) injury, unspecified
903.01	Axillary artery injury
903.02	Axillary vein injury
903.1	Brachial blood vessels injury
903.2	Radial blood vessels injury
903.3	Ulnar blood vessels injury
903.4	Palmar artery injury
903.5	Digital blood vessels injury
903.8	Injury to specified blood vessels of upper extremity, other
903.9	Injury to unspecified blood vessel of upper extremity

904 INJURY TO BLOOD VESSELS OF LOWER EXTREMITY AND UNSPECIFIED SITES

904.0	Common femoral artery injury
904.1	Superficial femoral artery injury
904.2	Femoral vein injury
904.3	Saphenous vein injury
904.40	Unspecified popliteal vessel(s) injury
904.41	Popliteal artery injury
904.42	Popliteal vein injury
904.50	Unspecified tibial vessel(s) injury
904.51	Anterior tibial artery injury
904.52	Anterior tibial vein injury
904.53	Posterior tibial artery injury
904.54	Posterior tibial vein injury
904.6	Deep plantar blood vessels injury
904.7	Injury to specified blood vessels of lower extremity, other
904.8	Injury to unspecified blood vessel of lower extremity
904.9	Injury to blood vessels, unspecified site

905-909 Late Effects of Injuries, Poisonings, Toxic Effects, and Other External Causes

After exiting the acute phase of a closed head injury, the victim faces daunting problems that may be lifelong, including functional cognitive deficits involving working memory, behavioral, affective disorders requiring antipsychotics and antidepressants, and impaired visuospatial ability. Skull fracture injuries pose a higher degree of neuropsychological dysfunction than head trauma without skull fracture. Studies have shown that the ability to find employment is affected by the patient's physical functioning from time of admission to discharge, cognitive functioning, behavioral functioning from admission to discharge, and injury severity as reflected by the initial Glasgow Coma Scale, the highest Glasgow Coma Scale, and duration of coma.

Late effects of musculoskeletal injuries include bursitis, traumatic arthritis, joint instability, synovitis, and tenosynovitis.

Late effects of injury to peripheral nerves are quite common, as recovery is very unpredictable. Expert and technically perfect microsurgical repair of a damaged nerve does not predict a full recovery since sensation may not be regained.

Late effects of spinal cord injury include paralysis, loss of bowel and bladder control, muscular atrophy and limb contracture.

Late effects of burns include scarring, joint immobility, nerve, and psychological damage.

Radiation can result in burns, paralysis, and tissue death.

905 LATE EFFECTS OF MUSCULOSKELETAL AND CONNECTIVE TISSUE INJURIES

905.0	Late effect of fracture of skull and face bones
905.1	Late effect of fracture of spine and trunk without mention of spinal cord lesion
905.2	Late effect of fracture of upper extremities
905.3	Late effect of fracture of neck of femur
905.4	Late effect of fracture of lower extremities
905.5	Late effect of fracture of multiple and unspecified bones
905.6	Late effect of dislocation
905.7	Late effect of sprain and strain without mention of tendon injury
905.8	Late effect of tendon injury
905.9	Late effect of traumatic amputation

906 LATE EFFECTS OF INJURIES TO SKIN AND SUBCUTANEOUS TISSUES

906.0	Late effect of open wound of head, neck, and trunk
906.1	Late effect of open wound of extremities without mention of tendon injury
906.2	Late effect of superficial injury
906.3	Late effect of contusion
906.4	Late effect of crushing
906.5	Late effect of burn of eye, face, head, and neck
906.6	Late effect of burn of wrist and hand
906.7	Late effect of burn of other extremities
906.8	Late effect of burns of other specified sites
906.9	Late effect of burn of unspecified site

✔5th Needs fifth-digit   **OK** Valid three-digit code

907 LATE EFFECTS OF INJURIES TO THE NERVOUS SYSTEM

907.0   Late effect of intracranial injury without mention of skull fracture

907.1   Late effect of injury to cranial nerve

907.2   Late effect of spinal cord injury

907.3   Late effect of injury to nerve root(s), spinal plexus(es), and other nerves of trunk

907.4   Late effect of injury to peripheral nerve of shoulder girdle and upper limb

907.5   Late effect of injury to peripheral nerve of pelvic girdle and lower limb

907.9   Late effect of injury to other and unspecified nerve

908 LATE EFFECT OF OTHER AND UNSPECIFIED INJURY

908.0   Late effect of internal injury to chest

908.1   Late effect of internal injury to intra-abdominal organs

908.2   Late effect of internal injury to other internal organs

908.3   Late effect of injury to blood vessel of head, neck, and extremities

908.4   Late effect of injury to blood vessel of thorax, abdomen, and pelvis

908.5   Late effect of foreign body in orifice

908.6   Late effect of certain complications of trauma

908.9   Late effect of unspecified injury

909 LATE EFFECTS OF OTHER AND UNSPECIFIED EXTERNAL CAUSES

909.0   Late effect of poisoning due to drug, medicinal or biological substance

909.1   Late effect of toxic effects of nonmedical substances

909.2   Late effect of radiation

909.3   Late effect of complications of surgical and medical care

909.4   Late effect of certain other external causes

909.5   Late effect of adverse effect of drug, medical or biological substance

909.9   Late effect of other and unspecified external causes

910 SUPERFICIAL INJURY OF FACE, NECK, AND SCALP, EXCEPT EYE

910.0   Face, neck, and scalp, except eye, abrasion or friction burn, without mention of infection

910.1   Face, neck, and scalp except eye, abrasion or friction burn, infected

910.2   Face, neck, and scalp except eye, blister, without mention of infection

910.3   Face, neck, and scalp except eye, blister, infected

910.4   Face, neck, and scalp except eye, insect bite, nonvenomous, without mention of infection

910.5   Face, neck, and scalp except eye, insect bite, nonvenomous, infected

910.6   Face, neck, and scalp, except eye, superficial foreign body (splinter), without major open wound or mention of infection

910.7   Face, neck, and scalp except eye, superficial foreign body (splinter), without major open wound, infected

910.8   Other and unspecified superficial injury of face, neck, and scalp, without mention of infection

910.9   Other and unspecified superficial injury of face, neck, and scalp, infected

911 SUPERFICIAL INJURY OF TRUNK

911.0   Trunk abrasion or friction burn, without mention of infection

911.1   Trunk abrasion or friction burn, infected

911.2   Trunk blister, without mention of infection

911.3   Trunk blister, infected

911.4   Trunk, insect bite, nonvenomous, without mention of infection

911.5   Trunk, insect bite, nonvenomous, infected

911.6 Trunk, superficial foreign body (splinter), without major open wound and without mention of infection

911.7 Trunk, superficial foreign body (splinter), without major open wound, infected

911.8 Other and unspecified superficial injury of trunk, without mention of infection

911.9 Other and unspecified superficial injury of trunk, infected

912 SUPERFICIAL INJURY OF SHOULDER AND UPPER ARM

912.0 Shoulder and upper arm, abrasion or friction burn, without mention of infection

912.1 Shoulder and upper arm, abrasion or friction burn, infected

912.2 Shoulder and upper arm, blister, without mention of infection

912.3 Shoulder and upper arm, blister, infected

912.4 Shoulder and upper arm, insect bite, nonvenomous, without mention of infection

912.5 Shoulder and upper arm, insect bite, nonvenomous, infected

912.6 Shoulder and upper arm, superficial foreign body (splinter), without major open wound and without mention of infection

912.7 Shoulder and upper arm, superficial foreign body (splinter), without major open wound, infected

912.8 Other and unspecified superficial injury of shoulder and upper arm, without mention of infection

912.9 Other and unspecified superficial injury of shoulder and upper arm, infected

913 SUPERFICIAL INJURY OF ELBOW, FOREARM, AND WRIST

913.0 Elbow, forearm, and wrist, abrasion or friction burn, without mention of infection

913.1 Elbow, forearm, and wrist, abrasion or friction burn, infected

913.2 Elbow, forearm, and wrist, blister, without mention of infection

913.3 Elbow, forearm, and wrist, blister infected

913.4 Elbow, forearm, and wrist, insect bite, nonvenomous, without mention of infection

913.5 Elbow, forearm, and wrist, insect bite, nonvenomous, infected

913.6 Elbow, forearm, and wrist, superficial foreign body (splinter), without major open wound and without mention of infection

913.7 Elbow, forearm, and wrist, superficial foreign body (splinter), without major open wound, infected

913.8 Other and unspecified superficial injury of elbow, forearm, and wrist, without mention of infection

913.9 Other and unspecified superficial injury of elbow, forearm, and wrist, infected

914 SUPERFICIAL INJURY OF HAND(S) EXCEPT FINGER(S) ALONE

914.0 Hand(s) except finger(s) alone, abrasion or friction burn, without mention of infection

914.1 Hand(s) except finger(s) alone, abrasion or friction burn, infected

914.2 Hand(s) except finger(s) alone, blister, without mention of infection

914.3 Hand(s) except finger(s) alone, blister, infected

914.4 Hand(s) except finger(s) alone, insect bite, nonvenomous, without mention of infection

914.5 Hand(s) except finger(s) alone, insect bite, nonvenomous, infected

914.6 Hand(s) except finger(s) alone, superficial foreign body (splinter), without major open wound and without mention of infection

✔5th Needs fifth-digit   **OK** Valid three-digit code

914.7 Hand(s) except finger(s) alone, superficial foreign body (splinter) without major open wound, infected

914.8 Other and unspecified superficial injury of hand(s) except finger(s) alone, without mention of infection

914.9 Other and unspecified superficial injury of hand(s) except finger(s) alone, infected

915 SUPERFICIAL INJURY OF FINGER(S)

915.0 Abrasion or friction burn of finger, without mention of infection

915.1 Finger, abrasion or friction burn, infected

915.2 Finger, blister, without mention of infection

915.3 Finger, blister, infected

915.4 Finger, insect bite, nonvenomous, without mention of infection

915.5 Finger, insect bite, nonvenomous, infected

915.6 Finger, superficial foreign body (splinter), without major open wound and without mention of infection

915.7 Finger, superficial foreign body (splinter), without major open wound, infected

915.8 Other and unspecified superficial injury of finger without mention of infection

915.9 Other and unspecified superficial injury of finger, infected

916 SUPERFICIAL INJURY OF HIP, THIGH, LEG, AND ANKLE

916.0 Hip, thigh, leg, and ankle, abrasion or friction burn, without mention of infection

916.1 Hip, thigh, leg, and ankle, abrasion or friction burn, infected

916.2 Hip, thigh, leg, and ankle, blister, without mention of infection

916.3 Hip, thigh, leg, and ankle, blister, infected

916.4 Hip, thigh, leg, and ankle, insect bite, nonvenomous, without mention of infection

916.5 Hip, thigh, leg, and ankle, insect bite, nonvenomous, infected

916.6 Hip, thigh, leg, and ankle, superficial foreign body (splinter), without major open wound and without mention of infection

916.7 Hip, thigh, leg, and ankle, superficial foreign body (splinter), without major open wound, infected

916.8 Other and unspecified superficial injury of hip, thigh, leg, and ankle, without mention of infection

916.9 Other and unspecified superficial injury of hip, thigh, leg, and ankle, infected

917 SUPERFICIAL INJURY OF FOOT AND TOE(S)

917.0 Abrasion or friction burn of foot and toe(s), without mention of infection

917.1 Foot and toe(s), abrasion or friction burn, infected

917.2 Foot and toe(s), blister, without mention of infection

917.3 Foot and toe(s), blister, infected

917.4 Foot and toe(s), insect bite, nonvenomous, without mention of infection

917.5 Foot and toe(s), insect bite, nonvenomous, infected

917.6 Foot and toe(s), superficial foreign body (splinter), without major open wound and without mention of infection

917.7 Foot and toe(s), superficial foreign body (splinter), without major open wound, infected

917.8 Other and unspecified superficial injury of foot and toes, without mention of infection

917.9 Other and unspecified superficial injury of foot and toes, infected

918 SUPERFICIAL INJURY OF EYE AND ADNEXA

918.0	Superficial injury of eyelids and periocular area
918.1	Superficial injury of cornea
918.2	Superficial injury of conjunctiva
918.9	Other and unspecified superficial injuries of eye

919 SUPERFICIAL INJURY OF OTHER, MULTIPLE, AND UNSPECIFIED SITES

919.0	Abrasion or friction burn of other, multiple, and unspecified sites, without mention of infection
919.1	Other, multiple, and unspecified sites, abrasion or friction burn, infected
919.2	Other, multiple, and unspecified sites, blister, without mention of infection
919.3	Other, multiple, and unspecified sites, blister, infected
919.4	Other, multiple, and unspecified sites, insect bite, nonvenomous, without mention of infection
919.5	Other, multiple, and unspecified sites, insect bite, nonvenomous, infected
919.6	Other, multiple, and unspecified sites, superficial foreign body (splinter), without major open wound and without mention of infection
919.7	Other, multiple, and unspecified sites, superficial foreign body (splinter), without major open wound, infected
919.8	Other and unspecified superficial injury of other, multiple, and unspecified sites, without mention of infection
919.9	Other and unspecified superficial injury of other, multiple, and unspecified sites, infected

920-924 Contusion with Intact Skin Surface

The skin of the face is vulnerable to severe contusions due to its proximity to unyielding bone. Any blunt trauma to the face may be noticed immediately due to swelling and discoloration.

A black eye can result in permanent vision loss, cataracts, and infection, though these complications are rare.

Gastrocnemius and the quadriceps femoris are the muscle groups most prone to contusions. If a muscle is repeatedly contused, it may become predisposed to developing myositis ossificans in the area of injury.

Hematomas, a large extravascular clot of blood, may require surgical evacuation, though most resorb naturally.

920 CONTUSION OF FACE, SCALP, AND NECK EXCEPT EYE(S) **OK**

921 Contusion of eye and adnexa

921.0	Black eye, not otherwise specified
921.1	Contusion of eyelids and periocular area
921.2	Contusion of orbital tissues
921.3	Contusion of eyeball
921.9	Unspecified contusion of eye

✓5th Needs fifth-digit   **OK** Valid three-digit code

922 CONTUSION OF TRUNK

922.0	Contusion of breast
922.1	Contusion of chest wall
922.2	Contusion of abdominal wall
922.31	Contusion of back
922.32	Contusion of buttock
922.33	Contusion of interscapular region
922.4	Contusion of genital organs
922.8	Contusion of multiple sites of trunk
922.9	Contusion of unspecified part of trunk

923 CONTUSION OF UPPER LIMB

923.00	Contusion of shoulder region
923.01	Contusion of scapular region
923.02	Contusion of axillary region
923.03	Contusion of upper arm
923.09	Contusion of multiple sites of shoulder and upper arm
923.10	Contusion of forearm
923.11	Contusion of elbow
923.20	Contusion of hand(s)
923.21	Contusion of wrist
923.3	Contusion of finger
923.8	Contusion of multiple sites of upper limb
923.9	Contusion of unspecified part of upper limb

924 CONTUSION OF LOWER LIMB AND OF OTHER AND UNSPECIFIED SITES

924.00	Contusion of thigh
924.01	Contusion of hip
924.10	Contusion of lower leg
924.11	Contusion of knee
924.20	Contusion of foot
924.21	Contusion of ankle
924.3	Contusion of toe
924.4	Contusion of multiple sites of lower limb
924.5	Contusion of unspecified part of lower limb
924.8	Contusion of multiple sites, not elsewhere classified
924.9	Contusion of unspecified site

925 CRUSHING INJURY OF FACE, SCALP, AND NECK

925.1	Crushing injury of face and scalp
925.2	Crushing injury of neck

926 CRUSHING INJURY OF TRUNK

926.0	Crushing injury of external genitalia
926.11	Crushing injury of back
926.12	Crushing injury of buttock
926.19	Crushing injury of other specified sites of trunk
926.8	Crushing injury of multiple sites of trunk
926.9	Crushing injury of unspecified site of trunk

927 CRUSHING INJURY OF UPPER LIMB

927.00	Crushing injury of shoulder region
927.01	Crushing injury of scapular region
927.02	Crushing injury of axillary region

927.03	Crushing injury of upper arm
927.09	Crushing injury of multiple sites of upper arm
927.10	Crushing injury of forearm
927.11	Crushing injury of elbow
927.20	Crushing injury of hand(s)
927.21	Crushing injury of wrist
927.3	Crushing injury of finger(s)
927.8	Crushing injury of multiple sites of upper limb
927.9	Crushing injury of unspecified site of upper limb

928 CRUSHING INJURY OF LOWER LIMB

928.00	Crushing injury of thigh
928.01	Crushing injury of hip
928.10	Crushing injury of lower leg
928.11	Crushing injury of knee
928.20	Crushing injury of foot
928.21	Crushing injury of ankle
928.3	Crushing injury of toe(s)
928.8	Crushing injury of multiple sites of lower limb
928.9	Crushing injury of unspecified site of lower limb

929 CRUSHING INJURY OF MULTIPLE AND UNSPECIFIED SITES

929.0	Crushing injury of multiple sites, not elsewhere classified
929.9	Crushing injury of unspecified site

930-939 Effects of Foreign Body Entering Through Orifice

Instances of foreign bodies in orifices are one of the most common reasons for emergency department visits. Foreign bodies in the eye are particularly common and only a physician should remove a foreign body in the eye because of the danger of damaging the eye. If the foreign body is not removed, or is improperly removed, infection and permanent vision loss can result.

Children frequently aspirate foreign bodies into the right main bronchus. Often, the act is not observed, and the child may present with pneumonia or a lung abscess if the foreign body has been present for a long time. Hypoxia may result for objects obstructing the breath. Typically, the foreign body is located by use of the flexible bronchoscope and removed in the operating room with a rigid bronchoscope.

Ingested foreign bodies generally do not cause problems unless impacted for some reason. An impacted foreign body may erode through the walls of the organ in impacted and cause mediastinitis in the chest cavity or peritonitis in the abdominal cavity.

930 FOREIGN BODY ON EXTERNAL EYE

930.0	Foreign body in cornea
930.1	Foreign body in conjunctival sac
930.2	Foreign body in lacrimal punctum
930.8	Foreign body in other and combined sites on external eye
930.9	Foreign body in unspecified site on external eye

✔5th Needs fifth-digit   **OK** Valid three-digit code

931 FOREIGN BODY IN EAR OK

932 FOREIGN BODY IN NOSE OK

933 FOREIGN BODY IN PHARYNX AND LARYNX

933.0 Foreign body in pharynx
933.1 Foreign body in larynx

934 FOREIGN BODY IN TRACHEA, BRONCHUS, AND LUNG

934.0 Foreign body in trachea
934.1 Foreign body in main bronchus
934.8 Foreign body in other specified parts of trachea, bronchus, and lung
934.9 Foreign body in respiratory tree, unspecified

935 FOREIGN BODY IN MOUTH, ESOPHAGUS, AND STOMACH

935.0 Foreign body in mouth
935.1 Foreign body in esophagus
935.2 Foreign body in stomach

936 FOREIGN BODY IN INTESTINE AND COLON OK

937 FOREIGN BODY IN ANUS AND RECTUM OK

938 FOREIGN BODY IN DIGESTIVE SYSTEM, UNSPECIFIED OK

939 FOREIGN BODY IN GENITOURINARY TRACT

939.0 Foreign body in bladder and urethra
939.1 Foreign body in uterus, any part
939.2 Foreign body in vulva and vagina
939.3 Foreign body in penis
939.9 Foreign body in unspecified site in genitourinary tract

940-949 Burns

Burns are classified by the degree of the burn (first degree through fourth degree) and the type of burn such as thermal, chemical, radiation, light, and electrical. The muscles, nerves, bones, blood vessels, respiratory system functions, temperature regulation, joint function, fluid/electrolyte balance, physical appearance and psychological functioning are all affected by a major burn injury.

An outline of the characteristics of the three degrees follows:

Degree	Color	Swelling	Pain	Skin Layer(s)	Eschar
1	Pink	Mild	Intense	Epidermis	None
2	Red	Moderate	Intense	2nd layer; minor if <15% body in adult, or <10% in child	None
3	White, brown, yellow, black	Severe	None	Full thickness, deep	Eschar

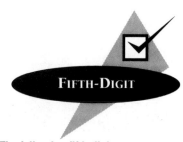

FIFTH-DIGIT

The following fifth-digit subclassification is for use with category 941:

0 face and head, unspecified site

1 ear [any part]

2 eye (with any other parts of face, head, and neck)

3 lip(s)

4 chin

5 nose (septum)

6 scalp [any part]

7 forehead and cheek

8 neck

9 multiple sites [except with eye] of face, head, and neck

The following fifth-digit subclassification is for use with category 942:

0 trunk, unspecified site

1 breast

2 chest wall, excluding breast and nipple

3 abdominal wall

4 back [any part]

5 genitalia

9 other and multiple sites of trunk

The following fifth-digit subclassification is for use with category 943:

0 upper limb, unspecified site

1 forearm

2 elbow

3 upper arm

4 axilla

5 shoulder

6 scapular region

9 multiple sites of upper limb, except wrist and hand

The impact of burn injuries is magnified according to the amount of body surface burned. Children have much smaller thresholds for what is considered severe. Radiation burns are the most dangerous burns, though they may have a more benign appearance than a third degree thermal burn.

Category 948 classifies the extent of body surface affected by the burn and is useful as an adjunctive set of codes in assessing morbidity and mortality in burn centers. It may also be used when no further information is available, as in a patient who is briefly brought to an emergency department, stabilized, and transported to a specialty unit.

940 BURN CONFINED TO EYE AND ADNEXA

940.0	Chemical burn of eyelids and periocular area
940.1	Other burns of eyelids and periocular area
940.2	Alkaline chemical burn of cornea and conjunctival sac
940.3	Acid chemical burn of cornea and conjunctival sac
940.4	Other burn of cornea and conjunctival sac
940.5	Burn with resulting rupture and destruction of eyeball
940.9	Unspecified burn of eye and adnexa

941 BURN OF FACE, HEAD, AND NECK

941.0 ✔5th Burn of face, head, and neck, unspecified degree
941.1 ✔5th Erythema due to burn (first degree) of face, head, and neck
941.2 ✔5th Blisters with epidermal loss due to burn (second degree) of face, head, and neck
941.3 ✔5th Full-thickness skin loss due to burn (third degree nos) of face, head, and neck
941.4 ✔5th Deep necrosis of underlying tissues due to burn (deep third degree) of face, head, and neck without mention of loss of a body part
941.5 ✔5th Deep necrosis of underlying tissues due to burn (deep third degree) of face, head, and neck with loss of a body part

942 BURN OF TRUNK

942.0 ✔5th Burn of trunk, unspecified degree
942.1 ✔5th Erythema due to burn (first degree) of trunk
942.2 ✔5th Blisters with epidermal loss due to burn (second degree) of trunk
942.3 ✔5th Full-thickness skin loss due to burn (third degree nos) of trunk
942.4 ✔5th Deep necrosis of underlying tissues due to burn (deep third degree) of trunk without mention of loss of a body part
942.5 ✔5th Deep necrosis of underlying tissues due to burn (deep third degree) of trunk with loss of a body part

943 BURN OF UPPER LIMB, EXCEPT WRIST AND HAND

943.0 ✔5th Burn of upper limb, except wrist and hand, unspecified degree
943.1 ✔5th Erythema due to burn (first degree) of upper limb, except wrist and hand
943.2 ✔5th Blisters with epidermal loss due to burn (second degree) of upper limb, except wrist and hand
943.3 ✔5th Full-thickness skin loss due to burn (third degree nos) of upper limb, except wrist and hand
943.4 ✔5th Deep necrosis of underlying tissues due to burn (deep third degree) of upper limb, except wrist and hand, without mention of loss of a body part
943.5 ✔5th Deep necrosis of underlying tissues due to burn (deep third degree) of upper limb, except wrist and hand, with loss of a body part

✔5th   Needs fifth-digit   **OK**   Valid three-digit code

944 BURN OF WRIST(S) AND HAND(S)

944.0 ✔5th Burn of wrist(s) and hand(s), unspecified degree

944.1 ✔5th Erythema due to burn (first degree) of wrist(s) and hand(s)

944.2 ✔5th Blisters with epidermal loss due to burn (second degree) of wrist(s) and hand(s)

944.3 ✔5th Full-thickness skin loss due to burn (third degree nos) of wrist(s) and hand(s)

944.4 ✔5th Deep necrosis of underlying tissues due to burn (deep third degree) of wrist(s) and hand(s), without mention of loss of a body part

944.5 ✔5th Deep necrosis of underlying tissues due to burn (deep third degree) of wrist(s) and hand(s), with loss of a body part

945 BURN OF LOWER LIMB(S)

945.0 ✔5th Burn of lower limb(s), unspecified degree

945.1 ✔5th Erythema due to burn (first degree) of lower limb(s)

945.2 ✔5th Blisters with epidermal loss due to burn (second degree) of lower limb(s)

945.3 ✔5th Full-thickness skin loss due to burn (third degree nos) of lower limb(s)

945.4 ✔5th Deep necrosis of underlying tissues due to burn (deep third degree) of lower limb(s) without mention of loss of a body part

945.5 ✔5th Deep necrosis of underlying tissues due to burn (deep third degree) of lower limb(s) with loss of a body part

946 BURNS OF MULTIPLE SPECIFIED SITES

946.0 Burns of multiple specified sites, unspecified degree

946.1 Erythema due to burn (first degree) of multiple specified sites

946.2 Blisters with epidermal loss due to burn (second degree) of multiple specified sites

946.3 Full-thickness skin loss due to burn (third degree nos) of multiple specified sites

946.4 Deep necrosis of underlying tissues due to burn (deep third degree) of multiple specified sites, without mention of loss of a body part

946.5 Deep necrosis of underlying tissues due to burn (deep third degree) of multiple specified sites, with loss of a body part

947 BURN OF INTERNAL ORGANS

947.0 Burn of mouth and pharynx

947.1 Burn of larynx, trachea, and lung

947.2 Burn of esophagus

947.3 Burn of gastrointestinal tract

947.4 Burn of vagina and uterus

947.8 Burn of other specified sites of internal organs

947.9 Burn of internal organs, unspecified site

948 BURNS CLASSIFIED ACCORDING TO EXTENT OF BODY SURFACE INVOLVED

948.0 ✔5th Burn (any degree) involving less than 10% of body surface

948.1 ✔5th Burn (any degree) involving 10-19% of body surface

948.2 ✔5th Burn (any degree) involving 20-29% of body surface

948.3 ✔5th Burn (any degree) involving 30-39% of body surface

948.4 ✔5th Burn (any degree) involving 40-49% of body surface

948.5 ✔5th Burn (any degree) involving 50-59% of body surface

948.6 ✔5th Burn (any degree) involving 60-69% of body surface

948.7 ✔5th Burn (any degree) involving 70-79% of body surface

948.8 ✔5th Burn (any degree) involving 80-89% of body surface

948.9 ✔5th Burn (any degree) involving 90% or more of body surface

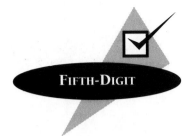

FIFTH-DIGIT

The following fifth-digit subclassification is for use with category 944:

0 hand, unspecified site

1 single digit [finger (nail)] other than the thumb

2 thumb (nail)

3 two or more digits, not including thumb

4 two or more digits including thumb

5 palm

6 back of hand

7 wrist

8 multiple sites of wrist(s) and hands

The following fifth-digit subclassification is for use with category 945:

0 lower limb (leg), unspecified site

1 toe(s) (nail)

2 foot

3 ankle

4 lower leg

5 knee

6 thigh (any part)

9 multiple sites of lower limb(s)

The following fifth-digit subclassification is for use with category 948 to indicate the percent of body surface with third degree burn; valid digits are in [brackets] under each code:

0 less than 10 percent or unspecified

1 10-19%

2 20-29%

3 30-39%

4 40-49%

5 50-59%

6 60-69%

7 70-79%

8 80-89%

9 90% or more of body surface

949 BURN, UNSPECIFIED SITE

949.0	Burn of unspecified site, unspecified degree
949.1	Erythema due to burn (first degree), unspecified site
949.2	Blisters with epidermal loss due to burn (second degree), unspecified site
949.3	Full-thickness skin loss due to burn (third degree nos), unspecified site
949.4	Deep necrosis of underlying tissue due to burn (deep third degree), unspecified site without mention of loss of body part
949.5	Deep necrosis of underlying tissues due to burn (deep third degree, unspecified site with loss of body part

950-957 Injury to Nerves and Spinal Cord

The body's nerves report to the central nervous system (CNS), which is composed of the brain and the spinal cord. Twelve pairs of cranial nerves originate in the brain, and 31 pairs of spinal nerves emanate from the spinal cord, developing major branches and associated complexes known as peripheral nerves. Every nerve has two roots: sensory and motor. The anatomical arrangement of the spinal nerve roots places the motor root anteriorly and the sensory root posteriorly.

Following is a table listing impairments due to injury to specific cranial nerves:

CRANIAL NERVES	IMPAIRMENT BY INJURY TO MOTOR ROOT
1st - Olfactory	Loss of smell
2nd - Optic	Traumatic blindness
3rd- Oculomotor	Ptosis of eyelid, double vision
4th -Trochlear	Unnatural rotation of eyeball, double vision
5th -Trigeminal	Eccentric jaw alignment, chewing
6th- Abducens	Unnatural rotation of eyeball (outwards); double vision
7th- Facial	Inability to move facial muscles of expression and animation
8th- Vestibulocochlear	Traumatic deafness; loss of balance
9th- Glossopharyngeal	Loss of taste; swallowing difficulty
10th- Vagus	Disturbance of innervation of heart, lungs, digestive organs
11th- Spinal accessory	Inability to rotate head
12th- Hypoglossopharyngeal	Loss of tongue mobility, thick speech or garbled speech

If a nerve is transected, expert and expeditious microsurgery is no guarantee that full functioning will return. Regeneration can lead to appropriate motor and sensory impulses or an aberrant response will manifest, such as crying crocodile tears involuntarily when sensing the smell of food.

950 INJURY TO OPTIC NERVE AND PATHWAYS

950.0	Optic nerve injury
950.1	Injury to optic chiasm
950.2	Injury to optic pathways
950.3	Injury to visual cortex
950.9	Injury to unspecified optic nerve and pathways

951 INJURY TO OTHER CRANIAL NERVE(S)

951.0	Injury to oculomotor nerve
951.1	Injury to trochlear nerve
951.2	Injury to trigeminal nerve
951.3	Injury to abducens nerve
951.4	Injury to facial nerve
951.5	Injury to acoustic nerve
951.6	Injury to accessory nerve
951.7	Injury to hypoglossal nerve
951.8	Injury to other specified cranial nerves
951.9	Injury to unspecified cranial nerve

952 SPINAL CORD INJURY WITHOUT EVIDENCE OF SPINAL BONE INJURY

Refer to category 806 for descriptions.

952.00	C1-C4 level spinal cord injury, unspecified
952.01	C1-C4 level with complete lesion of spinal cord
952.02	C1-C4 level with anterior cord syndrome
952.03	C1-C4 level with central cord syndrome
952.04	C1-C4 level with other specified spinal cord injury
952.05	C5-C7 level spinal cord injury, unspecified
952.06	C5-C7 level with complete lesion of spinal cord
952.07	C5-C7 level with anterior cord syndrome
952.08	C5-C7 level with central cord syndrome
952.09	C5-C7 level with other specified spinal cord injury
952.10	T1-T6 level spinal cord injury, unspecified
952.11	T1-T6 level with complete lesion of spinal cord
952.12	T1-T6 level with anterior cord syndrome
952.13	T1-T6 level with central cord syndrome
952.14	T1-T6 level with other specified spinal cord injury
952.15	T7-T12 level spinal cord injury, unspecified
952.16	T7-T12 level with complete lesion of spinal cord
952.17	T7-T12 level with anterior cord syndrome
952.18	T7-T12 level with central cord syndrome
952.19	T7-T12 level with other specified spinal cord injury
952.2	Lumbar spinal cord injury without spinal bone injury
952.3	Sacral spinal cord injury without spinal bone injury
952.4	Cauda equina spinal cord injury without spinal bone injury
952.8	Multiple sites of spinal cord injury without spinal bone injury
952.9	Unspecified site of spinal cord injury without spinal bone injury

953-957 Injury to Nerve Roots, Peripheral, and Superficial Nerves

A plexus or ganglion is a bundle of nerves that serves a particular region of the body. A plexus lies relatively deep in the body as opposed to superficial nerves, which are close to the surface of the skin.

Sympathetic nerves are under the conscious control of the body, whereas parasympathetic nerves are considered to be involuntary, allowing the body to carry on without distraction by routine functions such as breathing, heart beating, digesting, and staying oriented in space. These parasympathetic activities are considered the duties of the autonomic nervous system.

953 INJURY TO NERVE ROOTS AND SPINAL PLEXUS

953.0	Injury to cervical nerve root
953.1	Injury to dorsal nerve root
953.2	Injury to lumbar nerve root
953.3	Injury to sacral nerve root
953.4	Injury to brachial plexus
953.5	Injury to lumbosacral plexus
953.8	Injury to multiple sites of nerve roots and spinal plexus
953.9	Injury to unspecified site of nerve roots and spinal plexus

954 INJURY TO OTHER NERVE(S) OF TRUNK, EXCLUDING SHOULDER AND PELVIC GIRDLES

954.0	Injury to cervical sympathetic nerve, excluding shoulder and pelvic girdles
954.1	Injury to other sympathetic nerve, excluding shoulder and pelvic girdles
954.8	Injury to other specified nerve(s) of trunk, excluding shoulder and pelvic girdles
954.9	Injury to unspecified nerve of trunk, excluding shoulder and pelvic girdles

955 INJURY TO PERIPHERAL NERVE(S) OF SHOULDER GIRDLE AND UPPER LIMB

955.0	Injury to axillary nerve
955.1	Injury to median nerve
955.2	Injury to ulnar nerve
955.3	Injury to radial nerve
955.4	Injury to musculocutaneous nerve
955.5	Injury to cutaneous sensory nerve, upper limb
955.6	Injury to digital nerve, upper limb
955.7	Injury to other specified nerve(s) of shoulder girdle and upper limb
955.8	Injury to multiple nerves of shoulder girdle and upper limb
955.9	Injury to unspecified nerve of shoulder girdle and upper limb

956 INJURY TO PERIPHERAL NERVE(S) OF PELVIC GIRDLE AND LOWER LIMB

956.0	Injury to sciatic nerve
956.1	Injury to femoral nerve
956.2	Injury to posterior tibial nerve
956.3	Injury to peroneal nerve
956.4	Injury to cutaneous sensory nerve, lower limb
956.5	Injury to other specified nerve(s) of pelvic girdle and lower limb
956.8	Injury to multiple nerves of pelvic girdle and lower limb
956.9	Injury to unspecified nerve of pelvic girdle and lower limb

957 INJURY TO OTHER AND UNSPECIFIED NERVES

957.0	Injury to superficial nerves of head and neck
957.1	Injury to other specified nerve(s)
957.8	Injury to multiple nerves in several parts
957.9	Injury to nerves, unspecified site

✔5th   Needs fifth-digit   **OK**   Valid three-digit code

958-959 Certain Traumatic Complications and Unspecified Injuries

A potentially fatal air embolism, whether arterial or venous, may result from a penetrating and blunt chest trauma or from blast injuries. Signs are sudden cardiovascular collapse, air bubbles in arterial blood samples, air bubbles in retinal and coronary arteries, and frothy blood coming from a chest wound. Treatment must commence immediately.

A fat embolism is typically associated with fracture of one of the long bones, especially the femur. Children are vulnerable to throwing multiple fat emboli if subjected to blunt trauma such as in child abuse situations.

Secondary hemorrhage is usually arterial and most often associated with sepsis arising from traumatized tissues that have been repaired. Slipping of a ligature on repaired vessels is the second most frequent cause for secondary hemorrhage.

Posttraumatic wound infection, NEC includes injuries such as an infected, non-healing burn.

Traumatic shock sets in when the heart fails to deliver oxygenated blood and other nutrients to the body, usually because of a high rate of blood loss. The shock triggers other organ failure, with the kidney among the first affected. Blood volume must be restored as soon as possible to prevent the appearance of shock and its sequelae. Traumatic anuria runs a mortality rate of 60 percent.

Volkmann's ischemic contracture can appear in either the hand or the foot. In the hand, constriction of the radial artery produces the characteristic pronation and flexion. In the foot, a tibial fracture leading to an embolus or thrombus is more likely to be the causative agent.

Traumatic subcutaneous emphysema is tissue rupture that allows gas bubbles to form beneath the skin, a result of a high-pressure injury.

Compartment syndrome is an early complication of trauma, resulting from compression of nerves and tendons. Pain is extreme and is not easily relieved. Any compressive agent such as a cast or splint is immediately removed, though if removal is ineffective, the patient is surgically decompressed.

958 CERTAIN EARLY COMPLICATIONS OF TRAUMA

958.0	Air embolism as an early complication of trauma
958.1	Fat embolism as an early complication of trauma
958.2	Secondary and recurrent hemorrhage as an early complication of trauma
958.3	Posttraumatic wound infection not elsewhere classified
958.4	Traumatic shock
958.5	Traumatic anuria
958.6	Volkmann's ischemic contracture
958.7	Traumatic subcutaneous emphysema
958.8	Other early complications of trauma

959 INJURY, OTHER AND UNSPECIFIED

959.01   Head injury, unspecified
959.09   Injury of face and neck, other and unspecified
959.1   Injury, other and unspecified, trunk
959.2   Injury, other and unspecified, shoulder and upper arm
959.3   Injury, other and unspecified, elbow, forearm, and wrist
959.4   Injury, other and unspecified, hand, except finger
959.5   Injury, other and unspecified, finger
959.6   Injury, other and unspecified, hip and thigh
959.7   Injury, other and unspecified, knee, leg, ankle, and foot
959.8   Injury, other and unspecified, other specified sites, including multiple
959.9   Injury, other and unspecified, unspecified site

960-979 Poisoning by Drugs, Medicinal and Biological Substances

960 POISONING BY ANTIBIOTICS

960.0   Poisoning by penicillins
960.1   Poisoning by antifungal antibiotics
960.2   Poisoning by chloramphenicol group
960.3   Poisoning by erythromycin and other macrolides
960.4   Poisoning by tetracycline group
960.5   Poisoning of cephalosporin group
960.6   Poisoning of antimycobacterial antibiotics
960.7   Poisoning by antineoplastic antibiotics
960.8   Poisoning by other specified antibiotics
960.9   Poisoning by unspecified antibiotic

961 POISONING BY OTHER ANTI-INFECTIVES

961.0   Poisoning by sulfonamides
961.1   Poisoning by arsenical anti-infectives
961.2   Poisoning by heavy metal anti-infectives
961.3   Poisoning by quinoline and hydroxyquinoline derivatives
961.4   Poisoning by antimalarials and drugs acting on other blood protozoa
961.5   Poisoning by other antiprotozoal drugs
961.6   Poisoning by anthelmintics
961.7   Poisoning by antiviral drugs
961.8   Poisoning by other antimycobacterial drugs
961.9   Poisoning by other and unspecified anti-infectives

962 POISONING BY HORMONES AND SYNTHETIC SUBSTITUTES

962.0   Poisoning by adrenal cortical steroids
962.1   Poisoning by androgens and anabolic congeners
962.2   Poisoning by ovarian hormones and synthetic substitutes
962.3   Poisoning by insulins and antidiabetic agents
962.4   Poisoning by anterior pituitary hormones
962.5   Poisoning by posterior pituitary hormones
962.6   Poisoning by parathyroid and parathyroid derivatives
962.7   Poisoning by thyroid and thyroid derivatives
962.8   Poisoning by antithyroid agents
962.9   Poisoning by other and unspecified hormones and synthetic substitutes

963 POISONING BY PRIMARILY SYSTEMIC AGENTS

963.0   Poisoning by antiallergic and antiemetic drugs
963.1   Poisoning by antineoplastic and immunosuppressive drugs

✔5th   Needs fifth-digit   **OK**   Valid three-digit code

963.2   Poisoning by acidifying agents
963.3   Poisoning by alkalizing agents
963.4   Poisoning by enzymes, not elsewhere classified
963.5   Poisoning by vitamins, not elsewhere classified
963.8   Poisoning by other specified systemic agents
963.9   Poisoning by unspecified systemic agent

964 POISONING BY AGENTS PRIMARILY AFFECTING BLOOD CONSTITUENTS

964.0   Poisoning by iron and its compounds
964.1   Poisoning by liver preparations and other antianemic agents
964.2   Poisoning by anticoagulants
964.3   Poisoning by vitamin K (phytonadione)
964.4   Poisoning by fibrinolysis-affecting drugs
964.5   Poisoning by anticoagulant antagonists and other coagulants
964.6   Poisoning by gamma globulin
964.7   Poisoning by natural blood and blood products
964.8   Poisoning by other specified agents affecting blood constituents
964.9   Poisoning by unspecified agent affecting blood constituents

965 POISONING BY ANALGESICS, ANTIPYRETICS, AND ANTIRHEUMATICS

965.00   Poisoning by opium (alkaloids), unspecified
965.01   Poisoning by heroin
965.02   Poisoning by methadone
965.09   Poisoning by opiates and related narcotics, other
965.1   Poisoning by salicylates
965.4   Poisoning by aromatic analgesics, not elsewhere classified
965.5   Poisoning by pyrazole derivatives
965.61   Poisoning by propionic acid derivatives
965.69   Poisoning by other antirheumatics
965.7   Poisoning by other non-narcotic analgesics
965.8   Poisoning by other specified analgesics and antipyretics
965.9   Poisoning by unspecified analgesic and antipyretic

966 POISONING BY ANTICONVULSANTS AND ANTI-PARKINSONISM DRUGS

966.0   Poisoning by oxazolidine derivatives
966.1   Poisoning by hydantoin derivatives
966.2   Poisoning by succinimides
966.3   Poisoning by other and unspecified anticonvulsants
966.4   Poisoning by anti-Parkinsonism drugs

967 POISONING BY SEDATIVES AND HYPNOTICS

967.0   Poisoning by barbiturates
967.1   Poisoning by chloral hydrate group
967.2   Poisoning by paraldehyde
967.3   Poisoning by bromine compounds
967.4   Poisoning by methaqualone compounds
967.5   Poisoning by glutethimide group
967.6   Poisoning by mixed sedatives, not elsewhere classified
967.8   Poisoning by other sedatives and hypnotics
967.9   Poisoning by unspecified sedative or hypnotic

968 POISONING BY OTHER CENTRAL NERVOUS SYSTEM DEPRESSANTS AND ANESTHETICS

968.0   Poisoning by central nervous system muscle-tone depressants

968.1	Poisoning by halothane
968.2	Poisoning by other gaseous anesthetics
968.3	Poisoning by intravenous anesthetics
968.4	Poisoning by other and unspecified general anesthetics
968.5	Poisoning by surface (topical) and infiltration anesthetics
968.6	Poisoning by peripheral nerve- and plexus-blocking anesthetics
968.7	Poisoning by spinal anesthetics
968.9	Poisoning by other and unspecified local anesthetics

969 POISONING BY PSYCHOTROPIC AGENTS

969.0	Poisoning by antidepressants
969.1	Poisoning by phenothiazine-based tranquilizers
969.2	Poisoning by butyrophenone-based tranquilizers
969.3	Poisoning by other antipsychotics, neuroleptics, and major tranquilizers
969.4	Poisoning by benzodiazepine-based tranquilizers
969.5	Poisoning by other tranquilizers
969.6	Poisoning by psychodysleptics (hallucinogens)
969.7	Poisoning by psychostimulants
969.8	Poisoning by other specified psychotropic agents
969.9	Poisoning by unspecified psychotropic agent

970 POISONING BY CENTRAL NERVOUS SYSTEM STIMULANTS

970.0	Poisoning by analeptics
970.1	Poisoning by opiate antagonists
970.8	Poisoning by other specified central nervous system stimulants
970.9	Poisoning by unspecified central nervous system stimulant

971 POISONING BY DRUGS PRIMARILY AFFECTING THE AUTONOMIC NERVOUS SYSTEM

971.0	Poisoning by parasympathomimetics (cholinergics)
971.1	Poisoning by parasympatholytics (anticholinergics and antimuscarinics) and spasmolytics
971.2	Poisoning by sympathomimetics (adrenergics)
971.3	Poisoning by sympatholytics (antiadrenergics)
971.9	Poisoning by unspecified drug primarily affecting autonomic nervous system

972 POISONING BY AGENTS PRIMARILY AFFECTING THE CARDIOVASCULAR SYSTEM

972.0	Poisoning by cardiac rhythm regulators
972.1	Poisoning by cardiotonic glycosides and drugs of similar action
972.2	Poisoning by antilipemic and antiarteriosclerotic drugs
972.3	Poisoning by ganglion-blocking agents
972.4	Poisoning by coronary vasodilators
972.5	Poisoning by other vasodilators
972.6	Poisoning by other antihypertensive agents
972.7	Poisoning by antivaricose drugs, including sclerosing agents
972.8	Poisoning by capillary-active drugs
972.9	Poisoning by other and unspecified agents primarily affecting the cardiovascular system

973 POISONING BY AGENTS PRIMARILY AFFECTING THE GASTROINTESTINAL SYSTEM

973.0	Poisoning by antacids and antigastric secretion drugs
973.1	Poisoning by irritant cathartics

✔5th Needs fifth-digit   **OK** Valid three-digit code

973.2   Poisoning by emollient cathartics

973.3   Poisoning by other cathartics, including intestinal atonia drugs

973.4   Poisoning by digestants

973.5   Poisoning by antidiarrheal drugs

973.6   Poisoning by emetics

973.8   Poisoning by other specified agents primarily affecting the gastrointestinal system

973.9   Poisoning by unspecified agent primarily affecting the gastrointestinal system

974 POISONING BY WATER, MINERAL, AND URIC ACID METABOLISM DRUGS

974.0   Poisoning by mercurial diuretics

974.1   Poisoning by purine derivative diuretics

974.2   Poisoning by carbonic acid anhydrase inhibitors

974.3   Poisoning by saluretics

974.4   Poisoning by other diuretics

974.5   Poisoning by electrolytic, caloric, and water-balance agents

974.6   Poisoning by other mineral salts, not elsewhere classified

974.7   Poisoning by uric acid metabolism drugs

975 POISONING BY AGENTS PRIMARILY ACTING ON THE SMOOTH AND SKELETAL MUSCLES AND RESPIRATORY SYSTEM

975.0   Poisoning by oxytocic agents

975.1   Poisoning by smooth muscle relaxants

975.2   Poisoning by skeletal muscle relaxants

975.3   Poisoning by other and unspecified drugs acting on muscles

975.4   Poisoning by antitussives

975.5   Poisoning by expectorants

975.6   Poisoning by anti-common cold drugs

975.7   Poisoning by antiasthmatics

975.8   Poisoning by other and unspecified respiratory drugs

976 POISONING BY AGENTS PRIMARILY AFFECTING SKIN AND MUCOUS MEMBRANE, OPHTHALMOLOGICAL, OTORHINOLARYNGOLOGICAL, AND DENTAL DRUGS

976.0   Poisoning by local anti-infectives and anti-inflammatory drugs

976.1   Poisoning by antipruritics

976.2   Poisoning by local astringents and local detergents

976.3   Poisoning by emollients, demulcents, and protectants

976.4   Poisoning by keratolytics, keratoplastics, other hair treatment drugs and preparations

976.5   Poisoning by eye anti-infectives and other eye drugs

976.6   Poisoning by anti-infectives and other drugs and preparations for ear, nose, and throat

976.7   Poisoning by dental drugs topically applied

976.8   Poisoning by other agents primarily affecting skin and mucous membrane

976.9   Poisoning by unspecified agent primarily affecting skin and mucous membrane

977 POISONING BY OTHER AND UNSPECIFIED DRUGS AND MEDICINAL SUBSTANCES

977.0   Poisoning by dietetics

977.1   Poisoning by lipotropic drugs

977.2   Poisoning by antidotes and chelating agents, not elsewhere classified

977.3	Poisoning by alcohol deterrents
977.4	Poisoning by pharmaceutical excipients
977.8	Poisoning by other specified drugs and medicinal substances
977.9	Poisoning by unspecified drug or medicinal substance

978 POISONING BY BACTERIAL VACCINES

978.0	Poisoning by bcg vaccine
978.1	Poisoning by typhoid and paratyphoid vaccine
978.2	Poisoning by cholera vaccine
978.3	Poisoning by plague vaccine
978.4	Poisoning by tetanus vaccine
978.5	Poisoning by diphtheria vaccine
978.6	Poisoning by pertussis vaccine, including combinations with pertussis component
978.8	Poisoning by other and unspecified bacterial vaccines
978.9	Poisoning by mixed bacterial vaccines, except combinations with pertussis component

979 POISONING BY OTHER VACCINES AND BIOLOGICAL SUBSTANCES

979.0	Poisoning by smallpox vaccine
979.1	Poisoning by rabies vaccine
979.2	Poisoning by typhus vaccine
979.3	Poisoning by yellow fever vaccine
979.4	Poisoning by measles vaccine
979.5	Poisoning by poliomyelitis vaccine
979.6	Poisoning by other and unspecified viral and rickettsial vaccines
979.7	Poisoning by mixed viral-rickettsial and bacterial vaccines, except combinations with pertussis component
979.9	Poisoning by other and unspecified vaccines and biological substances

980-989 Toxic Effects of Substances Chiefly Nonmedicinal as to Source

As a general rule, the more known about the poisoning agent, the better the treatment plan and outcome. Poison Control Centers have been invaluable in supplying the health care professional with the exact composition of the thousands of poisonous substances. If the information is unknown, treatment must revolve around general supportive measures.

Treatment includes the use of corticosteroids and mannitol drips to minimize cerebral edema, dialysis to combat renal failure or to hasten the excretion of the poison, alkalinization or acidification of the urine, dialysis to remove lipid soluble substances from the blood, hemoperfusion, and chelating agents.

Poisoning defines when a wrong substance is ingested or the correct substance is taken in an incorrect dosage. There is a wide range of potentially toxic agents, as well as effects from ingesting poisonous substances or the incorrect amount of prescribed substances.

Category 988 excludes spoiled food that causes illness (food poisoning). The mistletoe berry is an example of poisonous flora belonging in this category.

980 TOXIC EFFECT OF ALCOHOL

980.0	Toxic effect of ethyl alcohol
980.1	Toxic effect of methyl alcohol
980.2	Toxic effect of isopropyl alcohol

✔5th   Needs fifth-digit   **OK**   Valid three-digit code

980.3   Toxic effect of fusel oil
980.8   Toxic effect of other specified alcohols
980.9   Toxic effect of unspecified alcohol

981 TOXIC EFFECT OF PETROLEUM PRODUCTS ＯＫ

982 TOXIC EFFECT OF SOLVENTS OTHER THAN PETROLEUM-BASED
982.0   Toxic effect of benzene and homologues
982.1   Toxic effect of carbon tetrachloride
982.2   Toxic effect of carbon disulfide
982.3   Toxic effect of other chlorinated hydrocarbon solvents
982.4   Toxic effect of nitroglycol
982.8   Toxic effect of other nonpetroleum-based solvents

983 TOXIC EFFECT OF CORROSIVE AROMATICS, ACIDS, AND CAUSTIC ALKALIS
983.0   Toxic effect of corrosive aromatics
983.1   Toxic effect of acids
983.2   Toxic effect of caustic alkalis
983.9   Toxic effect of caustic, unspecified

984 TOXIC EFFECT OF LEAD AND ITS COMPOUNDS (INCLUDING FUMES)
984.0   Toxic effect of inorganic lead compounds
984.1   Toxic effect of organic lead compounds
984.8   Toxic effect of other lead compounds
984.9   Toxic effect of unspecified lead compound

985 TOXIC EFFECT OF OTHER METALS
985.0   Toxic effect of mercury and its compounds
985.1   Toxic effect of arsenic and its compounds
985.2   Toxic effect of manganese and its compounds
985.3   Toxic effect of beryllium and its compounds
985.4   Toxic effect of antimony and its compounds
985.5   Toxic effect of cadmium and its compounds
985.6   Toxic effect of chromium
985.8   Toxic effect of other specified metals
985.9   Toxic effect of unspecified metal

986 TOXIC EFFECT OF CARBON MONOXIDE ＯＫ

987 TOXIC EFFECT OF OTHER GASES, FUMES, OR VAPORS
987.0   Toxic effect of liquefied petroleum gases
987.1   Toxic effect of other hydrocarbon gas
987.2   Toxic effect of nitrogen oxides
987.3   Toxic effect of sulfur dioxide
987.4   Toxic effect of freon
987.5   Toxic effect of lacrimogenic gas
987.6   Toxic effect of chlorine gas
987.7   Toxic effect of hydrocyanic acid gas
987.8   Toxic effect of other specified gases, fumes, or vapors
987.9   Toxic effect of unspecified gas, fume, or vapor

988 TOXIC EFFECT OF NOXIOUS SUBSTANCES EATEN AS FOOD
988.0   Toxic effect of fish and shellfish
988.1   Toxic effect of mushrooms

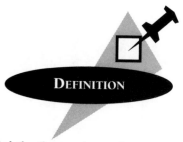

DEFINITION

Chelation therapy: the use of a compound that grasps the poisonous agent, rendering it inactive and no longer toxic.

Corticosteroid: an adrenal hormone that promotes an optimal speed for biochemical processes.

Hemo perfusion: blood perfusion through activated charcoal or an ion-exchange resin to remove a poison.

Mannitol: a natural substance that mitigates the chance of renal failure.

988.2	Toxic effect of berries and other plants
988.8	Toxic effect of other specified noxious substances
988.9	Toxic effect of unspecified noxious substance

989 TOXIC EFFECT OF OTHER SUBSTANCES, CHIEFLY NONMEDICINAL AS TO SOURCE

989.0	Toxic effect of hydrocyanic acid and cyanides
989.1	Toxic effect of strychnine and salts
989.2	Toxic effect of chlorinated hydrocarbons
989.3	Toxic effect of organophosphate and carbamate
989.4	Toxic effect of other pesticides, not elsewhere classified
989.5	Toxic effect of venom

Each of the 48 contiguous states in the United States harbour at least one species of venomous snake. The pit vipers (copperhead, cottonmouth, and rattlesnakes) and coral snakes are two venomous families widely spread in the United States. Approximately 8,0000 of the estimated 45,000 annual snakebites in this country are by poisonous snakes. Snake venoms are rated on a lethality index, with the Mojave rattlesnake having the highest index of any North American snake. Pit viper bites are associated with pain, swelling, and edema. Ecchymosis is common, ranging from moderate to severe. The patient may hemorrhage from the gums and develop hematemesis, melena, and hematuria. The coral snake bite generally produces nerve conduction damage and CNS damage. Annual fatalities are fewer than 15, most of which can be attributed to rattlesnake venom.

Survival often depends on the time it takes until medical help. If the patient is more than forty minutes from a hospital, an incision over the bite may be made and suction applied. Envenomation must be assessed whenever a patient presents at the medical center with a snake bite since about 20 percent to 30 percent of all pit viper bites do not involve venom injection, and about 50 percent from the same class as coral snakes does not involve venom injection. Protocol calls for treating snakebites without envenomation as puncture wounds. If envenomation does occur, the patient presents a complex poisoning picture. Depending on the type of snake, the patient may weaken several hours after the bite, experience difficulty salivating or speaking, or experience respiratory distress and cardiovascular failure in fatal cases).

Antivenom is needed in only 60 percent of pit viper bites. The young or elderly require antivenom for copperhead bites. Coral snake envenomation is not typically associated with pain or swelling and three vials of antivenom are routinely administered once envenomation by coral snake bite is determined.

Two lizards, the Gila monster and the beaded lizard, are poisonous. Treatment protocols are similar to those for pit viper bites, though there is no antivenom for these bites.

There are numerous venomous spider species in the United States. Most bites require only local care, although in cases of severe envenomation the

ↄ5th Needs fifth-digit   **OK** Valid three-digit code

victim must be hospitalized for supportive measures. Fatalities are few, with the greatest risk for children and the elderly.

989.6	Toxic effect of soaps and detergents
989.7	Toxic effect of aflatoxin and other mycotoxin (food contaminants)
989.81	Toxic effect of asbestos
989.82	Toxic effect of latex
989.83	Toxic effect of silicone
989.84	Toxic effect of tobacco
989.89	Toxic effect of other substances
989.9	Toxic effect of unspecified substance, chiefly nonmedicinal as to source

990-995 Other and Unspecified Effects of External Causes

990 EFFECTS OF RADIATION, UNSPECIFIED O K

A substance emitting ionizing radiation is capable of creating radiation sickness. Acute radiation sickness is classified as cerebral, gastrointestinal, or hematopoietic. The cerebral syndrome is fatal within a few hours of exposure to a dose in an amount greater than 30 Gy. The gastrointestinal syndrome involves a dose of at least 4 Gy, with death occurring within two or three weeks. The hematopoietic syndrome is also fatal, with neutropenia the contributing cause of death due to lowered immune resistance. The dose is 2 Gy to 10 Gy.

Recovery from a radiation accident depends on the size of the dose, the rate at which the dose is received, and the distribution of the dose over the body. While a large dose all at once over the entire body is fatal, the same dose administered therapeutically to a small area over a brief period of time may be repeated over time without fear of fatality. Therapeutic doses may cause radiation sickness, involving nausea, vomiting and diarrhea with malaise and tachycardia. These symptoms decline spontaneously, over time.

991 EFFECTS OF REDUCED TEMPERATURE

Accidental hypothermia results from conduction, convection, and radiation. Examples of conduction hypothermia are wet clothing and skin freezing upon metal contact. Convection injuries are from wind chill. The body core temperature can drop as low as 79°Fahrenheit. The rule is to resuscitate until the patient is warm. The extremities are at great risk of hypothermia, as well as the nose. They should be warm and dry at all times. While dry cold injury such as frostbite can result in gangrene, the gangrene is usually superficial, with a large reservoir of intact skin underneath the affected part. Wet cold injury is more pernicious, leading to wet gangrene. As the patient recovers from frostbite, the skin may slough from the affected part. This skin is treated with burn protocols.

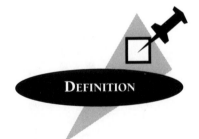

DEFINITION

GRAY (Gy): amount of energy absorbed from exposure to ionizing radiation.

991.0	Frostbite of face
991.1	Frostbite of hand
991.2	Frostbite of foot
991.3	Frostbite of other and unspecified sites
991.4	Effects of immersion of foot
991.5	Effects of chilblains
991.6	Effects of hypothermia
991.8	Other specified effects of reduced temperature
991.9	Unspecified effect of reduced temperature

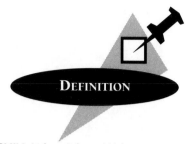

DEFINITION

Chilblain (pernio): a cold injury caused by exposure to cold damp conditions. There may be itching, blisters and ulcerations with encrusting.

Frostbite: a cold injury caused by exposure to dry and cold conditions, well below freezing.

Frostnip: a cold injury caused by exposure to damp and temperatures in freezing range.

Hypothermia: a disturbance of the body's ability to maintain life-sustaining temperatures and is associated with loss of the shivering reflex.

Trench foot: same as frostnip, with the foot as the site of the cold injury.

992 EFFECTS OF HEAT AND LIGHT

Heat related illnesses are arranged in order from the most deadly to mildest. Heat stroke has many names and is a major medical emergency, causing death in 10 percent of its victims.

Heat stroke is partitioned into two categories, equally dangerous — exertional and classic. Classic heat stroke victims typically are older, debilitated from chronic health problems, sedentary, and do not present with major systemic disorders. Exertional heat stroke, which may cause multiple systemic derangement, more often strikes younger, healthier individuals engaged in strenuous activity.

Both types of heat stroke must be treated immediately by immersing the patient in cold water. Water temperature must be monitored to prevent hypothermia. Stroke victims should be transported to the hospital, though prior to summoning help, the patient must be relieved from excessive temperature in the body core – greater than 104.9°Fahrenheit.

Heat exhaustion is excessive body core temperature in the range of 100.4°Fahrenheit to 104.9°Fahrenheit. The patient must be cooled and orally rehydrated, although there may be gastrointestinal distress necessitating intravenous administration of fluids. The patient generally recovers in two hours to three hours with appropriate support, though some cases are unresponsive and require hospitalization.

Heat syncope occurs from dehydration, lack of acclimatization to heat when undertaking exercise, and failure to undergo a cool-down period after exercise. Once the patient is prostrate, recovery is immediate.

Heat edema is the swelling of the extremities, typically the legs, in hot weather. Exercise and elevation of the affected parts lessens the swelling.

992.0	Heat stroke and sunstroke
992.1	Heat syncope
992.2	Heat cramps
992.3	Heat exhaustion, anhydrotic
992.4	Heat exhaustion due to salt depletion
992.5	Heat exhaustion, unspecified
992.6	Heat fatigue, transient
992.7	Heat edema
992.8	Other specified heat effects
992.9	Unspecified effects of heat and light

993 EFFECTS OF AIR PRESSURE

993.0   Barotrauma, otitic

Otitic barotrauma can affect aviators, divers, or tunnel workers. Symptoms include pain, hearing loss, rupture of the tympanic membrane, vertigo, and disorientation, which is perhaps the most dangerous manifestation since it can interfere with the ability to move to safety.

993.1   Barotrauma, sinus

Congestion in the sinuses is likely to cause pain and possibly nosebleeds if diving or swift ascent occurs

993.2   Other and unspecified effects of high altitude

     ✔5th   Needs fifth-digit   **OK**   Valid three-digit code

The higher the altitude, the thinner the atmosphere and the greater reduction in oxygen content. The effect is magnified by the proximity of the peak to the earth's poles. At 18,000 feet above sea level, the oxygen content of the atmosphere is reduced by 50 percent and the body must produce a greater number of red blood cells to carry oxygen. Given time to spend at various levels of ascent, most individuals can successfully adapt to the thinner atmosphere.

There are three levels of acute mountain sickness: mild, moderate, and severe. If the moderate degree should manifest, the victim must descend 1,000 feet, rest, and adapt. Climbers must take precautions against the severe form of this life-threatening condition, which requires immediate descent of 2,000-feet to 4000-feet. The moderate to severe forms can alter mental status, changes the degree of consciousness, and causes ataxia and shortness of breath with cyanosis, all of which can be fatal if the patient is not removed from the environment.

993.3   Caisson disease

Other common names for this disorder are the bends, and decompression sickness. Strictly speaking, "the bends" refers to the pain associated with decompression sickness, though it has become synonymous for the sickness.

Nitrogen gas dissolved in the tissue forms potentially lethal bubbles in the blood. Women, who have a higher proportion of fat, are at higher risk of decompression sickness than men.

993.4   Effects of air pressure caused by explosion
993.8   Other specified effects of air pressure
993.9   Unspecified effect of air pressure

994 EFFECTS OF OTHER EXTERNAL CAUSES
994.0   Effects of lightning

There are an estimated 750 lightning strikes of humans per year, with an associated mortality rate of 3 percent to 10 percent. Lightning strikes the highest points, so standing in a meadow, standing under a big tree, or carrying an umbrella, increase the chances of a strike. Electrical energy travels along the earth's surface and can enter the human by the leg closest to the strike and exits through the other leg.

The nerves, muscles, and blood vessels are excellent electrical conductors. Once an individual is struck, the results are typically cardiac arrest, respiratory arrest, vascular spasm, neurological damage, and autonomic instability, rather than burns and renal failure.

994.1   Drowning and nonfatal submersion

The great mortality risk in near drowning is posed by respiratory insufficiency leading to hypoxia and respiratory acidosis. These conditions are always addressed first, and aspiration is managed secondarily. Aspiration of seawater is rarely life threatening, although such aspiration

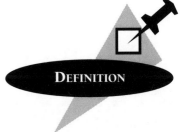

DEFINITION

Caisson disease: found in jobs that require working in a caisson, a watertight chamber used in underwater construction.

can cause mild elevations of sodium and chloride. Aspiration of large quantities of fresh water can cause massive increase of blood volume, life threatening electrolyte imbalance, and hemolysis leading to asphyxia and ventricular fibrillation.

The water temperature and duration of immersion are other factors when predicting survival from immersion. If an individual is exposed to cool water, over time hypothermia will set in, with its attendant problems. However, if the victim is suddenly tipped into cold water, the mammalian diving reflex reduces the body's oxygen need, thus increasing the chance of survival. The rule is to continue resuscitation efforts even if submerged for more than one hour.

994.2	Effects of hunger
994.3	Effects of thirst
994.4	Exhaustion due to exposure
994.5	Exhaustion due to excessive exertion
994.6	Motion sickness
994.7	Asphyxiation and strangulation
994.8	Electrocution and nonfatal effects of electric current

The extent of the injury by electric shock is a function of the amount of voltage delivered, current type, resistance to the current, and the length of contact to the current. If the skin is thick and dry, it will present greater resistance to the current, resulting in extensive burns, though only slight damage to internal organs. Of the two types of current, direct current is the least deadly since it throws the victim, cutting short the exposure to the current. Alternating current is three times more dangerous than direct current since the chances of tetanic contractions multiply threefold. Tetany is likely to occur when the "let-go reflex" is depressed, increasing the victim's length of contact with the current.

994.9	Other effects of external causes

995 CERTAIN ADVERSE EFFECTS NOT ELSEWHERE CLASSIFIED

995.0	Other anaphylactic shock not else where classifed

The key to understanding an allergy is to recognize that the previously sensitized individual has been re-exposed to the dose that begins the allergic reaction. Vasodilation and consequent loss of plasma into the tissues (productive of hives and angioedema) lead to hypovolemia. After receiving the "insult," the agitated system may present with reddened skin, pruritus, laryngeal edema, or bronchospasm. Shock can set in within a short time and, unless the process is arrested, the patient can die of vascular collapse.

995.1	Angioneurotic edema not elsewhere classified
995.2	Unspecified adverse effect of drug medicinal and biological substance, not elsewhere classified
995.3	Allergy, unspecified not elsewhere classified
995.4	Shock due to anesthesia not elsewhere classified

↙5th   Needs fifth-digit   **OK**   Valid three-digit code

Anesthetic drugs can cause vasodilation, which can lead to hypovolemic shock and vascular collapse. Patients are carefully monitored during anesthesia for any signs of inappropriate vasodilation.

Child and Adult Maltreatment

These codes address child and adult maltreatment. Emotional abuse is in a separate subcategory. Contusion codes on the trunk and lower extremities were increased to capture the characteristic marks of child physical abuse. The clinician may suspect elder abuse or neglect when the patient presents with withdrawal, dehydration, weight loss, and depression. An interview without the presence of the caregiver should be arranged to elicit more information. Battered women represent between 25 percent to 35 percent of all adult, female emergency department visits.

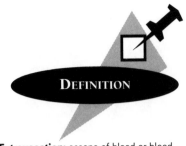

DEFINITION

Extravasation: escape of blood or blood components into the tissues.

Idiosyncratic: response unique to an individual.

Urticaria: another name for hives.

995.50	Child abuse, unspecified
995.51	Child emotional/psychological abuse
995.52	Child neglect (nutritional)
995.53	Child sexual abuse
995.54	Child physical abuse
995.55	Shaken infant syndrome
995.59	Other child abuse and neglect
995.6	Anaphylactic shock due to adverse food reaction

(Refer to Other anaphylactic shock, 995.0.)

995.60	Anaphylactic shock due to unspecified food
995.61	Anaphylactic shock due to peanuts
995.62	Anaphylactic shock due to crustaceans
995.63	Anaphylactic shock due to fruits and vegetables
995.64	Anaphylactic shock due to tree nuts and seeds
995.65	Anaphylactic shock due to fish
995.66	Anaphylactic shock due to food additives
995.67	Anaphylactic shock due to milk products
995.68	Anaphylactic shock due to eggs
995.69	Anaphylactic shock due to other specified food
995.7	Other adverse food reactions, not elsewhere classified
995.80	Adult maltreatment, usnpecified
995.81	Adult physical abuse
995.82	Adult emotional/psychological abuse
995.83	Adult sexual abuse
995.84	Adult neglect (nutritional)
995.85	Other adult abuse and neglect
995.86	Malignant hyperthermia
995.89	Certain adverse effects, not elsewhere classified, other

Hyperthermia and hypothermia due to adverse reaction to anesthesia result from a combination of muscle relaxant and inhalation general anesthetic. When an adverse reaction occurs, the operation must be stopped, and a reversal agent such as dantrolene must be administered. Family members should be tested for the same sensitivity.

996-999 Complications of Surgical and Medical Care, NEC

996 COMPLICATIONS PECULIAR TO CERTAIN SPECIFIED PROCEDURES

Patients may experience idiosyncratic reactions to the materials used in the prostheses, from lens implants to artificial skin. Prostheses can cause problems when displaced from the site of original insertion. Biliary stents may be dislodged.

Problems classified as mechanical, infectious, inflammatory, and "other" includes associated pain, embolism, hemorrhage, organ transplant rejections, and complications of reattached extremities or body parts. When the reason for an admission is linked to complications of medical or surgical care, the complication code is listed as the principal diagnosis, with any explanatory codes following. For example, a patient may be readmitted with sepsis following a previous medical contact. In this case, the coder must determine if the sepsis is linked to the previous contact since it may be attributable to either an infected line or postoperative infection.

996.00	Mechanical complication of unspecified cardiac device, implant, and graft
996.01	Mechanical complication due to cardiac pacemaker (electrode)
996.02	Mechanical complication due to heart valve prosthesis
996.03	Mechanical complication due to coronary bypass graft
996.04	Mechanical complication due to automatic implantable cardiac defibrillator
996.09	Mechanical complication of cardiac device, implant, and graft, other
996.1	Mechanical complication of other vascular device, implant, and graft
996.2	Mechanical complication of nervous system device, implant, and graft
996.30	Mechanical complication of unspecified genitourinary device, implant, and graft
996.31	Mechanical complication due to urethral (indwelling) catheter
996.32	Mechanical complication due to intrauterine contraceptive device
996.39	Mechanical complication of genitourinary device, implant, and graft, other
996.4	Mechanical complication of internal orthopedic device, implant, and graft
996.51	Mechanical complication due to corneal graft
996.52	Mechanical complication due to other tissue graft, not elsewhere classified
996.53	Mechanical complication due to ocular lens prosthesis
996.54	Mechanical complication due to breast prosthesis
996.55	Mechanical complications due to artificial skin graft and decellularized allodermis
996.56	Mechanical complications due to peritoneal dialysis catheter
996.59	Mechanical complication due to other implant and internal device, not elsewhere classified
996.60	Infection and inflammatory reaction due to unspecified device, implant, and graft
996.61	Infection and inflammatory reaction due to cardiac device, implant, and graft
996.62	Infection and inflammatory reaction due to other vascular device, implant, and graft
996.63	Infection and inflammatory reaction due to nervous system device, implant, and graft
996.64	Infection and inflammatory reaction due to indwelling urinary catheter
996.65	Infection and inflammatory reaction due to other genitourinary device, implant, and graft
996.66	Infection and inflammatory reaction due to internal joint prosthesis

✔5th   Needs fifth-digit   **OK**   Valid three-digit code

996.67	Infection and inflammatory reaction due to other internal orthopedic device, implant, and graft
996.68	Infection and inflammatory reaction due to peritoneal dialysis catheter
996.69	Infection and inflammatory reaction due to other internal prosthetic device, implant, and graft
996.70	Other complications due to unspecified device, implant, and graft
996.71	Other complications due to heart valve prosthesis
996.72	Other complications due to other cardiac device, implant, and graft
996.73	Other complications due to renal dialysis device, implant, and graft
996.74	Other complications due to other vascular device, implant, and graft
996.75	Other complications due to nervous system device, implant, and graft
996.76	Other complications due to genitourinary device, implant, and graft
996.77	Other complications due to internal joint prosthesis
996.78	Other complications due to other internal orthopedic device, implant, and graft
996.79	Other complications due to other internal prosthetic device, implant, and graft
996.80	Complications of transplanted organ, unspecified site
996.81	Complications of transplanted kidney
996.82	Complications of transplanted liver
996.83	Complications of transplanted heart
996.84	Complications of transplanted lung
996.85	Complications of bone marrow transplant
996.86	Complications of transplanted pancreas
996.87	Complications of transplanted organ, intestine
996.89	Complications of other transplanted organ
996.90	Complications of unspecified reattached extremity
996.91	Complications of reattached forearm
996.92	Complications of reattached hand
996.93	Complications of reattached finger(s)
996.94	Complications of reattached upper extremity, other and unspecified
996.95	Complications of reattached foot and toe(s)
996.96	Complications of reattached lower extremity, other and unspecified
996.99	Complications of other specified reattached body part

997 COMPLICATIONS AFFECTING SPECIFIED BODY SYSTEMS, NOT ELSEWHERE CLASSIFIED

Complications in the 997 category are organized according to body system. For example, urinary catheterization is an intervention or procedure and a urinary infection attributed to catheterization is coded with the 997.5 subcategory first and the appropriate urinary infection code secondarily. The more typical scenario with postoperative urinary tract infections is that following back, abdominal or pelvic surgery, the patient is unable to void and, thus, catheterized. The extended period of catheterization leads to a postoperative urinary tract infection, and is coded as such. In all cases, the medical record must clearly link the complication to the procedure. If unclear, the coder should ask the physician to document the existing link in an addendum to the report.

997.00	Unspecified nervous system complication
997.01	Central nervous system complication
997.02	Iatrogenic cerebrovascular infarction or hemorrhage
997.09	Other nervous system complications
997.1	Cardiac complications
997.2	Peripheral vascular complications

997.3	Respiratory complications
997.4	Digestive system complication
997.5	Urinary complications
997.60	Late complications of amputation stump, unspecified
997.61	Neuroma of amputation stump
997.62	Infection (chronic) of amputation stump
997.69	Other late amputation stump complication
997.91	Hypertension
997.99	Other complications affecting other specified body systems, NEC

998 OTHER COMPLICATIONS OF PROCEDURES, NOT ELSEWHERE CLASSIFIED

998.0	Postoperative shock, not elsewhere classified
998.11	Hemorrhage complicating a procedure
998.12	Hematoma complicating a procedure
998.13	Seroma complicating a procedure
998.2	Accidental puncture or laceration during procedure
998.3	Disruption of operation wound
998.4	Foreign body accidentally left during procedure, not elsewhere classified
998.51	Infected postoperative seroma
998.59	Other postoperative infection
998.6	Persistent postoperative fistula, not elsewhere classified
998.7	Acute reaction to foreign substance accidentally left during procedure, not elsewhere classified
998.81	Emphysema (subcutaneous) (surgical) resulting from a procedure
998.82	Cataract fragments in eye following surgery
998.83	Non-healing surgical wound
998.89	Other specified complications
998.9	Unspecified complication of procedure, not elsewhere classified

999 COMPLICATIONS OF MEDICAL CARE, NOT ELSEWHERE CLASSIFIED

Transfusion reactions, a major complication of medical care, is found in this category. Reaction to dialysis is another common cause of admission to acute care that falls under 999.9.

999.0	Generalized vaccinia as complication of medical care, not elsewhere classified
999.1	Air embolism as complication of medical care, not elsewhere classified
999.2	Other vascular complications of medical care, not elsewhere classified
999.3	Other infection due to medical care, not elsewhere classified
999.4	Anaphylactic shock due to serum, not elsewhere classified
999.5	Other serum reaction, not elsewhere classified
999.6	Abo incompatibility reaction, not elsewhere classified
999.7	Rh incompatibility reaction, not elsewhere classified
999.8	Other transfusion reaction, not elsewhere classified
999.9	Other and unspecified complications of medical care, not elsewhere classified

 5th Needs fifth-digit   **OK** Valid three-digit code